Gross Anatomy, Neuroanatomy, and Embryology for Medical Students

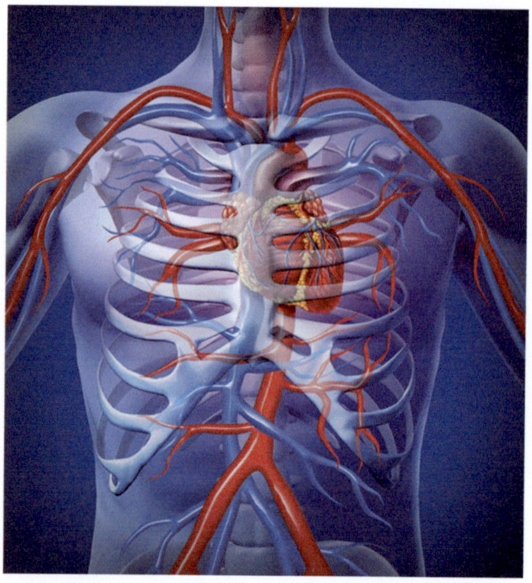

Jonathan Leo

Gross Anatomy, Neuroanatomy, and Embryology for Medical Students

The Ultimate Survival Guide

Springer

Jonathan Leo
Kansas City University
Kansas City, AL, USA

ISBN 978-3-031-87150-4 ISBN 978-3-031-87151-1 (eBook)
https://doi.org/10.1007/978-3-031-87151-1

This Springer imprint is published by the registered company Springer Nature Switzerland AG
The registered company address is: Gewerbestrasse 11, 6330 Cham, Switzerland

Preface

The amount of material presented to first year medical students is overwhelming, leaving students in a quandary. Since you have not picked a specialty yet, you need to know a little bit about everything. Once you pick a specialty, say surgery of the inner ear, or evaluation of the lower limb in sports injuries, or delivering babies, you will obviously go far behind this book in learning the anatomy of your specialty. And at that point, you can be forgiven for not knowing all the anatomy of the body, but, in the meantime, all anatomy is fair game for your gross anatomy course, boards, and for your preceptors. At some point, your older self will know a whole lot more detail about your specialty, but conversely 20 years from now you might not remember everything about those regions you do not see every day. If you become an otolaryngologist, the anatomy of the foot will be a distant memory. And if you become an orthopedic surgeon, the intricacies of the inner ear might not be on the tip of your tongue.

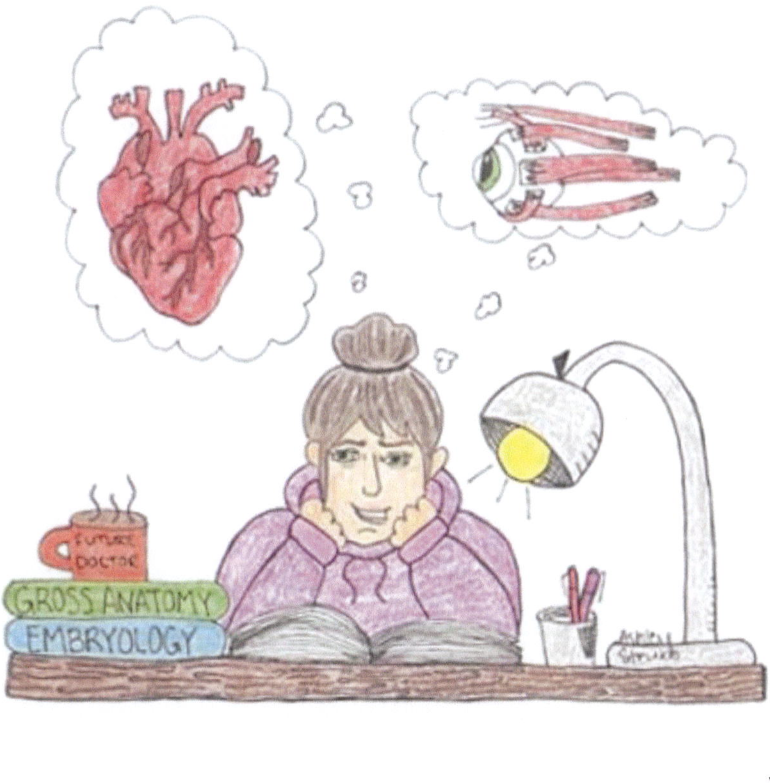

The tendency is for students to use brute force and attempt to simply "memorize" everything. But, there is a better way. During medical school, the trick is to focus on *understanding* all these complex topics and to think about long-term mastery. If you focus on mastery, the material is much more likely to "stick." Simply memorizing lists works for a test tomorrow but not 2 years later when you sit for board exams or walk into the exam room to see a patient.

One of the common coffee-break discussions among anatomy faculty members revolves around what to include in the first-year medical school curriculum. What we anatomists do not always acknowledge is that all our students are eventually going to specialize, so that at some point they can come back and tell us more about the details of their specialty than we know.

Whether or not a particular anatomical factoid should be included in a lecture or not can turn into hours of debate. Should we be teaching it in a first-year course, or leave it to their residency training? There are no "correct" answers to these questions. On the one hand, we do not want to leave out important concepts, but, on the other hand, we cannot teach everything. Somewhere in the middle is a happy medium, which is my goal with this book. The figures in the book are not exhaustive diagrams documenting every nook and cranny of a particular region, but instead they are simple diagrams focusing on one or two anatomical relationships that explain clinical scenarios.

The purpose of this text is obviously not an exhaustive deep dive into all gross anatomy. There are numerous other books that have done this. Likewise, it is not meant to be just a quick overview. Rather, it is meant to present each anatomical topic with clinical scenarios in mind. Hopefully, it will help first-year students with their coursework, and second-year students looking for a refresher before boards and rotations.

Everyone needs a study break now and then. I have added several *Historical Snippets* at the end of several chapters. They are short and only skim the surface of each topic. To me, they are interesting stories about famous people in medicine.

Thank you to Ashley Strube for the picture of the stressed-out student. And thanks to Jason Roney for the toe picture. Drs. Julia Alexander and Josheph Slusher graciously supplied the magnetic resonance imaging (MRIs) and other radiographs. And thanks to Margaret Russell and Jessice Morehouse for their comments and suggestions. Thanks to the historian Dr. Charles Hubbard who pointed me in the right direction with the story about Abraham Lincoln and the chicken bone. Finally, thanks to all my students for all the questions over the years. You do not realize it but every time you ask a question, the professor learns something also. And as anyone who has authored a book knows, the main reason to author a book is to learn something new. And a special thanks to Susan for hanging around all these years and being so supportive.

Kansas, AL, USA Jonathan Leo

Further Reading

Hanwell SM, Davies DC, Morris J, Parkin I, Whiten S, Atkinson M. et al. A core syllabus in anatomy for medical students – adding common sense to need to know. Eur J Anat. 2007;11(Suppl 1):3–18.

Contents

Part I

Gross Anatomy

1 The Head and Neck

Introduction

The head and neck region is typically considered the most complicated part of a gross anatomy course. There is more in this small space than either one of the limbs. As an undergraduate student you might have learned a mnemonic for the cranial nerves so that you could answer a question such as: Does cranial nerve (CN) V have, sensory, of both types of fibers? You can forget the mnemonics for the names of the cranial nerves, or for which nerves are motor, sensory, or both. These sayings will not get you far in medical gross anatomy. The pertinent point is not whether CN V is motor, sensory, or both—that is a given. The question is: How many of the fifty-one branches of CN V can you name? And which branches are motor, sensory, or both?

When studying the head, everything is organized around the cranial nerves and the skull. All the cranial nerves are important, but CNs V and VII cover so much territory that when you study the head, think of these two nerves as something like scaffolds to organize everything else around.

The Skull and Face

Architecture is the study of how to organize rectangles. The skull is like a house with many rooms. When studying the skull, it is helpful to think of the different regions of the skull as individual rooms with floors, ceilings, and walls. And in many cases the ceiling of one room is the floor of the room above it. For instance, the floor of the orbit is the ceiling of the maxillary sinus, and the floor of the maxillary sinus is the ceiling of the oral cavity. And between the various rooms, are doorways and hallways transmitting the nerves, arteries, and veins (Fig. 1.1).

The skull is the cranium plus the mandible. There are 22 bones that make up the skull. The neurocranium which holds the brain includes eight bones—the frontal, ethmoid, sphenoid, occipital, plus the two each of temporal and parietal. There are 14 that make up the face (viscerocranium). The *pterion* is the weakest point of the skull and represents the junction of the parietal, temporal, frontal, and sphenoid bones (Fig. 1.2). Fractures here can damage the middle meningeal artery. It is also a neurosurgical landmark. Broca's area is deep to it. Fracture of the ethmoid may lead to *rhinorrhea*—CSF draining into the nose (Table 1.1 and Fig. 1.3).

Skull Foramina

This is just an introduction as the details will be covered in each section. Think of the interior of the skull like a bowl with three sections: the anterior, middle, and posterior cranial fossae. We are going to start with the mnemonic SRO for <u>S</u>tanding <u>R</u>oom <u>O</u>nly. Nestled on the floor of the

J. Leo, *Gross Anatomy, Neuroanatomy, and Embryology for Medical Students*,
https://doi.org/10.1007/978-3-031-87151-1_1

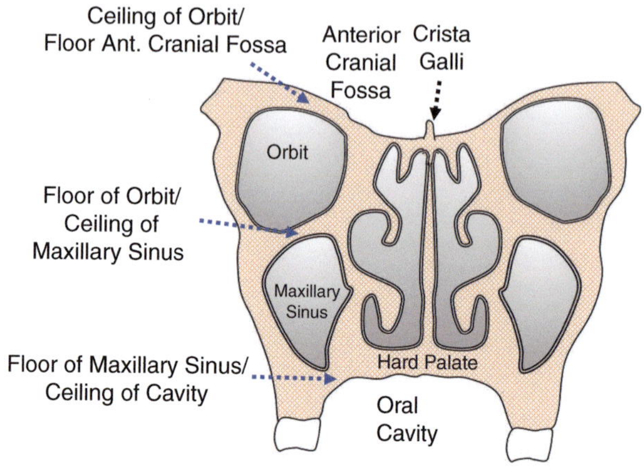

Fig. 1.1 How to think about the skull. The skull is a series of rooms with shared walls between the rooms. For instance, the floor of the orbit Is the ceiling of the maxillary sinus. Likewise, the hard palate is the ceiling of the oral cavity and the floor of the nasal cavity [21, 22]

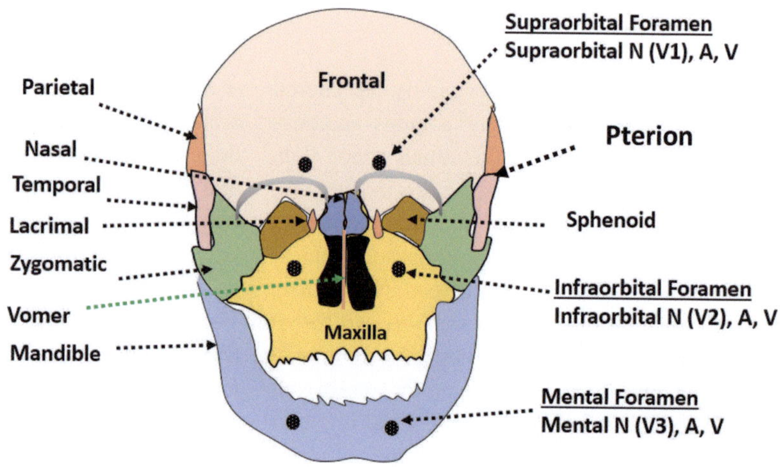

Fig. 1.2 Anterior view of the skull. Note the three openings lined up in a row: the supraorbital, infraorbital, and mental foramina. Each transmits an artery, nerve, and vein all named after the appropriate foramen [21, 22]

Table 1.1 Nerve supply to tongue

Cranial nerve	Modality
CN V (lingual nerve)	General sense to anterior two-thirds tongue
CN VII (chorda tympani)	Taste to anterior two-thirds tongue and parasympathetics to submandibular and sublingual glands
CN IX (sensory branch)	General sense and taste to posterior one-third of tongue
CN X (pharyngeal branch)	Motor to palatoglossus M
CN XII (motor branch)	Motor to genioglossus, styloglossus, and hyoglossus Ms

In summary there are five cranial nerves involved with the tongue

Muscle	Action
Cricothyroid	*Tenses Vocal Cords*
Lateral Cricoarytenoid	*Adducts Vocal Cords*
Posterior Cricoarytenoid	*Abducts Vocal Cords Opens Glottis*
Transverse and Oblique Arytenoids	*Adducts Vocal Cords*
Thyroarytenoids	*Adducts vocal cords*
Vocalis (Subset of Thyroarytenoids)	*Modifies Tension on Vocal Cords*

Fig. 1.3 Intrinsic muscles of the larynx. The posterior cricoarytenoid is the only muscle that opens the glottis [21, 22]

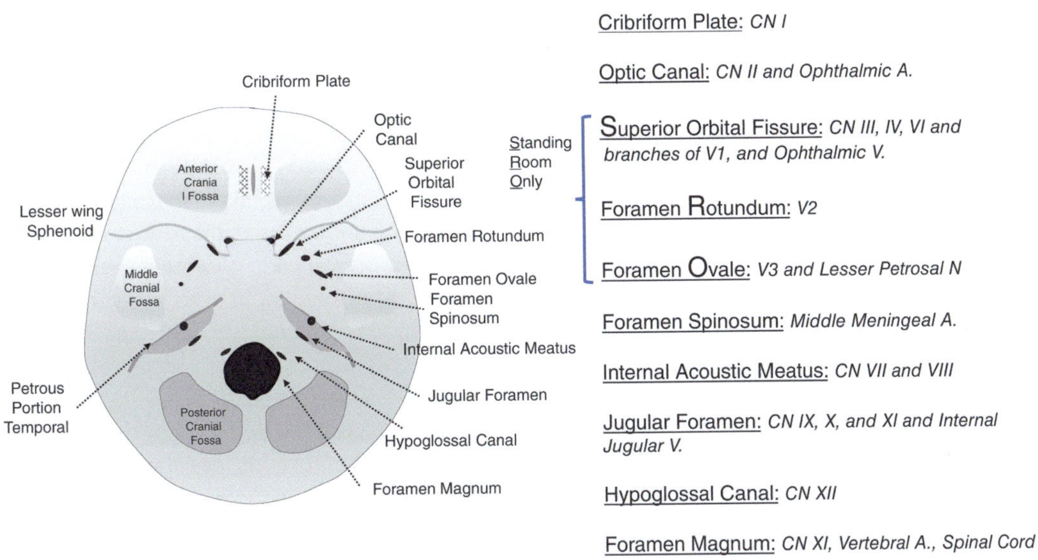

Fig. 1.4 The interior of the skull [21, 22]

middle cranial fossa is the trigeminal ganglion which sits in a space called *Meckel's cave*. Coming out of the ganglion are the three branches of the trigeminal nerve—V1, V2, and V3—which all exit the skull. V1 goes through the *superior orbital fissure*, V2 through *the foramen rotundum,* and V3 through *foramen ovale* (Fig. 1.4).

1. **S**uperior Orbital Fissure—V1
2. Foramen **R**otundum—V2
3. Foramen **O**vale—V3

We will delve into the details further on. But for now, note that next to the foramen ovale is the *foramen spinosum* with the *middle meningeal artery* entering the skull. Along the petrous portion of the temporal bone, we see the *internal acoustic meatus* which contains CNs VII and VIII. In the posterior fossa, the *jugular foramen* transmits CN IX, X, and XI. The *hypoglossal canal* transmits CN XII. In the center of the posterior fossa is the foramen magnum with the spinal cord, vertebral artery, and CN XI. Note that at this point CN XI enters the skull through the foramen magnum, it then *exits* the skull through the jugular foramen. In the anterior cranial fossa, we see the *crista galli* with the olfactory bulbs on either side.

Jugular Foramen Syndrome

Because CNs IX, X, and XI all travel through the jugular foramen, a mass in the foramen can lead to palsies of all three of these nerves (Vernet's Syndrome). The CN IX palsy will lead to a loss of sensation from the posterior one-third of the tongue and loss of the gag reflex. The CN X palsy will include dysphagia and dysarthria. The CN XI palsy will include paralysis of SCM and trapezius. In addition, if the mass is large enough it can also impinge on CN XII near the hypoglossal canal which would lead to a tongue deficit (Collet Syndrome). And if it expands even more, it could impinge on the sympathetic trunk traveling through the foramen magnum leading to Horner's syndrome (Villaret Syndrome). The internal jugular vein also travels with the nerves through the foramen, so that besides cranial nerve palsies, intracranial pressure can rise by blocking the internal jugular vein. For the nerve palsies given above, this was just the condensed version. Later in this chapter, each nerve is discussed in much more detail. This is a suitable time to point out a general concept when it comes to learning lesions. While I pointed out the names of the various syndromes above, knowing the exact name of the lesion or syndrome is not as important as knowing the relationships within a given neighborhood. In other words, when there is a lesion to one nerve, there is always a chance that the lesion will expand and comprise the neighboring structures. With lesions to the nerve, it is important to know which neighbors can also be affected. If you see a patient with a lesion to CN IX, X, and XI you will think about the jugular foramen, but if a month later there is a tongue deficit, then you know that the lesion has enlarged to hit a neighbor. It is much more important to understand, and have a visual representation of the relationships, than to memorize flashcards listing various syndromes.

Scalp

There is no structure in anatomy better suited to a mnemonic. The mnemonic for the scalp is SCALP (Fig. 1.5).

1. *Skin*. Hair Follicles are in the skin. Their associated sebaceous glands can become infected which will lead to redness and swelling around the cyst. There are no lymph nodes in the skin. The hair follicles also extend into the layer right below it.
2. *Connective Tissue*. This layer is made up of dense connective tissue connecting the skin to the underlying aponeurosis. A *caput succedaneum* typically results following a vacuum or forceps assisted vaginal delivery which leads to "molding" of the skull. Because the skull bones are not yet fused, the head can assume a V-shape corresponding to the vacuum shape. This will resolve on its own soon after birth. During this process vacuum was attached. The caput will have a soft, boggy-like feel to it that can move as the head position is changed. Keep in mind a caput succedaneum occurs *externally* to the pericranium.
3. *Aponeurosis*. In the front of the head is the frontalis muscle, and at the back of the head is the occipitalis muscle. The *galea aponeurotica* is a strong, tough ligament connecting these two muscles. All these structures together are referred to as the *occipitofrontalis muscle*. Anteriorly the ligament is attached to the upper eyelids. With lacerations, this layer is a landmark for determining how deep a laceration is. If the cut has penetrated this layer, especially in the coronal plane, then the patient will have a gaping wound because the aponeurosis will pull the two flaps apart. When suturing the wound, this will have to be considered. If the wound is only through the

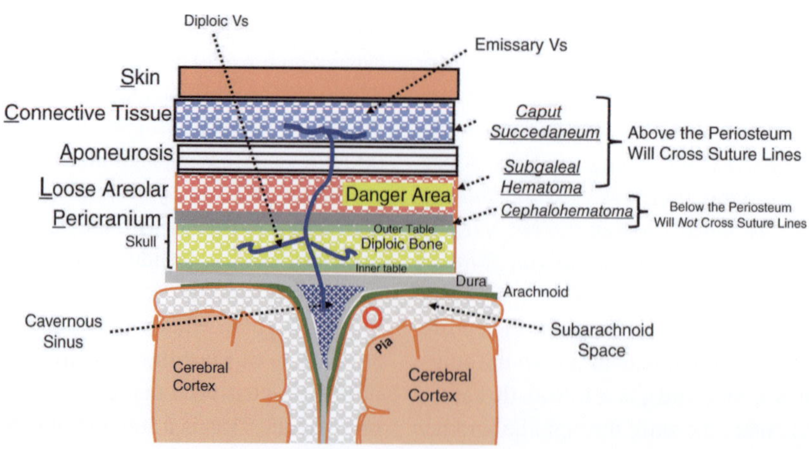

Fig. 1.5 The layers of the SCALP. Three pathologies, all of which can occur during delivery. Caput Succedaneum is a soft fleshy inflammation in the connective tissue layer. Subgaleal hematomas are found in the loose areolar layer. Cephalohematomas occur below the pericranium [21, 22]

skin and connective tissue, it will be "non-gaping" wound.

4. *Loose areolar layer.* Think of this layer as one large continuous space below the aponeurosis. It is sometimes referred to as the *danger area.* If you put your hand on your scalp and move the skin, this is the layer allowing for the movement. Traversing this layer are the scalp veins and diploic veins. Bleeding into this space can lead to a *subgaleal hematoma.* Blood in this layer can freely move from one point to another within the layer, and because this layer is still above the skull, the blood flow is not restricted by the suture lines. Subgaleal hematomas are life threatening and much more severe than the above-mentioned caput succedaneum. They can also result from superficial contusions to the scalp. Traumatic deliveries, or even excessive hair pulling can lead to blood pooling in this area. For instance, several hours after a patient receives a minor hit to the top of the head, they might develop black eyes. In this case the blood has moved from the site of the contusion to the corners of the eyes—remember the aponeurosis above it is connected to the upper eyelid. The black eyes in this case should not be confused with *Battle signs* (or Battle's Sign) which are indicative of major trauma to the skull such as the petrous portion of the temporal bone (basilar skull fracture). In this case blood can pool just posterior to the ear following a basilar skull fracture.
5. *Pericranium.* The pericranium or the periosteum is dense irregular tissue attached to the bone. During a difficult delivery, often with either forceps or a vacuum, shearing forces can lead to blood collecting between the periosteum and the skull bone forming a *cephalohematoma* (subperiosteal hematoma). It will usually take several hours to develop and will typically resolve over time. The most common site is over the parietal bone. The mass will not cross the suture lines and will not put pressure on the brain. *A cephalohematoma* occurs below the pericranium.

Deep to the periosteum is the bone tissue, made up of inner and outer tables sandwiching the diploic bone. Attached to the interior side of the skull is the dura mater, which in turn has two layers: the *periosteal* and *endosteal layers.* In several locations these two layers of dura separate from each other to make room for the venous sinuses such as the *superior and inferior sagittal sinuses.* The superficial veins from the scalp, and diploic veins from the skull bone also drain into these sinuses. Adherent to the dura is the arachnoid mater, and deep to the arachnoid mater is the subarachnoid space. Arteries perfusing the brain are found in the subarachnoid space. And just on top of the brain is the pia mater. The pia mater is tightly adherent to the brain surface, such that if you are touching an embalmed brain, or holding a brain in your hand, you are touching the pia mater. The subarachnoid space is between the pia and arachnoid layers.

The emissary veins run from the veins of the scalp, through the skull, to connect to the subdural sinuses. Infections can spread from the scalp through the veins to the subdural sinuses—the infection is moving from extracranial to intracranial.

Meninges

There are three layers of meninges between the brain and the skull. Starting deep and moving superficially, the deepest layer, adherent to the surface of the brain is the pia mater. The next layer is the arachnoid layer, and then against the skull is the dura. The dura is the thickest layer and can be pulled away from the surface of the skull. The arachnoid is a thin layer loosely adherent to the brain. It can easily be pulled away from the brain. The most important artery to the meninges is the middle meningeal artery. Most of the nerve innervation to the meninges travels on V1. However, in the middle cranial fossa, the area right around the foramen rotundum, travels on V2, while the area around the foramen ovale and moving laterally onto the skull travels on V3. The area right around the foramen magnum travels on the C1 and C2 spinal nerves (Fig. 1.6).

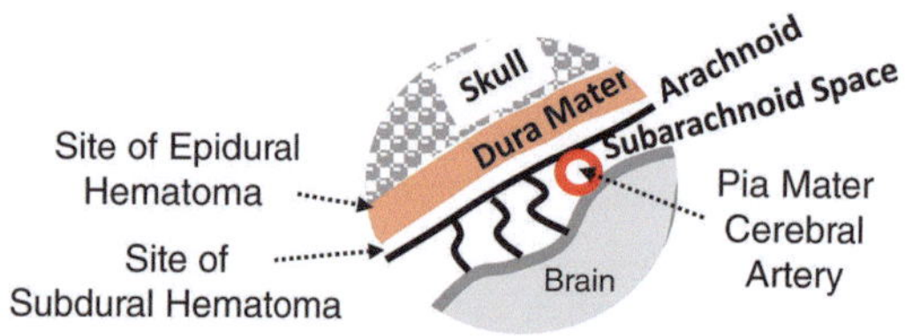

Fig. 1.6 Meninges. The pia mater is adherent to the brain. The arachnoid sits loosely atop the pia. The subarachnoid space is between the pia and arachnoid. The dura is tightly adherent to the skull. Epidural bleeds (Middle Meningeal A) are between the skull and dura mater. Subdural bleeds (Bridging Vs) are between the dura mater and arachnoid. The cerebral arteries are in the subarachnoid space. A rupture of an aneurysm will lead to blood in the subarachnoid space [21, 22]

Meningeal Irritation

There are two tests to check for meningeal irritation. *Kernig's sign* is elicited by having the patient lie supine with their hips and knees flexed. While keeping the hip flexed, the patient attempts to extend the leg. If there is pain or resistance this is a positive Kernig's sign and indicative of meningitis.

Brudzinski's sign is elicited by having the patient lie supine and then the examiner puts their hands behind the patient's neck and elevates the head towards the chest. If the patient flexes the hip and knee following this neck flexion this is a positive Brudzinski's sign.

Epidural Hematomas

The middle meningeal artery comes off the maxillary artery and enters the brain through the foramen spinosum. On its way superiorly it lies against the pterion which is the weakest part of the skull. A tear of the middle meningeal artery will lead to blood pooling between the dura mater and the skull—an epidural hematoma. In the classic scenario the patient passes out twice. For example, imagine a softball player getting hit in her head, who immediately passes out. As she is lying there, her teammates come running over, and she quickly regains consciousness. She seems all right and turns away the paramedics and other offers of assistance. However, an hour or two later, her condition rapidly deteriorates and she loses consciousness again. This is because the injury led to a tear of the middle meningeal artery and a slow accumulation of blood in her epidural space. This in turn led to a build-up of pressure on her brain which caused the loss of consciousness the second time. Imaging will reveal an elliptical or oval shaped mass of blood around the pterion.

Subdural Hematomas

Chronic subdural hematomas result from a slow bleed from the bridging veins draining into the superior sagittal sinus. In this scenario, the patient comes to the office complaining of a headache, nausea, vomiting, a difficult time sleeping, vertigo, etc. The patient is not sure why they feel like this, but on questioning you discover that several weeks ago they were in a minor car accident that rocked their head back and forth. This rocking motion tore the bridging veins. Imaging will reveal blood pooling in the subdural space all around one side or, in some cases, both sides of the brain. The image is sometimes said to resemble the shape of a banana. Alcohol and blood thinners increase the risk of a subdural bleed. Elderly patients with cerebral atrophy that stretches the bridging veins are prone to chronic subdural hematomas.

An acute subdural bleed has the same presentation, but the symptoms appear much sooner. An acute subdural hematoma is typically more severe than a chronic one. Treatment can require a craniotomy or a burr hole.

Common, External, and Internal Carotid Arteries

The common carotid artery travels in the carotid sheath with the internal jugular vein and the vagus nerve. A landmark for the common carotid artery is the *carotid tubercle* which is the anterior tubercle of the C6 vertebra. The common carotid artery runs anterior to the tubercle and the pulse

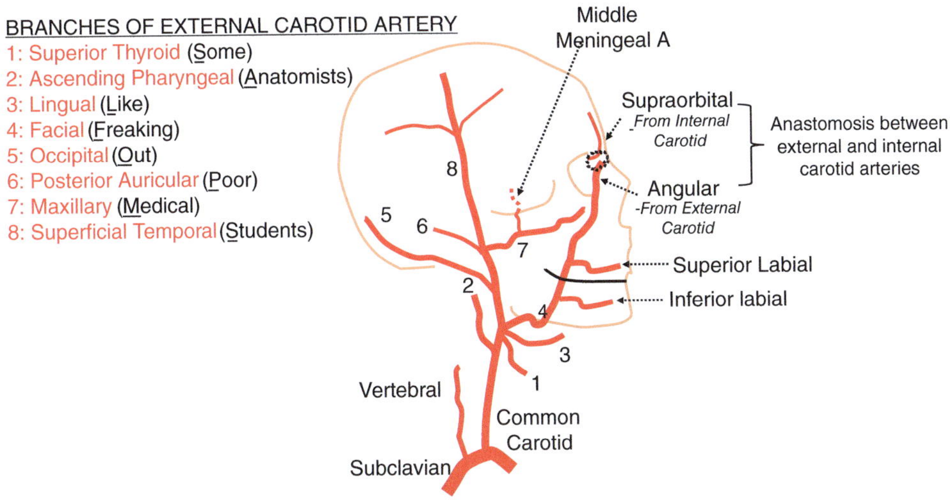

Fig. 1.7 Branches of the external carotid artery [21, 22]

can be felt here. Posterior to the tubercle is the vertebral artery crossing to enter the *foramen transversarium* of C6. The carotid artery typically splits at the level of C4 into the internal and external carotid arteries. The internal carotid is strictly intracranial with a few exceptions. The external carotid is strictly extracranial with one exception. The branches of the external carotid are (Fig. 1.7):

1. The *superior thyroid artery*. If you fill the external carotid artery with contrast material, all the branches can be seen ascending towards the head except for the superior thyroid artery which will be seen descending towards the thyroid gland. A branch of the superior thyroid artery is the *superior laryngeal artery* which pierces the thyrohyoid membrane with the *internal laryngeal nerve*.
2. The *ascending pharyngeal artery* is a small artery arising between the internal and external carotid arteries.
3. The *lingual artery* dives deep to the mandible to enter the oral cavity.
4. The *facial artery* travels through the submandibular gland as it approaches the mandible. Surgery of the gland here can damage the facial artery. It then crosses the mandible just in front of the masseter and heads towards the medial corner of the orbit. Just past its origin, it gives off a tonsillar branch to the palatine tonsils. On the way it gives off the superior and inferior labial arteries going to the superior and inferior lips. As the facial artery crosses the zygomaticus major it becomes the angular artery which travels to the corner of the eye, where it forms an anastomosis with the supraorbital artery, which is a branch of the frontal artery, which came from the internal carotid artery. The corner of the eye represents an anastomosis of the internal and external carotid systems. An increased pulse in the corner of the eye could be the result of a blockage of the internal carotid deep in the skull.
5. The *occipital artery* runs across the temporal bone and then runs between the trapezius and sternocleidomastoid. Close to the midline, its terminal branch runs with the greater occipital nerve to reach the posterior skull. It sometimes give a meningeal branch to the meninges in the region of the mastoid process.
6. The *posterior auricular artery* comes off the external carotid artery in the vicinity of the styloid process and runs between the external ear and the mastoid process. It gives a *posterior meningeal artery* that supplies the meninges in the posterior cranial fossa. Note on the posterior meningeal artery: Besides the ascending pharyngeal artery, the posterior

meningeal artery may arise from the vertebral artery, occipital artery, or posterior inferior cerebellar artery. If you are a neurosurgeon operating in this region, this would obviously be important, but for a primary care doctor this is not significant.

7. The *superficial temporal artery* runs anterior to the ear where its pulse can be felt. It runs with the auriculotemporal nerve. In cases of giant cell arteritis, biopsies of the superficial temporal artery can be taken. During the procedure, the auriculotemporal nerve can be damaged. The superficial temporal artery gives off the *transverse facial artery* which runs horizontally across the face.
8. The *maxillary artery* runs deep to the mandible to enter the infratemporal fossa where it gives off several branches. It then runs through the pterygopalatine fossa to enter the nasal cavity. It will be dealt with in more detail in each of those sections. It is an artery of the deep face, however one of its branches, the middle meningeal artery travels through the foramen spinosum to enter the middle cranial fossa and supply the meninges. Within the skull the middle meningeal artery divides into anterior and posterior divisions which leave an impression along the inner surface of the skull. In many cases the maxillary artery also gives off an *accessory meningeal artery* which travels through the foramen ovale to also enter the skull and supply the trigeminal ganglion.

A mnemonic for the branches of the external carotid artery is *Some anatomists like freaking out poor medical students.*

Venous Drainage Superficial Face and Neck

The *superficial temporal vein* drains into the *retromandibular vein*, which in turn divides into the anterior and posterior divisions. The posterior division turns into the *external jugular*, while the anterior division meets with the *facial vein* to form the *common facial vein.* The external jugular vein lies superficial to the sternocleidomastoid muscle. Increased pressure in the veins due to heart or lung pathology, for instance right-sided heart failure, can be seen as *jugular venous distension* (JVD) in the external jugular vein.

If you take a cross section through the mediastinum or the neck, there is a continuous venous channel serving as a landmark. The internal jugular vein travels in the neck where it runs into the right brachiocephalic vein, which in turn runs into the superior vena cava, which then turns into the right atrium of the heart. So, if you start superiorly and a take a cut at the T3 level on the right side, one can see the right brachiocephalic vein; if you move inferiorly to the superior mediastinum, on the right side will be the superior vena cava; and if you take a cut through the heart, on the right side is the right atrium. The right atrium forms the right border of the heart (Fig. 1.8).

Subclavian Vein Line

The subclavian vein passes in front of the anterior scalene muscle, while the subclavian artery passes posterior to the muscle. To access the vein, a needle is passed inferior to the clavicle from lateral to medial. One goal is to avoid piercing the apex of the lung.

Internal Jugular Vein Line

The *internal jugular vein* lies in a triangle formed by the two heads of the sternocleidomastoid and the clavicle. Within the triangle, the internal jugular vein is lateral to the common carotid artery. With a finger on the pulse of the artery, the needle is inserted laterally to the finger and the needle is moved inferolateral. In some cases, the needle will be inserted higher up in the neck (more superior) in which case the access is at the midpoint of the medial border of the sternocleidomastoid. The vein is still lateral to the artery at this point, so again the needle is placed lateral to the pulse of the artery.

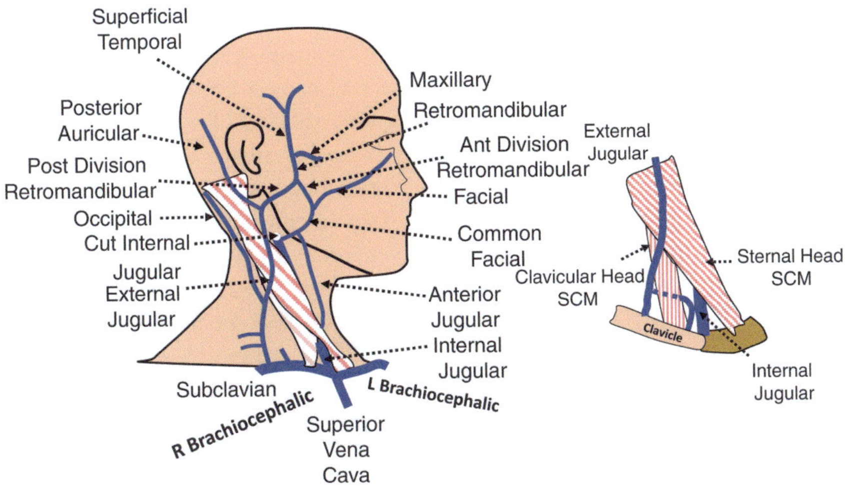

Fig. 1.8 The venous drainage of the face. The superficial temporal vein turns into the retromandibular vein which in turn divides into an anterior and posterior division. The posterior division goes down to the external jugular, while the anterior division goes down through the internal jugular vein. In the close-up of the neck, you can see the internal jugular vein between the two heads of the sternocleidomastoid muscle [21, 22]

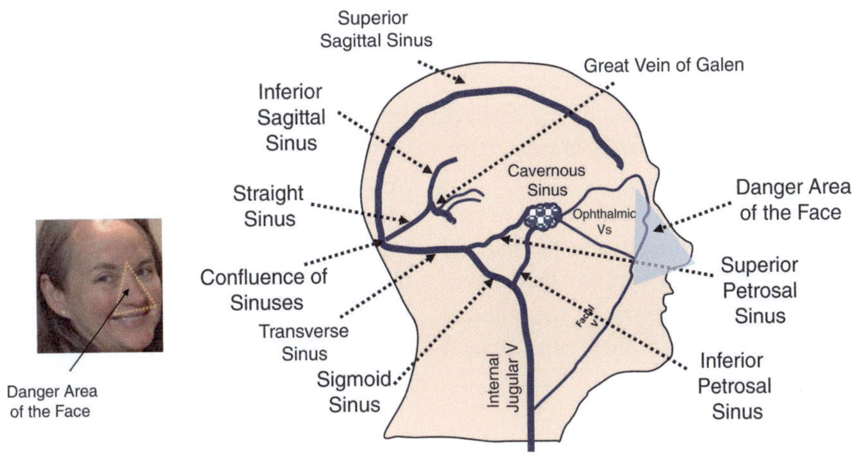

Fig. 1.9 Venous drainage of skull. The confluence of the sinus receives blood from the superior sagittal sinus and the straight sinus, and then drains into the transverse and sigmoid sinuses. From there it exits the skull through the internal jugular vein. The cavernous sinus receives blood from the danger area of the face via the deep veins. The cavernous sinus then drains via the superior and inferior petrosal sinuses [21, 22]

Venous Drainage of the Skull

Within the skull there are two layers of dura and in several regions these two layers separate to allow for venous drainage of blood. The *superior sagittal sinus* lies in the midline within the superior portion of the falx cerebri. Along the inferior portion of the falx cerebri is the *inferior sagittal sinus*, which in turn drains into the *straight sinus* (Fig. 1.9).

The straight sinus and superior sagittal sinus meet posteriorly in the midline at the *confluence of the sinuses*. The single confluence drains laterally to both the right and left sides as the transverse sinuses. Each transverse sinus then makes a right turn and descends as the sigmoid sinus to the jugular foramen to turn into the *internal jugular vein*. The cavernous sinus is a space around the sella turcica that receives venous blood from several areas and then drains via the *superior petrosal sinus* to the junction of the transverse sinus, and the *inferior petrosal sinus* to the junction of the sigmoid sinus and the internal jugular vein. It also receives venous drainage from the deep veins of the face.

Cavernous Sinus

The facial vein is valveless so infections can move in either direction. The danger area of the face is the triangle region around the nose that gets its name because an infection in the danger area of the face can track back along these veins into the cavernous sinus. For instance, take an individual on a walk in the woods who gets a small cut on the face from a tree limb and develops a superficial infection. What could have been just a minor issue, can now become a life-threatening condition if the infection travels back into the skull where it can lead to increased intracranial pressure.

Within the cavernous sinus are several important structures. Entering the sinus is the internal carotid artery which runs forward and then makes a 180° turn forming the genu of the internal carotid artery. In addition, there are several important cranial nerves running through here. The ophthalmic artery arises at the genu of the internal carotid artery. In the lateral wall of the sinus are CNs III, IV, V1 (ophthalmic nerve), and V2. Deeper in the sinus is CN VI (Abducens Nerve) hugging the genu of the internal carotid artery. An infection in the sinus will typically first compromise CN VI which will cause a medial strabismus, however as the infection spreads it will also affect the nerves on the lateral wall so that all the eye muscles will be affected, and the patient will develop complete ophthalmoplegia. In addition, V1 and V2 will be affected, but <u>*not*</u> V3 thus the muscles of mastication will be spared (Fig. 1.10). *Tolosa-Hunt syndrome* (THS) is an inflammatory condition of the cavernous sinus. The patients complain of pain around the eye, ophthalmoplegia, and loss of sensation from V1 and V2. Enlargement of the cavernous sinus is often seen on MRI in THS patients. The pathology can also involve the apex of the orbit.

Infratemporal Fossa

Where is the infratemporal fossa? The short answer is that it is the space behind the ramus of the mandible. And it contains most of the muscles of mastication. If you start with your hand on your mandible, you can feel the *masseter muscle*. To dissect the infratemporal fossa, you remove

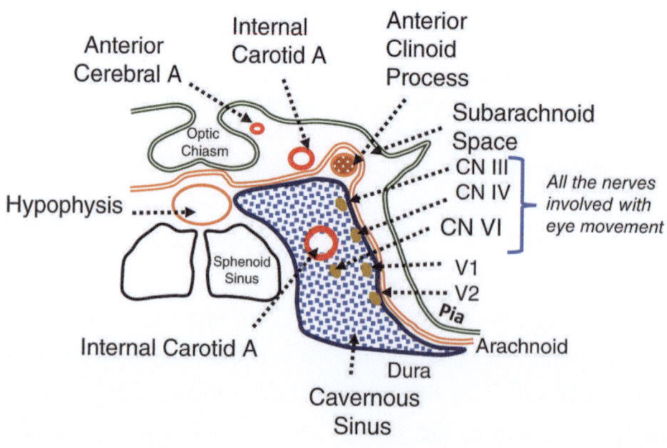

Fig. 1.10 Cavernous sinus. Running through the cavernous sinus are CNs III, IV, VI, and V1, and V2—or "all the cranial nerves associated with eye movements plus V1 and V2 but not V3." An infection in the cavernous sinus will typically first lead to a CN VI palsy, followed shortly by complete ophthalmoplegia [21, 22]

the masseter (which is outside of the IT fossa) and then remove the mandible to investigate the infratemporal fossa.

Think of the infratemporal fossa as a room. The ceiling is the greater wing of the sphenoid; the anterior wall is the infratemporal surface of the maxilla; the medial wall is the lateral pterygoid plate; the lateral wall is the mandible; and both the floor and posterior wall are open.

After removing the mandible, which is the lateral wall of the infratemporal fossa, the first muscle that you will notice in the fossa is the *medial pterygoid*. Both the masseter and the medial pterygoid form a sling holding the mandible. Acting together, they are elevators of the mandible (Fig. 1.11).

Just superior to the medial pterygoid is the *lateral pterygoid*, whose fibers run in an anterior to posterior direction. The lateral pterygoid has a superior and inferior head. The lateral pterygoid is the major muscle involved with elevation (closing the mouth) and protrusion of the mandible because via its attachment to the mandibular condyle it pulls the condyle anterior. It is innervated by CN V. If there is an injury to CN V and the patient is asked to protrude the jaw, then the mandible will deviate towards the weak side. In other words, a lesion to the right trigeminal nerve will lead to the jaw deviating to the right on attempted protrusion. This is because the functioning left lateral pterygoid will pull the jaw towards the right.

Also entering the infratemporal fossa at the anterosuperior corner is the *temporalis muscle,* which inserts onto the *coronoid process* of the mandible. Most of the temporalis muscle belly is found above the infratemporal fossa in the temporal fossa. The superior fibers of temporalis, running in a superior to inferior direction, will elevate the mandible, while the posterior fibers, running in an anterior to posterior direction will retract the mandible.

Infections, from tetanus for instance, or tumors of the muscles of mastication can lead to spasms of these muscles which are referred to as *trismus*. In some cases the patient will present with *lockjaw*.

Sphenoid Bone

The sphenoid bone is a single unpaired bone that is made up of a greater wing and lesser wing. It also houses the sella turcica with is bound by

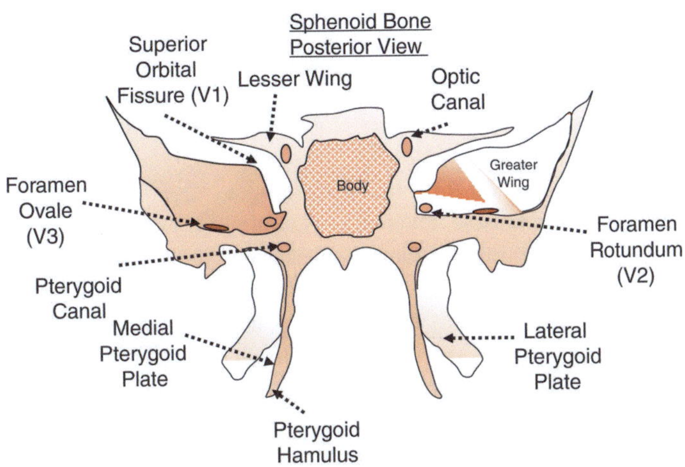

Fig. 1.11 Mandibular nerve. The mandibular nerve (V3) is seen entering the infratemporal fossa through the foramen ovale. The inferior alveolar nerve is entering the mandibular foramen. The chorda tympani Is a branch of the facial nerve joining the lingual nerve. The chorda tympani carries taste from anterior two-thirds of the tongue and parasympathetic fibers (dotted black line) to the submandibular ganglion. The parasympathetics from CN IX (dotted black line) travel on the auriculotemporal nerve to reach the parotid gland [21, 22]

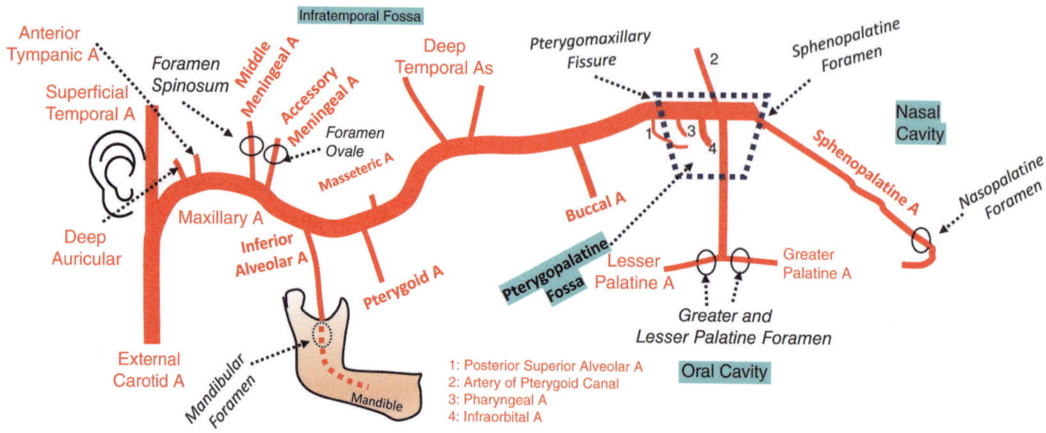

Fig. 1.12 The sphenoid bone. Note greater and lesser wings with the superior orbital fissure running between them. Foramen rotundum and foramen ovale are also seen on the greater wing. The descending medial and lateral pterygoid plates with the pterygoid hamulus on the medial pterygoid plate. The tensor veli palatini uses the pterygoid hamulus to make a sharp 90° turn as it enters the soft palate

anterior and posterior clinoid processes. It contains the three openings for the branches of the trigeminal nerve: (1) the superior orbital fissure, (2) the foramen rotundum, and (3) the foramen ovale. It has prominent articulations with the frontal, temporal, occipital, and parietal bones. Extending inferiorly is the pterygoid process with the medial and lateral pterygoid plates (Fig. 1.12).

Maxillary Artery

Crossing the infratemporal fossa from lateral to medial is the maxillary artery and its branches. For descriptive purposes, the artery can be divided into three sections based on their relationships to the lateral pterygoid muscle. The first part of the axillary artery is proximal to lateral pterygoid, the second part is behind the lateral pterygoid, and the third part is distal to lateral pterygoid. As the maxillary artery crosses the infratemporal fossa there are some branches that ascend towards the skull, and other branches that descend towards the mandible, nasal cavity, and the oral cavity (Fig. 1.13).

The first two branches off the maxillary artery are small and hard to find. The first one is the *deep auricular artery* which travels to the external ear. The second one is the *anterior tympanic artery* which travels with the chorda tympani through the *petrotympanic fissure* to supply the middle ear. Again, these are small and hard to find.

The next two branches which are easier to see are the *middle meningeal* and *accessory meningeal* arteries. The exact branching pattern of these meningeal arteries is variable. In some cases, they emerge as two distinct branches, while in other cases there is a single artery coming off the maxillary which then splits into two branches. Both these arteries ascend towards the skull. The middle meningeal artery travels through the foramen spinosum and enters the middle cranial fossa, while the accessory meningeal artery travels through foramen ovale to supply the trigeminal ganglion and then the meninges. The *inferior alveolar artery* is an example of a branch of the maxillary artery that descends. It travels with the inferior alveolar nerve towards the oral cavity to enter the mandible at the mandibular foramen to supply blood to the lower jaw. Right before it enters the mandibular foramen, it gives off a branch to the *mylohyoid muscle*. Likewise, the inferior alveolar nerve gives off a *nerve to mylohyoid* right before the entrance to the mandibular foramen.

Just past the inferior alveolar artery is another descending branch, the *pterygoid artery* which perfuses the pterygoid muscles. Moving along the maxillary artery are the *masseteric, deep tem-*

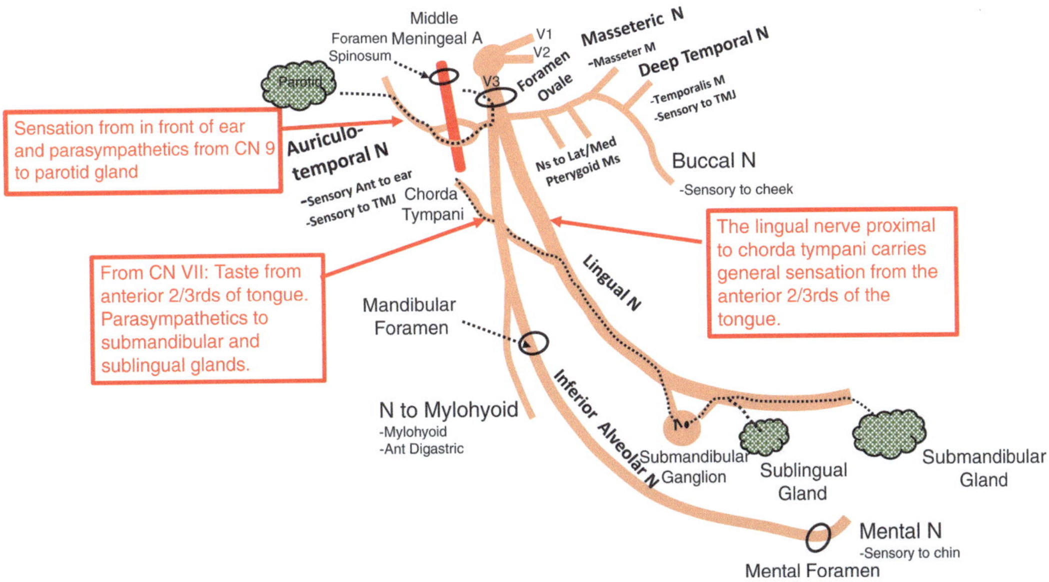

Fig. 1.13 Maxillary artery. The maxillary artery is seen traveling through the infratemporal fossa and giving off several branches such as infraorbital, middle meningeal, and deep temporal arteries. It then travels through the pterygomaxillary fissure to enter the pterygopalatine fossa. It continues across the pterygopalatine fossa and emerges through the sphenopalatine foramen as the sphenopalatine artery to enter the nasal cavity. It also gives off a descending palatine artery that approaches the palate and splits into a greater palatine artery heading towards the hard palate, and a lesser palatine artery heading to the soft palate [21, 22]

poral, and *buccal arteries.* Just before entering the pterygopalatine fossa the maxillary artery gives off the tiny *posterior superior alveolar arteries* which travel through the same named foramina in the maxilla to supply blood to the upper molars. The maxillary artery then passes through the *pterygomaxillary fissure* to enter the pterygopalatine fossa.

Mandibular Nerve (V3)

The nerve of the infratemporal fossa is the mandibular nerve which enters the fossae by traveling from the middle cranial fossa through the foramen ovale. It comes through foramen ovale as a large nerve trunk, and then right when it enters the fossa it splits into numerous branches. The motor nerves are all named for whichever muscle they are traveling to. For instance, the nerve fibers running to the lateral pterygoid are named the *nerve to lateral pterygoid.* The major sensory branches are as follows (Fig. 1.11):

1. The *auriculotemporal nerve* heads laterally towards the ear. On its way, it splits to go around the middle meningeal artery. As the nerve approaches the ear, it does a 90° turn and heads superiorly in front of the ear. After the nerve comes out of this 90° turn it is now running with the superficial temporal artery. Sensation from just in front of the ear is traveling on the auriculotemporal nerve, and the pulse felt in front of the ear is from the superficial temporal artery. The auriculotemporal nerve also carries sensory fiber from the external tympanic membrane.
2. The *inferior alveolar nerve* runs with the inferior alveolar artery to enter the mandibular foramen and run down the interior of the mandible. It is responsible for sensation from the lower teeth. In addition, right before it enters the mandibular foramen, it gives off a motor branch called the nerve to mylohyoid which in addition to supplying the mylohyoid muscle also supplies the anterior belly of the digastric. The terminal branch of the inferior

alveolar nerve exits the mental foramen and carries sensory information from the front of the jaw.

3. The *buccal nerve* is responsible for sensation from the inner surface of the cheek, gingiva of lower molars, buccal mucosa, and the skin over the anterior part of the buccinator. Remember, the skin on the cheek area below the eye and above the lip is infraorbital nerve. The buccal nerve gets a small patch of skin starting just above the corner of your mouth and coming down along the mandible. The dentist can block the nerve just near the third molar.
4. The *lingual nerve* travels down to the floor of the mouth and carries general sensory fibers from the anterior two-thirds of the tongue.

Temporomandibular Joint

There are two prominent points on the superior surface of the mandible, the *coronoid process,* and the *mandibular condyle.* The mandibular condyle articulates with the *mandibular fossa* on the zygomatic process of the temporal bone. The mandibular fossa is a weak point of the skull. The anterior portion of the condyle also articulates with the posteriorly facing *articular eminence* (Fig. 1.14).

The temporomandibular joint (TMJ) is unique because it has an articular disk in the middle of the joint. The disk is attached to the superior head of the lateral pterygoid and divides the temporomandibular joint into two spaces: a superior space above the articular disk—between the disk and the mandibular fossa, and an inferior space below the disk—between the disk and the condyle. The superior joint allows for protrusion and retraction, while the inferior joint allows for depression and elevation. The disk itself does not have any sensory fibers coming into it, however sensory fibers from the tissue around the joint travel on the auriculotemporal nerve. Lining the bony surfaces abutting the disk is fibrocartilage rather than hyaline cartilage. Hyaline cartilage is present in high stress areas, such as the knee, while fibrocartilage is better for long-term, high use areas such as the TMJ (Fig. 1.14).

Opening of the jaw is accomplished by the lateral pterygoid, digastrics, and mylohyoid muscles—but most importantly, the lateral pterygoid. Closing of the jaw is accomplished by the masseter, temporalis, and medial pterygoid muscles. When the jaw starts to open, the first movement is a hinge movement in the lower part of the joint. As the jaw continues to open, the mandible starts to move forward. This gliding movement now occurs at the upper joint, with the condyle sliding forward and coming to lie just inferior to the articular tubercle with the disk resting between the two structures. Preceding the gliding movement, the lateral pterygoid muscle pulls the disk anterior. Retraction is accomplished by the poste-

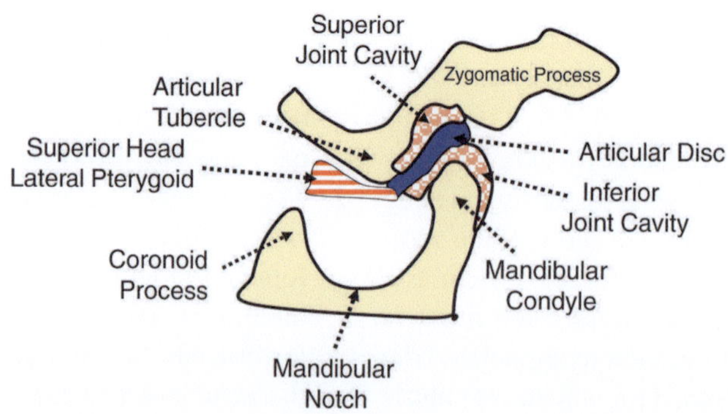

Fig. 1.14 TMJ. The temporomandibular joint is a synovial joint between the mandibular condyle and the mandibular fossa. The mandibular fossa is on the zygomatic process of the temporal bone. The anterior surface of the joint, is the posterior slope of the articular tubercle. Between the condyle and the fossa is the articular tubercle. The superior head of the lateral pterygoid is attached to the articular disc [21, 22]

rior fibers of the temporalis, while protraction is accomplished by the lateral pterygoid.

During excessive opening of the jaw, such as a big yawn, the condyle can move down the posterior slope, over the articular eminence and may come to lie on the anterior surface of the articular eminence where it becomes stuck. Keep in mind that during normal movements at the joint, the condyle is facing the posterior slope of the articular eminence, but in a dislocation the condyle has slipped forward and is now on the anterior slope of the eminence. The disk then comes to lie between the condyle and the tubercle and the disk acts like a door jamb holding the mandible in place. To reduce this dislocated joint, the mandible is typically pushed down so that the condyle moves away from the tubercle allowing the jaw to close.

Masticator Space

The mandible is held up by a sling formed by the masseter and the medial pterygoid muscles. The masseter is outside the mandible (superficial), and the medial pterygoid is medial to the mandible (deep), and working together, they elevate the mandible. Running down the superficial surface of the masseter and down around the submandibular gland and up the deep side of the medial pterygoid is the *masseteric fascia* surrounding the *masseteric space*. Within this space you can see the lateral pterygoid muscle, plus the various branches of the mandibular nerve (V3), and the maxillary artery. The *buccal nerve* can be seen traveling between the superior and inferior heads of the lateral pterygoid. The *inferior alveolar nerve* can be seen traveling to the mandible through the mandibular foramen. The *otic ganglion* is found on the medial side of V3 just after it enters the foramen ovale. Infections in the masseteric space can spread to other regions of the head and neck (Fig. 1.15). *Ludwig's Angina* refers to a bacterial infection in the submandibular, sublingual, and submental compartments. It often originates from an infected inferior molar and can lead to difficulty with swallowing, speaking, and breathing.

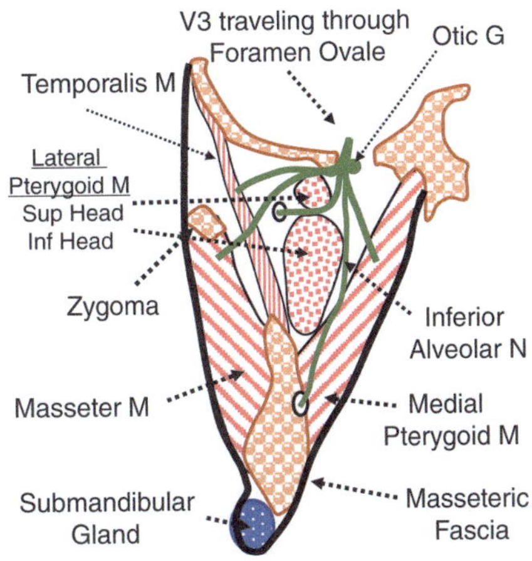

Fig. 1.15 V3 and foramen ovale. V3 comes through foramen ovale. It has muscular branches going to the muscles of mastication. The medial pterygoid and masseter muscles form a sling to support the mandible. The masseteric fascia covers this sling along with the submandibular gland. The inferior alveolar nerve is seen entering the mandibular foramen. The lateral pterygoid fibers run anterior to posterior, while the medial pterygoid fibers run superior to inferior [21, 22]

The Pterygopalatine Fossa

The pterygopalatine fossa is shaped like a chicken bucket, but it is about the size of a lifesaver hole. It is also like a train station with numerous train cars coming and going, to and from, all different corners of the city. There are seven doorways in the pterygopalatine fossa which connect the fossa to other rooms in the skull. When you study the pterygopalatine fossa, you are not just studying the skull, but also the nerves, arteries, and veins (Figs. 1.16, 1.17, and 1.18).

Pterygopalatine Fossa Doorways

1. Anterior through the *inferior orbital fissure* to the *orbit*
2. Lateral through the *pterygomaxillary fissure* to the *infratemporal fossa.*
3. Medially through the *sphenopalatine foramen* to the *nasal cavity*
4. Inferiorly through the *descending palatine canal* to the *oral cavity*

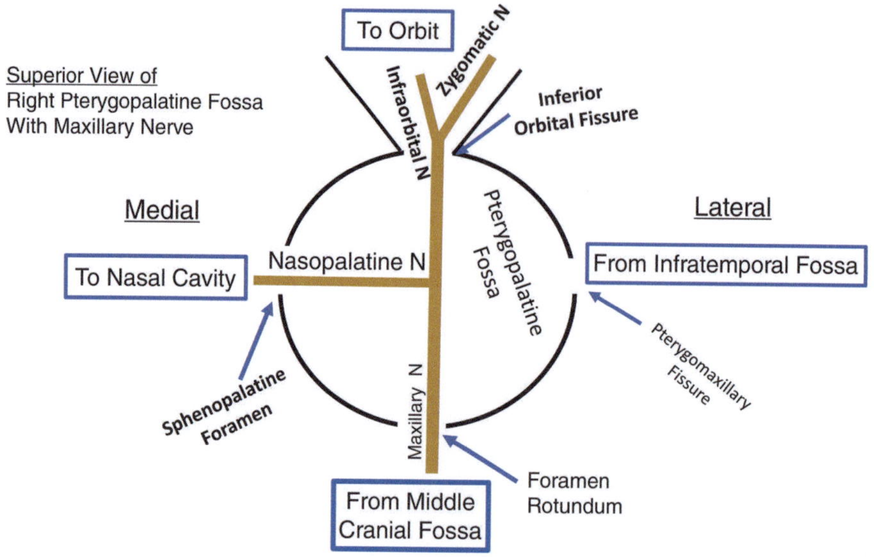

Fig. 1.16 Maxillary nerve. The maxillary nerve comes through the foramen rotundum and enters the pterygopalatine fossa. It continues through the fossa and emerges into the orbit as the infraorbital nerve, which gives off the zygomatic nerve. In the pterygopalatine fossa you can see the nasopalatine nerve heading through the sphenopalatine foramen to enter the nasal cavity [21, 22]

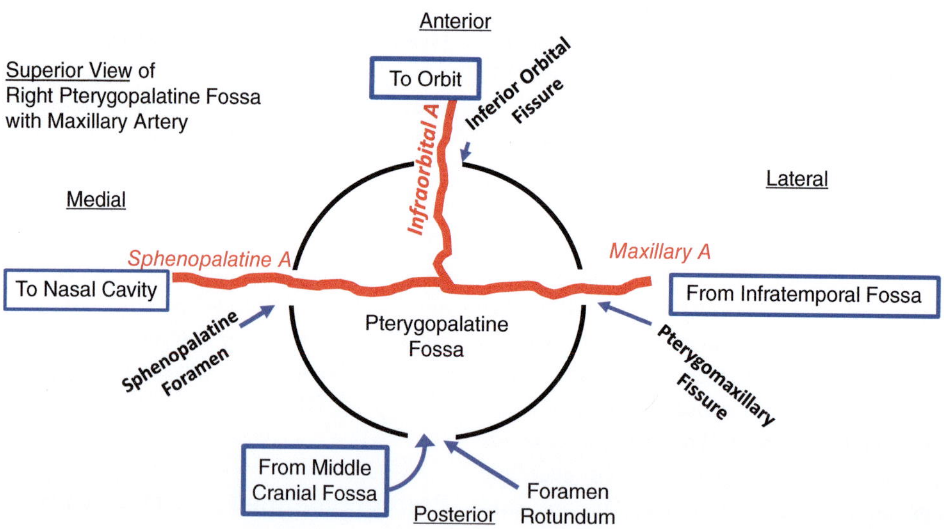

Fig. 1.17 Maxillary artery. Note the maxillary artery starting in the infratemporal fossa, coming through the pterygomaxillary fissure and entering the pterygopalatine fossa. It continues through the fossa and emerges into the nasal cavity as the sphenopalatine artery. In the pterygopalatine fossa you can see the infraorbital artery heading through the inferior orbital fissure to enter the orbit. There is no artery passing through the foramen rotundum [21, 22]

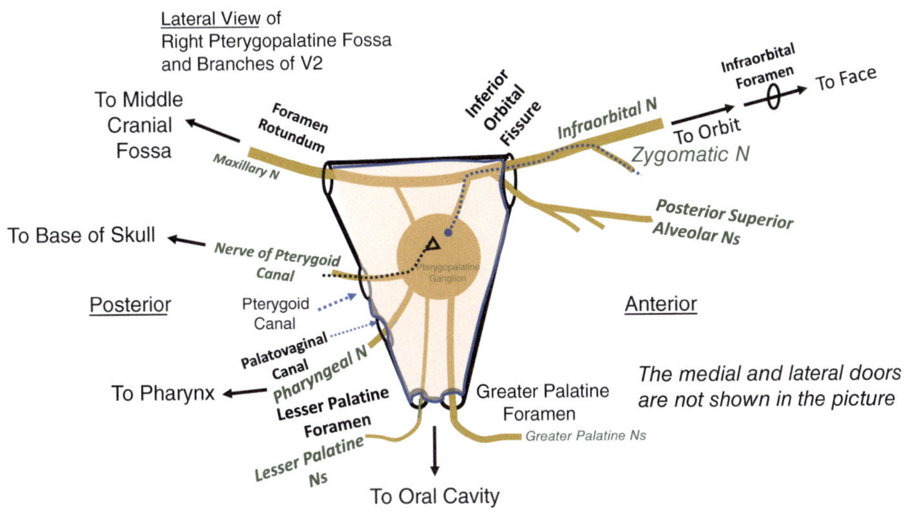

Fig. 1.18 Pterygopalatine fossa. The maxillary nerve is passing from the middle cranial fossa into pterygopalatine fossa and then moving through the inferior orbital fissure to enter the orbit. Hanging off V2 in the fossa is the pterygopalatine ganglion. Branches of V2 can be seen passing through various foramen into different regions of the skull. The greater and lesser palatine nerves descend and emerge onto the palate in the oral cavity. The nerve of the pterygoid canal is carrying preganglionic fibers from CN VII moving from the base of the skull through the pterygoid canal to enter the pterygopalatine fossa [21, 22]

There are three openings lined up in a column along the posterior wall.

1. Posterior through the *foramen rotundum* to the *middle cranial fossa*
2. Posterior through the *pterygoid canal* to the *base of the skull*
3. Posterior through the *palatovaginal canal* to the *pharynx*

As mentioned in the last section, the maxillary artery crosses the infratemporal fossa from lateral to medial. The medial doorway of the infratemporal fossa is the pterygomaxillary fissure. The maxillary artery travels through the pterygomaxillary fissure to enter the pterygopalatine fossa. It then continues across the pterygopalatine fossa and exits the fossa through the sphenopalatine foramen to enter the nasal cavity.

Within the fossa the maxillary artery gives off a descending palatine artery that descends through the *descending palatine canal* and then splits into two branches. (1) The *greater palatine artery* travels through the *greater palatine canal* to the hard palate, and the (2) *lesser palatine artery* travels through the *lesser palatine canal* to the soft palate. Along the posterior wall, the artery of the pterygoid canal travels back towards the base of the skull. And inferior to the pterygoid canal is the *palatovaginal canal* with a small artery traveling towards the pharynx. The palatovaginal canal is small, and you are most likely not expected to find it in the laboratory (Fig. 1.19).

The infraorbital artery enters the *inferior orbital fissure* to enter the orbit where it runs in the infraorbital grove, to the *infraorbital canal*, and to then emerge onto the face just inferior to the eye through the *infraorbital foramen.*

Coming off V2 within the pterygopalatine fossa, there are typically 2–3 small branches—the *posterior superior alveolar nerves*—moving anteriorly to enter the small *posterior superior foramina* in the maxilla. These nerves carry sensory fibers from the posterior superior teeth (the back upper molars).

Just before the *infraorbital nerve* enters the inferior orbital fissure, the *zygomatic nerve* branches off to supply the skin over the zygomatic process via the *zygomaticofacial* and *zygomaticotemporal* branches. Moving medially through the *sphenopalatine foramen*, is the *nasopalatine nerve* that crosses the superior surface of

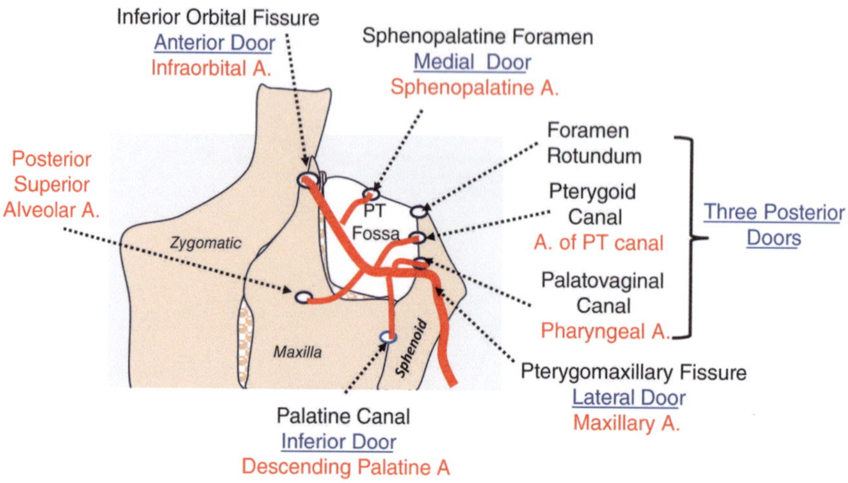

Fig. 1.19 Maxillary artery in the pterygopalatine fossa. The branches of the maxillary artery are passing through the various openings from the pterygopalatine fossa. Note the pterygomaxillary fissure is the lateral door of the pterygopalatine fossa but the medial door of the infratemporal fossa [21, 22]

the nasal cavity to run on the nasal septum forward to the *incisive foramen* (nasopalatine foramen).

Autonomics of Lacrimal Gland

Preganglionic parasympathetic fibers destined for the lacrimal gland start off as the *greater petrosal nerve* which is a branch of CN VII. The greater petrosal nerve leaves cranial CN VII in the vicinity of the geniculate ganglion and enters the pterygoid canal to travel to the pterygopalatine fossa where it synapses in the pterygopalatine ganglion. The post ganglionic fibers then travel on the zygomatic nerve to head towards the lacrimal gland. As they approach the lacrimal gland, they jump on the lacrimal nerve which is a branch of V1 (frontal nerve specifically). Thus, the postganglionic fibers to the lacrimal gland are taking advantage of both the *zygomatic nerve*, which is a branch of V2, and then the *frontal nerve* which is a branch of V1.

The *lacrimal reflex* refers to the fact that when the cornea is stimulated it can result in tear secretion. The afferent portion of the reflex is mediated by V1, while the motor portion is mediated by the autonomics of CN VII.

Facial Nerve

The facial nerve comes out of the brainstem and enters the skull by passing through the internal acoustic meatus. It then winds through the skull to eventually emerge through the stylomastoid foramen onto the face, just posterior to the parotid gland.

Facial Nerve, Muscles of Facial Expression and Parotid Gland

Once it comes out of the stylomastoid foramen it courses through the parotid gland dividing into five branches that supply the muscles of facial expression: **T**emporal, **Z**ygomatic, **B**uccal, **M**arginal Mandibular, **C**ervical, and **P**osterior auricular. **T**o **Z**anzibar **B**y **M**otor **C**ar, **P**lease. The posterior auricular nerve is also responsible for sensation from the concha bowl of the ear, and motor innervation to the occipitalis muscle (Fig. 1.20).

A parotid tumor or surgery on the parotid gland can damage branches of the facial nerve at this point. These branches of the facial nerve innervate the muscles of facial expression which are extremely thin muscles. Without going into

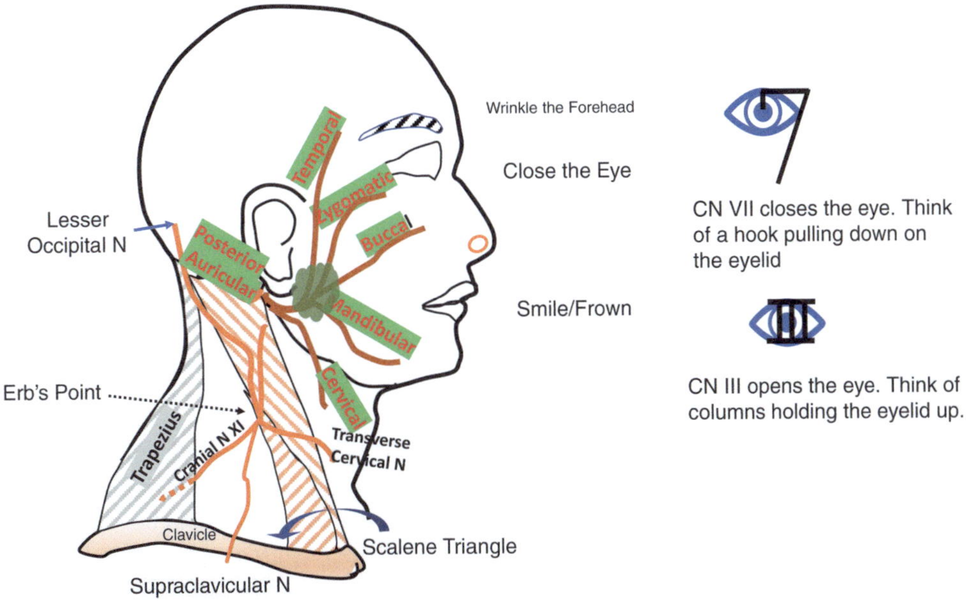

Fig. 1.20 To **Z**anzibar **B**y **M**otor **C**ar, **P**lease. Coming out of the stylomastoid foramen and winding through the parotid glad are the branches of the facial nerve: **T**emporal, **Z**ygomatic, **B**uccal, **M**andibular, **C**ervical, **P**osterior auricular. At the posterior border of sternocleidomastoid (Erb's Point) are several nerves: Lesser occipital, great auricular, transverse cervical, and supraclavicular. The accessory nerve can also be seen going posterior to trapezius [21, 22]

all the muscles of facial expression there are several important ones.

1. The *orbicularis oculi* is the sphincter surrounding the eye. Its primary function is closing the eye. It is also the efferent portion of the blink reflex. The afferent portion is V1 (ophthalmic nerve). For example, dust in the eye would be sensed by V1, and then the closing part of the eye blink would be CN VII acting on the orbicularis oculi.
2. The *orbicularis oris* is the sphincter around the mouth.
3. The *zygomaticus major* and *minor* elevate the corners of the upper lip. They are the most important muscles for laughing. A dimple on the cheek results from a splitting of the zygomaticus major.
4. The *frontalis* is involved in wrinkling your forehead. It is attached via an aponeurosis to the occipitalis.
5. The *buccinator* plays a significant role in eating, drinking, and the suckling reflex by keeping the cheek against the teeth. The buccinator is innervated by the *buccal branch of the facial nerve*, while the *buccal nerve* is a branch of V3 in the infratemporal fossa that carries sensory information from the cheek.
6. The *modiolus* is a point on each cheek, lateral to the lip where several muscles come together. There is little benefit on memorizing each muscle that comes to this point, but if you can picture the muscles, it makes sense: orbicularis oris, depressor anguli oris, levator anguli oris, platysma, buccinator, superior and inferior incisivus, and risorius.

The branches of CN VII on the face are straight forward. But prior to emerging on the face, the nerve travels through the facial canal within the petrous portion of the temporal bone. Think of the facial canal as a hallway with several doors. As the facial nerve travels through this hallway it gives off three branches. As a clinician, it is important to understand the pathway of CN VII within the facial canal.

In the canal these three branches all have different components of nerves in them. When you look at the nerve in lab, you can "see" the different branches, but you cannot "see" the different fibers. However you need to be able to visualize what types of fibers you find along these different branches. In other words, when you look at the greater petrosal nerve, it looks like any other nerve, but you need to know that it is a preganglionic parasympathetic nerve. Or when you look at the chorda tympani you need to know it has preganglionic parasympathetic fibers destined for the glands but that it also has special sensory fibers for taste (Figs. 1.20 and 1.21).

To understand the diverse types of fibers we are going to compare the facial nerve to a subway map (Fig. 1.22).

1. first branch is *the greater petrosal nerve* which carries preganglionic parasympathetic fibers (the grey line) destined for the pterygopalatine ganglion. It arises from the facial nerve within the facial canal. It exits through the hiatus for the greater petrosal nerve and runs in the groove for the greater petrosal nerve and then crosses foramen lacerum. It then travels through the pterygoid canal to enter the pterygopalatine fossa where the pterygopalatine ganglion is located. After synapsing in the pterygopalatine ganglion, one group of postganglionic fibers ascends to the lacrimal gland, other fibers descend to glands on the nasal mucosa, palate, and pharynx. Lesions to facial nerve of the pterygopalatine ganglion can result in ipsilateral dryness (xerostomia) of the paranasal sinuses, nasal cavity, and palate.
2. *nerve to stapedius* carries motor fibers (blue line) to the stapedius muscle which is involved in sound dampening. Damage to this nerve will result in hyperacusis.
3. *chorda tympani* is the third branch of the facial nerve within the facial canal. It carries sensory fibers from the anterior two-thirds of the tongue and parasympathetic fibers destined for the submandibular ganglion all four types of fibers mentioned above are present. It travels through the middle ear, exits through the petrotympanic fissure, and enters the infratemporal fossa where it joins the lingual nerve. The chorda tympani carries two types of fibers. It has preganglionic parasympathetic fibers (green line) destined for the submandibular ganglion and then to the submandibular and sublingual glands. It also conveys taste information from the anterior two-thirds of the tongue (Red Line).

As the facial nerve emerges from the stylomastoid foramen it has motor fibers to the muscles of

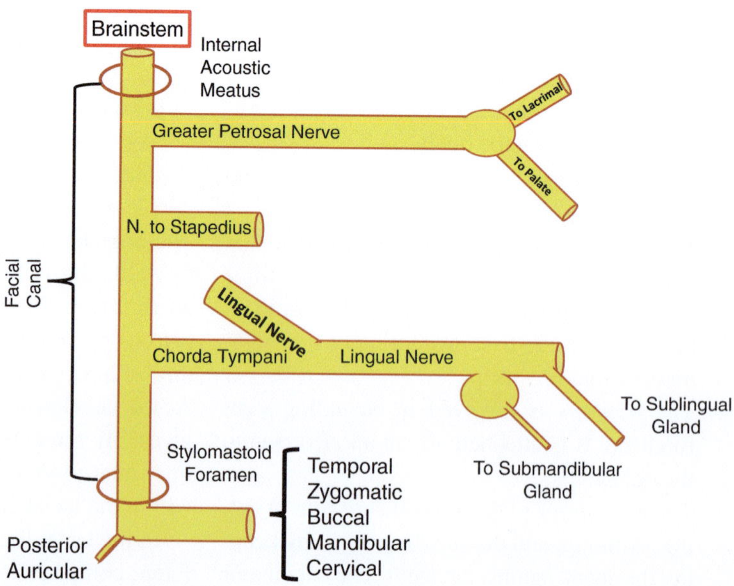

Fig. 1.21 Facial nerve and its branches [21, 22]

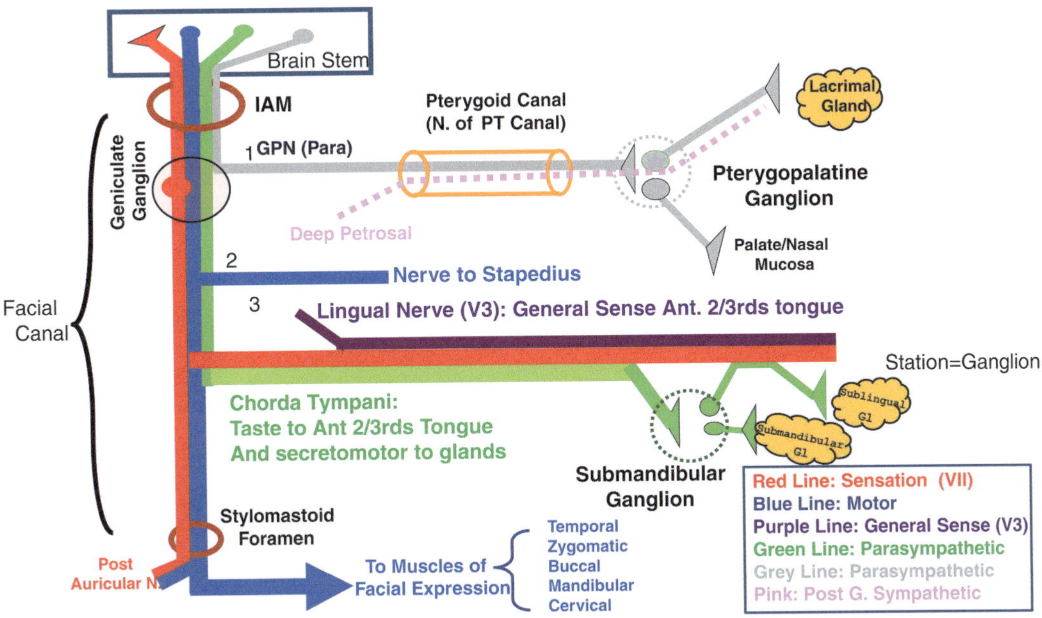

Fig. 1.22 Facial nerve pathway [21, 22]

facial expression (blue line) and sensory fibers to the external ear (red line).

The deep petrosal nerve (pink line) carries post ganglionic sympathetic fibers to the face—most importantly, the orbit. The deep petrosal nerve and greater petrosal nerve come together to form the nerve of the pterygoid canal, to enter the pterygopalatine fossa with the pterygopalatine ganglion.

There are several potential lesions to the facial nerve. On the diagram the lesions are placed at distinct parts of the nerve (Fig. 1.23).

Lesion A: With a parotid tumor or surgical complications of the parotid gland the facial nerve can be compromised. In this scenario, the patient will lose the muscles of facial expression on one side of the face, but since the nerve in the facial canal is intact there will be no deficit in hearing, taste, or glandular secretions from the lacrimal, submandibular, and sublingual glands. With a loss of facial muscles, the patient may drool from the corner of the mouth.

Lesion B represents classic Bell's palsy. In Bell's palsy, an infection of CN VII is thought to lead to inflammation and subsequent compression of the nerve in the canal. In this scenario, the patient will lose: the muscles of facial expression; taste from the anterior two-thirds of the tongue; secretions from the lacrimal gland which will lead to a dry eye; the submandibular and sublingual glands. Plus, because of the loss of the stapedius, they will complain that loud noises are aggravating. Loss of the submandibular and sublingual glands will not be obvious because the patient still receives secretions from the contralateral glands. They may also drool from the corner of their mouth.

While Bell's Palsy typically involves all the branches in the facial canal, it is possible for a tumor or other mass to only damage some of the branches. For instance, if there was a lesion to the facial nerve between the nerve to stapedius and the chord tympani, then the stapedius and lacrimal gland would be spared in this patient.

Lesion C is an acoustic neuroma. Because of the proximity of CNs VII and VIII as they enter the internal acoustic meatus, an acoustic neuroma which originates on CN VIII can also damage CN VII. This is rare but worth noting. The patient would have all the signs of the Bell's palsy patient, plus a hearing and balance deficit.

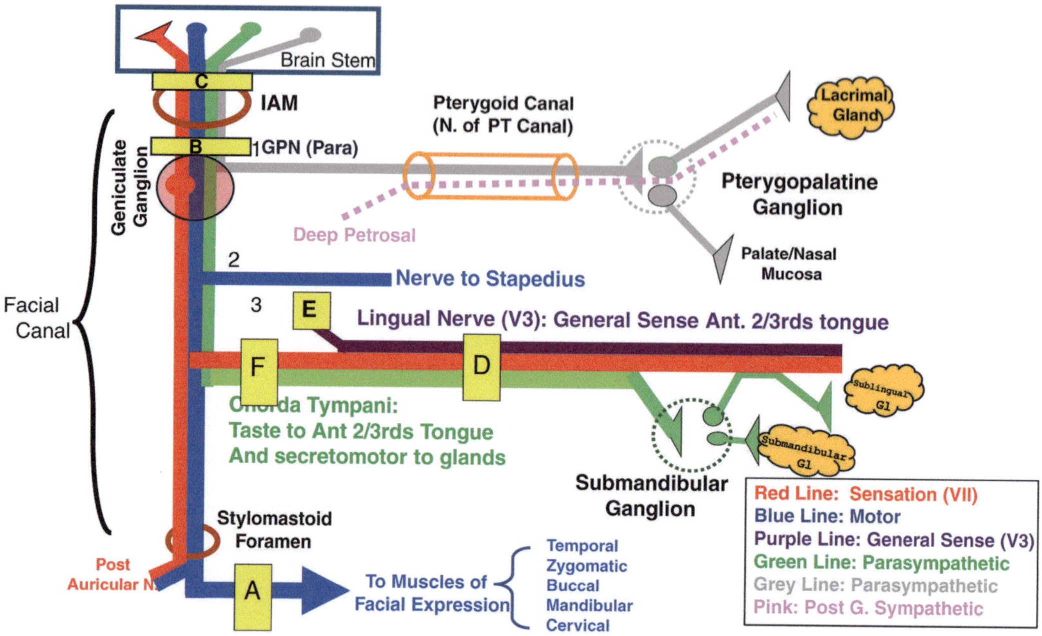

Fig. 1.23 Facial nerve pathway. Yellow Boxes indicate lesions. (See text for details [21, 22])

Lesion D. Another common injury involves the lingual nerve. The dentist needs to be careful of the lingual nerve when removing a wisdom tooth. If the lingual nerve is severed, then the patient will lose the following: taste to the anterior two-thirds of the tongue; the secretomotor fibers to the submandibular and sublingual glands; and general sense from the anterior two-thirds of the tongue. Remember the chorda tympani joins the lingual nerve, and the lingual nerve is a branch of V3 carrying general sense information from the tongue.

Lesion E is to the lingual nerve before the chorda tympani joins it, so taste and the glands would be spared, but the patient would lose general sensation from the anterior two-thirds of the tongue.

Lesion F is to the chorda tympani before it joins the lingual nerve so only taste and the glands would be affected.

Ramsay Hunt Syndrome

Ramsay Hunt Syndrome is caused by the varicella-zoster virus (shingles) and affects the facial nerve. After the herpes (varicella-zoster) virus infects nerves, it can remain dormant in the ganglion of sensory nerves for the life of the patient. With stress the virus can reactivate and lead to symptoms along the path of the nerve. With shingles, symptoms will be found following the dermatome of the infected nerve. If the facial nerve's geniculate ganglion is affected the symptoms will be found on the face. Patients will complain of pain in the ear and facial paralysis. Vesicles can also appear in the ear. In some cases, CN VIII is affected.

Buccal Nerve from CN V Versus Buccal Branch of CN VII

The terminology of the branches of CN V and CN VII can be confusing. Note that when talking about the branches of CN VII to the muscles of facial expression, we use the term *Temporal Branch*, *Zygomatic Branch*, or *Buccal Branch*. However, we have some branches of CN V which sound similar, such as *Zygomatic Nerve* and *Buccal Nerve* which carry sensory fibers. The <u>*buccal branch of CN VII*</u> is motor innervation to the buccinator muscle, while the buccal nerve is sensory to the cheek area. Likewise, the zygomatic branch of CN VII is a motor branch, while the zygomatic nerve (V2) is a sensory branch.

Temporal Bone

The *petrous portion of the temporal bone* is the strongest portion of the skull. The *internal auditory meatus* (IAM) is an opening on the petrous portion which transmits both CN VII and VIII. They both enter the IAM but quickly head in different directions. Cranial nerve VII does a 90° turn at the genu which is the site of the geniculate ganglion. Coming out of the geniculate ganglion is the greater petrosal nerve which leaves through the hiatus of the greater petrosal nerve and travels in the groove of the greater petrosal nerve to cross the foramen lacerum. The facial nerve then gives off the nerve to stapedius, and then the chorda tympani which crosses the malleus in the middle ear. The facial nerve finally exits the temporal bone at the stylomastoid foramen. Located on the temporal bone is the mastoid process with the mastoid air cells. Infections of the mastoid air cells can lead to inner ear deficits. Because of the potential for serious side effects, infections in this region are typically quickly treated. At one point in time, prior to the advent of antibiotics, mastoiditis was a significant cause of death in younger patients (Fig. 1.24). The word *temporal* refers to *time* and is used to refer to the area where the hair first turns grey, marking the passage of time.

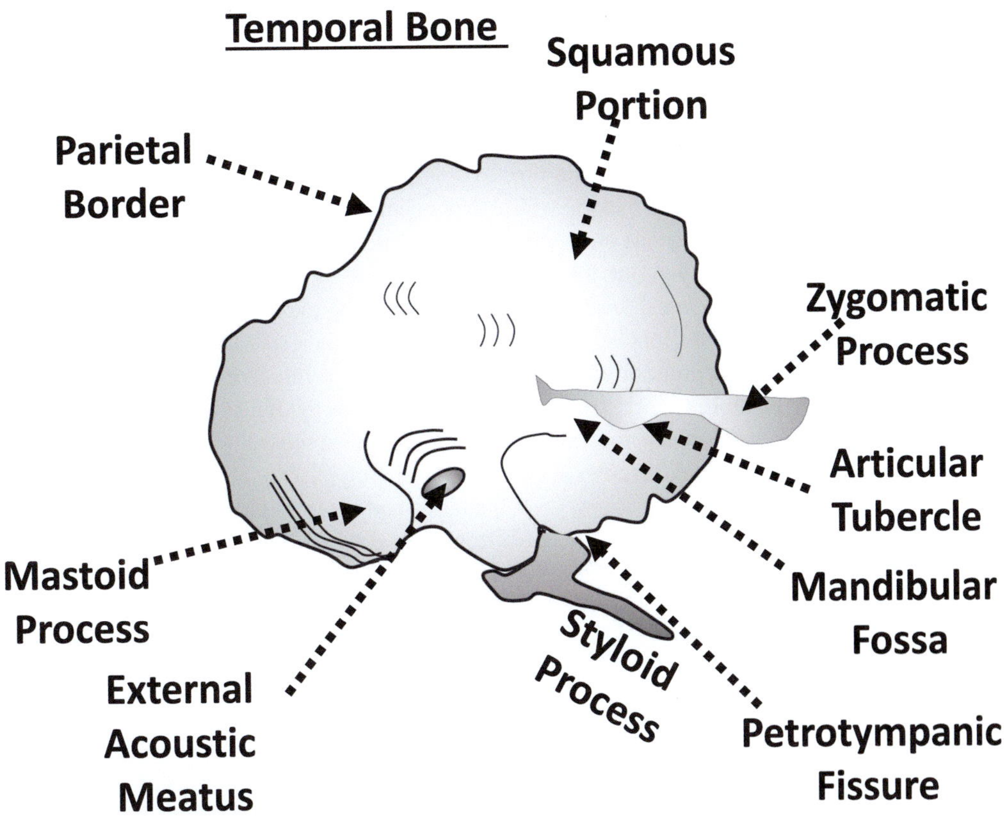

Fig. 1.24 Temporal bone (lateral view). The mandibular condyle sits in the mandibular fossa, posterior to the articular tubercle. When the Jaw opens, the mandible slides forward just inferior to the articular tubercle. The external acoustic meatus is the opening of the auditory tube. The petrotympanic fissure is an opening for the chorda tympani which is traveling on to the lingual nerve [21, 22]

Nasal Cavity

Before discussing the nasal cavity, it is important to understand the *ethmoid bone*, which is shaped like a cross. Start with a vertical line running down the middle. Superiorly, this line forms the *crista galli* which projects into the anterior cranial fossa and serves as an attachment point for the superior sagittal sinus. Running horizontally is another line which is part of the roof of the nasal cavity. On either side of the crista galli is the *cribriform plate* which has a series of small openings for the fibers connecting the olfactory epithelium to the olfactory bulb. Moving inferiorly, the center line continues into the nasal septum as the *perpendicular plate of the ethmoid.* Dropping down laterally, on each side are the labyrinths which house the ethmoid air cells (anterior, middle, and posterior). On the lateral side one also sees the *superior* and *middle concha* which are part of the ethmoid bone. The *inferior concha* is a separate bone (Concha means Keel in Latin).

The ethmoid bone contributes to both the nasal septum and lateral nasal wall. The *superior, middle, and inferior concha* form the lateral wall of the nasal cavity. The three conchae are something like bookshelves projecting out into the nasal cavity which are suspended over three spaces. The superior and middle concha are part of the ethmoid bone while the inferior concha is a separate bone. Underneath the superior concha is the *superior meatus*, underneath the middle concha is the *middle meatus*, and underneath the inferior concha is the *inferior meatus.* There is also a space above the superior meatus which is called the *sphenoethmoidal recess*. Staring superiorly and moving inferior (Fig. 1.25):

1. the highest opening is the *sphenoethmoidal recess* where the sphenoid sinus drains.
2. In the *superior meatus*, there is the opening of the posterior ethmoidal air cells.
3. In the *middle meatus* is a semicircular shaped opening called the semilunar hiatus. On the superior border of the hiatus is the *ethmoidal bulla*. On the inferior surface, there is a sharp line formed by the *uncinate process* (a projection of the ethmoid bone). Opening into the hiatus is the *ostium of the maxillary sinus*, which drains the maxillary sinus, along with the opening of the *frontonasal duct* which drains the frontal sinus and the anterior ethmoidal air cells. On the ethmoidal bulla are several small openings for the middle ethmoidal air cells.
4. Draining into the *inferior meatus* is the *nasolacrimal duct.*

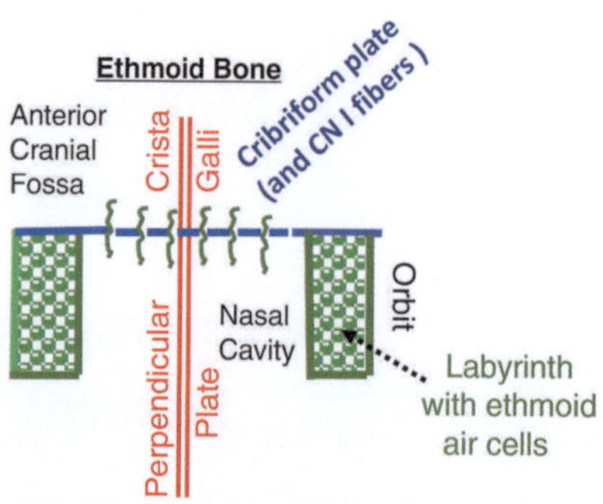

Fig. 1.25 Ethmoid Bone. It contributes to the boundaries of the nasal cavity, the anterior cranial fossa, and the orbit [21, 22]

The opening of the maxillary sinus is high up on the medial wall of the sinus resulting in a significant amount of fluid building up in the sinus before draining into the nasal cavity. A fluid filled sinus is a common spot for infections to take hold (sinusitis). If the infection bocks the ostium of the maxillary sinus the fluid can also back up into the frontal sinus via the frontonasal duct (Fig. 1.26).

Nasal polyps can also form in the various sinuses and the ethmoid air cells. If they become too large, they can herniate through various openings and then into various spaces. For instance, a polyp in the maxillary sinus can appear in the middle meatus, while a polyp in the anterior ethmoid air cells can appear in the sphenoethmoidal recess.

On the lateral nasal wall, at the superior posterior corner is the *sphenopalatine foramen* and coming through it is the *sphenopalatine artery* and *nasopalatine nerve* which travel onto the nasal septum and head anterior towards the *incisive foramen* to reach the anterior surface of the hard palate. In addition to the septum, the *sphe-*

nopalatine arteries and *nasopalatine nerves* also send branches to the lateral nasal wall.

Entering superiorly into the nasal cavity are the *anterior* and *posterior ethmoidal arteries* and *nerves* which drop down into the nasal cavity from the orbit. The anterior and posterior ethmoidal arteries come from the *ophthalmic artery*, and the anterior and posterior ethmoidal nerves come from the *nasociliary nerve* which is a branch of V1 (ophthalmic nerve). And finally, coming into the nasal cavity anteriorly at the nose are branches of the facial artery. Just inside the nose, at the vestibule, is *Kiesselbach's plexus* which is an anastomosis of these arteries. Nosebleeds are common in this region.

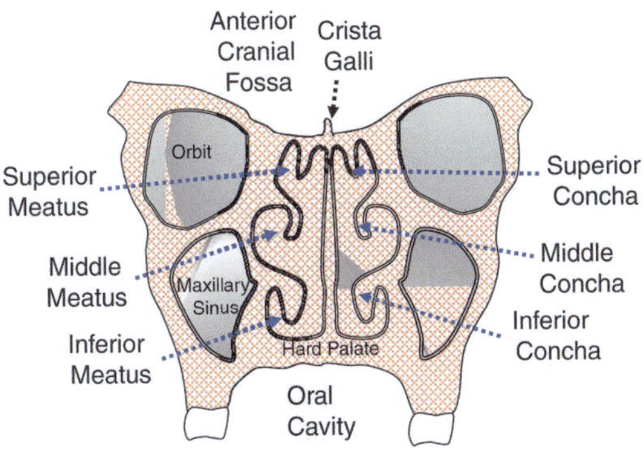

Fig. 1.26 Concha and meatuses. The concha are like three shelves pushing into the nasal cavity, which in turn creates three spaces—the meatuses. The floor of the orbit is the ceiling of the maxillary sinus. The hard palate is the ceiling of the oral cavity and the floor of the nasal cavity [21, 22]

The nasal septum is composed of the perpendicular plate of the ethmoid, the vomer (plowshare), and the nasal cartilage. "Broken noses" can lead to a deviated nasal septum.

The floor of the nasal cavity is the hard palate which is made up of the *palatine process of the maxilla* and the *horizontal plate of the palatine bone*. At the inferior border of the horizontal plate are the *greater* and *lesser palatine foramina*, which transmit the greater and lesser palatine nerves and arteries. The greater palatine arteries and nerves travel anterior to supply the hard palate. The lesser palatine arteries and nerves travel posterior along the soft palate and uvula.

The *greater* and *lesser palatine arteries* are both branches of *the descending palatine artery* which in turn comes from the maxillary artery in the pterygopalatine fossa. The greater and lesser palatine nerves are branches of V2 within the pterygopalatine fossa. From the pterygopalatine fossa, arteries and nerves descend into the oral cavity. At the superior border of the palatine bone is a notch, which is the *sphenopalatine foramen* (Fig. 1.27).

As air moves into the nasal cavity during inspiration, it travels superior to the palate. As it approaches the posterior portion of the palate it

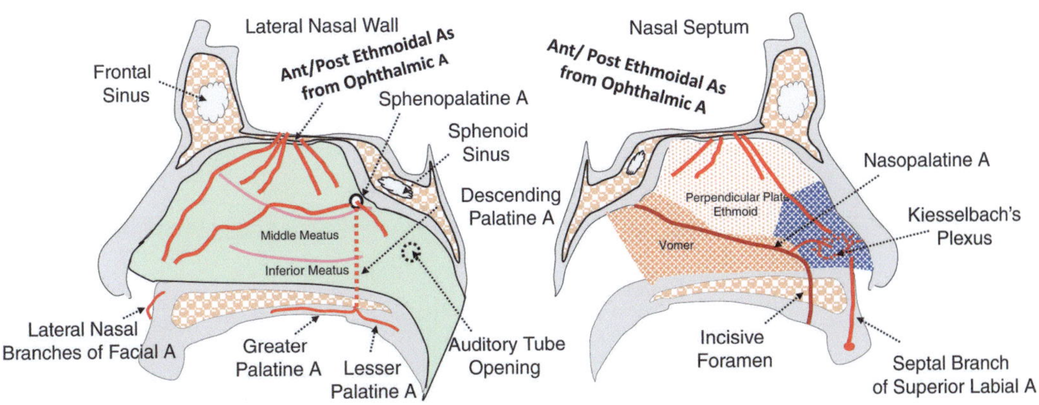

Fig. 1.27 Nasal Cavity. There are three arteries that contribute to the nasal cavity: (1) Descending from the ophthalmic artery are the anterior and posterior ethmoidal arteries, (2) emerging from the posterior superior corner at the sphenopalatine foramen is the sphenopalatine artery from the maxillary artery, (3) the facial artery sends branches into the vestibule. Kiesselbach's plexus is especially prone to nose bleeds [21, 22]

moves through two spaces, one on either side, called the *choanae*. As it moves through the choana, the air enters the nasopharynx. Choanal atresia is a rare condition where the infant has excessive growth of the bony structures in this area which block air flow into the lungs. The infant has a very difficult time breathing. Interestingly, when the infant is crying, the airflow improves. The condition is typically present right after delivery, and surgery, especially if it is bilateral, is required.

Oral Cavity

Palatine Bone

The *palatine bone* is shaped like a fishhook with a *perpendicular plate* and a *horizontal plate*. The horizontal plates from each side meet in the midline, and these two pieces, along with the palatine process of the maxilla, form the hard palate. It is not a perfect fishhook, as the top of the bone really has two pieces: laterally the *orbital process* contributes to the orbit, and medially the *sphenoidal process* contributes to the lateral nasal wall. Descending through the perpendicular plate are the *descending palatine artery*, the *greater palatine nerve*, and the *lesser palatine nerve*. At the junction of the horizontal plate of the palatine bone and palatine process of the maxilla is the *greater palatine foramen*. Slightly, posterior to the greater palatine foramen, but part of the palatine bone, is the *lesser palatine foramen* (Figs. 1.27 and 1.28).

The Tongue

There are many folds, ligaments, and muscles in the head: palatoglossus, palatopharyngeus, stylohyoid, hyoglossus, stylopharyngeus, glossoepiglotic, aryepiglottic, salpingopharyngeus, and the list goes on. When you first hear these names, they can sound overwhelming. But when you look at each one individually the name makes sense, as they are all named for their attachments. The lateral glossoepiglotic ligament, for example, runs from the tongue to the epiglottis.

If you look in the mirror, on each side of your mouth you will see a *palatoglossal arch* and the *palatopharyngeal arch*, with the *palatine tonsil* between them. There are numerous arches in this region which are formed by the mucous membrane of the oral cavity overlying either a muscle or a ligament. Whether it is a muscle or a ligament, it will be named for the two structures it connects.

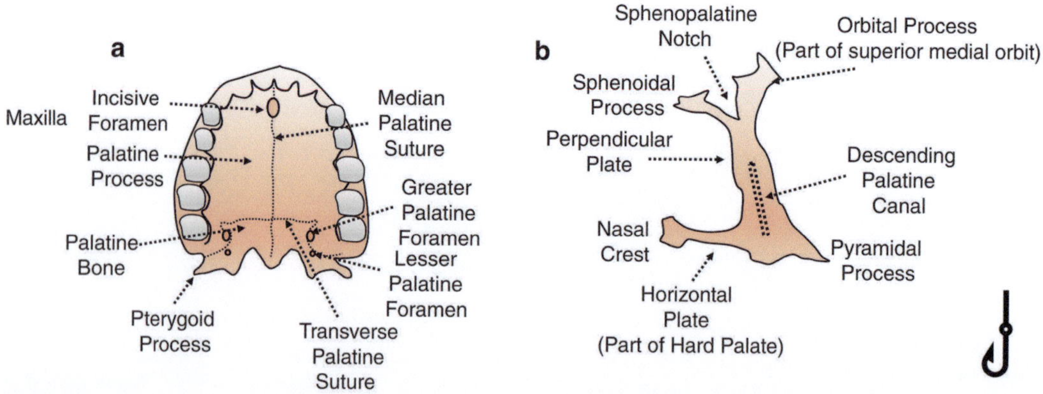

Fig. 1.28 Panel (**a**) The hard palate is made up of the larger palatine process of the maxilla and the horizontal plate of the palatine bone. The greater and lesser palatine foramina transmit the nerves arteries and veins of the same name which came from the pterygopalatine fossa and descended in the descending palatine canal. Panel (**b**) The palatine bone is shaped somewhat like a fishhook or a "**J**," with a descending perpendicular plate contributing to the lateral nasal wall, and a horizontal plate contributing to the hard palate [21, 22]

For instance, the palatoglossal arch is made by the underlying palatoglossal muscle which runs from palate to tongue, and the palatopharyngeal arch is made by the underlying palatopharyngeus muscle running from the palate to pharynx.

There are four extrinsic muscles of the tongue: *palatoglossus, styloglossus, genioglossus,* and *hyoglossus*. They are all innervated by the *hypoglossal nerve* (XII) except for palatoglossus which is innervated by the vagus nerve (X). All these muscles are named for where they start and where they end. The first part of the name is the giveaway. For instance, the styloglossus runs from the styloid process to the tongue. When looking from the lateral side towards the mouth, the styloglossus and hyoglossus muscles resemble a meat cleaver, with the styloglossus being the handle and the hyoglossus being the blade (Fig. 1.29). One cause of sleep apnea is relaxation of the genioglossus, which results in blockage of the upper airway.

The hypoglossal nerve emerges from the hypoglossal canal and wraps around the internal and external carotid arteries to enter the mouth just lateral to the hyoglossus muscle. When it crosses the external carotid artery it is near the lingual artery. However, the hypoglossal nerve runs superficial (lateral) to the hyoglossus muscle, while the lingual artery runs deep (medial) to the hyoglossus muscle (Fig. 1.29).

At the back of the tongue, running between the back of the tongue and the epiglottis are three ligaments. In the midline there is the single *median glossoepiglotic ligament*, and on either side are the two *lateral glossoepiglotic ligaments*. And then on either side of the median glossoepiglotic ligament are the vallecula. Each right and left *vallecula* is pouch or space where saliva can collect. Some have referred to this as the splash zone or flavor collector. The valleculae are important landmarks during intubation because the epiglottis is pulled anterior during the procedure.

The *frenulum* of the tongue attaches the inferior portion of the tongue to the floor of the mouth. In children it can sometimes be too tight, in which case it can be cut to allow more mobility for the tongue.

The *submandibular gland* lies in the submandibular triangle and is subdivided into two sections by the mylohyoid muscle. The *submandibular duct* travels anterior and medial to emerge on the *sublingual papilla* on either side of the *frenulum.* As it travels anterior, it crosses the lingual nerve. At the point where the two structures cross, the lingual nerve is lateral. The *sublingual gland* is located more medial and, rather than one large duct, it has a network of small ducts that enter on the medial side of the tongue. Both the submandibular and sublingual glands are innervated by postganglionic parasympathetic fibers from the submandibular ganglion, which in turn received preganglionic input from fibers traveling on the lingual nerve.

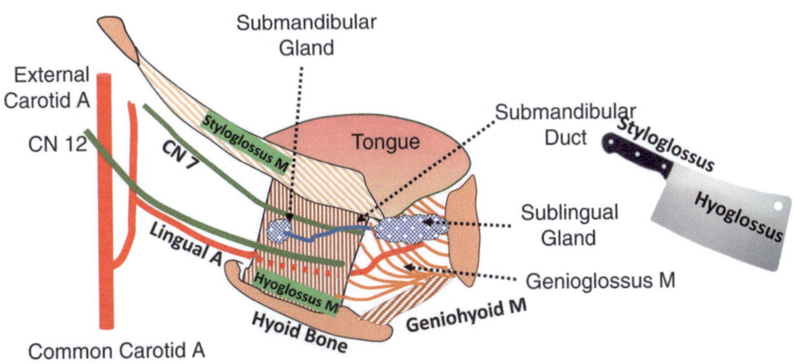

Fig. 1.29 Tongue. The styloglossus and hyoglossus together resemble a meat cleaver. The hypoglossal nerve runs lateral to the hyoglossus muscle. The lingual artery runs deep to the hyoglossus muscle. The lingual nerve is seen approaching the mouth from above. The submandibular gland is sending its duct to the sublingual caruncle. The geniohyoid runs from the genu of the mandible to the hyoid bone [21, 22]

In the infratemporal fossa the chorda tympani joins the lingual nerve. The lingual nerve is a branch of V3 that travels to the tongue and is responsible for general sense from the anterior two-thirds of the tongue. Note that the lingual nerve and lingual artery do not run together.

The glossopharyngeal nerve also comes out of the jugular foramen and travels to the posterior third of the tongue near the stylopharyngeus muscle. Besides innervating the stylopharyngeus, it is responsible for general sense and taste sensation from the posterior one-third of the tongue.

Eagle Syndrome

In some individuals, the styloid process or the stylohyoid ligament becomes elongated. This can compress the nearby glossopharyngeal nerve which leads to pain in the jaw area, difficulty swallowing, and a persistent feeling of something in the throat. This is referred to as Eagle syndrome (named after an otorhinolaryngologist) or Styloid syndrome. Surgical reduction of the styloid process can relieve the symptoms.

The floor of the mouth is formed by the mylohyoid and geniohyoid muscles. The mylohyoid is like a sheet running between the two sides of the mandible, while the geniohyoid is a strap muscle running from the genu of the mandible to the hyoid bone. The geniohyoid is innervated by a branch of C1 traveling on the hypoglossal nerve, while the mylohyoid is innervated by the nerve to mylohyoid which is a branch of the inferior alveolar nerve (Fig. 1.30).

The Tonsils

The palatine tonsils sit between the palatoglossal and palatopharyngeal folds. They receive a rich blood supply from branches of several arteries including the facial, maxillary, lingual, and ascending pharyngeal. However the most important supply comes from the tonsillar branch of the facial artery. The nerve to the tonsillar bed is the tonsillar branch of the glossopharyngeal nerve.

In addition to the palatine tonsils, there are several other locations for tonsillar tissue. The *pharyngeal tonsils* (adenoids) are in the upper regions of the pharynx, the *lingual tonsils* are on the posterior tongue, and the *tubal tonsils* are near the opening of the auditory tube. Together, this ring of tonsillar tissue is referred to as *Waldeyer's ring* because it forms a ring of tissues between the back of the mouth and the start of the pharynx.

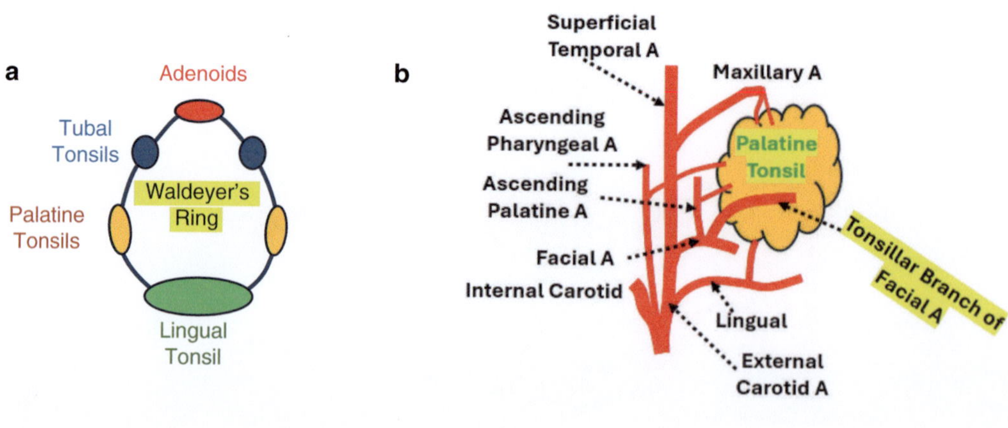

Fig. 1.30 The Tonsils. Panel (**a**) Waldeyer's ring is a ring of tonsillar tissue surrounding the back of the mouth. Panel (**b**) shows the rich blood supply to the palatine tonsils. The most important branch is the tonsillar branch of the facial artery [21, 22]

Palate

The palate is made up of the hard and soft palates. The hard palate is part of the maxilla. The uvulae is part of the soft palate. Several extrinsic muscles blend in with the soft palate. The *tensor veli palatini* arises from the pterygoid process and descends straight down vertically to wrap around the pterygoid hamulus to then run horizontally and blend in with the soft palate. It is shaped like an "L." When the muscle contracts it will pull the palate laterally to tense it. The *levator veli palatini* meanwhile runs from the temporal bone diagonally towards the midline to blend in with the soft palate and the levator from the other side. The two muscles together are shaped like a "V." The two levator muscles then form a sling so that when they contract, they will elevate the palate. While eating and drinking, the soft palate and uvula will elevate to prevent the contents in the oropharynx from moving into the nasal cavity. The levator veli palatini also arises from the cartilage of the auditory tube (pharyngotympanic tube or eustachian tube) and is involved in opening the airway to equalize pressure differences (Fig. 1.31). Some sources say that only the tensor veli palatini helps to open the pharyngotympanic tube while others say that both the tensor veli palatini and the levator veli palatini contribute to opening the pharyngotympanic tube. Suffice it to say, this is strictly an academic argument with little to do with clinical anatomy. I only point it out so that you do not get confused if you see different explanations of these two muscles and their role in opening the eustachian tube.

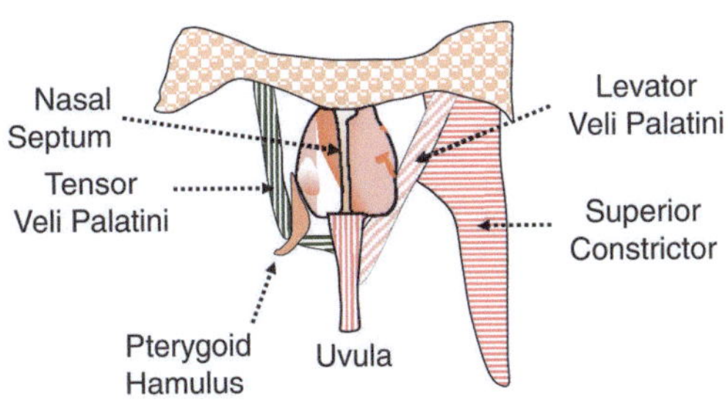

Fig. 1.31 Tensor and levator veli palatini. Note the levator veli palatini heads diagonally towards the midline to blend in with the soft palate. The tensor veli palatini descends vertically, and does a 90° turn around the pterygoid hamulus (hook) of the medial pterygoid plate and then heads horizontally to blend into the palate [21, 22]

Buccal Fat Pad

The buccal fat pad is a small pocket of fat sitting between the buccinator and the masseter muscle. Extensions of it come to lie under the zygomatic arch, It is pierced by the parotid duct. Weight loss does not typically affect the size of the buccal fat pad. For surgical reduction or removal of it, the surgeon gains access through the mouth.

Glossopharyngeal Nerve: Cranial Nerve IX

Right as the glossopharyngeal nerve exits through the jugular foramen, one can see the superior and inferior ganglion. They are both sensory ganglion (not autonomic). The superior ganglion has cell bodies for visceral sensation from the carotid sinus and body along with sensation from the pharynx and middle ear. The inferior ganglion has cell bodies associated with general sense and taste from the posterior one-third of the tongue. After emerging through the jugular foramen, between the internal jugular vein and the internal carotid artery, CN IX travels posterior to the styloid process and runs with the stylopharyngeus muscle between the superior and middle pharyngeal constrictors. It then travels deep to the hyoglossus muscle to enter the back of the tongue. Along its course it has several branches (Fig. 1.32).

1. Right as the glossopharyngeal nerve exits the jugular foramen, at the inferior ganglion, it gives off the *tympanic nerve* which contains parasympathetic fibers destined for the otic ganglion and the parotid gland. The tympanic nerve reenters the skull through the inferior tympanic canaliculus where it contributes to the tympanic plexus. The tympanic nerve carries sensation from the middle ear and the medial surface of the tympanic membrane. Emerging from the tympanic plexus is the lesser petrosal nerve that travels through the

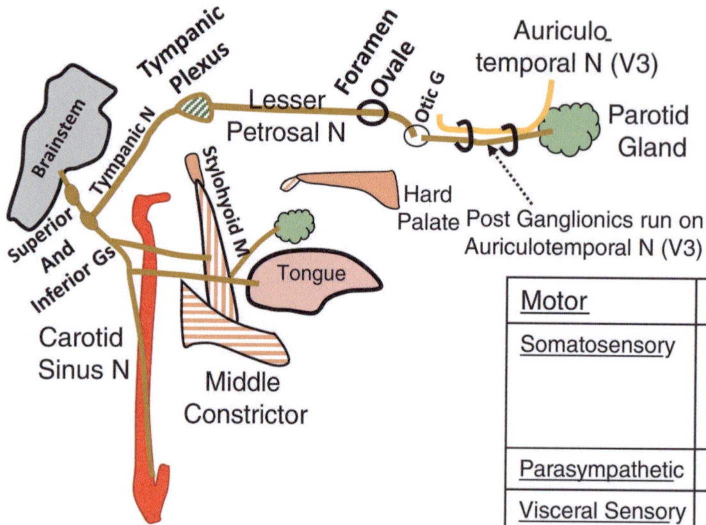

Motor	Stylopharyngeus
Somatosensory	Back of pharynx, Tympanic Membrane (Medial), Post 1/3 tongue: Taste/ General Sense
Parasympathetic	Parotid Gland
Visceral Sensory	Carotid Body and Sinus

Fig. 1.32 Glossopharyngeal nerve. The superior and inferior ganglion are located right as the nerve exits the brainstem. The first branch is the tympanic nerve which is sending preganglionic fibers to the otic ganglion. The postganglionic fibers then travel onto the parotid gland. The stylopharnygeal nerve supplies the stylopharyngeus muscle. The main nerve continues to the back of the tongue. On the way it sends a branch to the bed of the palatine tonsil [21, 22]

hiatus for the lesser petrosal nerve and travels on the floor of the middle cranial fossa in the groove for the lesser petrosal nerve. It then passes through the foramen ovale where it meets the otic ganglion. After the presynaptic parasympathetic fibers synapse in the otic ganglion, the post ganglionic fibers jump on the auriculotemporal nerve to travel to the parotid gland.

2. The *stylopharyngeal branch* send motor fibers to the stylopharyngeus muscle.
3. The *tonsillar branch* travels to the palatine tonsil where it lies posterior to the tonsil. It is responsible for sensation around the tonsil, the soft palate and arches, and the auditory tube. This is the nerve responsible for the afferent limb of the gag reflex. CN X is responsible for the efferent portion of the gag reflex. It can be injured during surgery on the palatine tonsil.4. The *carotid sinus branch* carries sensation from the carotid body and sinus.
5. The glossopharyngeal nerve continues to the back of the tongue where it is responsible for taste and general sensation from the posterior one-third of the tongue.

Orbit

The eye sits in the orbit but one of the first things to note is that the axis of the eye and the orbit are not the same. The orbit is a cone shaped structure pointing laterally. The medial wall of the orbit is more anterior than the lateral wall. Since we need the eye to look straight ahead, the axis of the eye is medially deviated which places the fovea lateral to the location of the optic nerve. The axis of the eye runs down through the macula where there is an abundance of cones. Medial to the fovea is the optic disc where the ganglion cells of the retina are converging. As they converge at the optic disc and travel down the optic nerve to the lateral geniculate body, they create a small blind spot in the temporal field of each eye (Fig. 1.33).

The six extraocular muscles are all appropriately named, and, except for the inferior oblique, they all originate from a *common tendinous ring*

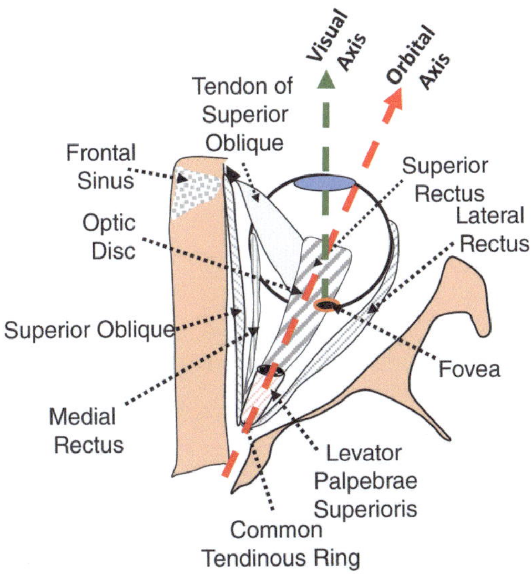

Fig. 1.33 Orbit. Note the origin of the four rectus muscles from the common tendinous ring. The medial wall of the orbit extends farther anteriorly than the lateral wall. The orbital axis is a line straight down the optic nerve to the tendinous ring. However, the eye is medially deviated so that the fovea is pointing straight ahead [21, 22]

that surrounds the optic nerve at the apex of the orbit. In a superior approach to the orbit, the *levator palpebrae superioris* is the first muscle you encounter. It inserts into the superior eyelid and is responsible for elevating the eyelid—opening the eye. Just deep to the levator palpebrae muscle is the superior rectus muscle.

Overview of Eye Muscles and Nerves

When you approach a patient with a deficit of an extraocular muscle, or see a test question, think of two parts to the scenario. The first part is when the patient is sitting in your office and you notice, or suspect, that something is amiss with the eyes. The second part of the exam is when you formally test the muscles by asking the patient to follow your finger as you move them through the test. We will first look at the actions of the eye muscles and their respective nerves. We will then look at how you would test the muscle and nerves. To do this we are going to look at two pictures to discuss the eye muscles.

Actions

The first picture shows the *actions* of the muscles (Fig. 1.34). This is the picture that you would see in a typical anatomy textbook. Anatomists like to talk about actions or functions. Note that medial rectus (MR) and lateral rectus (LR) each only have one action. The lateral rectus pulls the eye laterally (abduction), and medial rectus pulls the eyes medially (adduction). However, the other four muscles each have three actions. Superior oblique (SO) pulls the eye down and out, while inferior oblique (IO) pulls the eye up and out. And superior rectus (SR) pulls the eye up and in, while inferior rectus (IR) pulls the eye down and in. Yet, we also need to pay attention to the oft ignored intorsion and extortion movements. Intorsion is when the 12 o'clock position of your eye rotates towards your nose, and extortion is when it rotates away from the nose (Fig. 1.35).

Do not confuse intorsion and extortion with medial and lateral movements. Intorsion and extorsion involve the eyes rotating within the eye socket. While you are reading this, tilt your head to the right. If you did not have intorsion and extorsion, then your world (the page) would tilt, but you know that the world stays level. This is because your right eye intorted and your left eye extorted. As you walk down the street and your head moves this mechanism allows your eyes to compensate for head movements so that the world does not bob around and make you dizzy. When you look at the picture showing the actions of the muscles you can see that there are two interters (superior oblique and superior rectus), and two extorters (inferior oblique and inferior rectus) (Fig. 1.34).

The action picture for the eyes is important to understand because it explains what happens with the eyes when there is a nerve lesion.

Cranial Nerve Six Lesions

The eye is a democracy. To look straight ahead you need to have equal tension on medial and lateral rectus. If you have a deficit with the lateral rectus, then medial rectus will then take over and

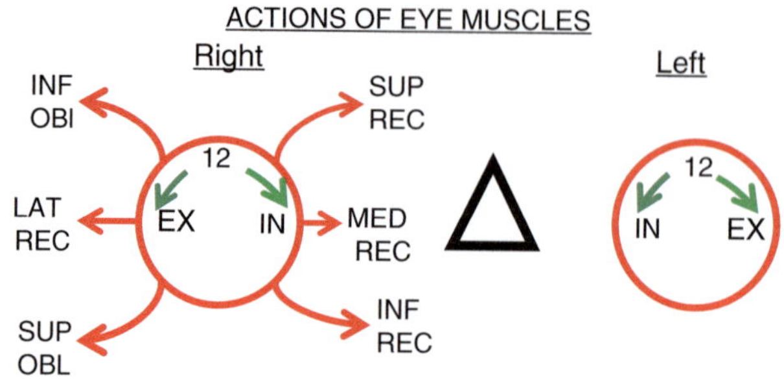

Fig. 1.34 Actions of eye muscles. The arrows show the actions of each muscle. For example, the medial rectus pulls the eye in, and the superior oblique moves the eye down, out, and intorts [21, 22]

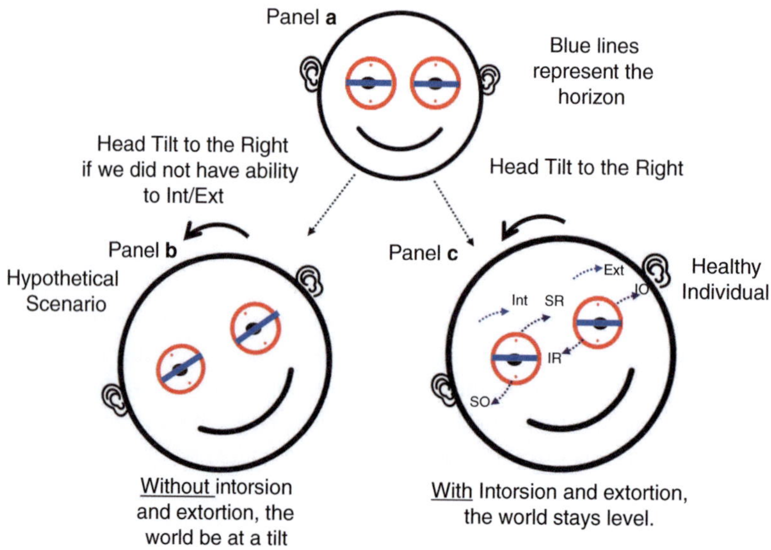

Fig. 1.35 Intorsion and Extortion. Panel (**a**), when you look straight ahead the world is level. When you tilt your head, you want the world to stay level. Panel (**b**) shows a hypothetical case (not a patient) of a person with no ability to intort or extort the eye. In this case the world will not be level when they tilt their head. Panel (**c**) show a healthy individual, with a head tilt to the right. The right eye responds by intorsion, and the left eye responds by extortion. Superior oblique (SO) and superior rectus (SR) are intorters; Inferior rectus and inferior oblique are extorters [21, 22]

move the eye medially. The patient will have a medial strabismus. If they have a deficit with medial rectus, then lateral rectus takes over and they have a lateral strabismus. The lateral rectus has been referred to as the "lover's muscle" in reference to a couple making sly motions with their eyes to each other.

As the fibers of CN VI exit the pons, they make a sharp 90° turn and head superiorly in the subarachnoid space. At this point, the fibers are traveling along the clivus on their way towards the posterior clinoid processes. As they approach the posterior clinoids, they make another 90° turn to travel horizontally under Gruber's ligament. From the point where CN VI slips under the dura and to the point where it enters the cavernous sinus is called Dorello's canal (The exact boundaries of Dorello's canal are debated and vary according to different authors, but these nuances are beyond the scope of this book.)

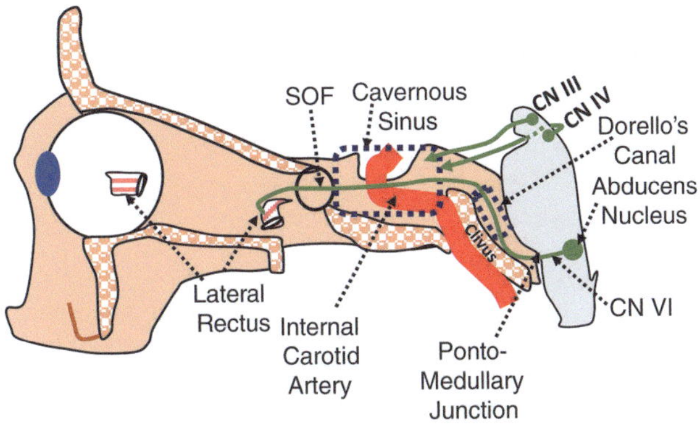

Fig. 1.36 Pathway of CN VI. The abducens nucleus sends fibers that emerge from the pontomedullary junction and run superiorly on the clivus. The fibers pierce the dura to enter Dorello's canal and then run to the cavernous sinus where they are lateral to the internal carotid artery. They then run through the superior orbital fissure (SOF) to enter the orbit. CN III is also seen exiting from the midbrain at the interpeduncular fossa. CN IV is seen exiting on the dorsal side of the midbrain and running to the cavernous sinus [21, 22]

As the fibers of CN VI emerge from the anterior cavernous sinus, they enter the apex of the orbit and the superior orbital fissure. The pathway of the CN VI fibers through these various divisions aid in understanding the various lesions:

Lesions of CN VI in the PNS:

1. Subarachnoid Space. Damage to the nerve in Dorello's canal typically results from increased intracranial pressure on the nerve between the clivus and the pons. Decreased intracranial pressure can also put pressure on the nerve. The deficit here is often secondary to a primary issue somewhere else in the CNS.
2. Cavernous Sinus: Infections, aneurysms, or carcinomas, can affect CN VI in the cavernous sinus. In addition, the optic nerve and CNs III, IV, and V1 and V2 can also be affected.
3. Superior Orbital Fissure (Rochen-Duvignead Syndrome): Tumors in the superior orbital fissure can also affect CN VI. The lesion here is like cavernous sinus lesions (Fig. 1.36).

Parkinson's Sign

Not to be confused with Parkinson's Syndrome, Parkinson's sign refers to lesion on CN VI at a very precise location. While a cavernous sinus lesion can compromise CNs III, IV, VI, and V1 and V2 leading to ophthalmoplegia and possibly Horner's Syndrome, there is also a more subtle deficit that can appear given a small lesion. Within the cavernous sinus, CN VI (6) travels towards the lateral rectus there is a small point where the postganglionic sympathetic fibers from the internal carotid artery briefly touch CN VI (6) . A small, isolated lesion at this point where these fibers emerge can lead to an ipsilateral CN VI palsy and an ipsilateral Horner's syndrome referred to as *Parkinson sign.* This is interesting, but rare (Fig. 1.37).

Cranial Nerve Three Lesions

A lesion to CN III will result in the loss of all the extraocular muscles except lateral rectus and superior oblique which will lead to the eye projecting down and out—a lateral strabismus. Because CN III has parasympathetic fibers, the patient will also have ptosis (droopy eyelid) and mydriasis (dilated pupil). *Duane Syndrome* is a rare congenital defect of CN VI that results in a reduced ability to abduct the eye. It is thought that the defect lies with miswiring of CN VI fibers to the muscle. It is not the muscle that is weak but the nerve. It is typically not present at birth but develops later in childhood. It can affect one eye or both eyes. *Moebius Syndrome* is a rare congenital defect that leads to deficits in the wiring of CNs VII and VI. It is present at birth and

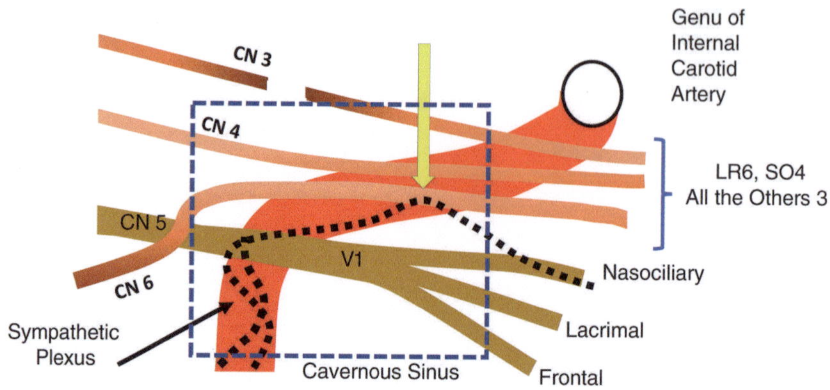

Fig. 1.37 Cavernous sinus and cranial nerves. Traveling through the cavernous sinus are cranial nerves 3, 4, 6, V1 and V2 (not shown). The postganglionic sympathetic fibers from the superior cervical ganglion are traveling up the internal carotid artery and jumping on CN V to go out on the nasociliary nerve to the long ciliary nerves. On the way, for just a moment, these fibers touch CN VI. A lesion here to CN VI can lead to an ipsilateral CN VI palsy and Horner's Syndrome [21, 22]

patients have facial paralysis (CN VII) and an inability to abduct the eye.

Cranial Nerve Four Lesions

With a lesion to the right CN IV the patient loses the right superior oblique, one of the two intorters of the right eye. With weakened intorsion, the right eye will now be extorted. With the right eye extorted, the patient now has two visual fields. To bring the world back to one visual field, the patient will lean away from the lesion side—in this case towards the left. This movement brings the right eye up to level, and since the muscles on the left are working the left eye will intort. Keep in mind that you cannot look at a patient's eyeball and see intorsion and extortion, but you can see their head tilt (Fig. 1.38).

Testing

The next picture focuses on the H test. This is the test used by clinicians to test the eye muscles. Naturally, this is the figure that you would see in a typical clinical exam textbook. While anatomists are interested in function, clinicians are more interested in how to test a muscle. To test the MR and LR, you ask the person to look medially or laterally. However, if you want to test the right SO, first you ask the patient to look left (adduction), and then once the eye is pulled in, you ask the person to look down. The only way the adducted eye can look inferiorly is with SO. The first part of the test, when the patient looked medially isolated the SO, so that the only way the patient can look down is with SO. The only way they look up is with IR. Ideally when you test the eye movements you keep on the H lines, and do not take the diagonal shortcuts (Fig. 1.39).

Oculomotor Nerve

The *oculomotor nerve* enters the orbit just lateral to the optic nerve and quickly divides into a *superior and inferior division*. The superior division travels between the levator palpebrae superioris and superior rectus. The inferior division travels lateral to the optic nerve and send branches to the medial rectus, inferior rectus, and inferior oblique.

Entering the back of the eye are the *short* and *long ciliary nerves*. There are some commonalities to these nerves and some differences. To explain these two nerves, we need to look at both CN III and CN V1 (ophthalmic nerve) (Fig. 1.40).

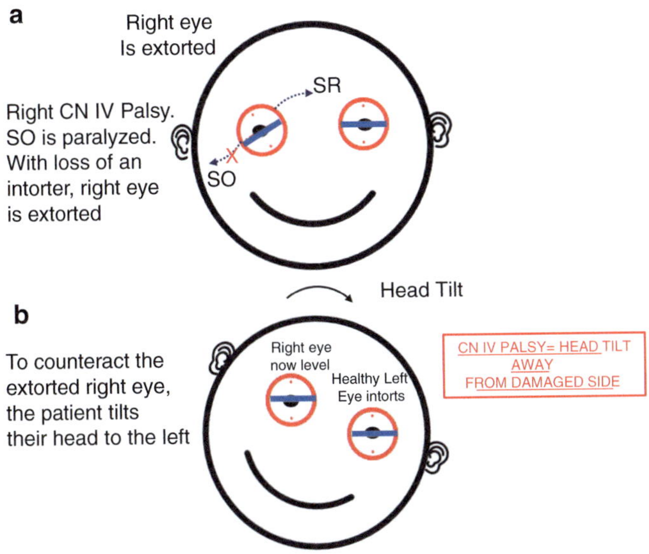

Fig. 1.38 Cranial nerve IV palsy. Panel (**a**) With a right fourth nerve palsy and loss of the superior oblique (SO), the right eye will be extorted. There is now a mismatch between the two visual fields. Panel (**b**) The patient responds by tilting their head to the left to bring the right eye up to level. Meanwhile, the left eye is working and is intorted so that that both eyes are now seeing the same visual field. The head tilt to the left compensates for the right fourth nerve palsy [21, 22]

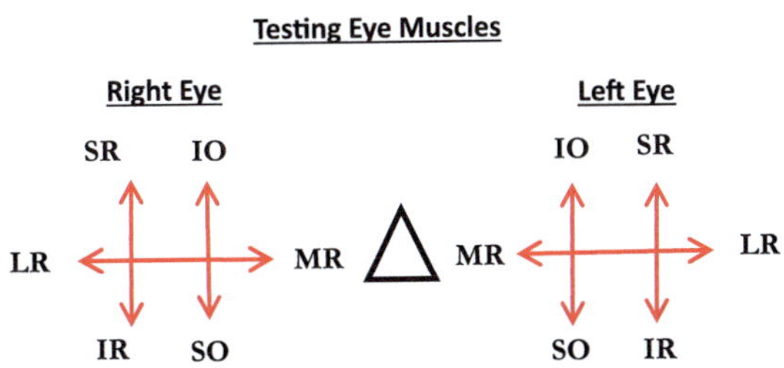

Fig. 1.39 Testing of eye muscles. Diagram of the H-test. To test superior oblique the patient first looks in and then down [21, 22]

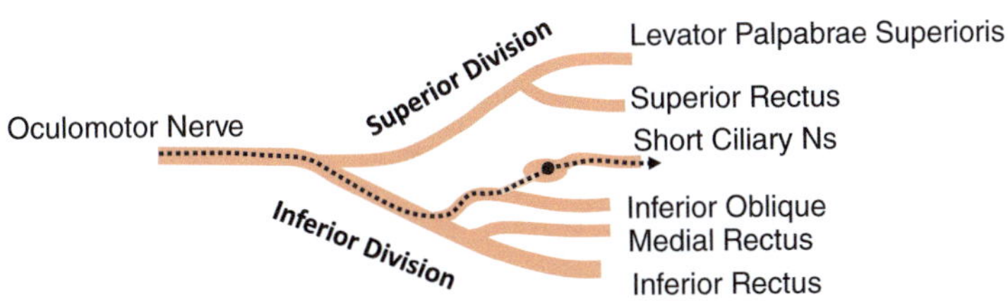

Fig. 1.40 CN III. The oculomotor nerve enters at the superior orbital fissure and splits into a superior and inferior division. The superior division innervates the levator palpebrae superioris and superior rectus. The inferior division innervates the inferior oblique, medial rectus, and inferior rectus. The ciliary ganglion hangs off the inferior division and is the site where the preganglionic fibers of CN III synapse with the postganglionic fibers. The postganglionic fibers innervate the constrictor pupillae, and the ciliary muscle [21, 22]

1. CN III is a motor nerve or an *efferent* nerve carrying motor fibers to the muscles mentioned above. As it enters the orbit it divides into superior and inferior divisions. The superior division supplies the levator palpebrae superioris and the superior rectus. The inferior division supplies the inferior oblique, inferior rectus, and medial rectus. In addition, the inferior division carries the parasympathetic fibers to the ciliary body and the pupillae constrictor.

   Coming out of the brain with CN III are preganglionic parasympathetic fibers that synapse on the ciliary ganglion which is attached to the inferior division of the oculomotor nerve. The *short ciliary nerves* can be seen coming off the ciliary ganglion. These are postganglionic parasympathetic fibers traveling to the constrictor pupillae to constrict the pupil, and to the ciliary muscle for accommodation. From the back of the eye, these autonomic fibers going to the dilator and sphincter pupillae travel between the sclera and the choroid. The ciliary ganglion is found between the optic nerve and the lateral rectus muscle. Trauma or surgery to the lateral orbit could affect the ciliary ganglion, which could lead to loss of the parasympathetic fibers and a dilated eye.
2. CN V1 (ophthalmic nerve) on the other hand is strictly an *afferent* or sensory nerve. One of the branches of CN V1 is the nasociliary nerve and coming off it are the *long ciliary nerves.* Sensation from the eyeball, such as a cotton swab touching the cornea, travels back along the short and long ciliary nerves. It seems logical that the long ciliary nerves would carry sensation, however it does not seem quite as logical for the short ciliary nerves to carry sensory fibers—remember they are coming off the ciliary ganglion and CN III. What happens is that the sensory information traveling on the short ciliary nerves jumps onto V1 via a communicating branch (Fig. 1.41).

Both the short and long ciliary nerves carry sensory fibers from the cornea. Keep in mind that CN III is a motor nerve so these sensory fibers in the short ciliary nerves quickly jump onto branches of V1 via the communicating branch. In addition, both sets of nerves carry sympathetic fibers (Fig. 1.40).

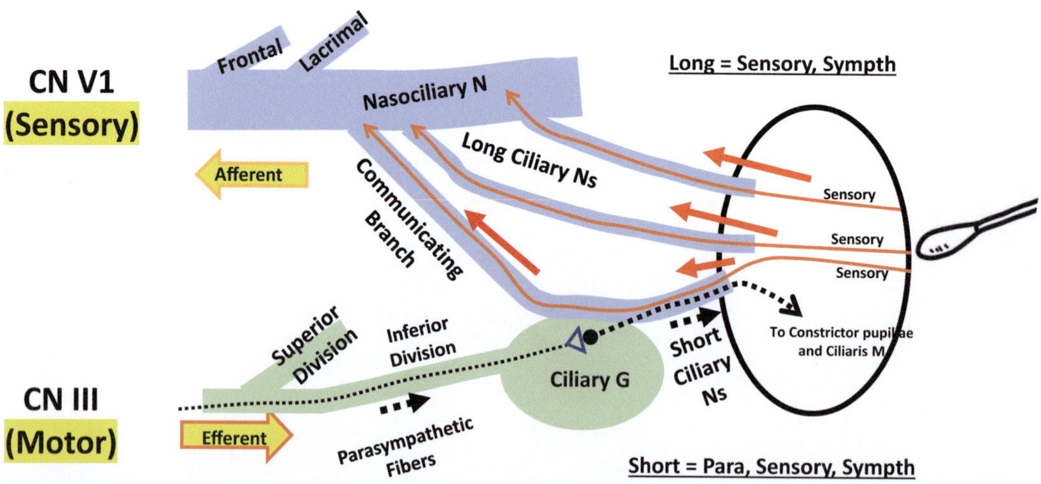

Fig. 1.41 Short and long ciliary nerves. CN III is a motor (efferent) nerve. The parasympathetic fibers on CN III travel on its inferior division, synapse in the ciliary ganglion and then travel on the short ciliary nerves to the constrictor. V1 is a sensory nerve (afferent). Sensation from the cornea travels on the short and long ciliary nerves to reach the nasociliary nerve. Note the communicating branch from the ciliary ganglion to the nasociliary nerve. Short ciliary nerves carry sensory and parasympathetic fibers. Long ciliary nerves carry sensory fibers. The sympathetic fibers are not shown; they travel on both long and short ciliary nerves [21, 22]

Ophthalmic Artery

The *ophthalmic artery* enters the eye at the optic canal. Within the orbit are several important branches (Fig. 1.42):

1. The *lacrimal artery* runs laterally and anteriorly to the lacrimal gland. It has a *recurrent branch* that travels through the superior orbital fissure to anastomosis with a branch of the middle meningeal artery. This represents an anastomosis between the internal and external carotid arteries.
2. *Anterior and posterior ethmoidal arteries* that travel medially to supply the ethmoid air cells and the superior portions of the nasal septum and lateral nasal wall.
3. *Posterior ciliary arteries* that enter the eye on either side of the optic nerve.
4. The *central artery of the retina* which travels deep inside the optic nerve.
5. The *supraorbital* and *supratrochlear arteries* exit the skull through the foramen of the same names and perfuse the skin over the forehead. Keep in mind that these are branches of the internal carotid artery that exit the skull. In the medial corner of the eye, they anastomosis with the angular artery which is a branch of the facial artery. The corner of the eye represents an anastomosis of the internal and external carotid systems. An increased pulse in the corner could be indicative of a blockage of the internal carotid artery and the body's response by having blood flow from the external carotid towards the brain.

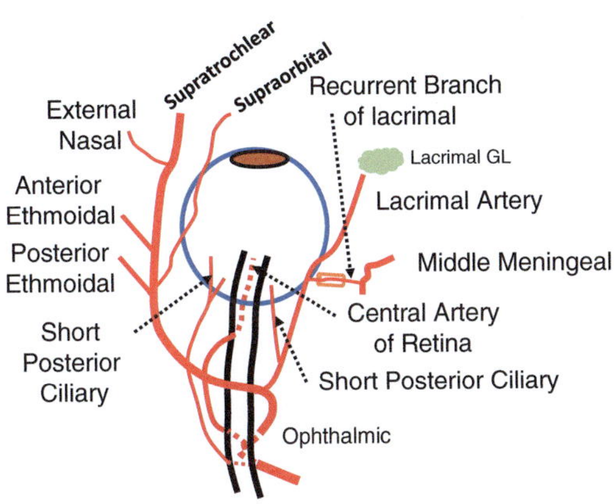

Fig. 1.42 Ophthalmic artery. The ophthalmic artery is a branch of the internal carotid artery that enters the orbit at the optic canal, lateral to the optic nerve. The lacrimal artery is a branch that heads to the lacrimal gland. The recurrent branch of the lacrimal anastomoses with the middle meningeal artery. The short posterior ciliary arteries enter the eye lateral to the optic nerve. The supraorbital and supratrochlear arteries emerge onto the face [21, 22]

Blood Supply to the Retina

The blood supply to the retina comes from the *ophthalmic artery,* however it comes from two different branches of the ophthalmic artery, and this branching pattern has important clinical significance. More proximally, the *central artery of the retina* comes off the ophthalmic artery and travels down the interior of the optic nerve to emerge onto the retina at the optic disc. From the disc region, branches of the central artery of the retina then fan out along the inner surface of the retina. Meanwhile, more distally, the *posterior ciliary arteries* are also branches of the ophthalmic artery, but these enter the eye at the external surface near the optic nerve and enter the choroid which has a rich blood supply. From the choroid, the blood perfuses the outer segments of the retina (Fig. 1.43).

An occlusion of the central artery of the retina will therefore block the blood to the internal surface of the retina causing the cells to die and the retina to turn cloudy. Meanwhile, the posterior ciliary arteries to the choroid are intact. Near the fovea, the internal surface of the retina is very thin, and the fibers at the fovea are pushed to the perimeter of the fovea allowing the practitioner to see blood in the choroid at the fovea. As a practitioner when you look into this patient's eye, you can see the blood perfusing the external retina at the fovea, but not the area around the fovea, leading to the name: "Cherry Red Spot."

V1: The Ophthalmic Nerve

The *ophthalmic nerve* (V1) leaves the middle cranial fossa through the superior orbital fissure and enters the orbit where it divides into three branches, think NFL:

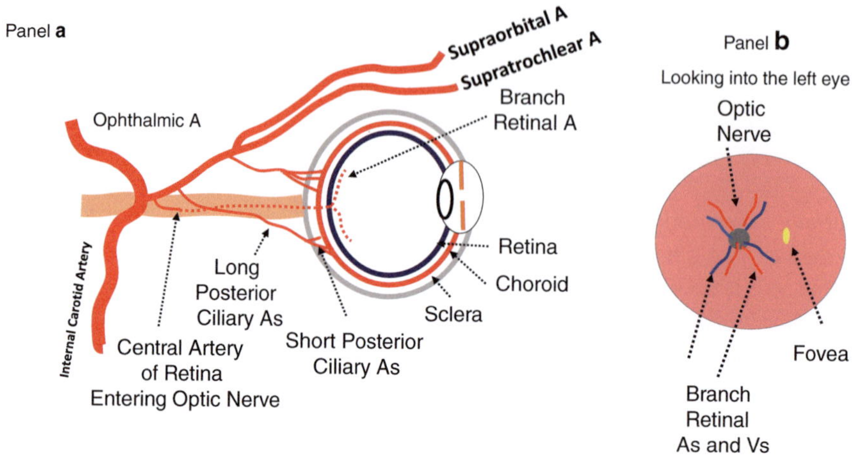

Fig. 1.43 Arteries to retina. In panel (**a**), the ophthalmic artery is a branch of the internal carotid artery. The blood supply to the inner retina comes from the central artery of the retina which enters the optic nerve and emerges onto the retina at the optic canal where it divides into retinal artery branches. The outer portions of the retina are supplied by the short ciliary arteries. Panel (**b**) is an anterior view—looking into the eye—showing the central artery of the retina emerging onto the retina and giving off the branch retinal arteries [21, 22]

1. The *nasociliary nerve* enters the orbit deep to the tendinous ring and just lateral to the optic nerve. It immediately crosses the optic nerve from lateral to medial to head towards the medial side of the orbit, where it gives off the *anterior and posterior ethmoidal nerves* that carry sensory information from the superior nasal cavity and the dorsum of the nose. It also gives off the *long ciliary nerves* that carry general sensory information from the cornea. There is also a *communicating branch* running from the oculomotor nerve to the nasociliary to provide a conduit for the sensory information on the short ciliary nerves to jump from CN III to CN V1 (ophthalmic nerve).
2. The *frontal nerve* travels superior to the levator palpebrae superioris and divides into two branches, the supraorbital and supratrochlear nerves that leave the skull through the same named foramen.
3. The *lacrimal nerve* carries sensory information from the lateral corner of the eye in the region of the lacrimal gland. However, running with it are postganglionic fibers from the pterygopalatine ganglion (CN VII) that innervate the lacrimal gland (Fig. 1.44).

Superior Orbital Fissure

There are three doorways at the back of the orbit that allow the nerves, arteries, and veins to approach the eye. Because there is an overlap between some of the doors, the diagram of this region resembles a Ven diagram. The main door is the *superior orbital fissure,* however the *tendinous arch* forms another door that overlays the medial part of the superior orbital fissure. There are some structures that come through just the superior orbital fissure—and not the tendinous ring—while there are other structures that come through the tendinous ring and the superior orbital fissure.

1. Coming through just the superior orbital fissure are the <u>L</u>acrimal, <u>F</u>rontal, and <u>T</u>rochlear nerves—think **LFT**. The superior division of the superior ophthalmic vein also comes through here.
2. Coming through the tendinous ring and the superior orbital fissure are the superior and inferior divisions of the oculomotor nerve, the abducens nerve, and the nasociliary nerve—think **36N**.

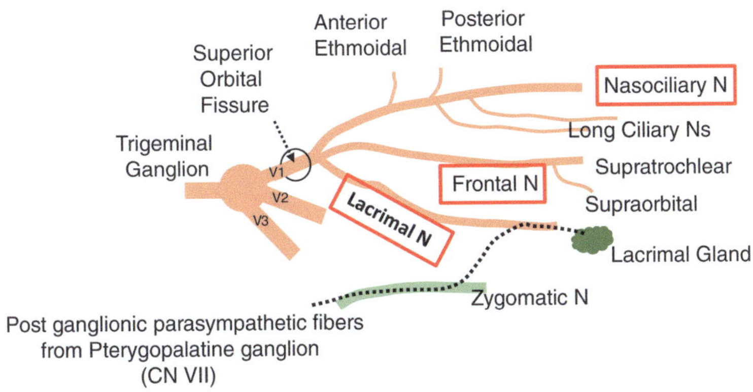

Fig. 1.44 V1. ophthalmic nerve (V1). There are three main branches: nasociliary, frontal, and lacrimal. The nasociliary nerve gives off the anterior and posterior ethmoidal nerves and the long ciliary nerves. The frontal nerve gives off the supraorbital and supratrochlear nerves that travel through the same named foramen to reach the skin over the orbit. Parasympathetic fibers from the pterygopalatine ganglion (CN VII) travel on the zygomatic nerve and then the lacrimal nerve to reach the lacrimal gland [21, 22]

3. In the medial corner of the superior orbital fissure there is a small space, outside of the tendinous ring that transmits the inferior ophthalmic vein.

In addition to the superior orbital fissure, there is the *optic canal* with the optic nerve and the ophthalmic artery. Note that the ophthalmic artery and ophthalmic vein do not run together.

Inferior Orbital Fissure

The *inferior orbital fissure* is located on the floor of the orbit. The *infraorbital artery* and nerve move from the pterygopalatine fossa through the inferior orbital fissure (the anterior door of the pterygopalatine fossa) to run in the *infraorbital groove*, then the *infraorbital canal*, and to then emerge through the *infraorbital foramen* and onto the face as the infraorbital nerve and artery. Once the nerve and artery come through the infraorbital foramen, they supply the skin between the lower eyelid and the upper lip. The inferior orbital fissure also contains the *zygomatic nerve* (Fig. 1.45 and Table 1.2).

Orbit Bones

The roof of the orbit is the *frontal bone* and *lesser wing of the sphenoid*; the floor is the *maxilla, palatine, and zygomatic* bones; the medial wall is the *ethmoid, maxilla, palatine, lacrimal, sphenoid,* and *zygomatic bones*; the lateral wall is the *zygomatic bone* and *greater wing of the sphenoid*. It is shaped like an ice cream cone with the optic canal at the apex, and the base opening onto the face. *Blowout fractures* of the orbit result from trauma to the eye that leads to fractures of these walls. The rim surrounding the base is usually spared. Inferior blowout fractures are the most common blowout fractures, and they usually occur in the vicinity of the infraorbital groove with the orbital contents herniating into the maxillary sinus. The inferior rectus muscle can also be compressed. The "buckling theory" proposes that the pressure on the eye leads to the boney orbit buckling. In many cases the fracture is nondisplaced because while the bone fractures it returns to its original position. This is referred to as a "trapdoor fracture." Remember the floor of the orbit is the ceiling of the maxillary sinus (Fig. 1.46).

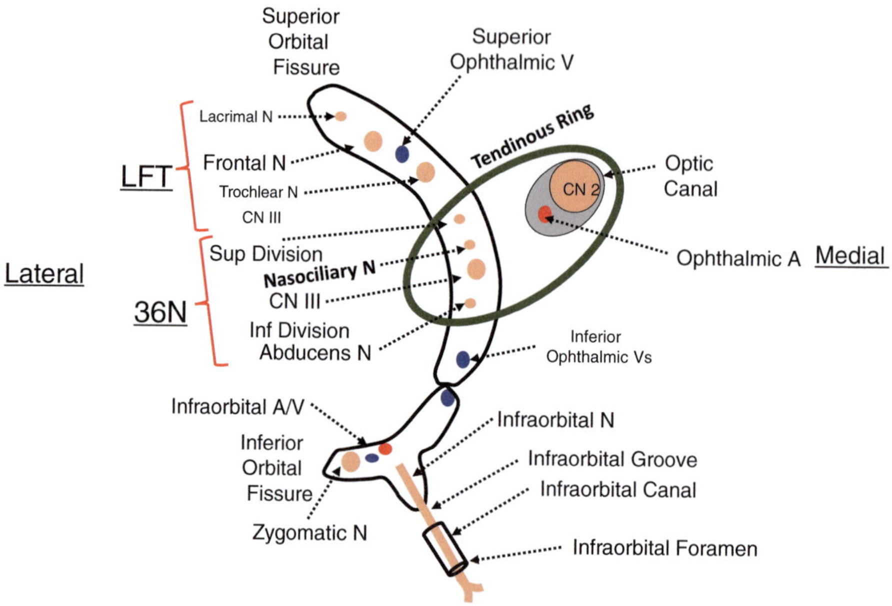

Fig. 1.45 LFT, 36N. Emerging through the superior orbital fissure are the Lacrimal (V1), Frontal (V1), and Trochlear nerves (CN IV), along with the superior ophthalmic vein. Emerging (36N) through the superior orbital fissure ***and*** the tendinous ring are the two divisions of the oculomotor nerve (CN III), the abducens nerve (CN VI), and the nasociliary nerve (V1). Emerging through the inferior orbital fissure is the infraorbital nerve (V1), artery, and vein, and the zygomatic nerve (V2). Running through the optic canal are the optic nerve (CN II) and the ophthalmic artery [21, 22]

Table 1.2 Openings around the orbit

Structure	Contents
Superior orbital fissure	CNs III, IV, VI, V1, V2, and superior ophthalmic vein
Inferior orbital fissure	CN V2
Optic canal	CN II, ophthalmic artery
Cavernous sinus	CNs III, IV, VI, V1, V2, and internal carotid artery

Petroclival Region: AKA, the Back of the Orbit

The petroclival region, which is a small region at the back of the orbit, brings together several cranial nerves which have already been discussed. Gruber's Ligament is a small ligament which runs from the apex of the petrous bone to the surface of the clivus just below the posterior clinoid process. CN III runs over the ligament and CN VI runs under the ligament. CN IV is also coming into the side of the ligament. All these nerves are headed towards the superior orbital fissure. Laterally, one can see the trigeminal ganglion living in Meckel's cave. Coming out of the trigeminal ganglion are the three branches of the trigeminal nerve. V1 is traveling through the superior orbital fissure, V2 through the foramen rotundum, and V3 through the foramen ovale. The greater petrosal nerve can also be seen running under the ganglion on its way to the foramen ovale (Fig. 1.47).

The Maxilla

The maxilla is the bone between your lower eyelid and your upper lip. It contributes to the walls of the orbit, the oral cavity, and the nasal cavity, and it houses the maxillary sinus. On the medial side is the nasolacrimal duct running from the medial corner of the orbit to the oral cavity. Sinus infections can lead to pain emanating from the upper teeth since they can penetrate the maxillary

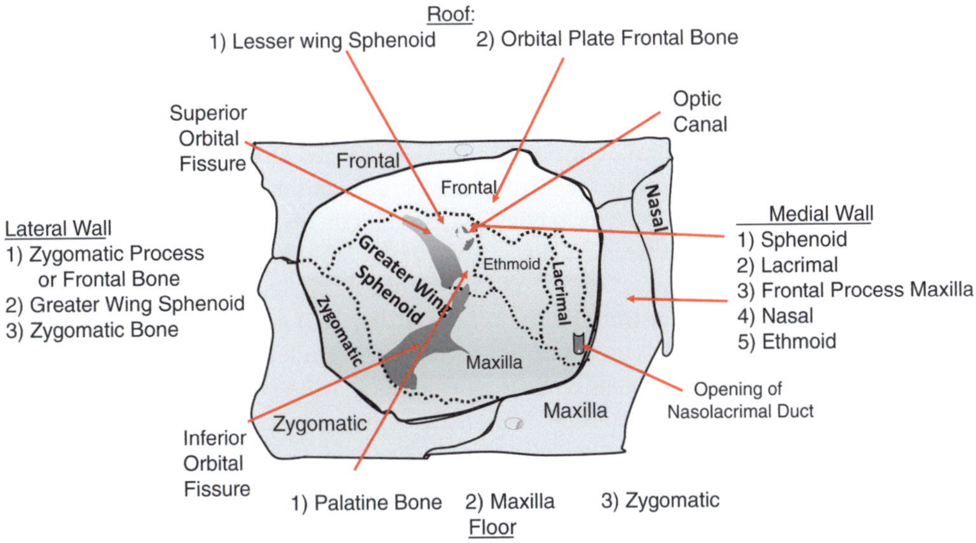

Fig. 1.46 Bones of the orbit. Note the openings of the superior orbital fissure, inferior orbital fissure, and the optic canal [21, 22]

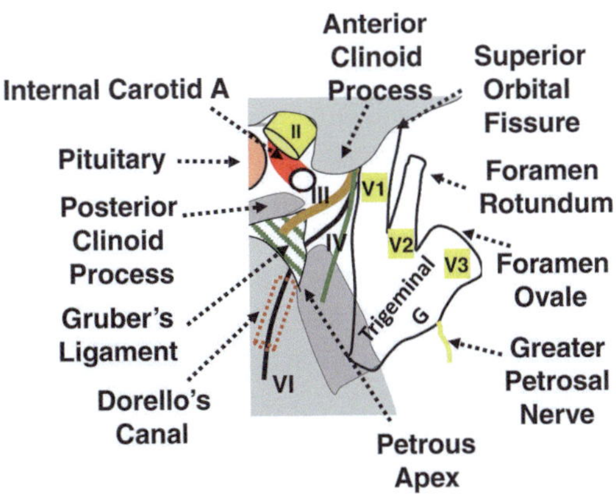

Fig. 1.47 Cranial nerves approaching posterior orbit (petroclival region.) Gruber's ligament runs from the petrous apex to the surface of the clivus just below the posterior clinoid process (spina sphenoidalis). CN III runs over the ligament. CN VI runs under the ligament. Prior to the ligament, CN VI is running in Dorello's Canal. The greater petrosal nerve runs under the trigeminal ganglion. To differentiate the nerves, they are different colors [21, 22]

sinus. The infraorbital nerve runs through the infraorbital groove, canal, and foramen to enter onto the face. Blowout fractures of the orbit can enter the maxillary sinus (Fig. 1.48).

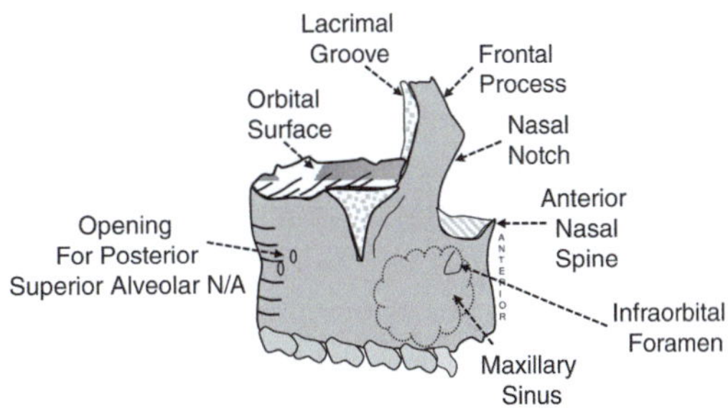

Fig. 1.48 The maxilla. The maxilla contributes to the orbit, and the nasal and oral cavities. It houses the maxillary sinus [21, 22]

Ear

For audition, the all-important membrane in the ear is the basilar membrane. Here is an analogy, imagine going to the beach, and with a sand shovel you dig two straight parallel channels going out to the ocean. The channels stretch to the water's edge and allow water to come into them. On top of each channel, you then lay a piece of paper. With this arrangement, you have two channels connected to the ocean, each with a piece of paper lying on the water's surface. Out on the ocean, there are motorboats, canoes, sailboats, fish jumping, and people swimming; activities that each create a distinctive wave pattern that reaches the two pieces of paper in the channels in the sand. Not only are the patterns different, but the timing of how the waves arrive at each channel vary depending on where the activity is occurring. If the activity is occurring on the right side, then the waves will hit the right channel before hitting the left channel. If the vibrations are coming from directly in front of you, they will reach each channel at the same time.

With your eyes closed and your hands on each piece of paper, just by feeling the vibrations of the paper you can interpret all the different activities occurring out on the ocean, and you can tell where everything is located. The two pieces of paper represent the basilar membranes inside your inner ear. Even with your eyes closed, the vibrations of the basilar membranes can sense the locations of the motorboat, the sailboat, and the rowboat. All the anatomy around these two membranes is designed to allow them to function properly. I digressed for a moment, but back to the anatomy.

The external ear is designed to act like a funnel to capture and direct sound waves into your external ear canal. Dogs and cats with their big wide ears are better at this than we are. As the sound waves move into the external ear canal, they eventually reach the tympanic membrane and vibrate it. When looking into the external ear at the tympanic membrane with an otoscope, the light creates a *cone of light* stretching from the *umbo* anteriorly and inferiorly to the edge of the tympanic membrane. On the right ear the cone of light would be in the 4–5 o'clock position, while on the left ear it would be in the 7–8 o'clock position. Swimmer's ear or *otitis externus* is an infection in the external ear canal.

The *tympanic membrane* is the only membrane in humans that is surrounded by air on both sides. It forms the medial wall of the external ear canal, and lateral wall of the middle ear. Most of the membrane is the *pars tensa*, while the smaller superior portion is the *pars flaccida*. These two regions are separated by the neck of the malleus. The *manubrium* (handle) of the malleus attaches to the pars tensa and ends in the *umbo*. The umbo is in the center of the eardrum and is the point where the bottom of the manubrium attaches. It only takes a miniscule amount of energy to vibrate the tympanic membrane. The amplitudes are in the picometer to nanometer range (smaller than a hydrogen atom). With excess fluid in the middle ear, the most common site to make an incision for drainage is the anterior inferior quadrant of the eardrum (Fig. 1.49).

On the other side of the tympanic membrane (the medial side) is the middle ear with the three ossicles. The malleus touches the tympanic membrane, and it will vibrate with the membrane. The malleus then vibrates the incus, and then the stapes. The stapes in turn contacts the oval window, which for the purposes of this book is our stopping point. The joints between the ossicles are hyaline lined synovial joints. The tympanic membrane translates the sound waves into mechanical energy—the movement of the ossicles. The surface area of the tympanic membrane is three times larger than the surface area of the oval window. This differential allows for amplification of the wave between the tympanic membrane and oval window.

At the *oval window,* the wave moves from an air-filled cavity into a fluid filled cavity thus the wave is translated from mechanical energy into hydraulic motion. We will leave it to the neuroanatomy, histology, and physiology books to continue with the pathway of vibrations through the inner ear.

However, in the middle ear, we have some important structures.

1. The *chorda tympani* nerve can be seen crossing the handle of the malleus on its way to eventually exit the *petrotympanic fissure* and enter the infratemporal fossa, where it joins with the lingual nerve. Infections in the middle ear can compromise the chorda tympani.
2. The *tendon of the tensor tympani* can also be seen entering the middle ear and making a 90° turn to insert on the malleus to tense the tympanic membrane during movements such as swallowing, chewing, and talking.
3. The smallest muscle in the body is the *stapedius* which can be seen in the middle ear

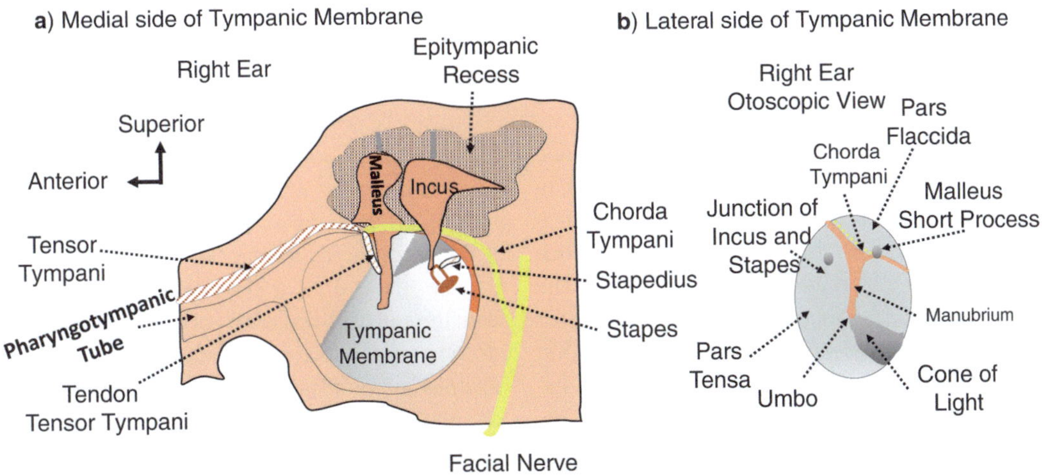

Fig. 1.49 Two views of the Tympanic Membrane. Panel (**a**) is from within the middle ear, looking laterally at the medial (interior) surface of the membrane. The malleus, incus, and stapes are all in view. The stapedius is attached to the stapes. The tensor tympani is running parallel to the pharyngotympanic tube to attach to the malleus. The chorda tympani can be seen crossing the malleus. Panel (**b**) is looking into the ear at the lateral side of the tympanic membrane. The cone of light is facing anterior. There are several impressions of structures located on the other side of the membrane such as the malleus and the junction of the incus and stapes [21, 22]

attaching to the stapes. Its job is to protect the inner ear in the presence of sudden, loud noises. The *acoustic reflex* refers to the stapedius and tensor tympani firing in response to loud noises. Both muscles stiffen the ossicular chain—the stapedius by fixing the stapes (CN VII) and the tensor tympani (CN V3) by stiffening the malleolus. The stapedius is the more important of the two muscles involved in the reflex. Testing the acoustic reflex is rare these days. If a patient reports that loud noises are bothersome, then the acoustic reflex is most likely affected—Bell's Palsy for instance.

The roof of the middle ear is the *tegmen tympani* which is part of the petrous portion of the temporal bone. This is a very thin bone separating the ear from the middle cranial fossa. With dissections of the ear, this bone is removed to investigate the ear. When you do this, you will also see the greater petrosal nerve in this region. Because the bone is so thin, a defect in it can allow CSF to move from the subarachnoid space into the ear which will be evident on an ear exam.

Otosclerosis is an abnormal growth where the stapes joins with the surrounding bone. *Cholesteatoma* is an abnormal growth of skin that can erode structures in the middle ear such as the ossicles and tympanic membrane. Chronic otorrhea is a predisposing factor. Surfer's ear comes from long-term exposure to cold water that leads to the development of a bony protuberance (exostoses) in the external ear.

The malleus and the incus project superiorly into the *epitympanic recess*. The middle ear also connects to the pharynx via the *eustachian tube* or *pharyngotympanic tube* which allows for equalization of pressures between the middle ear and ambient pressure. In adults, the eustachian tube descends diagonally, medially, and inferiorly from the middle ear to pharynx, which allows drainage to descend into the pharynx. In children the pathway is horizontal, which is not as efficient for drainage leaving children more susceptible to infections. Young children with chronic ear infections are candidates for tubes placed in the tympanic membrane to allow the middle ears to drain.

When a snorkeler or a scuba diver is descending, the ambient pressure rises and pushes on the tympanic membrane. Left to its own devices the tympanic membrane would rupture. But by holding their nose and blowing, this raises the pressure in the diver's pharynx, and in turn the middle ear via the eustachian tube. This increased pressure on the medial side of the tympanic membrane pushes the membrane open to allow the pressure to equalize. As the diver descends, they will have to continually equalize. The *tensor veli palatini* and *levator veli palatini* act on the soft palate which in turn acts on the opening of eustachian tube which sits right superior to the soft palate. Some experienced divers can master the movement of the eustachian tube without holding their nose.

The middle and inner ear are housed within the petrous portion of the temporal bone. In the laboratory, with a superior approach to the ear, the roof of the system is typically carefully pried off to look inside the middle and inner ear at the various structures.

There are several nerves that are responsible for sensation of the external ear. The tragus and the medial portion of the ear are supplied by the auriculotemporal nerve. The auriculotemporal nerve is also responsible for sensation from the external tympanic membrane. Just posterior to the tragus is the concha bowl, which is supplied by branches of CNs VII and X. The glossopharyngeal nerve is responsible the medial surface of the tympanic membrane. The posteroinferior portion of the external ear is supplied by the great auricular nerve (Fig. 1.50).

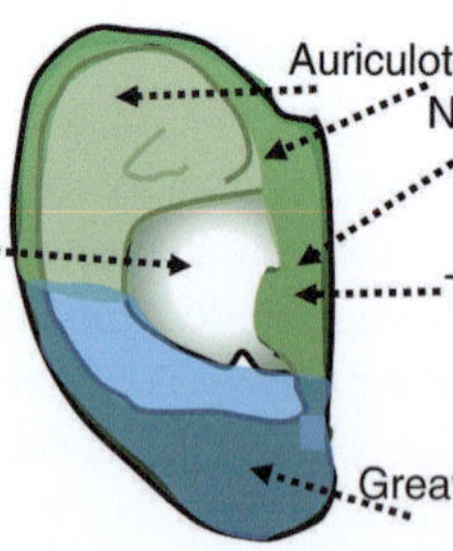

Fig. 1.50 Nerve supply to external ear. The tragus and superior portion of the ear are innervated by the auriculotemporal nerve. The earlobe and posteroinferior portion are innervated by the great auricular nerve. The skin anterior to the ear is also innervated by the auriculotemporal nerve. The concha bowl is innervated by branches of CN VII and X. Pathology in areas served by these nerves can lead to ear pain - secondary otalgia. A cough following aggravation of the tympanic membrane is due to stimulation of the vagus nerve [21, 22]

Neck

Triangles of the Neck

The main divisions of the neck are into the *anterior* and *posterior triangles*. If we start with the neck as a square, there are four sides: the midline of the neck, the mandible, the trapezius, and the clavicle. If we draw a diagonal line on one side from the superior-posterior corner to the anterior-inferior corner this represents the sternocleidomastoid and divides the neck up into the anterior and posterior triangles. In addition, each of these two larger triangles can be subdivided into several smaller triangles (Fig. 1.51).

Anterior Triangle

1. The *muscular triangle* contains the strap muscles of the neck and ansa cervicalis.
2. The *submandibular triangle* is bounded by the mandible and the anterior and posterior bellies of the digastric muscle. It contains numerous structures. The submandibular gland is located here. The submandibular nodes located here drain the inferior lateral teeth, and the lateral tongue.
3. The *carotid triangle* is bounded by the sternocleidomastoid, the posterior digastric and the superior belly of the omohyoid. It contains the internal carotid artery, the internal jugular vein, and the vagus nerve in the carotid sheath. In addition, the hypoglossal nerve is traveling across the region (Figs. 1.51 and 1.52).
4. There is only one *submental triangle,* located in the midline, which is bounded by the anterior digastric muscles and the hyoid bone. It contains the submental nodes which drain the anterior tongue and the two front teeth.

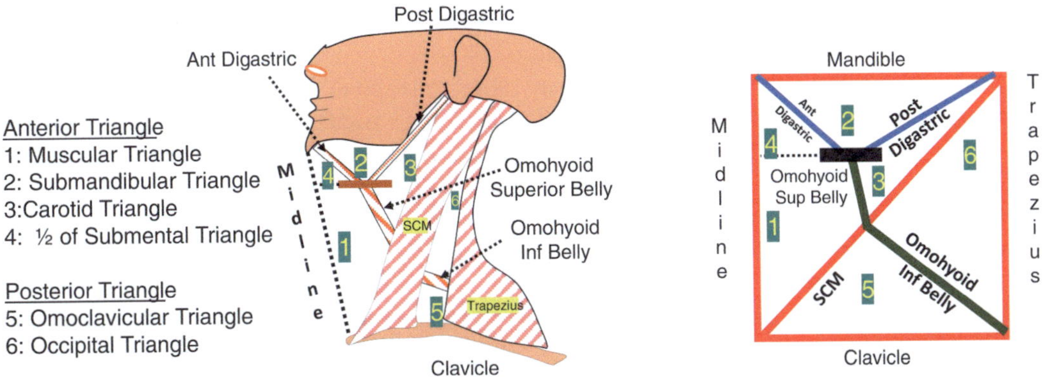

Fig. 1.51 Neck Triangles. The four borders of the square are: anterior = midline; posterior = trapezius; inferior = clavicle; Superior = mandible. Drawing a line—the SCM—from corner to corner gives you the anterior and posterior triangles. In the anterior triangle are the muscular, submandibular, and carotid triangles. In the posterior triangle are the omoclavicular (subclavian) and occipital triangles. All of these are paired triangles. The only single or unpaired triangle is the submental bounded by the right and left anterior digastric muscles and the hyoid bone [21, 22]

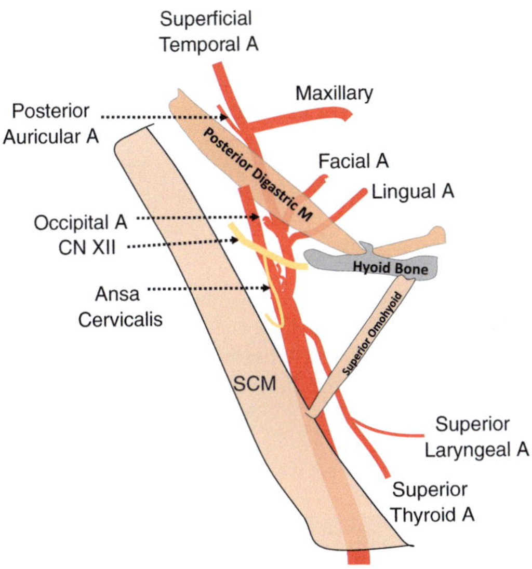

Fig. 1.52 Branches of the external carotid artery. In the carotid triangle the superior thyroid, ascending pharyngeal (not shown), occipital, lingual, and facial all come off the external carotid. Superior to the posterior digastric the occipital comes off. The two terminal branches of the external carotid are the superficial temporal and maxillary [21, 22]

Posterior Triangle

1. The *omoclavicular triangle* (AKA: subclavian triangle, or supraclavicular triangle) is bounded by the clavicle, the sternocleidomastoid, and the inferior belly of omohyoid. The anterior corner of the anterior triangle is a danger area meaning that there are important structures in this area.
2. The *occipital triangle* contains the accessory nerve emerging from the posterior border of sternocleidomastoid and traveling to the anterior border of the trapezius.

Ansa Cervicalis

The *ansa cervicalis* comes from C1, C2, and C3 and forms a loop from which branches emerge to innervate the strap muscles of the neck. It is found in the carotid triangle anterior to the internal jugular vein. Branches of C1 also travel for a moment with the hypoglossal nerve to travel to the geniohyoid and thyrohyoid muscles.

Fascia of the Neck

When dissecting the anterior neck, the platysma is the first muscle encountered. It is extremely thin and is found within the superficial fascia of the neck. It does not extend into the posterior triangle. It is involved with tensing the skin and is sometimes referred to as the "shaving muscle."

Platysmaplasty involves tightening the platysma to remove the creases and wrinkles of the neck. The deep cervical fascia of the neck is divided into investing, prevertebral, and pretracheal fascia.

1. The *investing fascia* is the most superficial layer of the deep cervical fascia, and it surrounds the sternocleidomastoid anteriorly, and the trapezius posteriorly.
2. The *pretracheal fascia* splits into two layers: a muscular layer surrounds the strap muscles of the neck, and the visceral layer surrounds the thyroid gland, trachea, and esophagus. Behind these structures the pretracheal fascia joins with the *buccopharyngeal fascia.* Inferiorly it blends in with the fibrous pericardium of the heart.
3. The *prevertebral layer* surrounds the vertebral vertebrae and the deep muscles.

Anterior to the prevertebral layer is the *retropharyngeal space* which allows movement of the neck structures. However, this space also allows infections to spread. An infection in the retropharyngeal space can spread to the superior mediastinum. The retropharyngeal space is subdivided into two spaces by the alar fascia (Figs. 1.53 and 1.54). Some books refer to the retropharyngeal space, not as being divided by the alar fascia, but just the compartment anterior to the alar fascia, with the danger area being posterior to the alar fascia [14].

Nerve Point of Neck

The nerve point of the neck is found halfway along a line paralleling the posterior border of the sternocleidomastoid going from the mastoid process to the sternoclavicular head. There are four sensory nerve branches, all of which come from the C5–6 roots:

1. The *transverse cervical nerve* crosses laterally in front of the sternocleidomastoid to reach the midline of the neck.
2. The *great auricular nerve* crosses the sternocleidomastoid with the external jugular vein and ascends towards the ear.

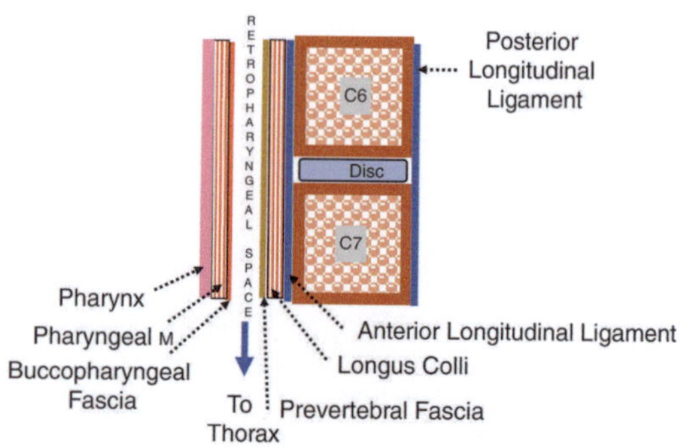

Fig. 1.54 "Danger space." The retropharyngeal space is between the buccopharyngeal and prevertebral fascia. An infection here can travel to the thorax [21, 22]

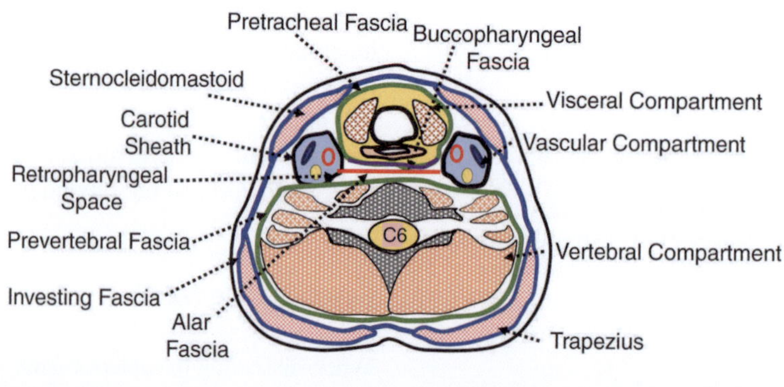

Fig. 1.53 Fascial compartments of the neck. The trapezius and sternocleidomastoid muscles are surrounded by the investing fascia. The prevertebral fascia surrounds the vertebral muscles and vertebral column. The carotid sheath surrounds the internal carotid artery, internal jugular vein, and the vagus nerve. The pretracheal and buccopharyngeal fascia surround the thyroid gland, trachea, and esophagus. The retropharyngeal space is between the visceral and vertebral compartments. The alar fascia separates the retropharyngeal space into two divisions [21, 22]

3. The *supraclavicular nerve* heads inferiorly towards the clavicle deep to the platysma.
4. The *lesser occipital nerve* runs along the anterior border of the trapezius towards the back of the ear.

While some refer to the nerve point and Erb's point as the same structure they are different points. Erb's point is a deeper structure that corresponds to the location of the upper trunk of the brachial plexus just before it passes deep to the clavicle. Lesions in this region lead to Erb's palsy, or upper trunk injuries.

Accessory Nerve

In one sense, it is a misnomer to call the *accessory nerve* a cranial nerve as it arises from spinal cord segments C1-C5. Rootlets coming out of the spinal cord merge together and ascend parallel to the spinal cord to enter the posterior cranial fossa through the *foramen magnum.* The accessory nerve then does a U-turn and leaves the skull through the *jugular foramen.* As it enters the neck it supplies the sternocleidomastoid and continues to cross the posterior triangle on its way to the trapezius muscle. The accessory nerve typically enters the posterior triangle just above the nerve point in the neck found along the posterior border of the sternocleidomastoid muscle. As it crosses the posterior triangle it is deep to the skin and superficial fascia. The platysma does not come back into the posterior triangle, so it does not cover the accessory nerve (Fig. 1.55).

Because of its long and superficial path, CN XI is susceptible to trauma during surgery in the posterior triangle. Bilateral action of the two sternocleidomastoid muscles elevates the chin by pulling the mastoid processes inferiorly (extension at the atlantooccipital joint). When the sternocleidomastoid on one side is active this will pull the mastoid process on that side inferiorly which leads to the chin deviating to the opposite side. If the accessory nerve is injured on one side, for instance the right, when the patient is asked to elevate the chin, it will point towards the right—the left side is working and moves the chin to the right.

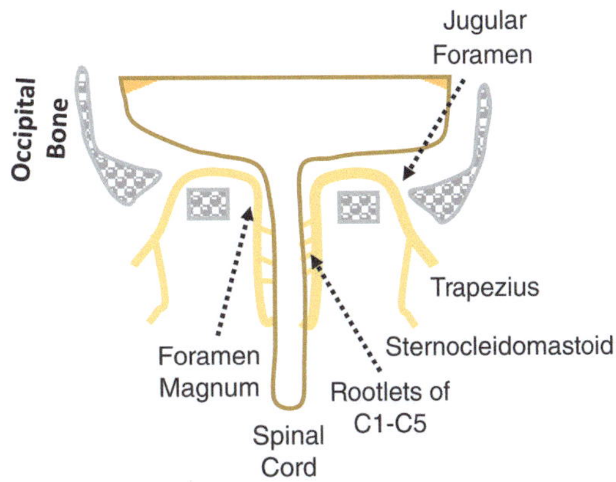

Fig. 1.55 CN XI. The accessory nerve arises from rootlets of the C1–C5 spinal cord and ascends into the foramen magnum to enter the skull with the spinal cord. In the skull, the accessory nerve does a U-turn and exits through the jugular foramen to innervate the sternocleidomastoid and trapezius muscles [21, 22]

Scalene Triangle and Thoracic Outlet Syndrome

In the anterior corner of the posterior triangle, several major structures are emerging from the thorax making this a clinically important region. This is where thoracic outlet syndrome occurs. If we zoom in on this region, we can see how the relationships of the various structures dictate the clinical symptoms.

Words of warning: Thoracic outlet syndrome is slightly controversial so do not be surprised if you see slight variations from one book to another. Even the name can be debated with some referring to it as thoracic inlet syndrome—is it a doorway into the thorax or out of the thorax? It can result from the presence of a cervical rib, tight anterior scalene muscle, space-occupying lesions, or trauma such as a clavicle fracture.

Both the anterior and middle scalene muscles are attached to the first rib. Between the anterior and middle scalene muscles, you can see the subclavian artery and the roots of the brachial plexus. Lesions here will lead to a reduced pulse in the upper limb, along with tingling in the fingers and weakness of the hand muscles. The muscle weakness in the hand is a combination of ulnar nerve

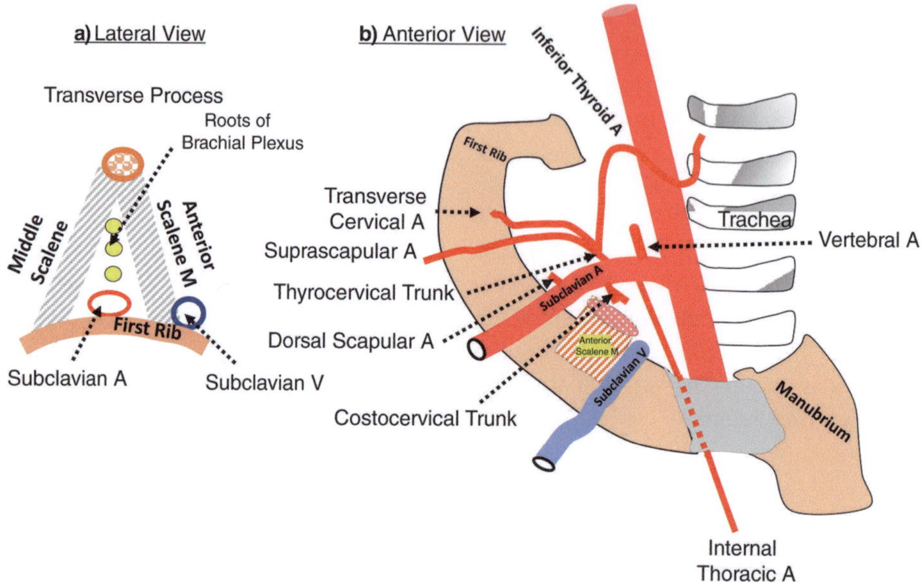

Fig. 1.56 Scalene muscles and the neck. In panel (**a**), the lateral view shows the scalene triangle between the anterior and middle scalene triangle. In panel (**b**) the subclavian artery is going over the first rib to become the axillary artery. The branches of the subclavian artery are shown. The anterior scalene is between the subclavian artery and vein [21, 22]

and median nerve deficits. Note that the subclavian vein is anterior to the anterior scalene (along with the phrenic nerve) (Fig. 1.56).

Subclavian Artery

On the right side, the *subclavian artery* runs from the bifurcation of the brachiocephalic trunk to the lateral border of the first rib. On the left side, the sublclavian artery is a branch from the aortic arch. On both sides, it can be divided into three parts based on the location of the anterior scalane muscle. The first part is proximal to the muscles, the second part is posterior to it, and the third part is distal to the muscle (Fig. 1.53).

First Part

1. The *vertebral artery* travels superiorly in the foramen transversarium of C1–C6 to enter the skull at the foramen magnum where it will eventually form the basilar artery. The basilar artery lies along the clivus which is formed by the union of the sphenoid and occipital bones. The *clivus* forms a diagonally running slope which the basilar artery and the pons are resting on.
2. The *internal thoracic artery* descends along the posterior border of the sternum where it eventually splits into the *musculophrenic* and *superior epigastric arteries*. Along the way it gives off the *anterior intercostal arteries.*
3. The *thryocervical trunk* gives off *the suprascapular, inferior thyroid, and transverse cervical arteries.*
   (a) The *suprascapular artery* heads posterior towards the scapula where it runs with the suprascapular nerve. Both these structures approach the *suprascapular notch.* The open superior end of the notch is closed off by the *superior transverse scapular ligament* creating a tunnel. The nerve passes through the tunnel, inferior to the ligament. The artery passes superior to the ligament (Navy under the bridge, Army above it). The artery contin-

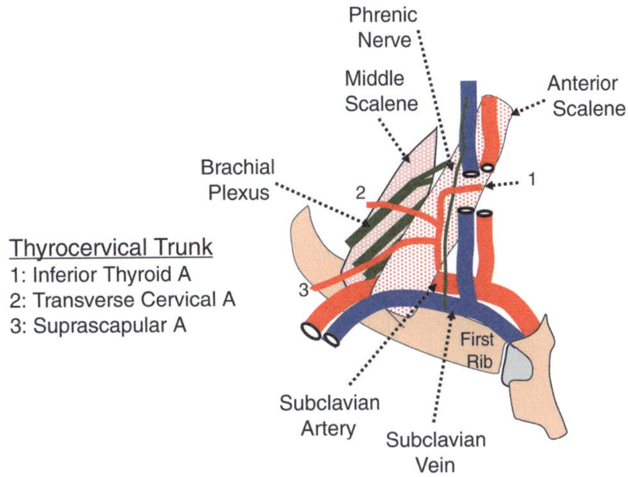

Fig. 1.57 Scalene triangle. The scalene triangle is between the first rib and the anterior and middle scalene muscles. The subclavian artery and brachial plexus are in it. The subclavian vein and phrenic nerve run in front of the anterior scalene. The three branches of the thyrocervical trunk can be seen [21, 22]

ues deep to the supraspinatus muscle, travels though the supraglenoid notch (the notch connecting the supraspinous and infraspinous fossas) to continue deep to the infraspinatus muscle in the infraspinous fossa.

(b) The *inferior thyroid artery* runs superior between the esophagus and trachea to reach the thyroid gland where it anastomosis with the superior thyroid artery. The inferior thyroid artery also gives off an *ascending cervical artery* which ascends towards the head. In some cases it arises as a direct branch of the thyrocervical trunk.

(c) The *transverse cervical artery* crosses the phrenic nerve and the anterior scalene muscle to reach the trapezius (Fig. 1.57).

Second Part

1. The *costocervical trunk* has two branches: (1) *superior intercostal artery* and (2) *deep cervical artery*.
   (a) The *superior intercostal artery* lies just lateral to the stellate ganglion. It runs along the neck of the first rib and gives off branches to the first and second intercostal spaces.
   (b) The *deep cervical artery* ascends posterior to the brachial pexus and between the transverse processes and the spinous processes, superfical to the semispinalis cervicis to anastomosis with the descending branch of the occipital artery.

Third Part

1. The *dorsal scapular artery* runs posterior towards the superior angle of the scapula where it dives deep to the levator scapulae and then descends along the medial border of the scapula to reach the inferior angle. It anastomoses with the *circumflex scapular artery* which comes through the triangular notch, and the *suprascapular artery* which comes through the notch connecting the supraspinous and infraspinous fossae.

Pharynx and Larynx

The pharynx is a muscular tube responsible for transporting air down into the lungs, and for food down into the esophagus. It has three circular sphincters and two strap muscles. Think of this arrangement as three cups stacked on top of each other with two straws. The constrictors make up the tube, so each muscle starts at a bony prominence on one side and runs in a circular direction to meet the same muscle coming around from the other side. They meet at the pterygomandibular raphe in the midline. The superior constrictor is attached to the medial pterygoid plate and the mandible, the middle constrictor to the hyoid bone, and the inferior constrictor to the thyroid cartilage. Running from the *torus tubarius* and merging into the superior constrictor like a straw is the *salpingopharyngeus*. And, like a straw, running from the styloid process and merging into the pharyngeal wall between the middle and inferior constrictor is the *stylopharyngeus* (Fig. 1.58).

The pharynx is subdivided into three divisions, the *nasopharynx* is posterior to the nasal cavity, the *oropharynx* is posterior to the oral cavity, and the *laryngopharynx* is posterior to the larynx (Fig. 1.59).

The *epiglottis* is an oval shaped piece of cartilage extending to the base of the tongue where three ligaments connect the tongue to the epiglottis. In the midline is the single *median glossoepiglotic ligament* and on each side are the *lateral glossoepiglotic ligaments.* Between the median glossoepiglotic ligament and each lateral glossoepiglotic ligament is a space called the *vallecula.*

Larynx

The two essential pieces of the larynx are the paired vocal cords. When studying the larynx everything can be related to the vocal cords. The

Muscle	Function
Salpingopharyngeus	*Elevate Pharynx*
Stylopharyngeus	*Elevates Larynx and Pharynx*
Superior Constrictor	*Constriction*
Middle Constrictor	*Constriction*
Inferior Constrictor	*Constriction*

Fig. 1.58 Pharyngeal muscles. Three muscles resemble three cups, and two resemble two straws [21, 22]

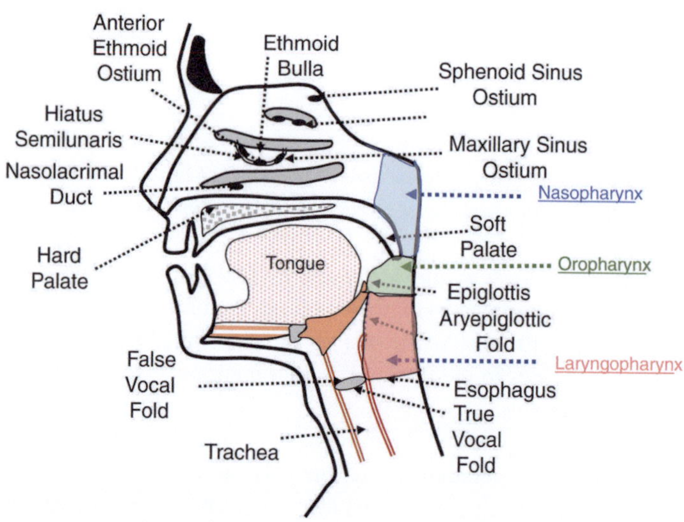

Fig. 1.59 Pharynx. The pharynx is composed of the nasopharynx, oropharynx, and laryngopharynx. The nasolacrimal duct starts at the medial corner of the eye and allows fluid to drain into the inferior meatus. The sphenoid sinus opens above the superior concha. The maxillary sinus opens into the hiatus semilunaris in the middle meatus, which is at the base of the ethmoid bulla [21, 22]

structures around the vocal cords are designed to either move the cords or to protect them. The space between the vocal cords is the glottis. During inspiration, the glottis needs to be open, while during phonation the glottis is closed. All the muscles, cartilage, and nerve innervation can be examined considering their effects on vocal cord movement.

The *thyroid cartilage* is shaped like a triangle with one of its points facing anteriorly as the *thyroid prominence*. Thyroid means "shield" and it protects the larynx and serves as an attachment point for various supporting structures and muscles. Flaring out from the midline prominence on each side are the laminae forming the two sides of the triangle. The third side of the triangle, which is posterior, is open. Running from the superior surface of the thyroid up to the hyoid is the *thyrohyoid membrane*. There are four extensions of the thyroid cartilage, two superior horns and two inferior horns. Attached to the inferior border of the thyroid cartilage is the *cricothyroid membrane* (Fig. 1.60).

The *cricoid cartilage* resembles a class ring with the signet facing posterior. In contrast to the thyroid cartilage, which is open posteriorly, the cricoid is a continuous ring. Sitting on top of the cricoid cartilage are the *arytenoid cartilages* (ladle in Latin). And where the cricoid and each arytenoid meet, there is a synovial joint that allows movement of the arytenoid. The arytenoids are shaped like a triangle with their anteriorly facing *vocal processes,* and laterally facing *muscular processes*, serving as attachments for the lateral cricoarytenoid muscles and the posterior cricoarytenoid muscles. Sitting on top of the arytenoids are the *corniculate* cartilages and encapsulated in the aryepiglottic folds are the *cuneiform* cartilages. These two small, and hard to identify cartilages play a role in supporting the aryepiglottic folds.

The quadrangular membrane lays down like a sheet running from the epiglottis to the *vestibular folds* (false folds) and covers the laryngeal structures. Inferior to the vestibular folds are the *true vocal folds* housing the vocal ligaments. The true vocal folds appear as thin sharp white line, while the false folds resemble just a loose outpocketing of tissue. Between the true and false folds are the small slit-like *ventricles* which continue laterally into the *saccules*.

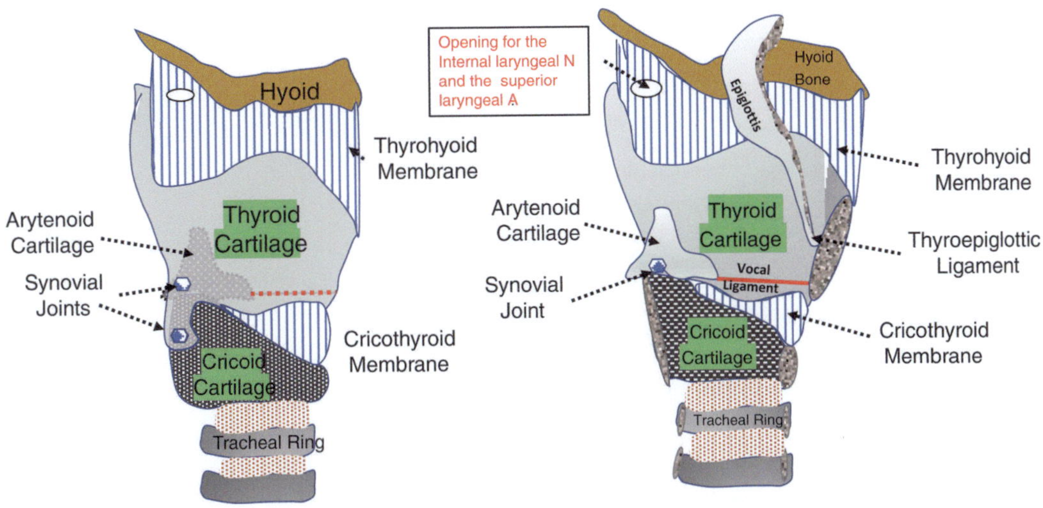

Fig. 1.60 Larynx. The arytenoid cartilages sit on top of the cricoid cartilages, with a synovial joint between the two structures. The vocal ligament runs from the arytenoid cartilage to the thyroid cartilage. Between the thyroid cartilage and cricoid cartilage is the cricothyroid membrane. Between the thyroid cartilage and hyoid bone is the thyrohyoid membrane. The epiglottis runs from the thyroid cartilage and ascends behind the hyoid bone and the tongue [21, 22]

1. At the synovial joints between the cricoid and arytenoid cartilages, the *cricoarytenoid joints*, you can see how the *lateral cricoarytenoid* pulls the muscular processes anteromedial, which in turn moves the vocal processes medially to close the glottis (Fig. 1.59).
2. Also attached to the muscular processes are the *posterior cricoarytenoids* which will pull the muscular processes posteromedial which in turn moves the vocal processes laterally to open the glottis. This is the only muscle that opens the glottis (Fig. 1.60).
3. Just behind the arytenoids and running from one arytenoid to another are the *transverse arytenoids* which help to close the glottis (Fig. 1.61).
4. Superficial to the transverse arytenoids are the *oblique arytenoids* which also help to close the glottis.
5. The oblique arytenoids continue superiorly as the *aryepiglotticus* muscles which contribute to closing the laryngeal inlet. The laryngeal membrane overlying the aryepiglotticus muscles make up the *aryepiglottic folds.*
6. Along the sides of the aryepiglottic folds are the *thyroarytenoid muscles* which contribute to opening of the laryngeal inlet (Fig. 1.3).

A Note on Terminology

Some anatomy textbooks will differentiate the terms *glottis* and *rima glottidis* from each other and they will define the word "glottis" as the vocal cords plus the opening between them, while the term "rima glottidis" is used for just the space between the vocal cords. Other authors will use the terms "glottis" and "rima glottidis" as synonyms referring to the space between the vocal cords. In the world of clinical medicine, and likewise with many researchers, the term glottis refers to the opening between the vocal cords.

Cricothyrotomy

An emergency airway opening—*cricothyrotomy*—will be made through the cricothyroid membrane. For instance, if a child swallows a marble, or other small toy, it can get stuck in the glottis and then block air from entering the lungs. An emergency opening would be made in the midline through the cricothyroid membrane. Making an opening in the thyrohyoid membrane would not allow air to enter the

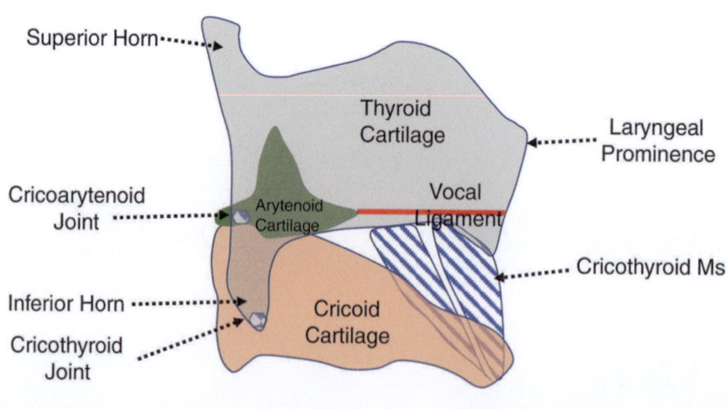

Fig. 1.61 Larynx. The arytenoid cartilage is sitting on top of the cricoid cartilage. Running from the vocal process of the arytenoid to the thyroid cartilage is the vocal ligament. The cricothyroid muscles are the only extrinsic muscle of the larynx. When they contract, the vocal ligament is stretched, which raises the pitch. There is a synovial joint between the inferior horn of the thyroid cartilage and the cricoid cartilage, and there is another one between the arytenoid and cricoid cartilages [21, 22]

lungs. During this procedure, to find the incision site an understanding of the relationships of the thyroid cartilage, hyoid bone, cricoid cartilage, and the cricothyroid membrane is essential. One issue to be wary of is the presence of a *thyroid ima artery*. In approximately 3–4% of us, there is a small thyroid ima artery arising from the brachiocephalic trunk and running in the midline to supply the thyroid gland. A midline incision can compromise this thyroid ima artery.

Tracheotomy

A tracheotomy (tracheostomy) is a surgical procedure that involves placement of a tracheostomy tube between the tracheal rings and into the trachea. It is a short wide tube that can be connected to a ventilator, or it may be left open. Depending on the patient's status, it can be removed, and the hole will heal, or it can remain in place. If it remains in place, a device can be attached to the tube allowing the patient to speak, or they can learn to speak by placing a finger over the hole.

Cranial Nerve X and the Larynx and Pharynx

Cranial nerve X is the main nerve supply to the larynx and pharynx, and it has motor, sensory, and parasympathetic fibers. During surgery on neck structures, such as a thyroidectomy, these nerves can be damaged (Fig. 1.62).

Cranial nerve X contains motor, sensory, and parasympathetic fibers, and is the main nerve supply to muscles of the pharynx and larynx. The first branch of the vagus nerve is the *auricular branch* which is responsible for some sensation from around the auricle and from the concha bowl (posterior to tragus). The second branch is the *pharyngeal branch* which goes to all the muscles of the pharynx and soft palate except for tensor veli palatini (CN V) and stylopharyngeus (CN IX). With lesions to the pharyngeal nerve the uvula will deviate away from the side of the lesion when the patient is asked to say "Aaaahhhhh."

The next branch is the *superior laryngeal nerve* which splits into internal and external branches. The *internal branch of the superior laryngeal nerve* is responsible for sensation

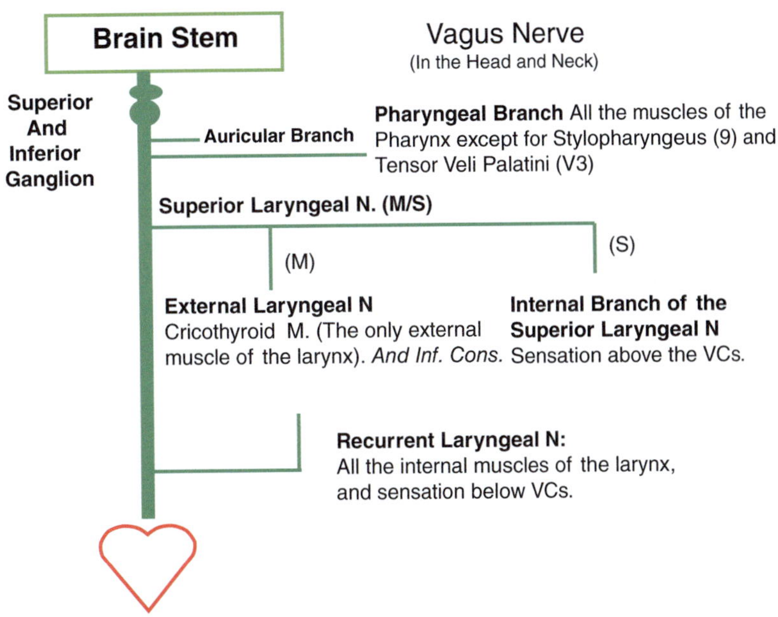

Fig. 1.62 The vagus nerve [21, 22]

above the vocal cords. A fish bone or chicken bone caught in the throat can lodge in the piriform recess and lead to aggravation of the internal branch of the superior laryngeal nerve. The internal laryngeal nerve runs with the superior laryngeal artery (a branch of superior thyroid artery). The internal branch is responsible for sensation from the internal surface of the laryngopharynx. Pathology in this region can lead to ear pain—referred pain due to the auricular branch of vagus.

The *external branch of the superior laryngeal nerve* goes to the only external muscle of the larynx—the *cricothyroid muscle*. It runs with the superior thyroid artery and can be injured during thyroid surgery. A lesion to the external branch will lead to a monotone voice, with a higher pitch than normal and a "breathy" voice.

The *recurrent laryngeal nerve* branches off the vagus nerve in the thorax and ascends in the neck. On the right, it makes a loop around the subclavian artery at the T1–T2 level, and on the left, it runs around the aortic arch at the T4–T5 level. As it travels superiorly in the neck it is found between the trachea and esophagus—the tracheoesophageal space. As the nerve crosses the cricothyroid joint it becomes the inferior laryngeal nerve. As it approaches the inferior constrictor it divides into an anterior branch which is the motor supply to all the laryngeal muscles except for the cricothyroid muscle, and a posterior branch to supply sensation below the vocal cords. One of the muscles the anterior branch supplies is the posterior cricoarytenoid, which is responsible for opening the glottis. It runs with the inferior thyroid artery.

In summary there are two ways one can refer to the nerves supply of the larynx. If you look closely, they both mean the same thing.

1. *All the muscles* of the larynx are supplied by the recurrent laryngeal nerve, except for the cricothyroid, which is supplied by the external laryngeal nerve. *or,*
2. All *the internal* muscles of the larynx are supplied by the recurrent laryngeal nerve, while the only *external muscle* of the larynx is supplied by the external laryngeal nerve (Fig. 1.63).

Arteries to Larynx and Pharynx

The *superior thyroid artery* is the first branch of the external carotid artery, and it is the only branch of the external carotid artery that descends towards the neck, which can serve as a helpful landmark on an angiogram of the external carotid branches. All the other branches of the external carotid artery ascend towards the head. On its way to the thyroid gland, the superior thyroid artery gives off a *superior laryngeal artery* which joins the internal branch of the superior laryngeal nerve. Both the superior laryngeal artery and the internal laryngeal nerve then pierce the thyrohyoid membrane.

As the superior thyroid artery continues its descent towards the thyroid gland it runs with the external laryngeal nerve. As it approaches the

Fig. 1.63 Muscles of the pharynx and the soft palate [21, 22]

Muscle	Nerve	Action
Levator Veli Palatini	*CN X*	*Elevates soft palate, opens auditory tube*
Tensor Veli Palatini	*CN V (V3)*	*Tenses soft palate, opens auditory Tube*
Uvulae	*CN X Pharyngeal Branch*	*Elevates uvula*
Palatoglossus	*CN X*	*Elevates root of tongue*
Palatopharyngeus	*CN X Pharyngeal Branch*	*Constricts isthmus*

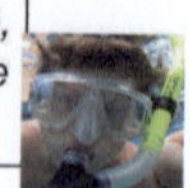

thyroid gland, it divides into anterior and posterior branches, which form an anastomosis with the *inferior thyroid artery* which is a branch of the thyrocervical trunk (Fig. 1.61).

As the two recurrent laryngeal nerves run superiorly, they cross the inferior thyroid artery. During their course, the two nerves are close to each other right behind (posterior to) the trachea. Because of how close they are, they can both be injured at the same time. A horse voice and difficulty with swallowing could be indicative of an aortic aneurysm (Fig. 1.61 and 1.64).

With a unilateral injury to the recurrent laryngeal nerve the affected vocal cord will typically assume a paramedian (off-center) position. This allows the patient to breathe, but phonation is compromised. In these individuals, during phonation when you want the vocal cords centered in the midline, the vocal cord on the healthy side will compensate for the injured side and adduct past the midline to meet the damaged vocal cord (Figs. 1.64 and 1.65).

With a bilateral injury,as time goes on the position of the cords can change. Right after the injury, both cords can assume a paramedian position. This allow the patient to breathe, but speaking is difficult. In some cases, eventually the two cords assume a medial position and meet in the midline, resulting in a situation where they cannot breathe. Surgery is warranted in this case (Fig. 1.65).

Parasympathetic Hitchhikers

Cranial nerves III, VII, IX, and X all have a parasympathetic component. Of these four nerves, three of them—III, VII, and IX—have parasympathetic fibers that hitchhike on branches of CN V to travel to their targets. They have all been discussed with their respective sections earlier in the chapter. The discussion below focuses on the greater and lesser petrosal nerves. The greater petrosal nerve is a parasympathetic branch of CN VII that runs in the groove for the greater petrosal nerve in the temporal bone. It then crosses foramen lacerum to join with the deep petrosal nerve (sympathetic fibers) to form the nerve of the pterygoid canal (Fig. 1.66).

Cranial nerve IX leaves the skull through the jugular foramen. It quickly gives off the tympanic nerve, which enters the middle ear to form

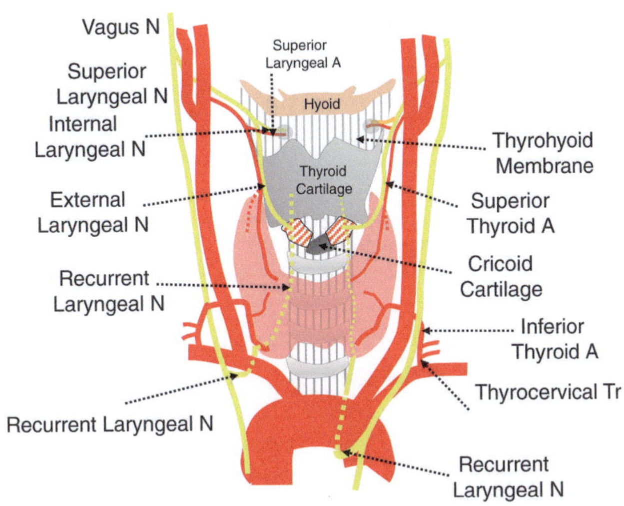

Fig. 1.64 Larynx nerves and arteries. The superior laryngeal nerve splits into the internal and external branches. The internal branch runs with the superior laryngeal artery and pierces the thyrohyoid membrane. The external branch runs with the superior thyroid artery. The right recurrent laryngeal nerve wraps around the subclavian artery. The left recurrent laryngeal nerve wraps around the aortic arch. The thyrocervical trunk gives off the inferior thyroid artery [21, 22]

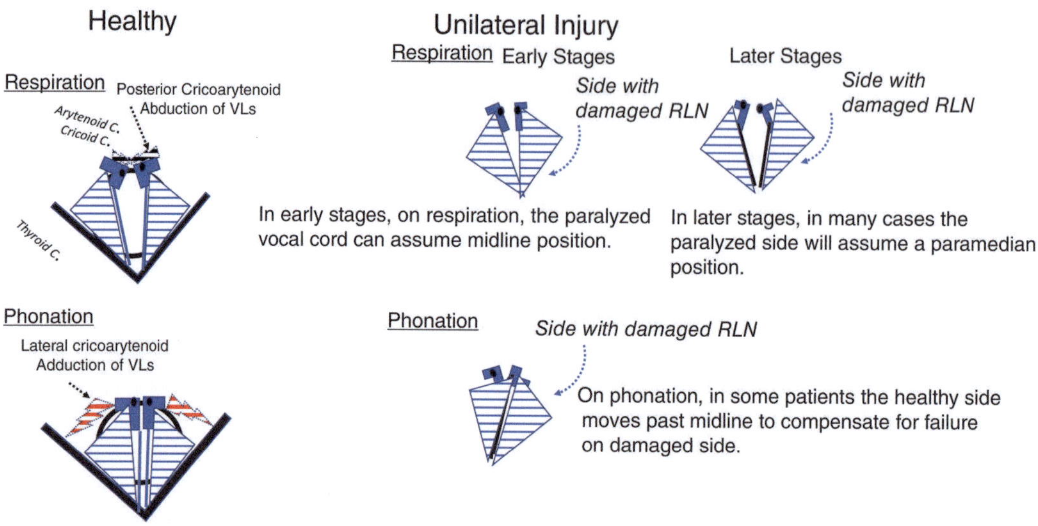

Fig. 1.65 Recurrent laryngeal nerve injury. In the healthy person, the glottis opens during respiration and closes during phonation. With a unilateral recurrent laryngeal nerve injury, in some patients the vocal cords will assume a median or paramedian position. On phonation the vocal cord on the healthy side will move past the midline. In other patients, the cord can remain adducted on the damaged side. If this happens on both sides then asphyxiation is possible [21, 22]

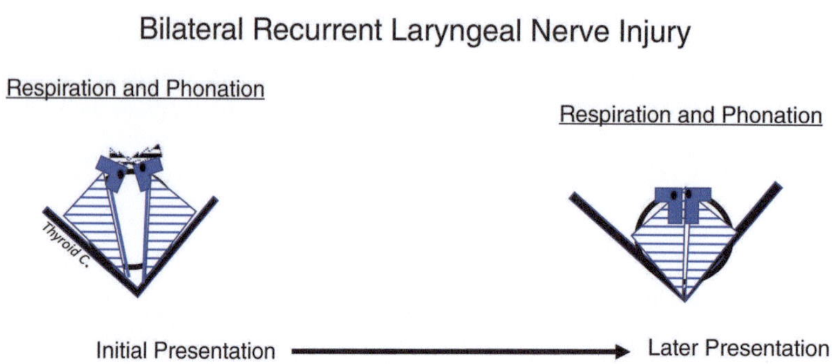

Fig. 1.66 Bilateral recurrent laryngeal nerve injury. In the early stages of bilateral recurrent laryngeal nerve injury, the glottis opens during respiration and phonation. In the later stages, in some patients, the vocal cords will be adducted, leading to a closed glottis, potential asphyxiation, and an emergency [21, 22]

the tympanic plexus. From the tympanic plexus the lesser petrosal nerve then leaves the skull through the *hiatus for the lesser petrosal nerve,* runs in the *groove of the lesser petrosal* and travels through the *foramen ovale* to reach the *otic ganglion* in the infratemporal fossa. From the otic ganglion the postganglionic parasympathetic fibers travel to the parotid gland on the auriculotemporal nerve (V3) (Figs. 1.67 and 1.68).

Parotid Gland

The parotid gland sits in front of the ear. The parotid duct comes out of the gland and crosses the check to drain into the mouth opposite the upper second molar. *Sialolithiasis* refers to stones that get caught in the parotid duct. Mumps is a viral infection of the parotid gland. Mumps can often go along with an infection of the testes—*orchitis*.

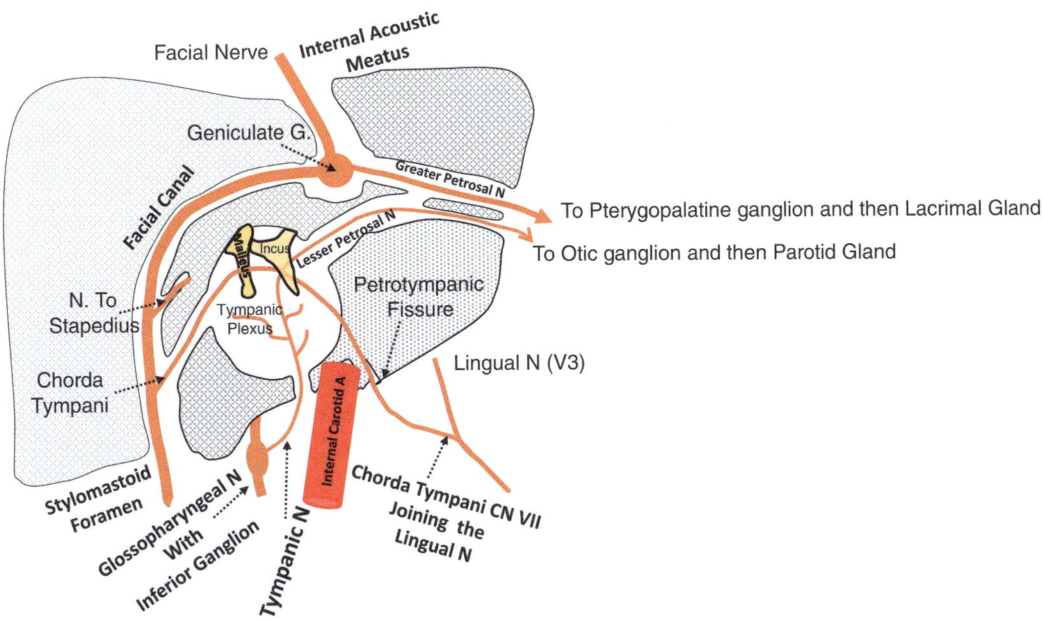

Fig. 1.67 Parasympathetics of Cranial Nerves VII and IX. As CN IX leaves the skull through the jugular foramen it gives off the tympanic nerve which enters the middle ear and contributes to the tympanic plexus. It then leaves the middle ear as the lesser petrosal which travels to the parotid gland via the otic ganglion. The greater petrosal is the first branch of cranial nerve VII and travels to the pterygopalatine ganglion and then to the lacrimal gland [21, 22]

Frey Syndrome, Crocodile Tears, and Confused Parasympathetic Fibers

The parasympathetic fibers in the head are very thin, delicate fibers. In some injuries to the head, these fibers can be severed. When the fibers regrow, they can become confused and end up innervating the wrong target leading to unwanted parasympathetic responses.

If the auriculotemporal nerve and its parasympathetic fibers are cut during surgery, these fibers can regrow and may connect to the sweat glands and blood vessels such that in the presence of food the patient sweats in the region of the parotid gland, and the skin in this area becomes red (Frey Syndrome). This can occur during surgery of the salivary glands, a neck lift, and diabetes mellitus. *Frey Syndrome* was originally named after the Polish Neurologist Lucja Frey-Gottesman (1889–1942). Its more modern name is *Auriculotemporal Nerve Syndrome* (Its more recent name). (Fig. 1.69).

If the facial nerve is damaged in the facial canal, either at the geniculate ganglion or proximal to the ganglion, this can lead to degeneration of the greater petrosal nerve. Sitting close to the greater petrosal nerve is the lesser petrosal nerve. And the parasympathetic fibers on the lesser petrosal nerve can end up forming connections to the pterygopalatine ganglion and thus innervating the lacrimal gland. Salvation is the normal response to food in the vicinity, however in the case of patients with aberrant nerve innervation, food in the vicinity leads to lacrimal gland stimulation and crying. The term *crocodile tears* comes from the myth that crocodiles cry before eating their food. Note that the exact mechanism behind the clinical presentation of crocodile tears and which nerves are involved in the regeneration are debated. But the exact mechanism does not change the diagnosis (Fig. 1.70).

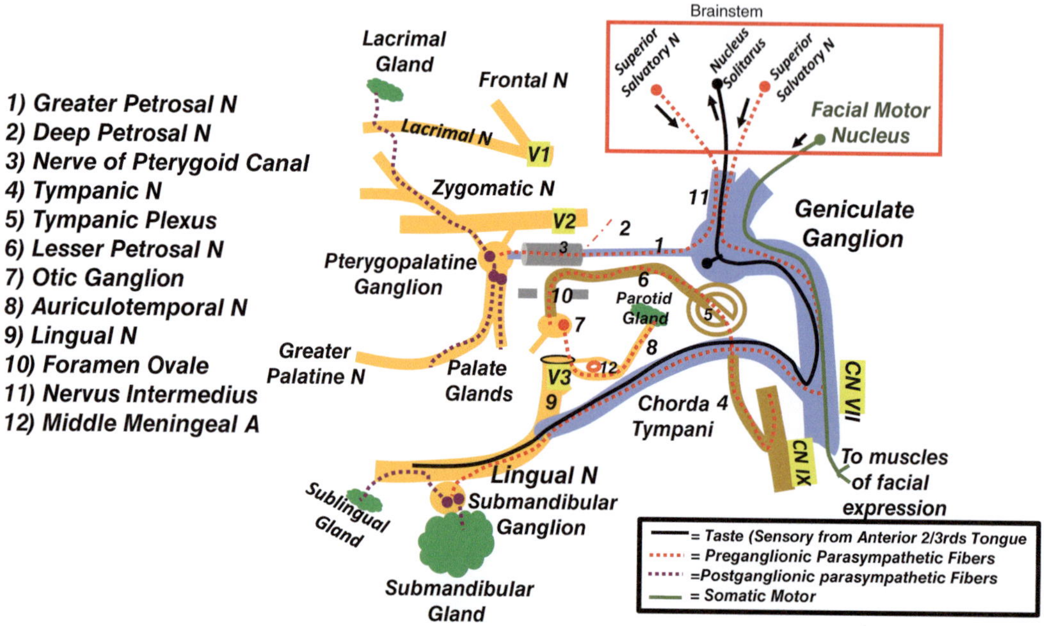

Fig. 1.68 Parasympathetics to glands. Both CN VII and CN IX have parasympathetic fibers that use CN V to travel to their targets. CN VII has the greater petrosal nerve (parasympathetic) that meets the deep petrosal nerve (sympathetic) to form the nerve of the pterygoid canal (parasympathetic and sympathetic) that travels to meet the pterygopalatine ganglion in the pterygopalatine fossa. After synapsing in the PT ganglion, the post ganglionic parasympathetic fibers jump on the zygomatic nerve (V2) and then jump onto the lacrimal nerve (V1) to reach the lacrimal gland. They also travel on the greater and lesser petrosal nerves to the glands on the palate. In addition, CN VII has the chorda tympani with preganglionic fibers that joint the lingual nerve (V3) to reach the submandibular ganglion. In addition, the chorda tympani has taste fibers from the anterior two-thirds of the tongue. CN IX has the tympanic nerve, which meets the tympanic plexus, which gives off the lesser petrosal nerve that exits the skull through foramen ovale to meet the otic ganglion. The post ganglionic parasympathetic fibers then jump on auriculotemporal to reach the parotid gland [21, 22]

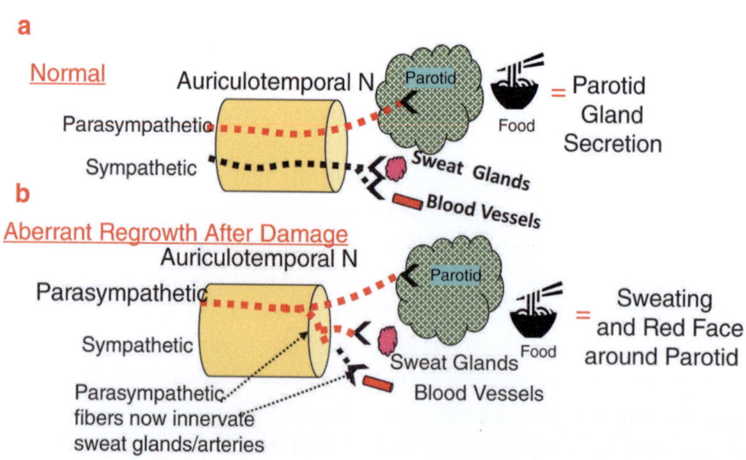

Fig. 1.69 Frey's Syndrome. Normally (Panel **a**) the parasympathetic fibers innervate the parotid gland and in the presence of food, the parotid will send secretions into the mouth. After injury (Panel **b**) to the auriculotemporal nerve, the parasympathetic fibers regrow but get confused and now innervate the sweat glands and arteries. This leads to redness (vasodilation) and sweating in front of the ear [21, 22]

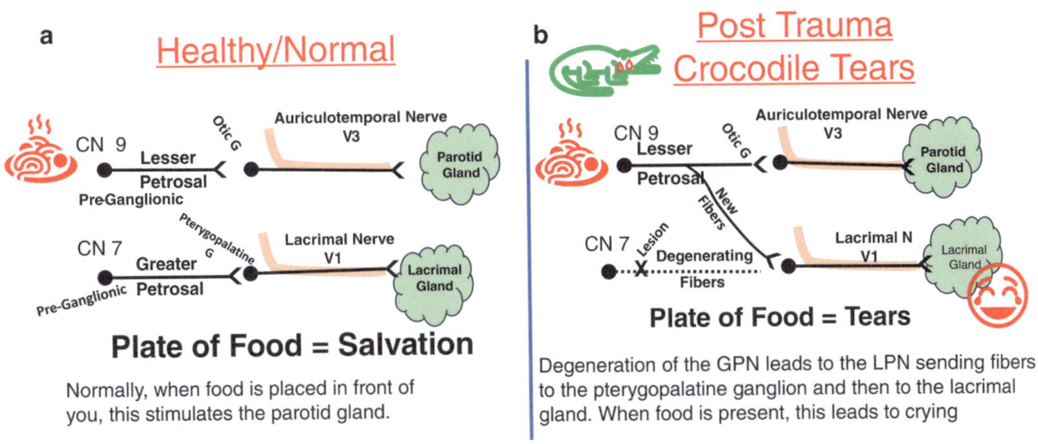

Fig. 1.70 Crocodile tears [21, 22]

Aortic Arch, Carotid and Vertebrobasilar Systems

When discussing the major arteries coming out of the aorta it helps to tie them in with the brain and upper limbs. This is an overview of the organization of these arteries. The details of each are addressed within different sections of the book. The three branches arising from the aortic arch are the (1) *brachiocephalic trunk* which goes onto divide into the right common carotid and right subclavian arteries; (2) the *left common carotid artery*; and (3) *the left subclavian artery*. The common carotid arteries travel in the neck to divide into the internal and external carotids. The internal carotid artery travels through the carotid canal to enter the skull where it will divide into the *middle* and *anterior cerebral arteries* (Fig. 1.71).

The *external carotid artery* goes on to perfuse the face and the skull. The *vertebral arteries* come off the subclavian arteries to enter the skull through the foramen magnum where they come together to form the single *basilar artery*. Just before they join, they give off the *posterior inferior cerebellar arteries*. At the top of the basilar artery there are the *right* and *left superior cerebellar arteries* and the *right* and *left posterior cerebral arteries*. Between them is CN III. The *posterior communicating arteries* connect the posterior cerebral arteries with the internal carotid arteries (Fig. 1.53). Aneurysms of the posterior communicating artery often compress CN III. T*rigeminal neuralgia* is thought to result from compression from the superior cerebellar artery on the trigeminal nerve just as it emerges from the trigeminal ganglion.

Thyroid Gland

The thyroid gland is a bilobed gland in the neck that secretes T3 and T4 which is under direct control by the anterior pituitary which in turn is part of the hypothalamic/pituitary axis. The hypothalamus releases Thyrotropin releasing hormone (TRH) which tells the anterior pituitary to release thyroid stimulating hormone which tells the thyroid gland to release T3 and T4. Under the microscope the thyroid gland is characterized by the presence of numerous follicles. The follicle cells on the periphery of a follicle synthesize thyroglobulin and secrete it into the lumen of the follicle where it is stored. Iodide comes from the bloodstream and enters the follicle where it transforms into iodine which in turn binds to the thyroglobulin to form T3 and T4 which is released into the bloodstream. Most of the T4 will be converted to T3 by the target cells (Fig. 1.71).

Triiodothyronine (T3) and thyroxine (T4) increase the metabolic rate by increasing heat production and the consumption of oxygen. Excess levels of T3 and T4 (hyperthyroidism) result in a metabolic rate that is too high, leading

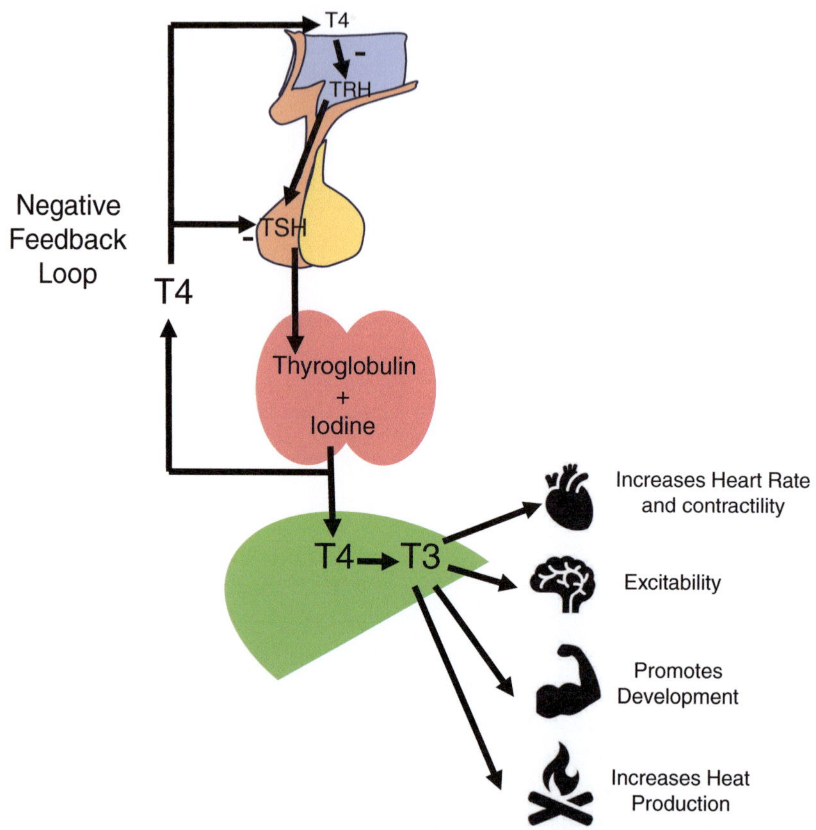

Fig. 1.71 T3 and T4 production. The hypothalamus releases thyroid releasing hormone (TRH) which tells anterior pituitary to release thyroid stimulating hormone (TSH). TSH tells thyroid gland to secrete T3 and T4, both of which affect the heart, brain, and muscle. They also increase heat production and oxygen consumption [21, 22]

to weight loss, cardiovascular changes, and irritability. *Graves' disease* is the result of an overactive thyroid gland due to an autoimmune disease. These individuals have abnormal antibodies to thyroid stimulating hormone receptors. The overactivity of the thyroid gland is evidenced by the presence of larger than normal follicular cells and depleted levels of colloid—the thyroid gland is working overtime to transform thyroglobulin into T3 and T4.

Goiter is a larger than normal thyroid gland. It can be caused by an iodine deficiency, hyperthyroidism or hypothyroidism. It can compress structure in the neck such as the larynx, trachea, recurrent laryngeal nerve, or esophagus.

The *parafollicular cells* of the thyroid gland produce *calcitonin* which decreases calcium levels in the blood stream. Calcitonin increases the activity of osteoblasts leading to bone deposition which moves calcium from the blood into bone. It also decreases the activity of osteoclasts. In humans, calcitonin plays a nonexistent to negligible role in calcium regulation as shown by the fact that removal of a thyroid gland does not affect calcium regulation. In some other animals, calcitonin is more important.

Parathyroid Glands

The parathyroid glands are four small glands that sit right behind the thyroid gland and are involved in calcium regulation via *parathyroid hormone* (PTH). Think of the bones as a reservoir for calcium that can either store calcium when it is in excess or release calcium when it is needed. The kidney also plays a role in calcium regulation by controlling the amount of calcium that is excreted or retained.

The most prominent cells of the parathyroid glands are the *principal cells* (sometimes called chief cells) which serve as calcium sensors. Calcium receptors on these cells detect low levels of calcium levels in the blood and via intracellular IP3 and G proteins release PTH. In bone, PTH stimulates osteoclasts to break up bone tissue with the subsequent release of calcium into the bloodstream. And in the kidney, PTH acts on the tubular network to increase the absorption of calcium so that the body retains calcium, and it also acts on the kidney tubules to release phosphate into the tubular lumen. Besides the principal cells, there are also *oxyphil cells*, which increase in number with age.

Calcitonin, on the other hand, is released by C cells of the thyroid gland and it has the opposite effect of PTH. Whereas PTH increases osteoclast activity, calcitonin inhibits osteoclast activity; and whereas PTH increases calcium resorption by the renal tubular network, calcitonin inhibits renal absorption of calcium,

If PTH levels are low (hypoparathyroidism), the balance of calcium shifts towards bone and away from the rest of the body. This excess calcium in the bones leads to increased mineralization. And at the same time, the lower levels of calcium in the rest of the body leads to abnormal muscle contractions. Conversely, if PTH levels are high (hyperparathyroidism) then calcium is released from the bone and deposited in other organs such as the kidney and cartilage (Fig. 1.72).

Hyperparathyroidism

Ninety-eight percent of the calcium in the body is found in bone. Of the remaining 2%, half of that is inactive, so it is just a small amount of the free calcium that is available for physiological effects. An increase in parathyroid hormone will lead to increased serum calcium (hypercalcemia) and decreased levels of phosphate (hypophosphatemia). A mnemonic for remembering the symp-

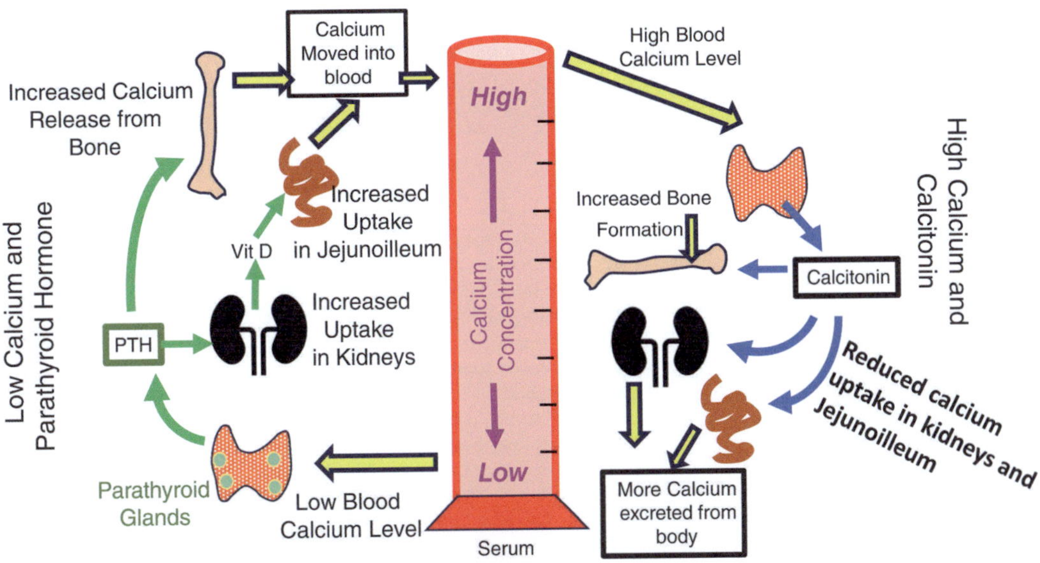

Fig. 1.72 Regulation of blood calcium levels. When calcium in the blood is low, parathyroid glands secrete parathyroid hormone (PTH) which leads to increased uptake by kidneys and jejunoilleum, and increased calcium release by the bones. High calcium in the blood leads to the release of calcitonin by the thyroid glands which leads to increased bone deposition and reduced calcium uptake by the kidneys and jejunoilleum

toms of hypercalcemia is Stones, Bones, Groans, Thrones, and Psychic Disturbances. In short, the patient can present with renal stones, abdominal discomfort, constipation, pancreatitis, and hallucinations. The osteoclasts are more active which increases serum calcium. In addition, PTH stimulates the ENaC channels to increase absorption of calcium from the renal tubules leading to increased levels of serum calcium. In addition, PTH increases the absorption of vitamin D in the GI tract. Besides masses of the parathyroid glands, low levels of calcium and vitamin D can lead to increased levels of PTH.

Most (90%) cases of hypercalcemia come from hyperparathyroidism or a malignancy.

Hypoparathyroidism

In contrast to elevated levels of PTH, low levels of PTH are most often caused by autoimmune destruction or surgical removal of the parathyroid gland. In these cases, the bone will absorb more calcium and release phosphate into the blood.

Subclavian Steal Syndrome

Subclavian steal syndrome involves the upper limb stealing blood from the brain. To discuss the syndrome, you need to visualize the three main branches arising from the aorta and know where they are going. In subclavian steal syndrome there is a blockage of the subclavian artery close to its origin which is prior to the start of the vertebral artery. This blockage prevents blood from flowing down to the upper limb, but the vertebral artery comes to the rescue. To keep blood flowing to the upper limb, blood comes down the vertebral artery to move past the blockage. While this benefits the upper limb, it causes problems for the brain because the vertebrobasilar system now receives less blood, leading to syncope and ataxia. Some patients with subclavian steal syndrome will present with neck pain and contralateral long tract deficits (Fig. 1.73).

In addition, in an elderly patient who complains of feeling dizzy when they turn their head—backing out of the garage for instance—this could be the result of temporary occlusion of the vertebral artery which leads to reduced blood flow to the brainstem centers responsible for balance. This is sometimes referred to as *Bowhunter's Syndrome*, because of the head movement involved with turning the head to aim an arrow.

Cervical artery dissection refers to the layers of the arteries traveling to the head (carotid and vertebral) separating and allowing blood to pool between the layers—like water getting between the layers of plywood. This creates a pseudoan-

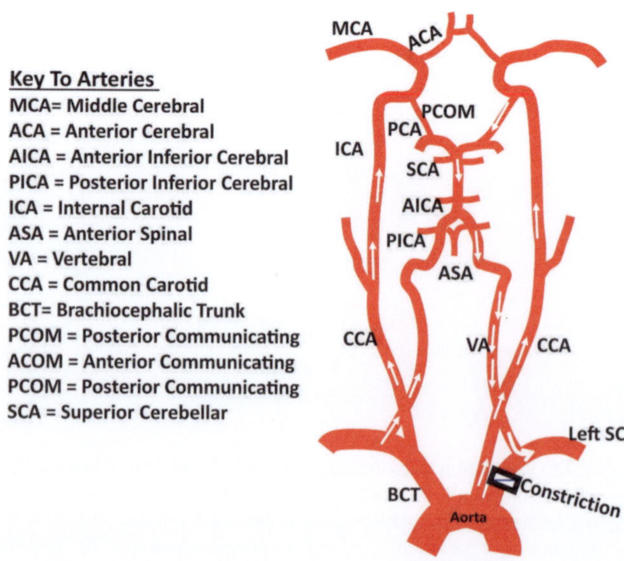

Fig. 1.73 Subclavian steal syndrome. There is a blockage of the subclavian artery proximal to the vertebral artery. The blood now comes down from the vertebrobasilar system to enter the subclavian artery distal to the constriction—the subclavian "steals" the blood from the brain [21, 22]

eurysm and can lead to headaches, pain around the face and eyes, and double vision. It can eventually lead to a stroke.

Le Fort Fractures

Le Fort fractures are fractures that separate the midface from the skull and can be classified as Type 1, II, or III. All these subtypes involve a fracture of the pterygoid plate. Without going into all the minute details, the fracture line in Type I is a horizontal line sitting between the oral and nasal cavities just above the palate. This results in a floating palate, malocclusion of the teeth, and difficulty speaking, Type II is slightly higher with the fracture line forming a triangle around the nasal cavity with the apex making its way into the inferior portion of the orbit, Type III is higher and goes through the middle of the orbit and into the base of the skull. One way to remember the different subtypes is: Speak no evil, see no evil, hear no evil. Type I affects speaking, Type II also affects seeing, and Type III also affects hearing (Figs. 1.74 and 1.75).

Lymphatics of the Head and Neck

The lymphatics of the head and neck are complicated for two reasons: (1) there are numerous nodes in this region, and (2) sources vary on how to organize the nodes. The goals for a student is to have a general overview of how the system works, but to also know the more clinically relevant nodes.

Think of the lymphatics in this region as something like a funnel. The center of the funnel is the deep cervical chain running along the internal jugular vein. At the top, the wide part of the funnel fans out to encompass the various regions of the face. Out on the wide part of the funnel are various lymph nodes draining specific regions, and these nodes will then typically drain into nodes closer to the deep cervical nodes, and then these drain into the deep cervical chain. Most of these outer nodes are appropriately named, such as parotid, preauricular, posterior auricular, submental, and submandibular, for instance.

Towards the base of the deep cervical chain is the *juguloomohyoid node*, which is just inferior to the junction of the inferior and superior bellies of omohyoid. These nodes drain the tongue.

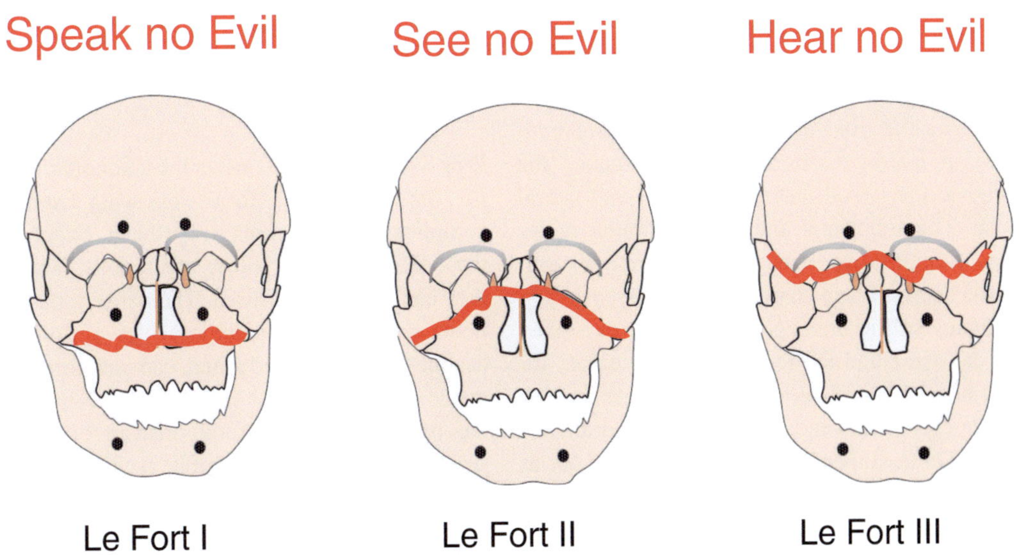

Fig. 1.74 Le Fort fractures. La Fort fractures are midfacial fractures. Le Fort I is just above the upper teeth and affects speaking. Le Fort II is through the inferior orbit and affects vision. Le Fort III is through the mid orbit and affects hearing. This is just a brief description [21, 22]

Jugulodigastric (tonsillar): Face, Pharynx, Tonsil
Juguloomohyoid: Tongue
Submental: Lower lip, apex of tongue
Submandibular: Cheek, side of nose, lower lip

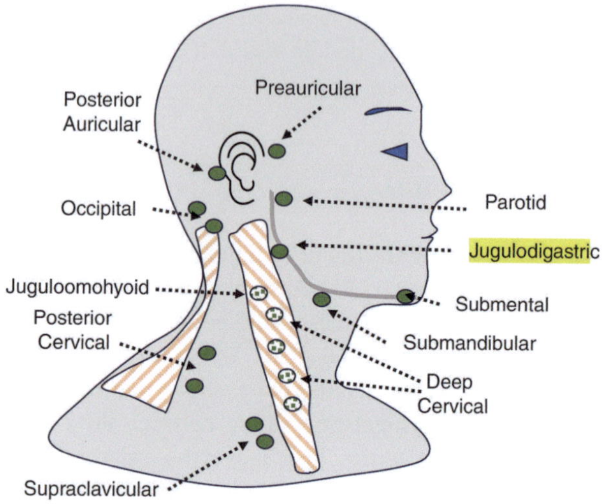

Fig. 1.75 Lymphatics of head and neck [21, 22]

Keep in mind that a malignant cell traveling through the lymphatic system might travel through one node or several different nodes on its way to the right lymphatic duct or thoracic duct. And the nodes are appropriately termed, such that the first node the cell moves through is the *primary node*, then the *secondary node*, and then the *tertiary node*. Each node acts as a fence or a barrier to slow down the passage of the malignant cell. The more fences, or nodes, the better. As an example of drainage patterns, take the submental and submandibular nodes. The *submental nodes* drain the lower lip, floor of the mouth, the incisors, and the front of the tongue. The *submandibular nodes* drain the lateral tongue, the gingiva, the lateral teeth, the cheek, and lateral nose. The submental and submandibular nodes then drain into the juguloomohyoid nodes—part of the deep cervical chain.

Many of the drainage patterns are explained by the name and the location of the region, for instance the buccal nodes drain the cheek and the lower eyelid, and the occipital nodes drain the scalp. On the other hand, some nodes are not as self-explanatory, for importance the *parotid nodes* drain the external ear, temple, forehead, and scalp.

The deep cervical nodes in turn drain into the jugular trunk, which on the right drains into the right lymphatic duct, and on the left into the thoracic duct.

Self-test

To test your knowledge of the autonomic fibers in the head and neck, try and label as many of the structures in Fig. 1.76. The answers are on Fig. 1.77.

And one more way to test yourself is to look at the nerves listed in the right column of Fig. 1.78 and ask yourself where the cell bodies of origin are. The key is on the left side.

Historical Snippet: Lucja Frey and Frey Syndrome

Frey Syndrome occurs when the autonomic fibers in the face are torn following surgical complications or trauma to the head. Eventually these torn autonomic fibers can regrow, however they can become confused. The parasympathetic fibers on the auriculotemporal nerve, normally destined for the parotid gland, can now form connections with the sweat glands of the scalp. When the patient is shown food, instead of parotid secretions, they now exhibit facial sweating, often from in front of their ear.

The syndrome was first described by Lucja Frey (1889–1942), a polish neurologist. During the German occupation of Poland, Frey was sent to the Lwów ghetto and forced to work as a physician. She was murdered along with many of her relatives and patients in 1942.

1)
2)
3)
4)
5)
6)
7)
8)
9)
10)
11)
12)

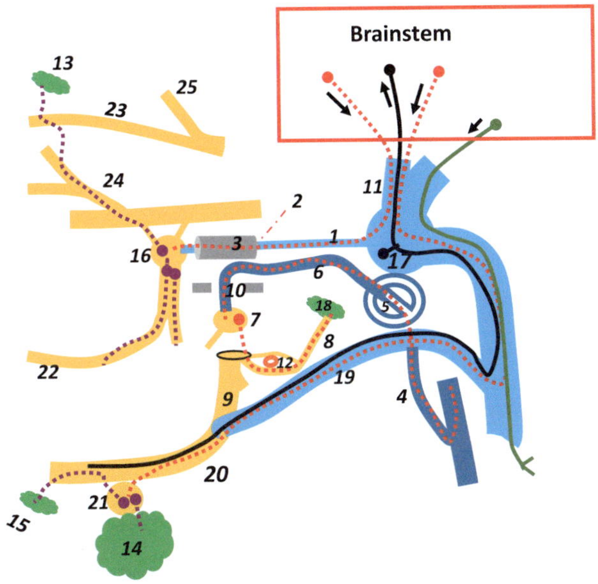

13)
14)
15)
16)
17)
18)
19)
20)
21)
22)
23)
24)
25)

Fig. 1.76 Parasympathetics to glands. This is a self-test. See how many of the tags you can identify. The key is on the next figure [21, 22]

1) Greater Petrosal N
2) Deep Petrosal N
3) Nerve of Pterygoid Canal
4) Tympanic N
5) Tympanic Plexus
6) Lesser Petrosal N
7) Otic Ganglion
8) Auriculotemporal N
9) Lingual N
10) Foramen Ovale
11) Nervus Intermedius
12) Middle Meningeal A

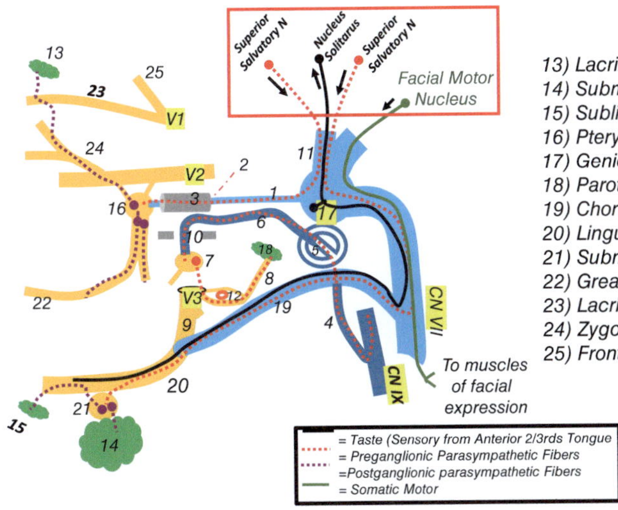

13) LacrimalGland
14) Submandibular Gland
15) Sublingual Gland
16) Pterygopalatine G
17) Geniculate G
18) ParotidGl
19) Chorda Tympani
20) Lingual N
21) Submandibular G
22) Greater Palatine N
23) Lacrimal N
24) Zygomatic N
25) Frontal N

Fig. 1.77 Parasympathetics to glands. Both CN VII and CN IX have parasympathetic fibers that use CN V to travel to their targets. CN VII has the greater petrosal nerve (parasympathetic) that meets the deep petrosal nerve (sympathetic) to form the nerve of the pterygoid canal (parasympathetic and sympathetic) that travels to meet the pterygopalatine ganglion in the pterygopalatine fossa. After synapsing in the PT ganglion, the post ganglionic parasympathetic fibers jump on the zygomatic nerve (V2) and then jump onto the lacrimal nerve (V1) to reach the lacrimal gland. They also travel on the greater and lesser petrosal nerves to the glands on the palate. In addition, CN VII has the chorda tympani with preganglionic fibers that joint the lingual nerve (V3) to reach the submandibular ganglion. In addition, the chorda tympani has taste fibers from the anterior two-thirds of the tongue. CN IX has the tympanic nerve, which meets the tympanic plexus, which gives off the lesser petrosal nerve that exits the skull through foramen ovale to meet the otic ganglion. The post ganglionic parasympathetic fibers then jump on auriculo-temporal to reach the parotid gland [21, 22]

Where are the Cell Bodies of origin for fibers in the?	Key
1) Greater Petrosal N	1) Superior Salvatory N
2) Deep Petrosal N	2) Superior Cervical G
3) Nerve of Pterygoid Canal	3) Superior Salvatory N, Superior Cervical G
4) Chorda Tympani	4) Geniculate G, Superior Salvatory N
5) Lingual nerve proximal to chorda tympani	5) Trigeminal G
6) Lesser Petrosal Nerve	6) Inferior Salvatory N
7) Auriculotemporal Nerve	7) Trigeminal G, Otic G
8) Lacrimal nerve	8) Trigeminal G, Pterygopalatine G
9) Greater Palatine Nerve	9) Pterygopalatine G, Trigeminal G

Fig. 1.78 The cell body game. The questions are on the left. The answers are on the right. Use the previous figure to visualize the answers

Further Reading

1. Barry BJ, Whitman MC, Hunter DG, Engle EC. Duane syndrome. In: Adam MP, Ardinger HH, Pagon RA, et al., editors. GeneReviews; 2019. Available at https://www.ncbi.nlm.nih.gov/books/NBKX90/.
2. Betti C, Milani GP, Lava SA, Bianchetti MG, Bronz G, Ramelli GP, Simonetti BB, Bergman MM. Auriculotemporal Frey syndrome no associated with surgery or diabetes: systematic review. Eur J Pediatr. 2022;181:2127–34.
3. Carroll M, Schade D. A practical approach to hypercalcemia. Am Fam Physician. 2003;67(9):1959–66.
4. Chen CE, Liao ZZ, Lee Y, Liu C, Tang C, Chen R. Scalp trauma in an adult. J Emerg Med. 2017;53(5):e85–8.
5. Chuang DC, Fang F, Chang TN, Lu JC. Thoracic outlet syndrome: past and present—88 surgeries in 30 years at Chang Gung. Plast Reconstr Surg Glob Open. 2016; Available at: PMC. nih.gov
6. Coskun Ö, Chatzioglou GN, Öztürk A. Henry Gray (1827–1861): the great author of the most widely used resource in medical education. Childs Nerv Syst. 2020. Available at: doi:https://doi.org/10.1007/s00381-0200047-48-7.
7. Earwood JS, Rogers TS, Rathjen A. Ear pain Diagnosing common causes and uncommon causes Amer Fam Physc. 2018;97(1):20-7.
8. Ebner RN, Ayerza R, Aghetoni F. Sixth nerve palsy + ipsilateral Horner's syndrome = Parkinson's syndrome. Saudi J Ophthalmol. 2015;29:63–6.
9. Ellis H. Anatomy of a head injury. Neurosurgery. 2007;25(12):505–7.
10. Esling JH. States of the glottis. In: Encyclopedia of language and linguistics. 5th ed. 2006. Available at: https://doi.org/10.1016/B0-08-044854-2/05098-7.
11. Ezer H, Banerjee AD, Thakur JD, Nanda A. Dorello's canal for laymen: a lego-like presentation. J Neurol Surg. 2012;73:183–9.
12. Gray H. Anatomy: descriptive and surgical. Toronto: Strathearn Books; 1858.
13. Hartl DM. Recurrent laryngeal nerve paralysis: current concepts and treatment: part II causes, diagnosis, and management. Ear Nose Throat J. 2000;80:918–27.
14. Hayes B. The anatomist: a true story of Gray's anatomy. New York: Ballantine Books; 2008.
15. Hiatt JL, Gartner LP. Textbook of head and neck anatomy. Philadelphia: Wolters Kluwer; 2010.
16. Hrelec C, Zhang E. Anatomy and physiology of phonation. Int J Head Neck Surg. 2021;12(4) https://doi.org/10.5005/jp-journals-10001-1511.
17. Ikeda AK, Burke AB. Le Fort fractures. Semin Plast Surg. 2021;35(4):250–5.
18. Khonsary SA, Ma Q, Villablanca P, Emerson J, Malkasian D. Clinical functional anatomy of the pterygopalatine ganglion, cephalgia, and related dysautonomias: a review. Surg Neurol Int. 2013;4(6):S422–8.
19. Kirchner JA. Semon's law a century later. J Laryngol Otol. 1981;96:645–57.
20. Landers T, Maino K. Clarifying Erb's point as an anatomic landmark in the posterior triangle. Dermatol Surg. 2012;38:954-57.
21. Leo J. Medical neuroanatomy for the boards and clinic: finding the lesion. 2nd ed. Cham: Springer; 2024.
22. Leo J. Clinical anatomy and embryology: a guide for the classroom, clinic, and clinic. 2nd ed. Cham: Springer; 2024.
23. Luers JC, Huttenbrink KB. Surgical anatomy and pathology of the middle ear. J Anat. 2015;238:338–53.
24. Lydiatt DD, Bucher GS. The historical Latin and etymology of selected anatomical terms of the larynx. Clin Anat. 2010;23(2):131–44.
25. Maciejewska I, Dziewiatkowski J, Spodnik E. Lucja Frey: a pioneering physician in tragic times. Clin Anat. 2007;20(6):588–90.
26. Moore K, Dalley AF, Agur A. Clinically oriented anatomy. 7th ed. Baltimore: Lippincott Williams and Wilkin; 2014.
27. Nicholson L. Caput succedaneum and cephalohematoma: the Cs that leave bumps on the head. Neonatal Netw. 2007;26(5):277–81.
28. Taylor WB, Vandergriff CL, Opatowsky MJ, Layton KF. Bowhunter's syndrome diagnosed with provocative digital subtraction cerebral angiography. Proc of Baylor Univ Med Cent. 2012;25(1):26–7.
29. Thiagarajah C, Kersten RC. Medial wall fracture: an update. Craniomaxillofac Trauma Reconstr. 2009;2(3):135–46.
30. Woodburne RT, Burkel WE. Essentials of human anatomy. 9th ed. Oxford University Press; 1994.

2 The Thorax

Anterior Thoracic Wall

Breasts

The *mammary glands* are located anterior to the pectoralis major and serratus anterior muscles. Between the breast tissue and the pectoralis major is the retromammary space. The retromammary space allows movement of the breast on the chest wall. The *suspensory ligaments* (Cooper's Ligaments) of the breast are connective tissue connecting the skin to the deep layer of the superficial fascia. The ligaments are like the spokes of a wheel running from the periphery to the center which results in the formation of compartments within the breast that house the ducts and lobules. Carcinoma can lead to the blockage of the lymphatic vessels in one or more compartments which gives a "dimpling" or "orange-peel" appearance to the breast. If one of the compartments is infected and needs to be drained, an incision should remain localized to that segment. In other words, a radial incision that runs parallel to the suspensory ligaments, would be better than a semicircular incision which cuts across the suspensory ligaments.

The glands or lobules are housed in these compartments. The glands drain via the small lactiferous ducts to the main lactiferous ducts, which are found within a compartment, and then to the lactiferous sinuses which open onto the nipples at the areola.

Regarding lymphatic drainage of the breast, the lateral side (75%) of the breast drains towards lymph nodes in the vicinity of the armpit, while the medial side (remaining 25%) drains to the parasternal nodes along the sternum.

Now for the details. The nodes around the armpit are subdivided into several distinct groups, all of which are appropriately named. The *central group* is deep in the armpit and forms the top of a tripod receiving drainage from the *anterior, posterior,* and *lateral nodes*. After receiving drainage from these regions, the central group drains to the apical group which is just below the clavicle—not surprisingly this group is sometimes referred to as the *infraclavicular group* (Fig. 2.1).

These axillary nodes can also be organized into three distinct levels, all based on their location to pectoralis minor. Level 1 is distal to pectoralis minor, level II is posterior to pectoralis minor, and level III is proximal to pectoralis minor. It is much easier to remember the numbering format than the naming format. Remember that the axillary artery is also divided into three parts based on the pectoralis minor (Fig. 2.1).

J. Leo, *Gross Anatomy, Neuroanatomy, and Embryology for Medical Students*,
https://doi.org/10.1007/978-3-031-87151-1_2

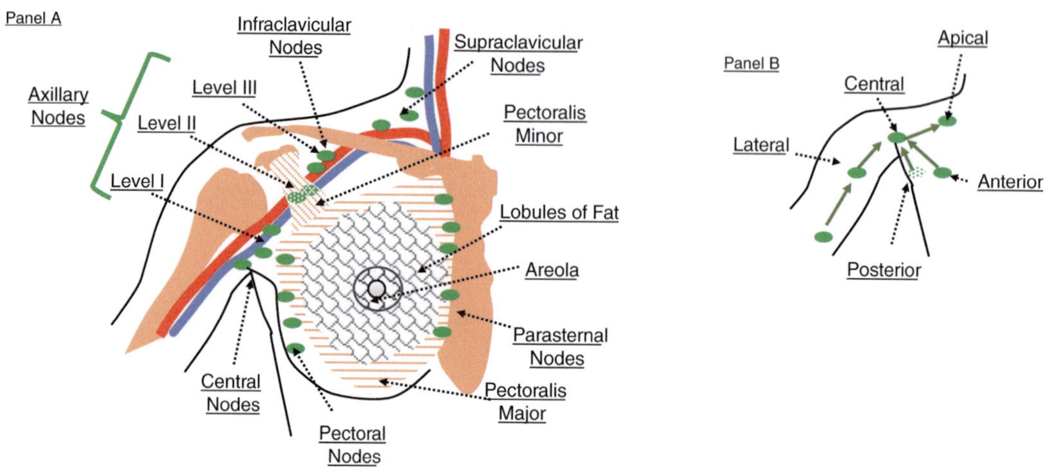

Fig. 2.1 Lymphatic drainage of breast. Panel (**a**) shows the lateral side of the breast (75%) draining to the axillary nodes which then drain Into the infra and supraclavicular nodes. The pectoralis minor is a landmark and divides the axillary nodes into three levels. The remaining medial side (25%) drains into the parasternal nodes. Panel (**b**) shows the lateral, posterior, and anterior nodes all draining into the central nodes which in turn drains into the apical nodes [5, 6]

Neurovascular Supply to the Breast

For clinical scenarios, the most important blood supply to the breast is the *lateral thoracic artery* supplying the lateral side of the breast. This artery runs with the long thoracic nerve. Radical mastectomies that damage this nerve will paralyze the serratus anterior resulting in a winged scapula and difficulty in abducting the upper limb from 90° to straight over the head. The breast also receives blood from the anterior and posterior intercostal arteries. The nerves to the breast also come from the intercostal nerves (T4–T6).

Anterior Thoracic Wall Muscles

The musculature of the anterior thoracic wall is formed by the three intercostal muscles lying between the ribs and the transversus thoracis. They are all innervated by intercostal nerves.

1. The *external intercostal muscles* pass from the lower border of one rib to the upper border of the rib below. Their fibers are oriented as the "hands in the pocket" direction.
2. The *internal intercostal muscles* run from the inferior surface of a costal groove to the superior border of the rib below at right angles to the external intercostal muscles.
3. The *innermost intercostal muscles* run from the superior surface of a costal groove to the superior border of the rib below in the same orientation as the internal intercostal muscles.
4. The origin of the small *transverse thoracis* is on the posterior inferior portion of the sternum and the xiphoid process. Its fibers run laterally and ascend to reach ribs 2–6.

Neurovascular Organization of the Anterior Thoracic Wall

The *costal grooves* are located on the inferior surface of the ribs. Each groove houses a neurovascular bundle containing an intercostal vein, artery, and nerve. These bundles are situated between the internal intercostal and innermost intercostal muscles (Fig. 2.2).

1. The *intercostal nerves* arise from the spinal nerves. They start posteriorly and wrap around

to end on the anterior thoracic wall. Note the terminology here, there are no *anterior* or *posterior* intercostal nerves, just intercostal nerves.

2. However, the *intercostal arteries* are given the prefix of either anterior or posterior. For the first two spaces, the posterior intercostal arteries come from the superior intercostal artery which is a branch of the costocervical trunk. The posterior intercostal arteries in the remaining spaces (3–9) arise from the abdominal aorta and wrap around the thoracic wall in the costal groove where they meet with the anterior intercostal arteries. In the first six intercostal spaces the anterior intercostal arteries are branches of the internal thoracic arteries as they descend posterior to the sternum. The internal thoracic eventually gives off a *musculophrenic artery* which in turn gives off the anterior intercostal arteries to enter spaces 7–9.

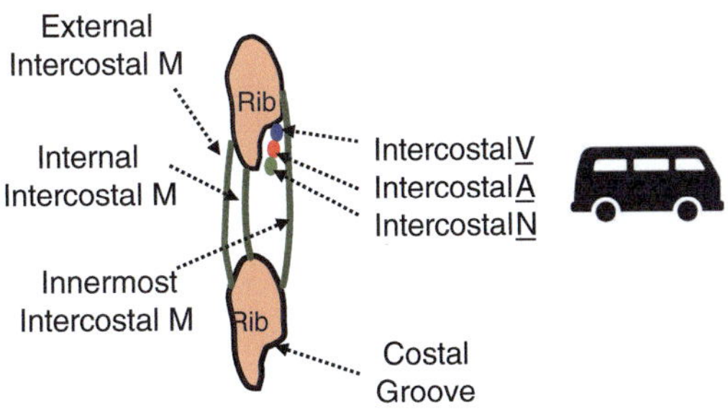

Fig. 2.2 Ribs and neurovascular structures. The intercostal veins, arteries and nerves travel in the costal groove on the inferior surface of the ribs [5, 6]

Mediastinum

The dividing line for the *mediastinum* is a horizontal line referred to as the transverse thoracic plane, or TTP. The TTP starts anteriorly at the junction of the second rib with the manubrium and body of the sternum (sternal angle) and runs posterior to the junction of the T4 and T5 vertebrae. Above the line is the *superior mediastinum*, and below the line are the *anterior, middle, and posterior mediastinum* (Fig. 2.3).

1. The superior border of the *superior mediastinum* is an ascending diagonal line running from the sternal notch upwards to the T1 vertebra. Within the superior mediastinum is the aorta, superior vena cava, trachea, esophagus, vagus nerve, and left recurrent laryngeal nerve. The thoracic duct drains into the venous circulation at the angle between the left internal jugular and left subclavian vein and is found within the superior mediastinum.

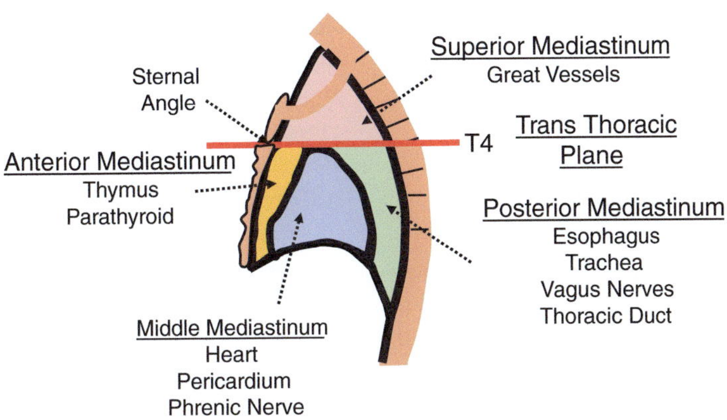

Fig. 2.3 The important dividing line for the mediastinum runs from the sternal angle to the junction of the T4 and T5 vertebrae. The superior mediastinum is above the line, and the anterior, middle, and posterior mediastinum subdivisions are below the line. The anterior mediastinum includes the thymus and parathyroid. The middle mediastinum includes the heart, pericardium, and phrenic nerves. The posterior mediastinum includes the esophagus, trachea, and vagus nerves [5, 6]

2. The *anterior mediastinum* is between the body of the sternum and the fibrous pericardium of the heart. In children it contains the thymus. During adolescence it is replaced by adipose tissue. In adults the anterior mediastinum is a site for tumors—either thymomas or lymphomas. In addition, a thyroid goiter can expand inferiorly and enter the anterior mediastinum. Teratomas can also be found in the anterior mediastinum.
3. The *middle mediastinum* contains the heart and the pericardium, the ascending aorta, the superior vena cava, azygos vein, the pulmonary trunk, pulmonary veins, phrenic nerves, vagus nerves, and the inferior vena cava. Also in middle mediastinum is the trachea which bifurcates at the level of (in the cadaver at T4/T5).
4. The *posterior mediastinum* contains the esophagus, thoracic aorta, azygous vein, hemiazygos vein, thoracic duct, splanchnic nerves, and vagus nerves. The sympathetic trunk is posterior to the pleura and the mediastinum, but the thoracic splanchnic nerves emerge from the sympathetic trunk and move anteriorly into the posterior mediastinum. Note that while I mentioned above that the sympathetic trunk is just behind the posterior mediastinum, some authors list it as being in the posterior mediastinum. In other words, from one textbook to another the location of the sympathetic trunk, being in either the posterior mediastinum or just behind it, varies. However, it is a debate over semantics and not critical for clinical medicine.

The Pericardium and Sinuses

There are three layers of *pericardium*. The thick, tough outermost layer is the fibrous pericardium. It is a cone shaped structure attached to the diaphragm inferiorly via the *pericardiophrenic ligaments*, and the adventitia of the great vessels superiorly. The *phrenic nerve* and *pericardiacophrenic vessels* are located just lateral to the fibrous pericardium.

Deep to the fibrous pericardium, is the serous pericardium which is subdivided into two layers, the parietal and visceral layers. The parietal and visceral layers are continuous and encase the pericardial space. The visceral layer is attached to the heart and is reflected onto the parietal layer which is attached to the fibrous layer. The parietal layer is reflected around the great vessels to create two compartments. One compartment contains the aorta and pulmonary trunk, and the second compartment contains the superior vena cava, the inferior vena cava, and the four pulmonary veins. This in turn makes two spaces. The *transverse pericardial sinus* is posterior to the aorta and pulmonary trunk, and anterior to the superior vena cava. The *oblique sinus* is posterior to the heart and bound by the four pulmonary veins (Fig. 2.3).

Accumulation of fluid in the pericardial space—between the visceral and parietal layers—can lead to *cardiac tamponade*. Patients will typically present with bulging neck veins, hypotension, and distant heart sounds.

The Heart

The right atrium receives oxygen poor blood from both the superior and inferior vena cava. The coronary sinus also delivers oxygen poor blood from the heart muscle itself to the right atrium. From the right atrium, the blood travels through the tricuspid valve into the right ventricle. The tricuspid valve is composed of three cusps which are connected via *chorda tendineae* to the papillary muscles. The combination of chorda tendineae and papillary muscles prevent the valve cusps from backflowing into the right atrium during contraction. From the right ventricle, blood moves through the semilunar valve into the pulmonary trunk on its way to the lungs to pick up oxygen, and it then returns to the left atrium. From the left atrium, blood moves through the mitral valve into the left ventricle. From the left ventricle, blood moves from through the aortic semilunar valve to the ascending aorta (Fig. 2.4).

The great vessels emerge from the heart and enter the superior mediastinum. There are several important relationships in this area.

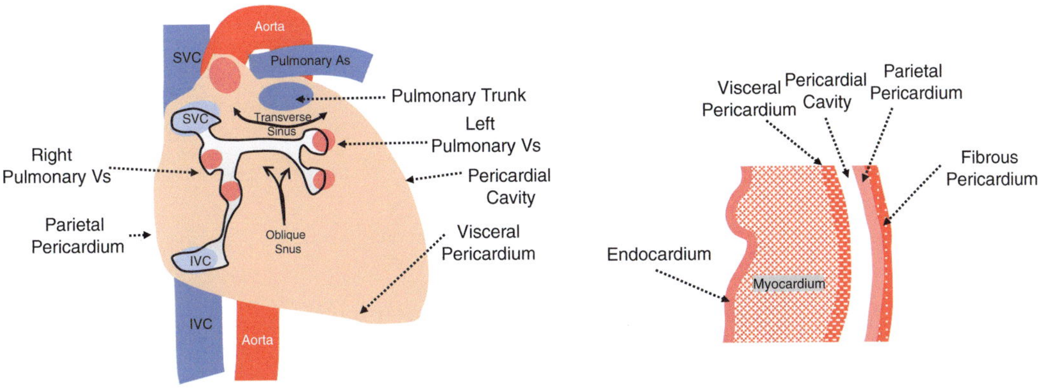

Fig. 2.4 Pericardial cavity and sinuses. The visceral pericardium is adherent to the heart. It connects and folds back on the parietal pericardium to form the pericardial cavity. The fibrous pericardium is a thick layer outside the heart attaching to the diaphragm inferiorly. The oblique pericardial sinus is bounded by the pulmonary arteries. The transverse pericardial sinus is anterior to the SVC, but posterior to the aorta and pulmonary trunk [5, 6]

1. The *right brachiocephalic vein* enters the superior vena cava heading towards the right border of the heart.
2. The *left brachiocephalic vein* crosses anterior to the aorta and the aorta's three large branches. This is at the T3 level.
3. The *ascending aorta* comes out of the heart at the T4 level just to the left of the superior vena cava. The right pulmonary artery passes deep to the aorta.
4. The *right and left internal jugular veins* are lateral to the common carotid arteries. A central line is placed into the internal jugular vein by going lateral to a finger on the pulse of the common carotid.

Blood Supply to the Heart

The blood supply to the heart comes from the right and left coronary arteries which are the first branches coming off the aorta. The openings of the right and left coronary arteries are below the upper extensions of the cusps of the aortic valve. The right coronary descends in the atrioventricular groove towards the inferior border of the heart where it is turns around to travel posteriorly to the crux of the heart (the intersection between the atrioventricular and interatrial grooves) (Figs. 2.5, 2.6 and 2.7).

1. The first branch of the right coronary artery is the *right conus branch* to the pulmonary conus.
2. The next branch is the *sinoatrial nodal branch* which travels posterior to the superior vena cava to reach the sinoatrial node. In some cases, it can arise from the left coronary artery.
3. As the right coronary artery reaches the inferior border it gives off a *marginal branch*. The right coronary artery supplies most of the right ventricle, a small portion of the left ventricle, and the posterior one third of the interventricular septum.
4. As the right coronary artery reaches the posterior surface of the heart it gives off the *posterior interventricular artery*. Often coming from the posterior interventricular is the *atrioventricular nodal artery*.

The *left coronary artery* is short and quickly splits into a

1. A *circumflex branch* that runs towards the left side in the atrioventricular groove and which eventually meets up with the right coronary artery at the crux. The circumflex gives off the *left marginal artery* and the *posterior ventricular branch of left coronary artery*.
2. The *anterior interventricular branch*, also known as the left anterior descending,

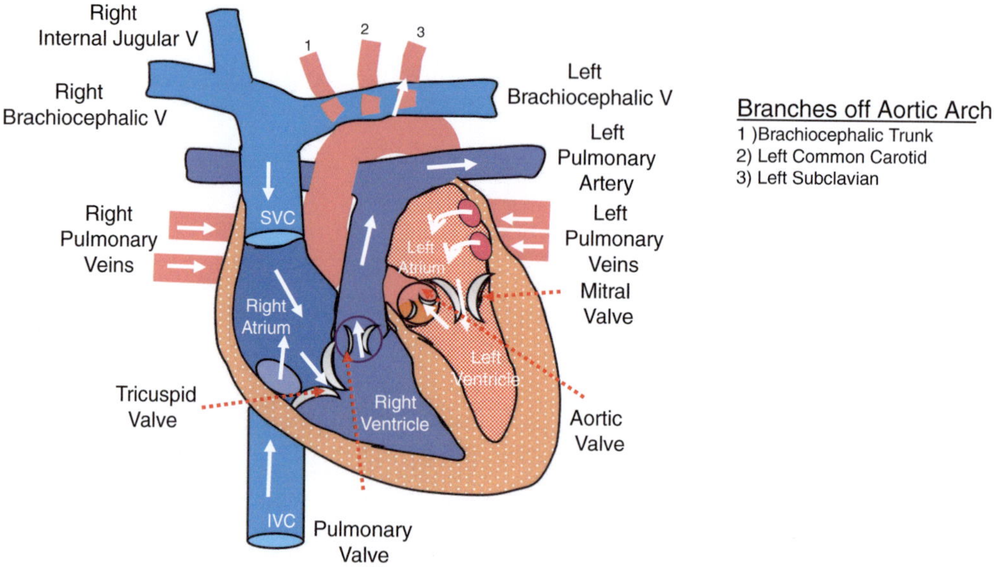

Fig. 2.5 Interior of the heart. Blood enters the right atrium from the SVC and IVC. It then passes through the tricuspid valve to enter the right ventricle. From the right ventricle it moves through the pulmonic valve into the pulmonary trunk to pulmonary arteries to lungs. After picking up O^2 in the lungs it comes back to the left atrium; then through the mitral valve into left ventricle; then out the left ventricle through the aortic valve to aorta. Note the left brachiocephalic vein crosses the midline from left to right to reach the SVC. The right brachiocephalic vein does not cross the midline. The three branches off the aorta arise behind the left brachiocephalic vein [5, 6]

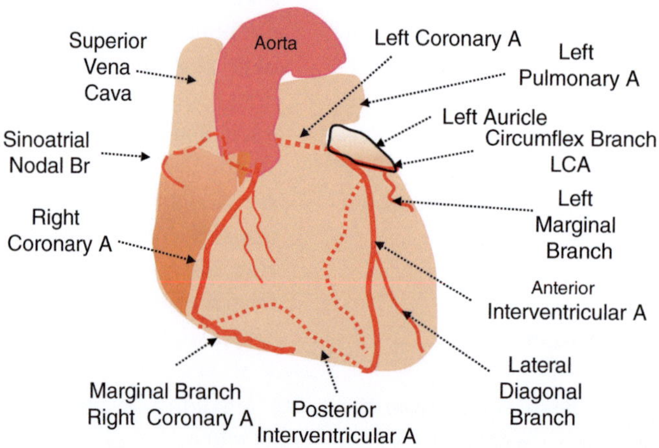

Fig. 2.6 Blood supply to heart. The right coronary artery (RCA) descends in the coronary sulcus. It gives off the marginal branch which supplies the inferior border. The RCA continues posterior. The posterior interventricular artery typically arises from the RCA. The left coronary artery is much shorter than the RCA as it quickly divides into the circumflex and the anterior interventricular artery. The circumflex gives off a left marginal branch [5, 6]

Left Coronary Artery

Anterior Interventricular A	**Anterior 2/3rds of interventricular septum**, Anterior wall of left vetricle
Left Circumflex A	Posterior wall of left vetricle
Left Marginal A	Left vetricle

Right Coronary Artery

Right Conus Branch	Pulmonary Conus
Sinoatrial Nodal Br	Sinoatrial node
Right Marginal A	Right ventricle and right atrium, reachesapex
Posterior Interventricular A	**Posterior 1/3 of interventricular septum**

Fig. 2.7 Coronary arteries. If you can picture the location of the vessels on the heart surface this should all make sense. The interventricular septum receives its supply from two branches. The anterior two-thirds of the septum is from the anterior interventricular branch of the left coronary artery, while the posterior one-third is from the posterior interventricular artery, a branch of the right coronary artery [5, 6]

or LAD, or widow maker, descends towards the apex and supplies most of the left ventricle and left atrium. It also supplies most of the interventricular septum (anterior two-thirds). As it passes down the anterior surface of the heart it gives off several diagonal branches of the anterior interventricular artery.

Heart dominance refers to whether an individual heart receives most of its blood from either the right or left coronary arteries. To determine whether an individual is right or left dominant the pertinent question is: Where does the posterior interventricular artery come from? Most individuals are right dominant, in which case the posterior interventricular artery arises from the right coronary artery. However, in some individuals, the circumflex artery which is a branch of the left coronary artery gives off the posterior interventricular artery, making this an example of a left dominant heart. And in some cases, the anterior interventricular artery continues around the apex, turns, and ascends in the interventricular groove as the posterior interventricular artery, which is also an example of a left dominant individual.

Venous Drainage of the Heart

Most of the venous drainage of the heart enters the *coronary sinus* which then drains into the right atrium. The coronary sinus is found on the posterior surface of the heart and runs with the circumflex artery. Running on the anterior surface, with the anterior interventricular artery, is the *great cardiac vein* which turns posterior to turn into the coronary sulcus to meet the coronary sinus. Running with the posterior interventricular artery in the posterior interventricular sulcus, is the *middle cardiac vein* which also drains into the coronary sinus. And running on the right border of the heart with the right marginal artery and draining into the coronary sinus is the *small cardiac vein*. The coronary sinus in turn drains into the right atrium. In addition, besides the vessels mentioned above, which all drain into the coronary sinus, there are several small *anterior cardiac veins* which drain directly into the right atrium. At the opening of the coronary sinus, there is a small valve, the *valve of the coronary sinus*. Also draining into the coronary sinus, close to its origin, is the *oblique vein of the left atrium* (Fig. 2.8).

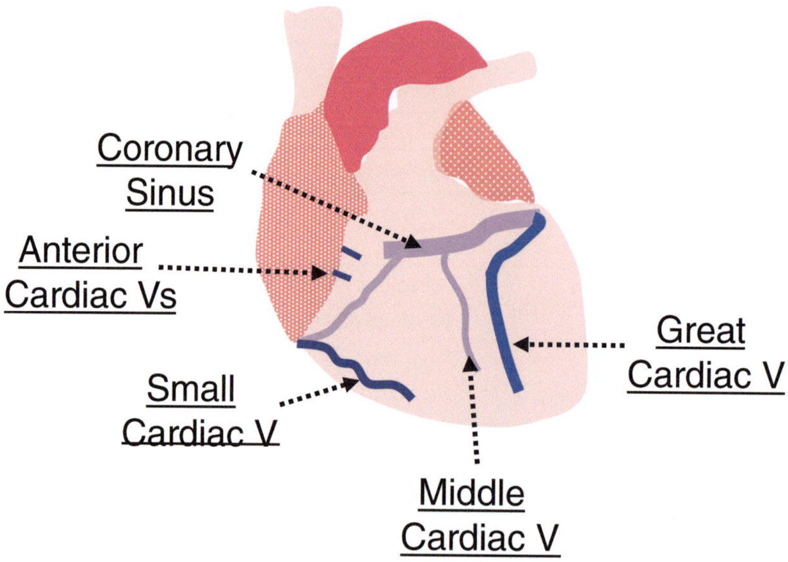

Fig. 2.8 Venous drainage of the heart. The great cardiac, middle cardiac, and small cardiac veins all drain into the posteriorly located coronary sinus. The anterior cardiac veins drain directly into the right atrium [5, 6]

Nerves to the Heart

The internal conducting system of the heart starts at the *sinoatrial node* which is found in the vicinity of the opening of the superior vena cava. Impulses then travel to the *atrioventricular node* (AV node) which is found near the septal leaflet of the tricuspid valve and the opening of the coronary sinus. At the AV node there is a slight delay of the impulse to allow the atria to completely empty before the contractions are over. From the AV node the impulses then travel down through the bundle of His fibers in the *interventricular septum* towards the apex. There are two branches of the bundle of His, the *right and left bundle branches*. From the apex the impulse then travels along *Purkinje fibers* on the ventricular walls.

The right and left vagus nerves provide the parasympathetic nerve supply to the heart. They both travel in the carotid sheath with the common carotid artery and internal jugular vein to enter the thorax. The left vagus nerve travels over the aortic arch, where it gives off the recurrent laryngeal, and then continues towards the heart. The right vagus nerve gives off the recurrent laryngeal which travels around the subclavian artery.

The sympathetic efferent nerves to the heart come from the inferior and middle cervical ganglion. The superficial cardiac plexus is situated on the aortic arch, while the deep cardiac plexus is under the aortic arch. These plexuses are a combination of parasympathetic and sympathetic fibers. Afferent sensations from the heart travel on the sympathetic nerves to the T1–4 levels which are the same levels responsible for shoulder pain. This is why a patient during a heart attack will complain of pain in the left shoulder.

The Interior of the Heart

The right atrium is characterized by a line of demarcation referred to as the *crista terminalis* which represents the division between the smooth and rough portions of the right atrium. Remember the smooth portion of the atrium developed from the sinus venosus, while the rough portion or pectinate muscle came from the primitive atrium. This interior line, the crista terminalis can also be seen on the exterior of the right atrium where it is referred to as the sulcus terminalis. If you follow the crista terminalis up to the superior pole this is the location of the sinoatrial node.

You can also see the superior vena cava and inferior vena cava draining into the right atrium. The coronary sinus drains into the right atrium near the opening of the inferior vena cava. Along the atrial septum one can see the fossa ovalis, and the limbus of the fossa ovalis.

Moving through the tricuspid valve into the right ventricle one can see the rough portion of the ventricular musculature referred to as the trabeculae carneae. The cusp or leaflets of the tricuspid valve are connected via chordae tendineae to the papillary muscles. Because there are three leaflets, there are three papillary muscles, the anterior, posterior, and septal. In addition, there is a specialized portion of papillary muscle that is referred to as the septomarginal trabecula, or moderator band, which connects the interventricular septum to the papillary muscle. This septomarginal trabecula is a useful landmark for the right ventricle when looking at the heart with an ultrasound. Branches of the right bundle branch travel in the septomarginal trabecula to coordinate the action of the tricuspid valve.

In the left atrium one can see the four pulmonary veins draining into the posterior wall. In the left ventricle there are only two leaflets with two papillary muscles. There is no septomarginal trabecula in the left ventricle.

In the left atrium is a small appendage known as the left atrial appendage (LAA) which is an outpouching of the atrial wall whose appearance has been likened to a windsock. Its exact purpose is unknown, but one theory is that it acts like a reservoir for excess blood when pressure rises in the left atrium. In some cases, this can lead to blood pooling in the left atrium which can lead to clotting and a thromboembolism. The left atrial appendage can be surgically removed.

Running from the left superior pulmonary vein to the opening of the LAA is a small ridge of tissue. In some cases, during an echocardiogram it can be mistaken for a thrombosis leading to the patient being mistreated with an anticoagulant such as coumadin. It is unknown when or who coined the term, but this ridge is sometimes referred to as the "Coumadin ridge."

Borders of the Heart

To know your way around a cross section through the neck or thorax, a good starting place is drawing a line on the right side going down through the right side of the heart. The line will progress down through the right internal jugular vein, which meets with the right subclavian vein, and then down into the right brachiocephalic vein, which then drains into the *superior vena cava*, and then down into the right atrium. Thus the right side is made of three venous structures: internal jugular vein, right brachiocephalic, and superior vena cava, and then the right atrium. When you look at a cross section think of this line running down from the neck into the thorax (Fig. 2.9).

The borders of the heart are represented by a trapezoid with vertical lines running from the costal cartilages of rib 3–6 on the right and ribs 2 to the 5th intercostal space on the left. Horizontal lines then connect the corners to outline the superior and inferior borders. The inferior border of the heart runs from rib 6 to rib 5, crossing behind the sternum. The superior border closes the trapezoid running from rib 2 on the left to rib 3 on the right.

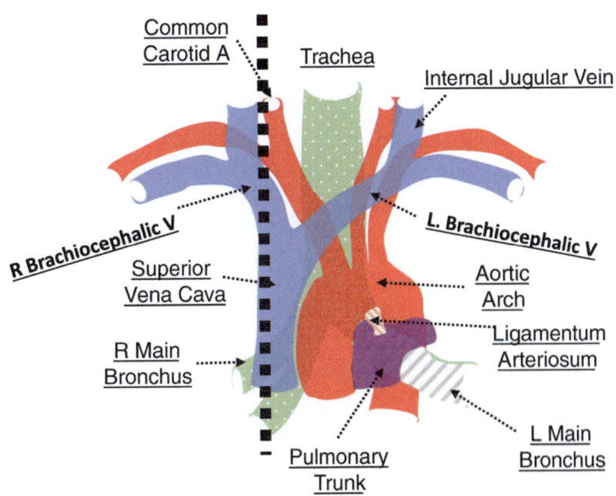

Fig. 2.9 Heart outflow. Note the three great vessels lined up in a row: (1) superior vena cava, (2) aorta, and (3) pulmonary trunk. The right and left brachiocephalic veins join to form the superior vena cava. The left brachiocephalic vein crosses in front of the three branches coming off the aorta [5, 6]

The right border of the heart is the right atrium which is located just to the right of the sternum. The anatomic base of the heart is the posterior surface (not the diaphragmatic surface) and is the left atrium. Just posterior to the base is the esophagus. A transesophageal echocardiogram involves an endoscope placed in the esophagus to visualize the heart (Figs. 2.10 and 2.11).

The anterior surface of the heart is mostly formed by the right ventricle, so a stab wound to the left of the sternum, between ribs 2 and 5 would penetrate the right ventricle. Continuing to

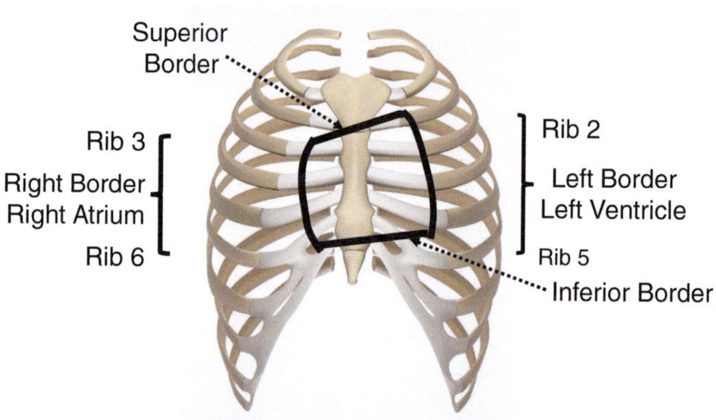

Fig. 2.10 Borders of the heart. The right border runs from the costal cartilages of rib 3 to rib 6 just to the right of the sternum. The left border runs from rib 2 to the fifth intercostal space on the left side. The right border is the right atrium, the left border is the left ventricle. Hidden from this view is the base of the heart (posterior) which is the left atrium. The right ventricle forms the inferior border and apex of left ventricle. The superior border is the right and left atria [5, 6]

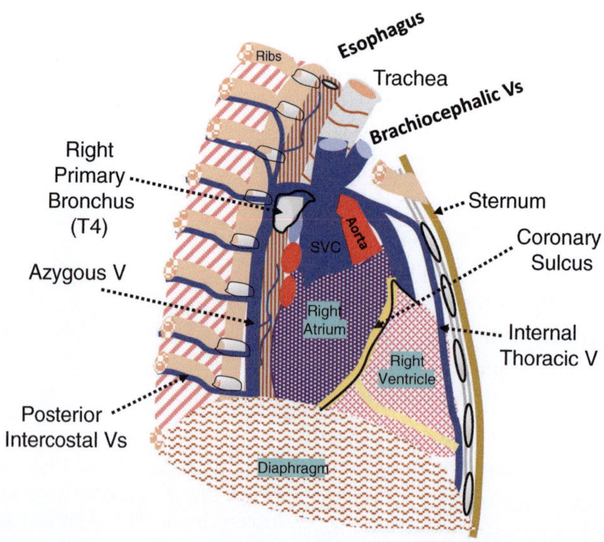

Fig. 2.11 Posterior mediastinum. The azygous vein is ascending behind the esophagus, arches over the right primary bronchus and enters the superior vena cava (SVC). The posterior Intercostal veins drain into the azygous vein. The base of the heart is the left atrium, just anterior to the esophagus. The anterior border of the heart is the right ventricle. The internal thoracic vein drains just posterior to the sternum. The trachea is bifurcating at T4/T5 [5, 6]

the left from the sternum across the right ventricle, at the left border of the heart one can see the edge of the left ventricle. While most of the anterior surface is the right ventricle, all the way on the left side, at the left border, the left ventricle makes an appearance.

Heart Valve Projections and Auscultation Sites

The atrioventricular valves are located between the atria and ventricles. The mitral valve is located on the left side, and tricuspid valve is on the right side. During ventricular systole they prevent blood from the ventricles from moving back into the atria—during ventricular systole (contraction) these doors should remain closed. During diastole they will be open.

The semilunar valves, which are the aortic and pulmonic valves, are between the ventricles and the outflow tracts. Both the aortic and pulmonic valves each have three cusps. Due to the development of these structures and the rotation of the truncus arteriosus, the cusps are situated such that in the pulmonic valve there is an anterior cusp, while the aortic valve has a posterior cusp. Each valve then has a right and left cusp. The cusps are crescent moon shaped. The edge of each cusp is referred to as the *lunula*, and in the middle of each lunula is a *nodule*. When the valves close, the three nodules will all meet in the center. The heart valves are located posterior to the sternum (Fig. 2.12).

The aortic and pulmonic valves are situated close to each other at the third costal cartilage. The aortic valve is slightly lower and to the right of the pulmonic valve. The tricuspid and mitral valves are lower down, near where the fourth costal cartilages meets the body of the sternum. However, when auscultating the valves, the sounds for each valve are not heard directly over the valve. For example, the aortic valve is located just to the right of the sternum, but the sound of the aortic valve is heard on the right at the second intercostal space.

Erb's point is located at the third intercostal space on the left. It is the location of aortic and pulmonic valves.

The pulmonic valve is heard to the left at the second intercostal space. The tricuspid valve is heard just to the left of the sternum at the fifth costal cartilage. The mitral valve is heard at the apex of the heart at the fifth intercostal space on the left in the midclavicular line (Fig. 2.13).

At the beginning of systole, as pressure in the ventricles increases, the AV valves close producing the first heart sound S1. As the pressure in the ventricles rises, the aortic and pulmonic valves open allowing blood to enter the aorta and pulmonary trunk. As the pressure rises in the great vessels, it will eventually be greater than the pressure in the ventricles at which point the aortic and pulmonic valves close producing the second heart sound S2.

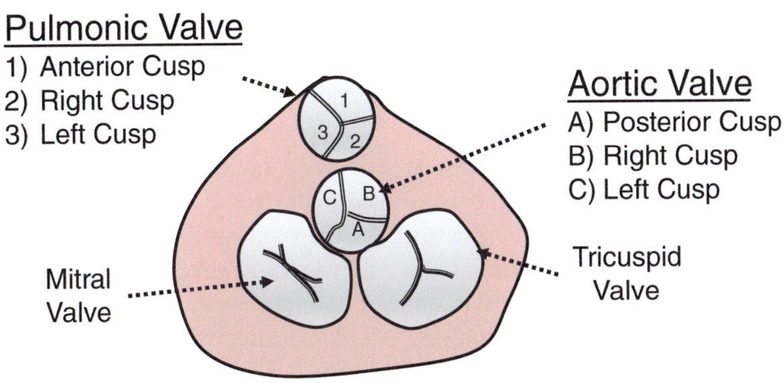

Fig. 2.12 Heart valves. There are three cusps each in the aortic and pulmonic valves. Both have right and left cusps, while the pulmonic has an anterior cusp, and the aortic valve has a posterior cusp. The pulmonic valve's anterior cusp is across from the pulmonic valve's posterior cusp [5, 6]

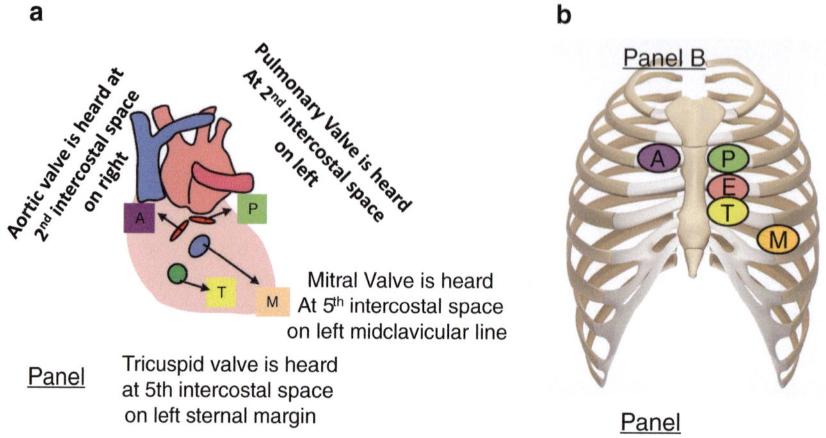

Fig. 2.13 Two representations of heart sound locations. Panel (**a**) shows the locations of the valves. The arrows show the locations of where the sounds are heard. Panel (**b**) shows the borders of the heart and the locations of the heart sounds relative to the ribs and sternum. An easy mnemonic is A PET Monkey. *E* Erb's point [5, 6]

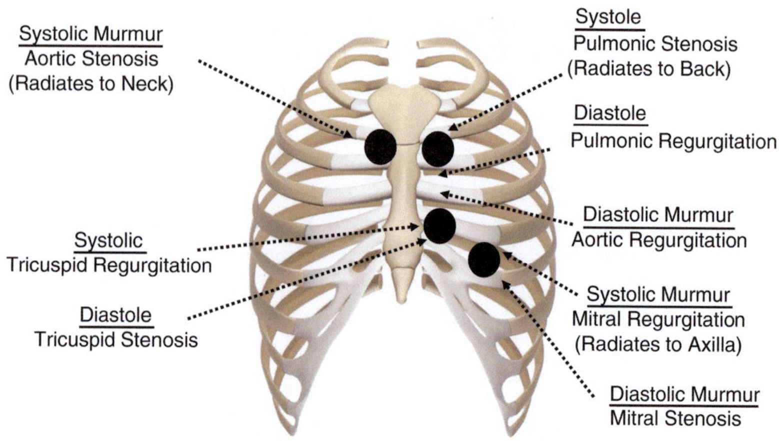

Fig. 2.14 Common locations for hearing heart murmurs [5, 6]

Disruptions of blood flow through the various valves can lead to murmurs that can be heard in either systole or diastole. Both the location of the murmur and whether it is heard at systole or diastole are important in determining which valve is affected. This disrupted flow typically results from either stenosis of the valve or regurgitation of the valve. Think of the valves like doors, a stenotic valve indicates a problem with opening the door—it does not open wide enough. And conversely, regurgitation is a problem with closing the door—it does not close all the way.

When a chamber, such as the left ventricle, is contracting and trying to push blood downstream, the outflow or downstream valve wants to remain open. At the same tie, the valve on the upstream side wants to be closed so that blood does not go in the reverse direction. If the outflow valve is stenotic then blood is ejected through a much smaller opening which will lead to a sound heard downstream of the valve. In contrast, if the upstream valve is not closed all the way—it is incompetent—then the valve will allow blood to flow in the reverse or retrograde direction. As the sound moves in a retrograde direction the sound will be heard outside the chamber (Fig. 2.14).

On the other hand, when a chamber is filling, it is the upstream valve that wants to be open, to allow blood to flow into the heart, while the downstream valve wants to be closed to allow the

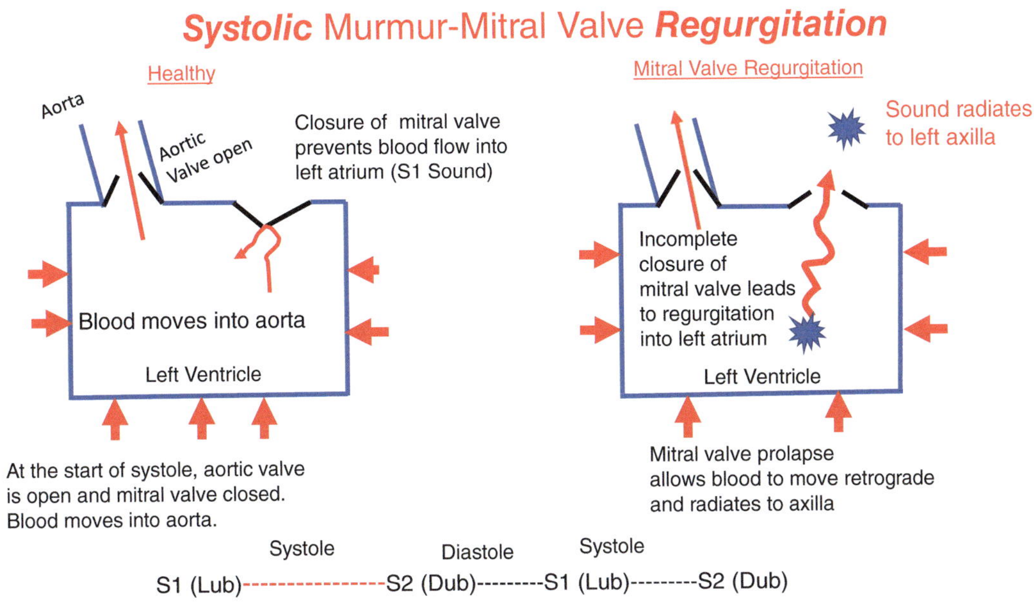

Fig. 2.15 Systolic murmur [5, 6]

chamber to fill. If the upstream valve is stenotic this will lead to blood coming through the valve at a higher pressure with the sound also heard in the chamber. In the specific examples below, we are going to focus on the left ventricle, with the mitral valve being the upstream valve, and the aortic valve being the downstream valve. Keep in mind we are focusing on the blood flow and the anatomy of murmurs, to understand just the basics at this point. We are not focusing on all the details about different heart murmurs. If you understand the basics, it will be easier to understand the nuances of heart murmurs when you get to your medical physiology course.

Systolic Murmurs

Mitral Valve Regurgitation

Take a systolic murmur resulting from mitral valve regurgitation as an example. In a healthy individual, during systole, the mitral valve will be closed, and the aortic valve will be open so that blood goes out the aortic valve but not the mitral valve. With mitral valve regurgitation, during systole, there is an incomplete closure of the mitral valve, which allows a small amount of blood to move through the mitral valve in a retrograde direction. The sound will then radiate to the left axilla and be heard throughout systole (pan systolic) (Fig. 2.15).

Aortic Stenosis

With aortic stenosis blood flow through the aortic valve is impeded in systole which leads to a sharper faster flow through the aorta resulting in the high-pitched sound radiating to the carotid arteries in the right neck (Fig. 2.16).

Diastolic Murmurs

Mitral Valve Stenosis

In a healthy individual, during diastole, the mitral valve remains open, while the aortic valve is closed. This allows the filling of the ventricle. With mitral stenosis the blood coming through the mitral valve is impeded and comes through the smaller opening faster and sharper which leads to a murmur heard at the apex—near the left fifth space in the mid-clavicular line (Fig. 2.17).

Aortic Regurgitation

With aortic regurgitation, the aortic valve is incompetent which allows blood to flow back

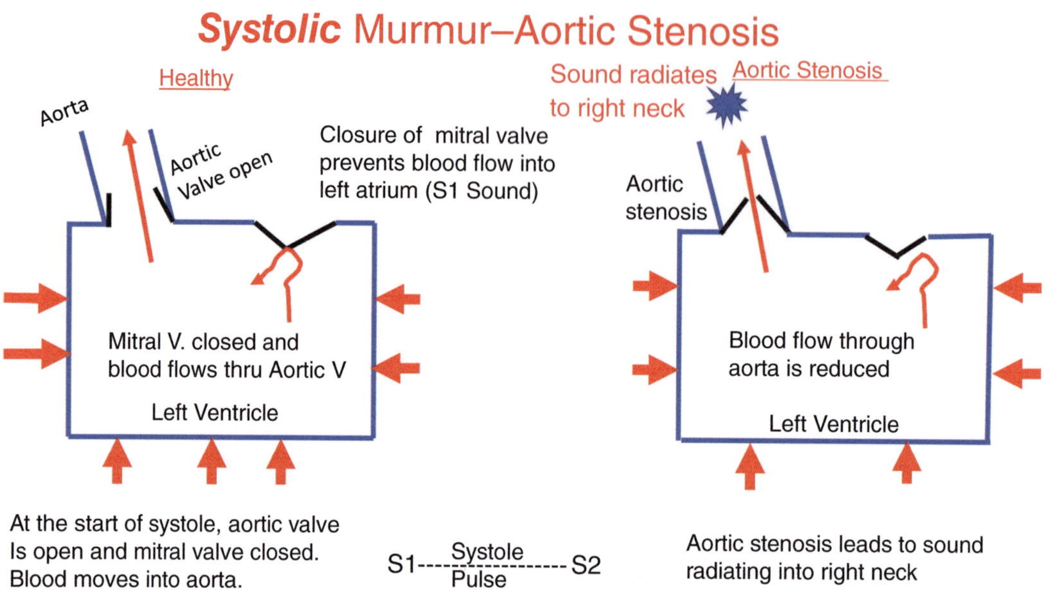

Fig. 2.16 Systolic murmur. Aortic stenosis [5, 6]

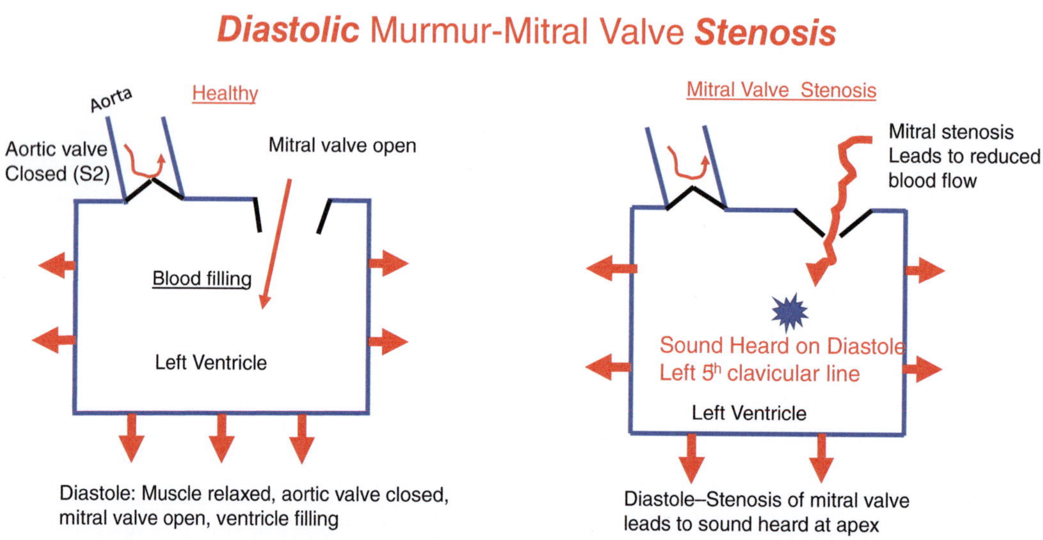

Fig. 2.17 Diastolic murmur. Mitral valve stenosis [5, 6]

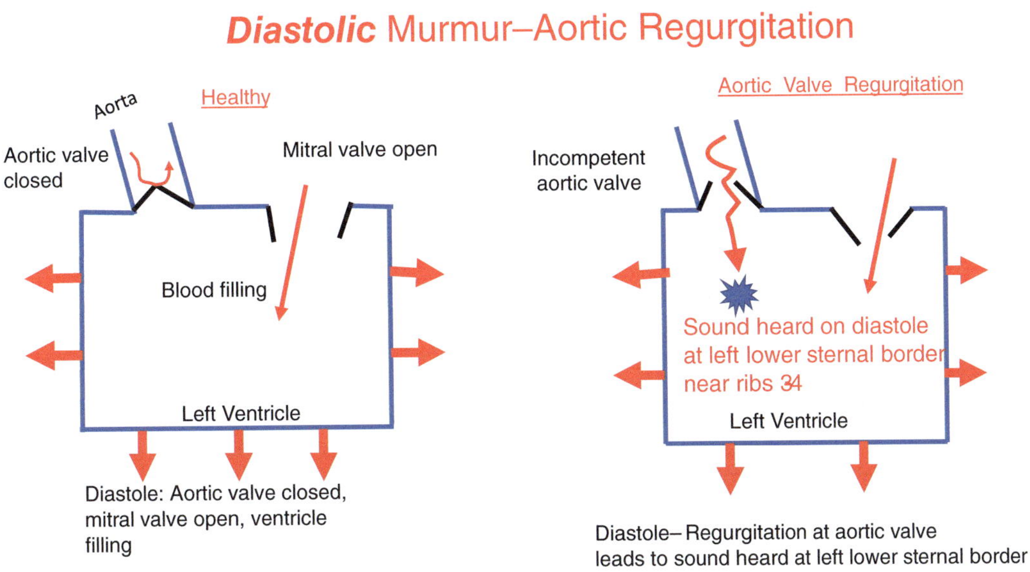

Fig. 2.18 Diastolic Murmur. Aortic regurgitation [5, 6]

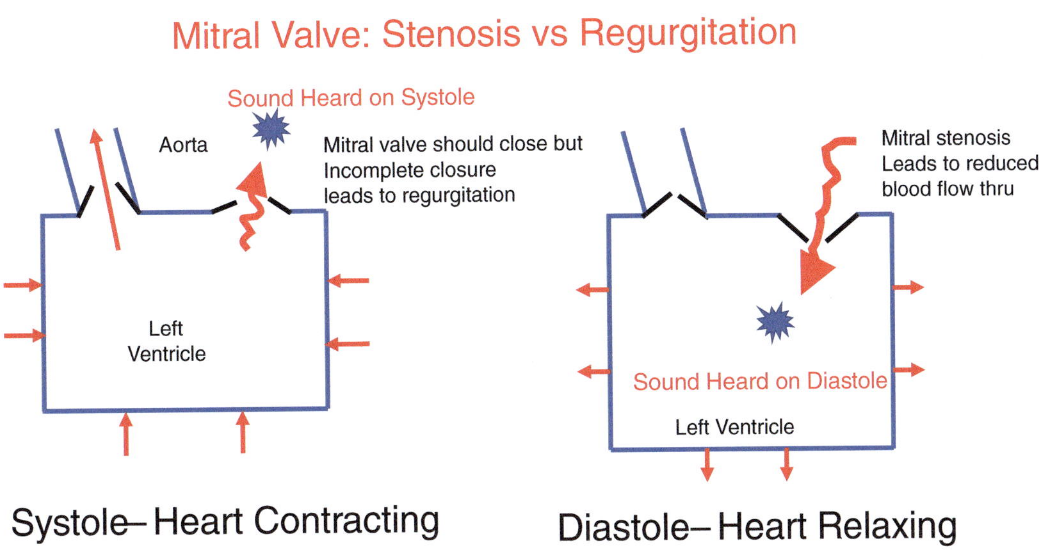

Fig. 2.19 Mitral valve: stenosis versus regurgitation [5, 6]

from the aorta into the left ventricle with the sound radiating to the left sternal border near ribs 3–4 (Fig. 2.18).

Mitral Valve Stenosis During Systole Versus Regurgitation During Diastole

With mitral valve regurgitation, the sound will be heard outside the heart—at the left axilla during systole. With mitral stenosis, the sound will be heard inside the heart during diastole (Fig. 2.19).

Putting all this together there are two steps to determine the nature of the murmur.

1. In step #1 ask if the murmur is above or below the midsternal line. If the murmur is above the line, then the murmur is either the aortic valve, or pulmonic valve.

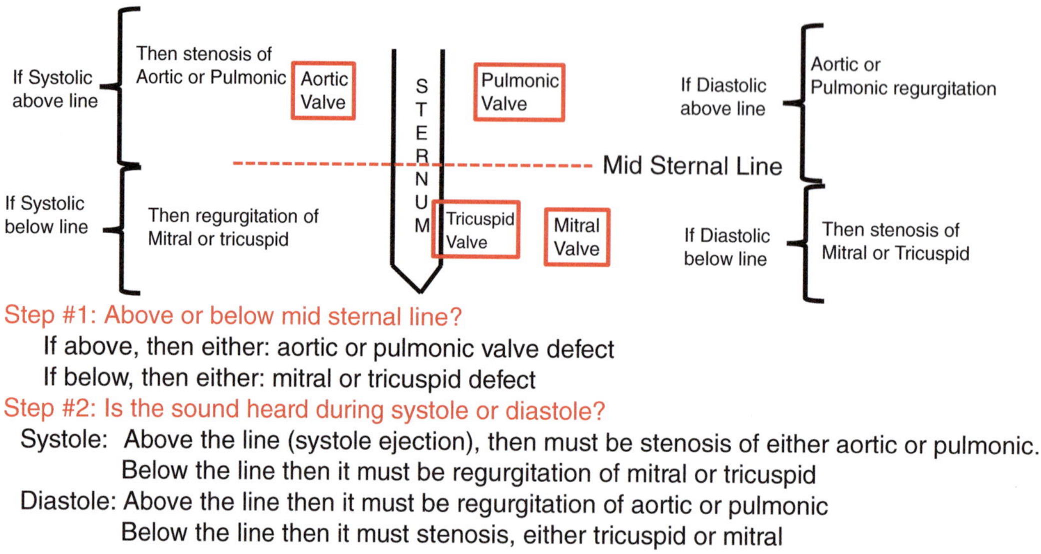

Fig. 2.20 Murmur detection [5, 6]

2. In step #2 ask if the sound is heard during systole or diastole. If the sound is heard above the line during systole, then it must be stenosis of the either the aortic or pulmonic valve. If it is heard below the line during systole, then it must be regurgitation of the mitral or tricuspid valve. If it is heard during diastole, and above the line then it must be regurgitation of the aortic or pulmonic. And if it is heard below the line during diastole then it must be stenosis of either the tricuspid or mitral valve (Fig. 2.20).

Esophagus

The esophagus transmits food from the oral cavity to the stomach and can be divided into thirds. The proximal one-third is made up of skeletal muscle, while the distal one-third is made up of smooth muscle, leaving the middle one-third composed of a combination of skeletal and smooth muscle. In the neck the esophagus passes behind the trachea. Once the trachea bifurcates, at the T4–T5 vertebral body level, the esophagus comes to lie posterior to the left atrium of the heart. It then travels through the diaphragm at the esophageal hiatus accompanying the right and left vagus nerves. Posterior to the esophagus is the thoracic aorta (Fig. 2.21).

There are several points along the esophagus as it travels from the mouth to the diaphragm where structures press on it and lead to constrictions.

1. The *cricopharyngeus* is the thickened inferior end of the inferior constrictor and forms the *pharyngoesophageal constriction.*
2. The aortic arch and the left main bronchus also cross the esophagus close to each other and from the *aortobronchial constriction.*
3. The last constriction is the *diaphragmatic constriction* at the esophageal hiatus that marks the entrance to the stomach.

Zenker's Diverticulum

As mentioned above, the start of the esophagus is the cricopharyngeus, which is a circular muscle that opens to allow the bolus to enter the esophagus but then quickly closes once the bolus passes through it so that the contents keep moving down the esophagus. These circular fibers meet the diagonally oriented fibers of the inferior constrictor. At this junction there is a small posteriorly located weak point in the pharyngeal wall referred to as *Killian's triangle.* In some cases, this weakness allows a bolus to herniate through which leads to *Zenker's diverticulum.* Food can

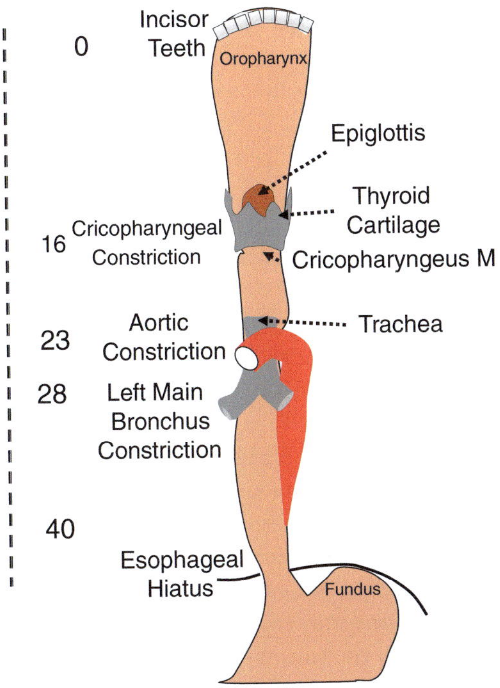

Site	Vertebral Level	Distance from central Incisor
Cricopharynx	C6	16 cm
Aortic Arch	T4	25 cm
L. Main Bronchus	T5	28 cm
Esophageal Hiatus	T10	40 cm

Fig. 2.21 Esophageal constrictions. The scale on the right shows the distance from the middle incisors. The first constriction is at the cricopharyngeus muscle. The next is where the aorta crosses in front of esophagus, and right below the aorta is the left main bronchus. The last constriction is the esophageal hiatus [5, 6]

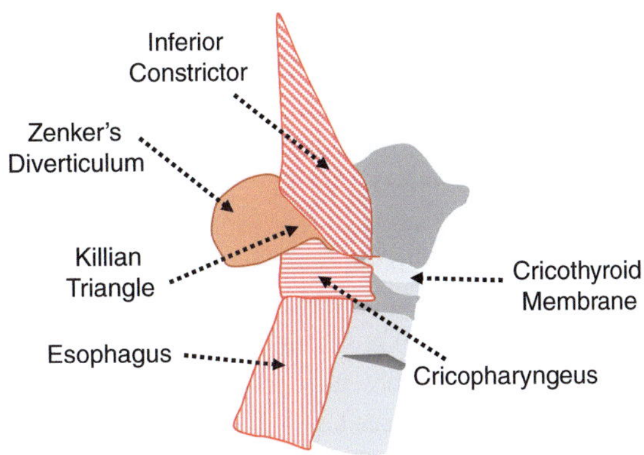

Fig. 2.22 Zenker's diverticulum. The mucosa and submucosa has herniated out of Killian's triangle between the inferior constrictor and the cricopharyngeus [5, 6]

become trapped in this outpocketing which will lead to bad breath and difficulty swallowing (Fig. 2.22).

At the junction with the stomach, the *phreno-esophageal ligament* runs from the esophagus to the diaphragm and is involved in coordinated movements that allow a bolus to move from esophagus into the stomach.

Thoracic Duct

The thoracic duct arises from the cisterna chyli at the level of T12 and passes through the diaphragm with the aorta at the aortic hiatus. Also passing though the aortic hiatus is the azygous vein. At this point, the thoracic duct is between the azygous vein and the aorta. It now enters the posterior mediastinum just to the right of the vertebrae and lateral to the esophagus. It continues its ascent lateral to the vertebrae and then starts to cross from the right to the left side at approximately the T7 level. It crosses posterior to the esophagus and aorta. It completes crossing the midline by T5 and then ascends on the left side towards the corner of the neck. As it approaches the neck it runs posterior to the aortic arch and the carotid sheath. It then arches over the subclavian artery to descend anteriorly to drain into the venous network where the left internal jugular and left subclavian veins come together (Pirogoff's angle). In the neck it lies close to the phrenic nerve, the thyrocervical trunk, and the sympathetic trunk.

If the thoracic duct is occluded in the upper thoracic regions, the duct can be surgically anastomosed with the azygous vein so that the lymphatic system can drain into the venous system.

Virchow's Node

Nestled in at the termination of the thoracic duct into the venous network is a large lymph node—the supraclavicular node or *Virchow's node*—that drains several areas. A malignant tumor in an abdominal organ is often asymptomatic, however one of the first signs that may be present is a swollen Virchow's node—referred to as Troisier's sign. This swollen node could be a sign of a primary tumor in the kidney, ovary, testes, breasts, a GI organ, or Hodgkin's lymphoma. Because of its proximity to the phrenic nerve, a swollen node can compress the nerve leading to dyspnea. In an understated comment, Shetty noted: "The clinician's interest is aroused when on a routine examination, he palpates a Virchow node."

A *Sister Mary Joseph Node* (or nodule) is a swollen node in the umbilicus that was first noticed by Sister Mary Joseph Dempsey (1856–1939), a nun and the surgical assistant to Dr. William Mayo in the early days of the Mayo Clinic. Dr. Mayo authored a paper about the finding and credited her with the finding. It is associated with advanced malignancies in the pelvis and indicates a poor outcome.

Ribs and Sternum

There are three parts to the sternum:

1. the *manubrium* is the widest part of the sternum and has a facet for articulation with the first rib laterally. The manubrium is slanted posteriorly and is located behind the clavicle which makes it impossible to palpate the first rib.

The clavicle articulates with the superior portion of the manubrium at the *sternoclavicular joint*. This joint connects the upper limb to the sternum and supports the shoulder. Within the joint cavity is a thick fibrous articular disc dividing the joint into two spaces. The anterior and posterior sternoclavicular ligaments strengthen the joint anterior and inferiorly. The *interclavicular ligament* runs superiorly across the sternal notch and connects the two clavicles. Moving laterally across the first rib the *costoclavicular ligament* (rhomboid ligament) runs from the costal cartilage of the first rib to the clavicle. Injuries to the joint are rare, but it can be injured in car accidents or sporting injuries. The posterior ligaments are much stronger than the anterior ligaments thus dislocations usually result in the clavicle being displaced anteriorly.

The right and left brachiocephalic veins pass posterior to the sternoclavicular joint and then form the superior vena cava also posterior to the manubrium.

2. The manubrium meets the *body of the sternum* at the *manubriosternal joint* forming the *sternal angle* which is easily palpated. The second rib forms a synovial joint via demifacets with the manubrium and sternum also at the sternal angle. The superior most portion of the manubrium is the sternal notch (jugular notch). Using the sternal angle and the second rib as a landmark, the examiner can then move their hands inferiorly to palpate and count ribs 3–7 which attach to the body of the sternum.
3. The inferior portion of the sternum articulates with the *xiphoid process*.

Rib 1 articulates with the manubrium. Anteriorly, ribs 2–10 end in costal cartilages which in turn articulate with the sternum. Ribs 1–7 are referred to as true ribs because their costal cartilage attaches directly to the sternum. Ribs 8–10 do not attach directly to the sternum and are referred to as false ribs. The costal cartilage of ribs 8–10 attach to the cartilage of the rib above. And ribs 11 and 12 are floating ribs as they do not attach to the sternum but instead end within the musculature of the posterior abdominal wall. *Costochondritis* is inflammation of the cartilage between the ribs and the sternum.

The Pleura

The lungs are surrounded by the pleura. The *visceral pleura* is adherent to the lungs and is reflected onto the surrounding structures as the *parietal pleura*. Between the visceral and parietal layers is the *pleural space*. As the parietal pleura passes over various regions it is given a name appropriate to that region. The pleura along the thoracic wall is termed the *costal pleura*, which in turn is divided into anterior, posterior, and lateral divisions. Above the first rib, the *superior costal pleura* meets with the *cupula* of the pleura. At the diaphragm, the costal pleura meets with the *diaphragmatic pleura*. And medially, the costal pleura meets with the *mediastinal pleura*. At the root of the lung, the pleura extends inferiorly as the *pulmonary ligament*. On the left side, the pleura is reflected laterally at the fourth costal cartilage and then continues inferiorly and lateral to the sternum past ribs 5 and 6. At the seventh rib, the pleura comes back medially. This diversion creates the *cardiac notch* which leaves a space just lateral to the sternum on the left where a needle can be inserted without going through the pleural space. Where the costal pleura meets the mediastinal and diaphragmatic pleura there are sharp lines of reflection. These lines are important landmarks and can be mapped onto the thoracic wall.

In the midclavicular line, the pleural reflection is at the 8th rib; at the mid-axillary line, at the 10th rib; and at the paravertebral line, at the 12th rib. At each of these locations, the lungs (during normal respiration) are located two levels higher.

Table 2.1 Pleura reflections and lung borders along the body wall

	Mid-clavicular line	Mid-axillary line	Paravertebral line
Lungs	Rib 6	Rib 8	Rib 10
Pleura	Rib 8	Rib 10	Rib 12

In other words, lungs are at ribs 6, 8, and 10, while the pleura is at ribs 8, 10, and 12 (Table 2.1).

In the mid-axillary line this space between ribs 8 and 10 is the *costodiaphragmatic space*. Effusions can be collected here. A pleural tap or *thoracocentesis* can be performed here with the needle passing just superior to a rib (which is on the inferior border of the intercostal space) to avoid the neurovascular bundle within the costal groove on the inferior surface of the rib. Where the costal parietal pleura meets the mediastinal parietal pleura the line of reflection creates the *sternocostal recess*. There are no spaces superiorly.

The Trachea

The trachea is about a four-inch-long tube descending from the larynx to the lungs. As air moves down the larynx and passes through the glottis it enters the trachea. The trachea is composed of approximately 20 cartilaginous C-shaped rings. The rings are open posteriorly so that the front of the trachea is round and rigid, while the back is flat and flexible (Fig. 2.23). Running between the ends of the rings, and completing the circular loop, is the trachealis muscle. Because the cartilage is not found posteriorly, this gives a bolus of food moving down the esophagus the ability to momentarily expand anteriorly into the trachea on its way to the stomach. On both sides of the trachea—between the esophagus and trachea—are the recurrent laryngeal nerves.

At approximately the T4–T5 vertebral body level (it can vary on size of individual) the trachea bifurcates into the two main stem bronchi. Foreign objects that travel down the trachea will enter the right main stem bronchus where they

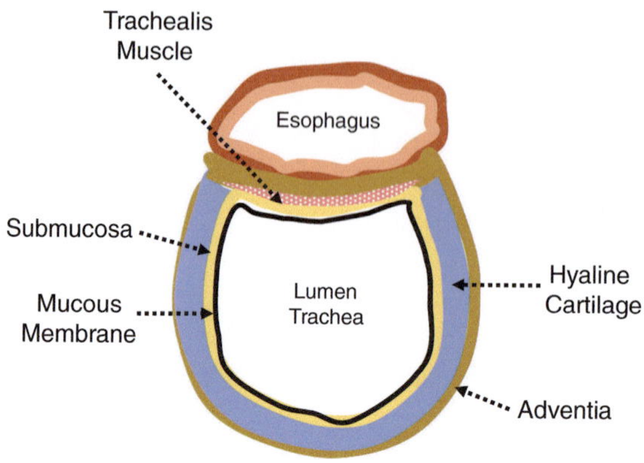

Fig. 2.23 Trachea and esophagus. The C-shaped cartilaginous rings are closed posteriorly by the trachealis muscle. This allows for expansion of the esophagus into the trachea when a bolus of food is moving to the stomach. The C-shaped rings keep the respiratory tract open. In the submucosa are the seromucous glands. Note that in front of the esophagus is the trachea. However, the trachea bifurcates at T4/T5, so below T%, with no more trachea, the heart (left atrium) is now in front of the esophagus [5, 6]

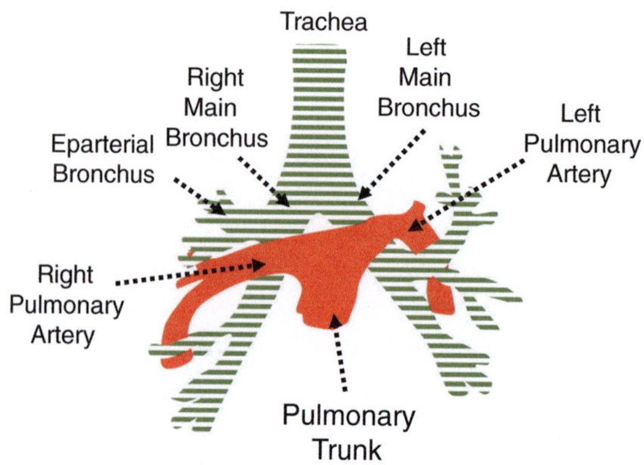

Fig. 2.24 Trachea, bronchi, and pulmonary artery. The right main bronchus is shorter, wider, and straighter (more vertical). Bronchi can be categorized into eparterial or hyparterial—whether above or below the pulmonary artery. The right upper bronchus is the eparterial bronchus. Coming off the right and left main bronchi are the secondary (lobar) bronchi, which in turn each give rise to tertiary bronchi [5, 6]

become lodged, due to the right main bronchus being wider, shorter, and more vertical.

Just above the aortic arch, the brachiocephalic trunk and left common carotid arteries are anterior to the trachea. The azygos vein can be seen arching over the right main bronchus. The right main bronchus divides into three lobar bronchi: superior, middle, and inferior. The superior lobar bronchi is sometimes referred to as the eparterial bronchus because it arches over the right pulmonary artery. The left main bronchus divides into two lobar bronchi: superior and inferior (Figs. 2.24 and 2.25).

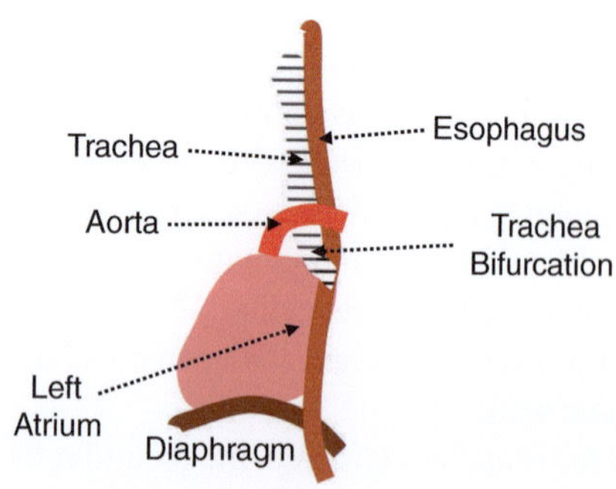

Fig. 2.25 Anterior relations of esophagus. Above T5–T6, anterior to the esophagus is the trachea. Since the trachea divides at T5–T6, anterior to the esophagus, below this level is the left atrium of the heart [5, 6]

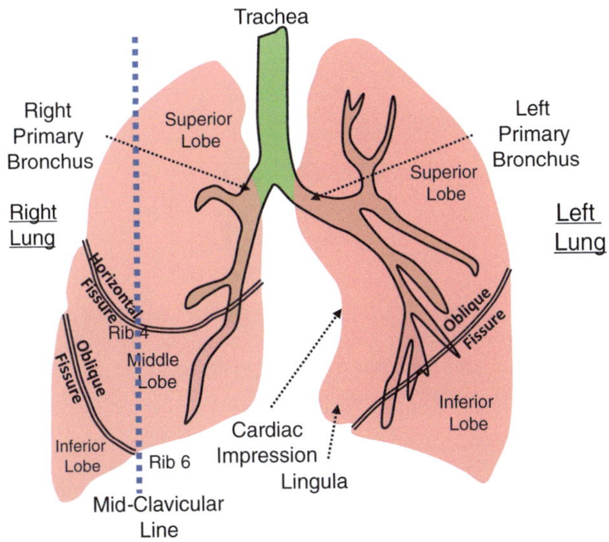

Fig. 2.26 Lungs. There are three lobes in the right lung and two on the left lung. The horizontal fissure runs parallel to the fourth rib. The oblique fissures intersect the inferior borders of the lung at the sixth rib. Thus, a stab wound in the right midclavicular line between ribs four and six would be in the middle lobe. The cardiac impression is formed by the impression of the heart. The lingula is part of the superior lobe of the left lung [5, 6]

The Lungs

The lungs assume the shape of the thorax. On the superior surface they resemble a cone and rise above the first rib and middle of the clavicle to the T1 vertebral body. Structures passing next to the lungs leave impressions on the lung tissue (Fig. 2.26).

1. On the right lung, the trachea and esophagus leave two distinct impressions on the medial surface. There is a prominent impression of the azygos vein which can be seen arching over the root of the lung. Anterior to the groove for the trachea is the impression made by the right brachiocephalic vein, which turns into the impression of the superior vena cava.
2. On the left lung, the trachea and esophagus together form one impression rather than two distinct impressions that one sees on the right. Anterior to this impression are the impressions of the subclavian artery and brachiocephalic vein. Just inferior to the root of the lung is a distinct impression of the esophagus—remember by this point the trachea has divided and disappeared into the lungs.

The right lung has three lobes, and the left lung has two lobes. On the right the *horizontal fissure* parallels rib 4 and separates the superior and middle lobes. The *oblique fissure* is found on both lobes and intersects the mid-clavicular line at rib 6. On the right, the oblique fissure separates the middle lobe from the inferior lobe. On the left side the oblique fissure separates the superior from inferior lobe. The lingual of the left lung is equivalent to the middle lobe of the right lung.

A stab wound on the right, in the mid-clavicular line, above rib 4, would go through the superior lobe. If the stab wound was between ribs 4 and 6 in the mid-clavicular line, then it would go through the middle lobe. Keep in mind that most of the inferior lobe lies posterior, so when listening for sounds from the inferior lobe one would typically place the stethoscope on the posterior surface. Likewise, the superior lobe faces anterior.

The bronchial arteries which are branches of the thoracic aorta supply the lungs.

The lymphatic drainage of the deep regions of the lung drains to the *bronchopulmonary nodes*, then into the *tracheobronchial nodes*, then into the *broncomediastinal nodes*. All the right lung

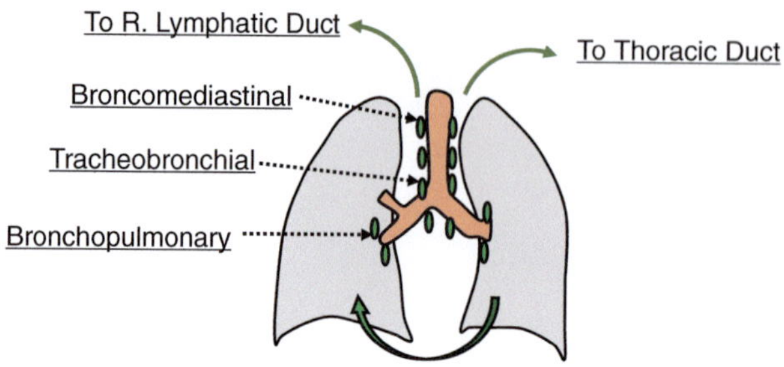

Fig. 2.27 Lymphatic drainage of the lung. The deep areas of the lung drain into the bronchopulmonary nodes, then into the tracheobronchial nodes, and then into the broncomediastinal nodes. On the right side the drainage is into the right lymphatic duct, and on the left into the thoracic duct. The lower left lung can drain across the midline to the right side [5, 6]

then drains into the *right lymphatic duct*. On the left, the superior and middle portions of the lung drain into the *thoracic duct*. However, the inferior portion of the left lung drains to the right and left side. Some portion of the left lower lung can cross over to the right side and then drain into the right lymphatic duct.

The superficial surface of the lung—corresponding to the visceral pleura drain to the hilar nodes which in turn drain into the tracheobronchial nodes (Fig. 2.27).

Pneumothorax

*Pneumothoraxe*s or collapsed lungs can be broken down into several distinct categories. For example, a stab wound or other penetrating injury of the chest wall that opens the pleura cavity is referred to as an *open pneumothorax* because it allows air from outside the wall to move into and out of the pleural cavity through the opening. However, injuries to the lung wall itself, such as a car accident, where the lung is thrown forward and tears the pleura leads to a *closed pneumothorax*. With a closed scenario, the abdominal wall itself is not damaged. The air then moves from the lung into the pleural cavity. A *spontaneous pneumothorax* is a type of closed pneumothorax that does not involve trauma. Instead, a bleb of lung tissue bursts, allowing air to move from the lungs into the pleural space (Figs. 2.28 and 2.29).

A *tension pneumothorax* is an emergency. Take a penetrating injury to the thoracic wall that creates a skin flap acing as a one-way valve. Air can enter the pleural cavity through the opening on inspiration, but it cannot exit through the flap on expiration. The pressure then builds up in the pleural space and pushes the heart towards the opposite side. Tracheal deviation to the opposite side will also be present. The heart will not move back and forth with each breath but will instead remain on the opposite side. Again, this is an emergency as the patient can have cyanosis, tachycardia, jugular venous distension, and hypotension. An x-ray at the end of inspiration can show the mediastinal shift. A line showing the edge of the pleural space will often be present. At first the air will concentrate on the superior lateral side of the thorax (Fig. 2.28).

Azygos Vein

The azygos vein is a bypass around the heart. If you think about the inferior vena cava in the abdominal region providing a conduit for structures along the posterior abdominal wall to drain, and the superior vena cava sitting above the heart to drain structures in the head, this leaves a gap behind the heart in the thoracic region. In other words, the presence of the heart takes the place of the inferior vena cava in the thoracic region, so something needs to take the place of the IVC. The azygos vein is a bypass around the heart, running from the IVC to the SVC. The azygos vein is found on the right side. On the left side, one can see a hemiazygos and accessory azygos vein.

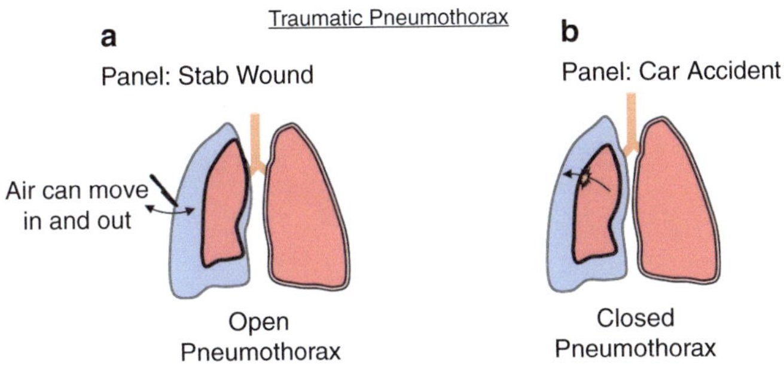

Fig. 2.28 Traumatic Pneumothorax. Panel (**a**) shows an open pneumothorax (chest wall is open) from a stab wound. Air enters the pleural space from outside the body. Panel (**b**) shows a closed pneumothorax (chest wall is not compromised) resulting from a car injury which resulted in the lung tissue rupturing and air moving from the lungs into the pleural space. In both cases the lung has collapsed. Not shown is a spontaneous closed pneumothorax which can result from a piece of lung tissue rupturing. A tension pneumothorax occurs when the air in the pleural cavity cannot escape and the pressure pushes the heart to the opposite side [5, 6]

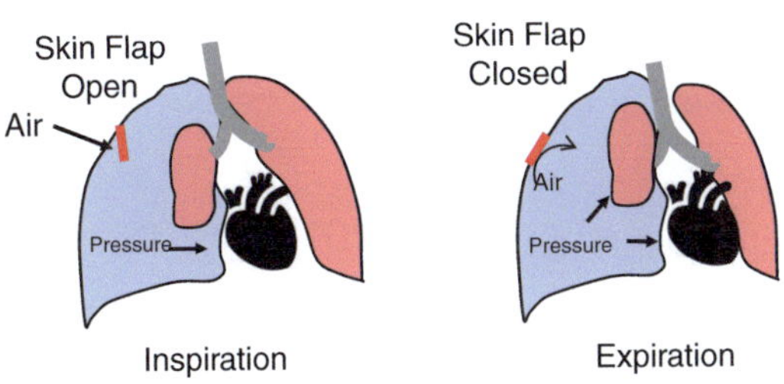

Fig. 2.29 Tension pneumothorax. There is a penetrating injury that allows air to move through the flap and into the lung. On expiration the flap is closed, and air cannot escape the pleura cavity. Pressure in the cavity increases and with each successive breath the lung moves further towards the opposite side and compresses the heart [5, 6]

This system allows the posterior body wall to drain into the venous system. The diagram below shows the specific pattern of drainage for the body wall; however, it is not necessary for a first-year medical student or allied health student to memorize the exact pattern of drainage pattern—there are more things to focus on with more clinical relevance than the pattern of drainage in this region (Fig. 2.30).

Stellate Ganglion

There are three cervical ganglia: the superior, middle, and inferior ganglion. Technically, when the inferior cervical ganglion fuses with the T1 ganglia, which is the case in most of us, this is referred to as the stellate ganglion, or cervicothoracic ganglia. When most people use the term "stellate ganglion" they are referring to the inferior ganglia. It typically sits just anterior to the C7 transverse process. In the anatomy lab, the best way to find it is, once the lungs are removed, start with the first part of the subclavian artery where it is medial to the anterior scalene. At this point you can find the costocervical trunk coming off the inferior portion of the subclavian artery, and the first branch of the costocervical trunk is the superior intercostal artery. The stellate ganglion is a star-shaped structure just near the superior intercostal artery. During a dissection, if the lung is present, the cupula will be pushing up against the stellate ganglion. To adequately see the stellate ganglion, it is necessary to remove the lung. The ansa subclavia is a small threadlike connection of nerve tissue that runs from the middle to the inferior cervical ganglion anterior to the subclavian artery (Figs. 2.31 and 2.32).

A stellate nerve block is sometimes used for the relief of pain or to ease the symptoms of Raynaud's disease (hyperhidrosis). A landmark often used for this nerve block is the transverse process of C6 (Chassaignac's Tubercle). The C7 transverse process is a bit too close to the dome of the pleura. If the nerve block hits the sympathetic fibers to the head and face, then the patient will develop Horner's syndrome such as a constricted pupil, loss of sweating, and drooping of the eyelid. Likewise, if the temperature in the

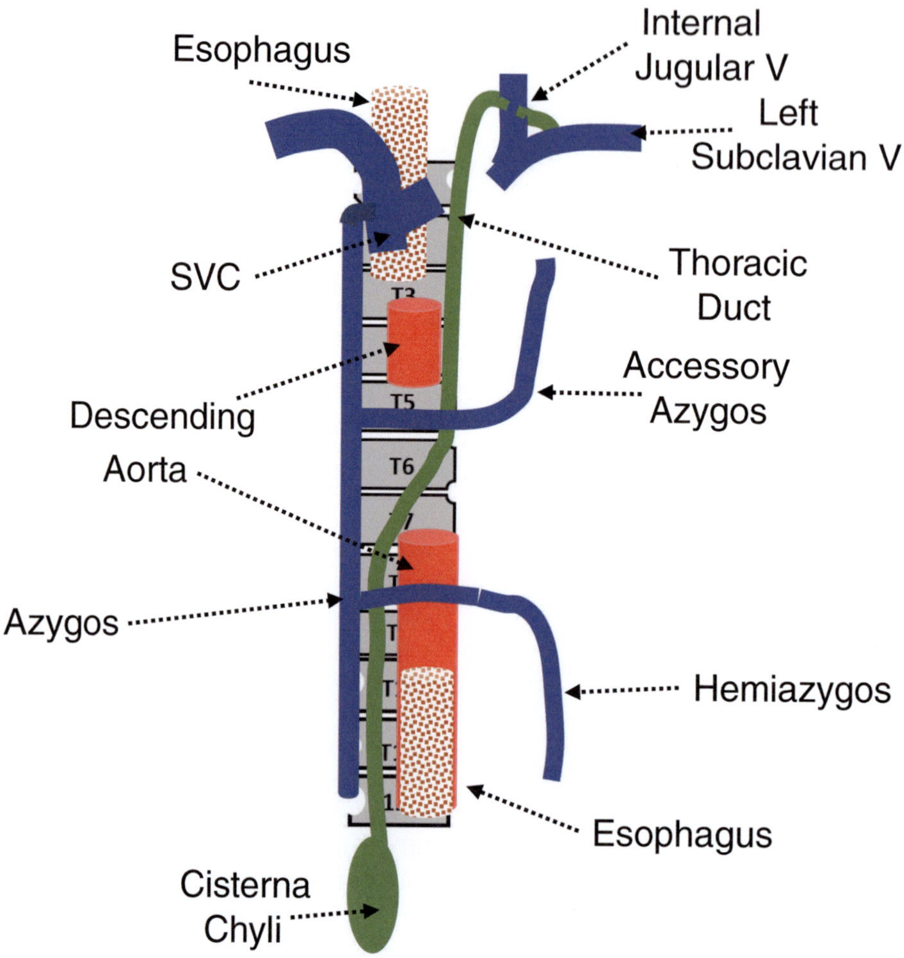

Fig. 2.30 Thoracic duct. The thoracic duct emerges from the cisterna chyli and travels through the aortic aperture of the diaphragm with the aorta and the azygous vein. It travels up on the right side of the vertebral bodies between the azygos and esophagus. At around T7 it starts to cross the midline, completing its cross by T5. It then ascends behind the aortic arch and the subclavian artery. It then does a loop to come around and meet the venous system at the junction of the left internal jugular vein and left subclavian veins [5, 6]

upper limb drops, then the block has successfully blocked the sympathetic supply to the upper limb.

Pericardiocentesis

If fluid builds up around the heart (cardiac tamponade), pericardiocentesis, a needle aspiration, can be used to remove the fluid. The needle is typically inserted at the left infrasternal angle and is directed towards the left shoulder—specifically the left mid-clavicular line. There is a significant risk with this blind approach. As imaging modalities have become more advanced, it is common to utilize several types of imaging to assist with the procedure.

Beck's Triad

Cardiac tamponade can result in three characteristic findings which all relate to anatomy. This increased pressure will reduce the heart's ability to

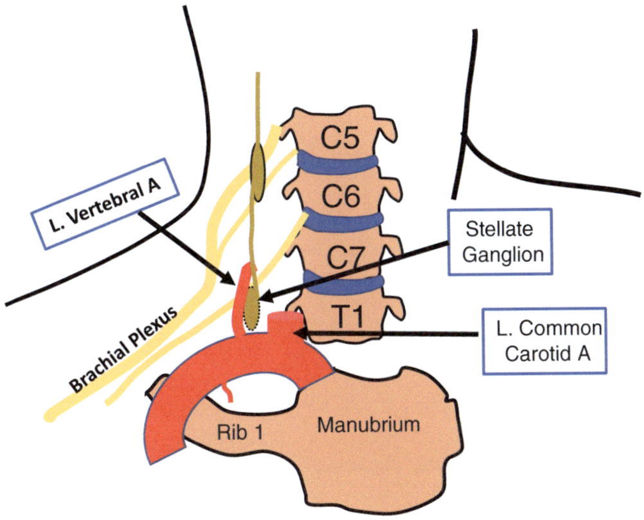

Fig. 2.31 Stellate ganglion. The stellate ganglion sits lateral to the common carotid artery and the transverse process of C7. It is also just posteromedial to the vertebral artery [5, 6]

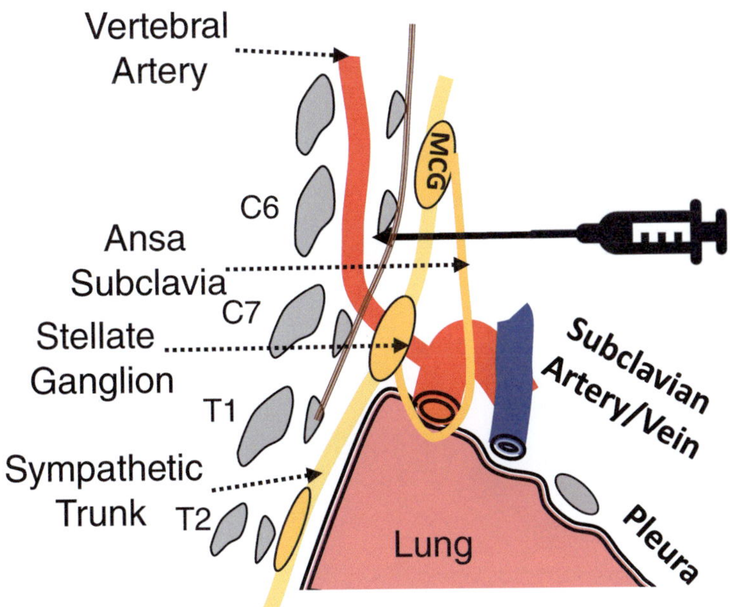

Fig. 2.32 Stellate ganglion. The stellate ganglion sits just superior to the apex of the lung across from the C7 transverse process. Ansa subclavia loops around the subclavian artery and connects the middle and inferior cervical ganglia. Needle approaches will often aim for C6 to avoid the lung [5, 6]

pump blood—the mean arterial pressure (MAP) will decrease. In turn, blood entering the heart will back up leading to increased pressure in the neck veins, and a bulging external jugular vein. This will also result in distant or muffled heart sounds. A straightforward way to think of Beck's Triad is the three D's: (1) Distant heart sounds, (2) Distended veins, and (3) Decreased MAP (Fig. 2.33).

Cross Sections Through Neck and Thorax

The following cross sections start at the T3 vertebral body and descend through the neck and into the mediastinum. Note that at the level of T3 one can see the left brachiocephalic vein crossing anterior to the three branches coming off the

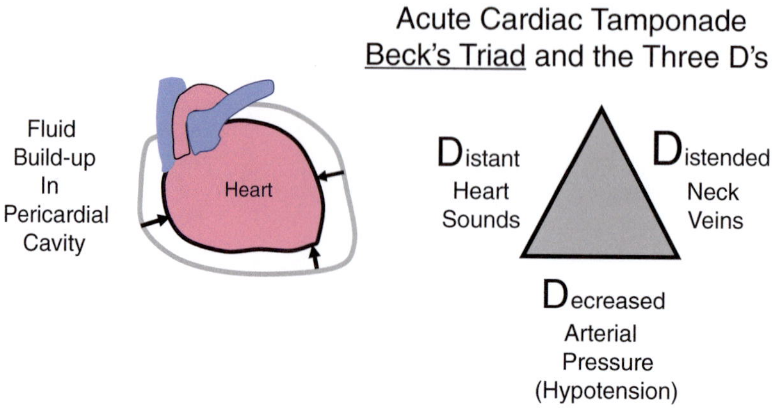

Fig. 2.33 Becks triad and the three D's. Fluid build up in the pericardial cavity will exert pressure on the heart reducing the heart's ability to pump blood out to the periphery. In addition, blood will back up on the venous side, leading to dilated veins in the neck [5, 6]

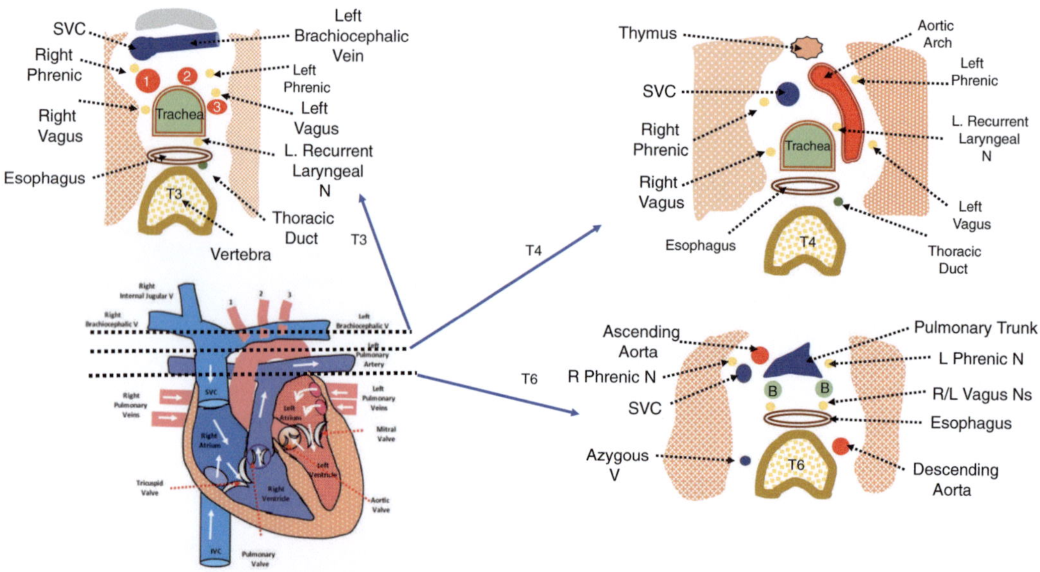

Fig. 2.34 Cross sections through mediastinum. There are three cuts through the mediastinum. Note that at T3, one can see the three branches of the aortic arch: (1) brachiocephalic trunk, (2) left common carotid, and (3) left subclavian. At T2, one can see the arch, and at T5, one can see the ascending and descending aorta. The trachea is present at T3 and T4. By T6 it has bifurcated into the two bronchi (B) [5, 6]

aorta. The phrenic nerves are more anterior compared to the vagus nerves. The esophagus is posterior to the trachea. Moving down to T4 one can now see the aortic arch. And on the right side is the SVC descending towards the right atrium. The thoracic duct is posterior to the esophagus. Moving down to T6, the trachea has now bifurcated into the right and left main bronchi. At this point we are below the aortic arch, and we see the ascending and descending aorta. In front of the bronchi is the pulmonary trunk about to give off the right and left pulmonary arteries (Figs. 2.34 and 2.35).

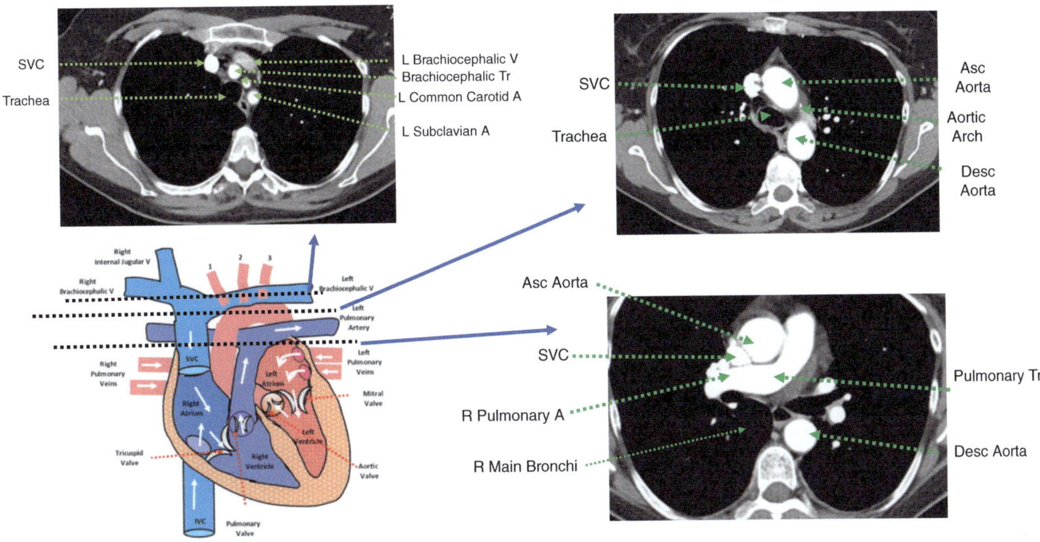

Fig. 2.35 Cross sections through mediastinum. Same as previous figure but now with MRI images [5, 6]

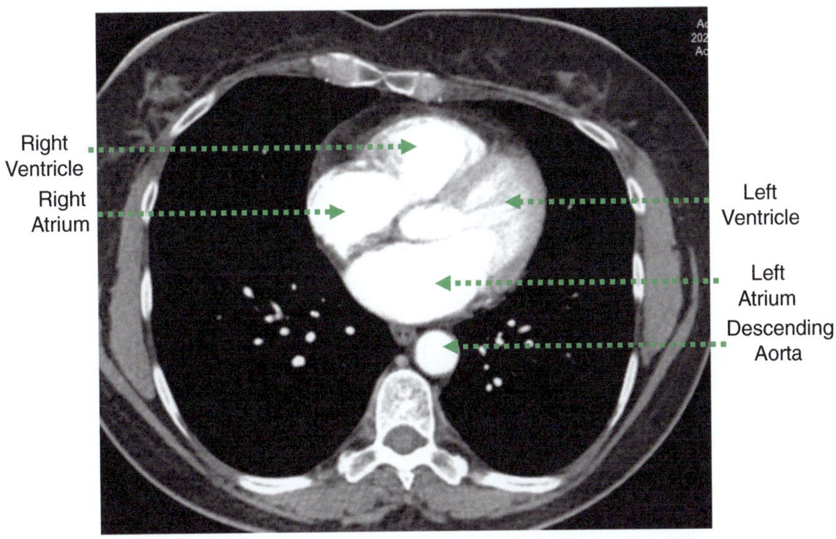

Fig. 2.36 Cross section MRI of heart. On the right side you can see the right atrium which is the right border of the heart. The base of the heart is facing posterior and is the left atrium. The anterior surface of the heart is the right ventricle. Note that the left ventricle makes an appearance on the left anterior side [5, 6]

Cross Section of Heart and Its Borders

When one looks at a cross section through the heart, you need to know the borders of the heart to make sense of the image. In the section below, on the right side we can see the right atrium. The base of the heart, which is posterior, is the left atrium. Most of the anterior surface is the right ventricle. While the left border is the left ventricle (Fig. 2.36).

Chest Tube Placement

Chest tubes are most often placed in the fifth intercostal space in the mid axillary line. To avoid the neurovascular bundle in the costal groove, the line is placed on the superior border of the fifth rib (Fig. 2.37).

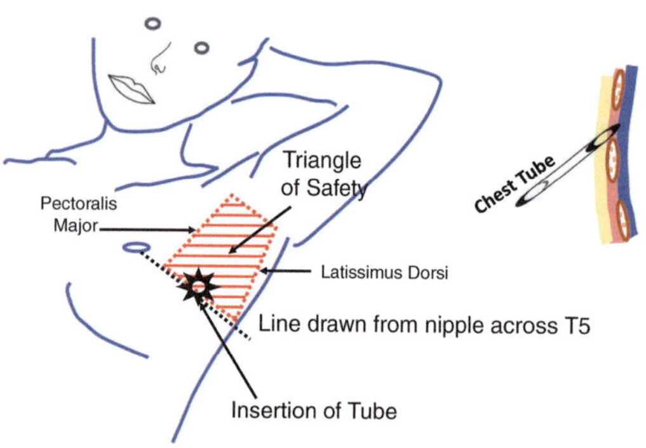

Fig. 2.37 Triangle of safety and intercostal chest drain. The triangle is bounded by the lateral border of pectoralis major and latissimus dorsi muscles. The apex is the axilla. The base is a line drawn laterally from the nipple [5, 6]

Historical Snippet: Gray's Anatomy

When medical professionals hear the word "Gray's" everyone knows the reference. In 1848, Henry Gray, a senior, and Henry Carter, a first-year student, overlapped as students at St. Georges Medical School in England. Back then, students started medical school when they were 18. The two Henries became friends during medical school and eventually collaborated on a paper about the spleen. Gray wrote the manuscript, and Carter, the artist, created 23 paintings. The paper went on to win the Astley Cooper Prize in Anatomy that year. After their early success, one project led to another, and another, until they finally agreed on writing a "Manual of Anatomy" for medical students (Fig. 2.38).

Their 1858 masterpiece was titled: *Anatomy: Descriptive and Surgical*, and included 363 figures. Henry Gray was only 31 years old. The medical world in the mid 1800s was quite different compared to now. As an example, here is a description from the first edition of Gray's Anatomy describing the surgical procedure on a

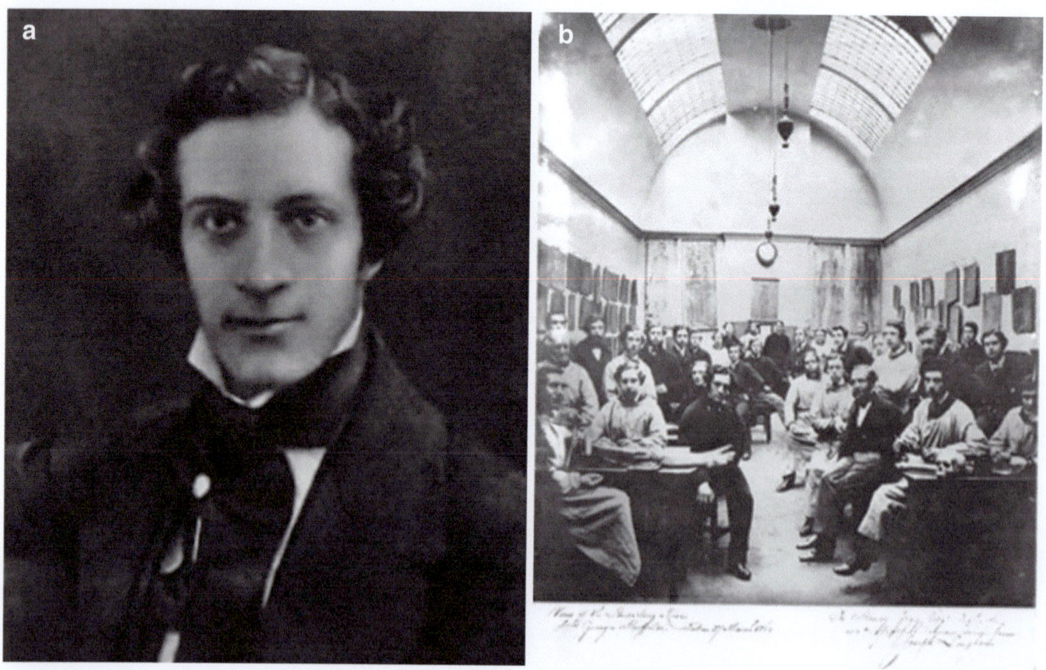

Fig. 2.38 Henry Gray, British Anatomist (1827–1861). Panel (**a**) is a portrait of Henry Gray. In panel (**b**) Gray is with his students in the anatomy lab. Gray is at the feet of the cadaver on the left

patient, not a cadaver, for tying a ligature on the first part of the axillary artery. It is a long-detailed description in the book but, in short, after Gray's directions for the skin incision along the clavicle, he states: "After tearing through the deep fascia with the fingernail, the internal jugular vein will be seen crossing the artery; this should be pressed aside, and the artery avoided." While a surgical procedure during Gray's career would have involved the use of chloroform as anesthesia, surgeons did not start using gloves until 1889, thus the use of the fingernails to clean away the deep fascia.

Henry Gray was 34 when he died in 1861 from smallpox which he contracted from a patient—his nephew. Gray had been working on a new book plus a new edition of the anatomy book. None of his papers survived, most likely because, following the death of a smallpox patient, anything that they had touched was immediately burned, including the sheets, towels books, papers, etc. Henry Carter, meanwhile, lived until he was 65. Some authors have pointed out that Henry Carter's pictures had just as much to do with their anatomy book's success as Gray's writing, and that Carter should have been given more credit than he has for the book's enormous influence on medicine.

Further Reading

1. Al-Saady NM, Camm AJ. Left atrial appendage: structure, function, and role in thromboembolism. Heart. 1999;82:547–55.
2. Galvan VG. Sister Mary Joseph's nodule. Ann Inter Med. 1998;128:410.
3. Hanifin C. Cardiac auscultation 101: a basic science approach to heart murmurs. JAAPA. 2010;23(4):44–8.
4. Hanna IR, Silverman ME. A history of auscultation and some of its contributors. Am J Cardiol. 2002;90:259–67.
5. Leo J. Medical neuroanatomy for the boards and clinic: finding the lesion. 2nd ed. Cham: Springer; 2024.
6. Leo J. Clinical anatomy and embryology: a guide for the classroom, clinic, and clinic. 2nd ed. Cham: Springer; 2024.
7. McKay T, Thomas L. Coumadin ridge in the left atrium demonstrated on three-dimensional transthoracic echocardiography. Euro J Echocardiogr. 2006;9:298–300.
8. Moore K, Dalley AF, Agur A. Clinically oriented anatomy. 7th ed. Baltimore: Lippincott Williams and Wilkin; 2014.
9. Peigh G, Majdani J. A novel approach to teaching cardiac auscultation. MedEdPublish. 2017; https://doi.org/10.15694/mep.2017.000095.
10. Tran J, Haussner W, Shah KS. Traumatic pneumothorax: a review of current diagnostic practices and evolving management. Clin Rev. 2021;61(5):517–28.
11. Tubbs RS, Shah NA, Sullivan BP, Marchase ND, Cömert A, Acar HI, Tekdemir I, Loukas M, Shoja MM. The costoclavicular ligament revisited: a functional and anatomical study. Rom J Morphol Embryol. 2009;50(3):475–9.

3 The Abdominal Cavity

Anterior Abdominal Wall

The anterior abdominal wall has two competing jobs. One is to keep the gastrointestinal tract and related organs inside the abdomen, and the second is to remain pliable enough to allow for the various trunk movements. When pressure in the abdominal cavity goes up, abdominal contents will look for a way out of the abdominal cavity at weak points in the wall.

Just deep to the skin, the fascia is divided into two layers. *Camper's fascia* is the fatty layer of fascia and *Scarpa's* is the deeper tough membranous layer (Fig. 1.1). Camper's fascia does not continue into the perineum. Scarpa's is continuous with Colle's fascia in the perineum, and with the *fascia lata* of the thigh (Fig. 3.1).

Most of the anterior wall is made up of four muscles. There are three layers of circular muscles running from posterior to anterior; plus, a long bilateral strap muscle running longitudinally in the midline. The three circumferential muscles are:

1. The *external abdominal oblique* runs from the external surface of ribs 5–12 and circles around the abdominal wall anteriorly to insert into the linea alba, pubic tubercle, and iliac crest. The orientation of the fibers can be mimicked by putting your hands in your pockets. The testes and spermatic cord pierce the external abdominal oblique at the *superficial inguinal ring*, which is superior to the inguinal ligament. The *inguinal ligament* is the curled-under edge of the external abdominal oblique. The *lacunar ligament* is a small, thickened piece that forms the medial wall of the femoral ring.
2. Deep to the external oblique is the *internal abdominal oblique* whose fibers run from the iliac crest, thoracolumbar fascia and ASIS to the linea alba. At the most anteromedial corner of the muscle, the fibers run posterior to the spermatic cord to contribute to the conjoint tendon which inserts into the *pecten pubis*.

1) Skin
2) Camper's Fascia
3) Scarpa's Fascia
4) External Abdominal Oblique M.
5) Internal Abdominal Oblique M.
6) Transversus Abdominus M.
7) Fascia Transversalis
8) Extraperitoneal fat
9) Parietal Peritoneum

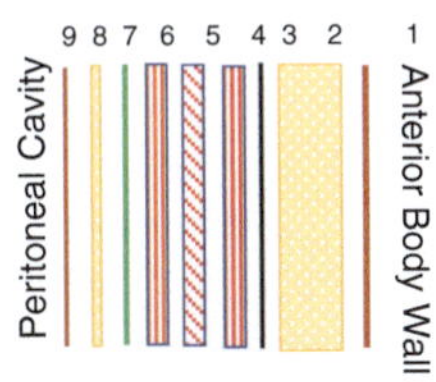

Fig. 3.1 Layers of Anterior Abdominal Wall [10, 11]

J. Leo, *Gross Anatomy, Neuroanatomy, and Embryology for Medical Students*,
https://doi.org/10.1007/978-3-031-87151-1_3

3. Deep to the internal oblique is the *transversus abdominis* running from the internal surfaces of the costal cartilages of ribs 7–12, iliac crest, thoracolumbar fascia, and inguinal ligament to the linea alba and via the conjoint tendon to the pecten pubis.

The *rectus abdominus* is the bilateral midline muscle with fibers running superior to inferior. The fibers are attached superiorly to the xiphoid process and the costal cartilages of ribs 5–7. Inferiorly the fibers are attached to the pubic symphysis and pubic crest. The muscle is interrupted by three to four tendinous intersections running laterally across the muscle. These tendinous intersections divide the muscle up into smaller sections, giving rise to the term in body builders of 4-pack or 6-pack. The lateral edge of the muscle is referred to as the *linea semilunaris*. The linea semilunaris is not a straight line but has a slight curve to it. Between the two halves of the rectus abdominus is the centrally located *linea alba*.

Rectus abdominus diastasis refers to a separation of the two sides of rectus abdominus in the midline located linea alba. This separation can allow an out pocketing of intestinal contents. It typically has an oval shape with the center being around the umbilicus and then narrowing superiorly and inferiorly.

Arcuate Line

The fibers from the three circular abdominal muscles, mentioned above, all have an interesting organization as they approach the linea semilunaris and rectus abdominus. Found behind the rectus abdominus, the *arcuate line* is a horizontal line inferior to the umbilicus and is an important landmark for the organization of these muscles. There are differences above the arcuate line versus below the arcuate line in how the three abdominal muscles circumnavigate their way around the rectus abdominus on their way to the midline (Arcuate means Bow in Latin).

Above the arcuate line the external abdominal oblique muscle passes anterior to the rectus abdominus. The internal abdominal oblique muscle splits to go around the rectus abdominus, and the transversus abdominus muscle runs posterior (behind) the rectus abdominus. Above the arcuate line, these circumferential muscles form a strong tough membrane on both sides of the rectus abdominus, referred to respectively, as either the *anterior layer of the rectus sheath*, or the *posterior layer of the rectus sheath*. Deep (or posterior) to the posterior layer of the rectus sheath is the *transversalis fascia* (Fig. 3.2).

Below the arcuate line there is a subtle difference in the organization of the layers. The fascia of all three muscles—the external oblique,

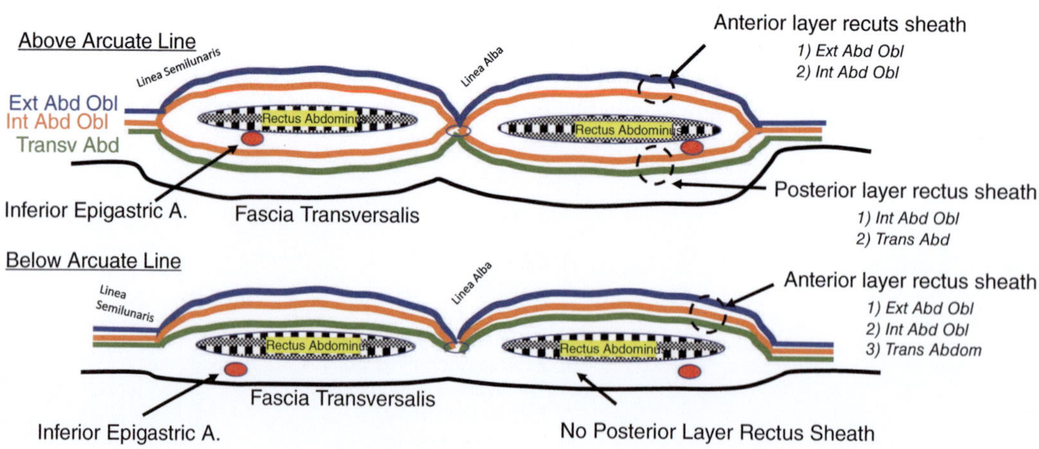

Fig. 3.2 Rectus Sheath. Note the relationship of the three muscles of the anterior abdominal wall and their relationship to the rectus abdominus above versus below the arcuate line. Note the location of inferior epigastric artery above and below the line [10, 11]

internal oblique, and transversus abdominus—all pass in front of rectus abdominus. Below the arcuate line, there is an anterior layer of the rectus sheath, but no corresponding posterior layer of rectus sheath. Below the arcuate line, the layer behind the rectus abdominus, is the fascia transversalis.

Anterior Abdominal Wall Hernias

Because of the potential weak spots in the abdominal wall, abdominal contents can herniate through the wall. *Epigastric* hernias are rare but will be found in the epigastric space. *Umbilical* hernias, also known as paraumbilical hernias, herniate through the umbilicus. *Hypogastric* hernias occur in the midline between the umbilicus and pubic symphysis. *Spigelian* hernias are found lateral to the rectus abdominus at the linea semilunaris, typically below the arcuate line. Spigelian hernias are more like a delamination, where the abdominal contents slip between layers of the abdominal wall, rather than a simple protrusion (Fig. 3.3). In many cases, the spigelian hernia lands between the external and internal abdominal oblique without piercing the external abdominal oblique. In some cases, it does not pierce the internal abdominal oblique. Incisional hernias occur along scars from prior surgeries where two pieces of the abdominal wall were sutured together.

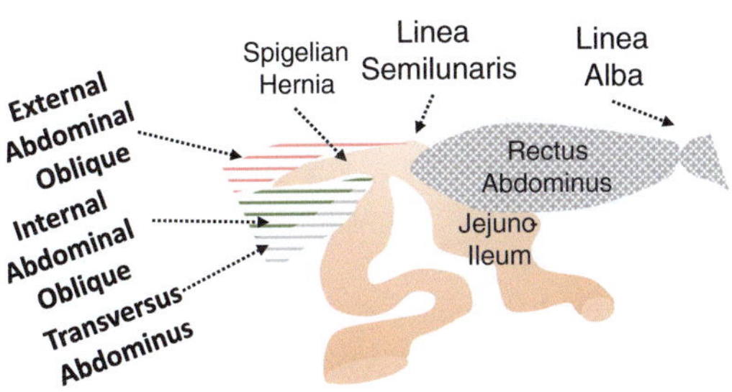

Fig. 3.3 Spigelian Hernia. Note that the abdominal contents are herniating out at the linea semilunaris. The hernia is more like a delamination of the layers where the contents sneak between the external and internal abdominal obliques [10, 11]

Blood Supply to Anterior Abdominal Wall

The blood supply to the anterior abdominal wall comes from descending branches that start in the thoracic, and ascending branches that start down in the pelvic area. Where these descending and ascending branches meet on the abdominal wall are important sites of anastomoses with significant clinical importance. There are two parallel tracts for the vessels, one is superficial to the fascia, and one is deeper.

1. Deep to the fascia, *the superior epigastric artery* comes off the internal thoracic artery near the xiphoid process and descends along the anterior abdominal wall towards the umbilicus. Meanwhile, the *inferior epigastric artery* is a branch of the external iliac artery right before it goes under the inguinal ligament, and it ascends towards the umbilicus. It passes upward along the anterior abdominal wall forming a fold of tissue called the *lateral umbilical ligament*. As the inferior epigastric artery travels up the anterior wall, initially it is found between the rectus abdominus and the fascia transversalis, but more superiorly it is found between the rectus abdominus and the posterior layer of the rectus sheath. The superior and inferior epigastric arteries form an anastomosis on the anterior abdominal wall. This is an anastomosis between branches of the subclavian artery and branches of the external iliac artery.
2. Superficial to the fascia *the thoracoepigastric veins* represent the joining of the lateral thoracic veins with the *superficial epigastric veins*. The thoracoepigastric veins, found on the anterolateral abdominal wall in the midclavicular line, drain into the lateral thoracic vein (which drains into the superior vena cava). Meanwhile the superficial epigastric veins drain into the great saphenous vein which in turn drains into the femoral vein located in the femoral triangle. These two veins meet on the lateral abdominal wall and represent an anastomosis between the superior vena cava and inferior vena cava. Swollen

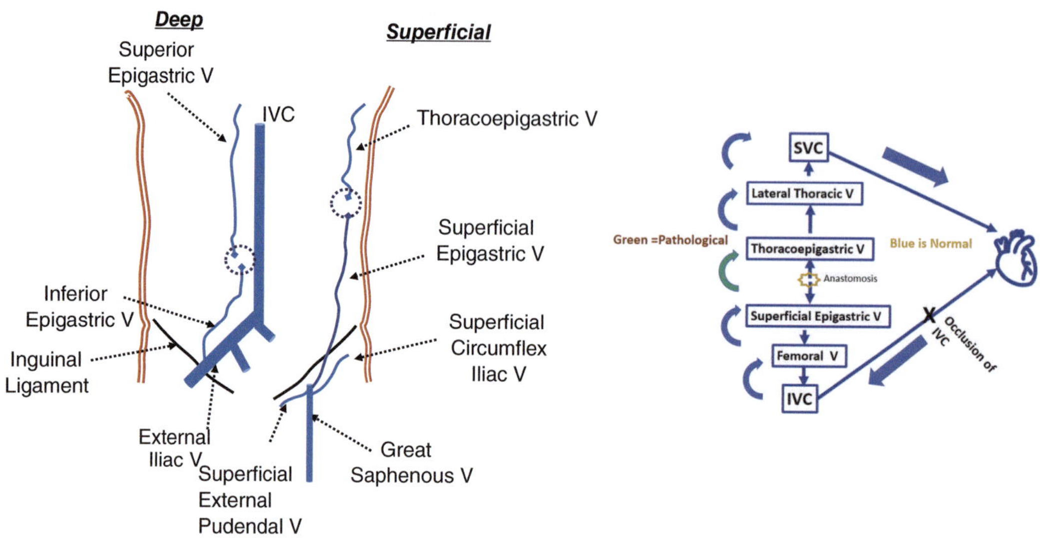

Fig. 3.4 Anterior Abdominal Wall Venous Drainage. Panel (**a**) On the patient's right side. The deep drainage is shown with the anastomosis between the inferior epigastric vein and the superior epigastric vein. On the patient's left side, the superficial drainage is shown between the superficial epigastric vein and the thoracoepigastric vein. Panel (**b**) shows how a blockage of the IVC could lead to dilated vessels of the anterior abdominal wall [10, 11]

veins in the lateral anterior wall could be due to a blockage of the inferior vena cava. Because these veins are superficial, when they become dilated it will be readily apparent on a physical exam (Fig. 3.4).

Paraumbilical Veins with Superficial Epigastric Veins

The *paraumbilical veins* are small veins around the umbilicus which ascend along the anterior wall to drain into the portal vein. The paraumbilical veins anastomose with the *superficial epigastric veins*. This is an anastomosis between portal vein and inferior vena cava. *Portal hypertension* will lead to these veins being dilated.

Inguinal Canal

During fetal development, the testes and ovaries start off in the abdominal region, and then migrate down towards their final adult locations. The ovaries remain in the pelvic cavity, but the testes will push through the anterior abdominal wall to migrate to the scrotum dragging with them all the structures they contact during their migration.

At the fifth month of development, the testes are sitting in the abdominal cavity right above the inguinal ligament behind the *fascia transversalis.* They eventually push through this fascia forming an opening called the *deep inguinal ring* which is just lateral to the inferior epigastric artery. Now that they have pushed through the fascia, they continue their migration anterior to the fascia transversalis (Fig. 3.5).

Moving anterior, the next layer is a muscle, *transversus abdominus* which starts from the AISIS, arches over the deep inguinal ring, runs medially behind the spermatic cord, and attaches to the pubic tubercle (Fig. 3.5).

In front of the transversus abdominus is the *internal abdominal oblique*, which from the ASIS and the lateral one-third of the inguinal ligament, passes anterior to the spermatic cord,

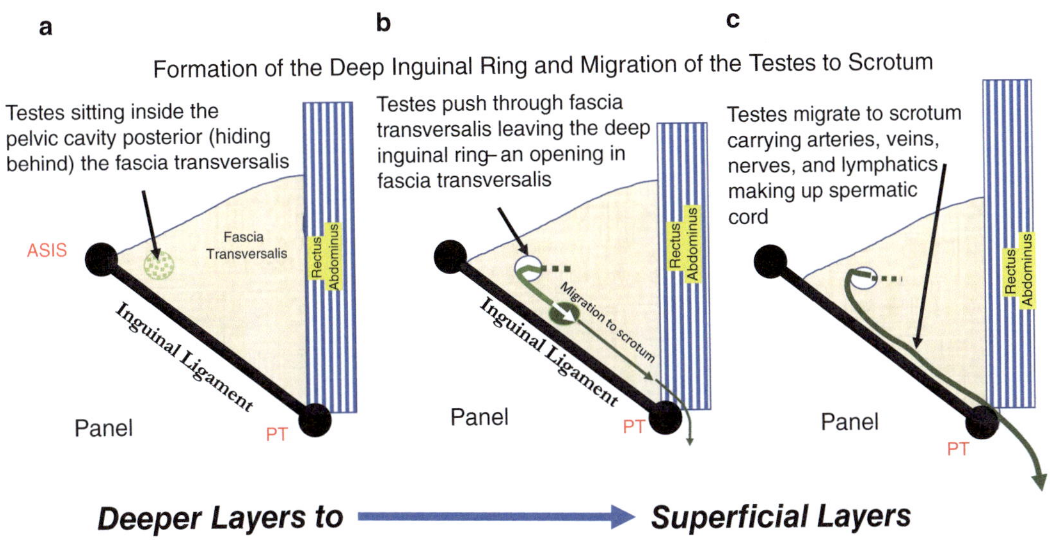

Fig. 3.5 In panel (**a**), at the fifth-month of fetal development, the testes are sitting behind (posterior to) the fascia transversalis. In panel (**b**), the testes have pushed through the fascia transversalis and formed the deep inguinal ring. The testes now descend parallel to the inguinal ligament, and anterior to the fascia transversalis forming the inguinal canal. In panel (**c**), the testes have migrated all the way to the scrotum [10, 11]

and then runs medially behind the spermatic cord, with the transversus abdominus to attach to the pubic tubercle. The combination of the two extensions of transversus abdominus and internal abdominal oblique that meet behind the spermatic cord near the pubic tubercle is referred to as the *conjoint tendon*, or "falx inguinalis."

The next layer is the external abdominal oblique with its fiber orientation of "hands in the pocket." Medial and superior to the pubic tubercle, the spermatic cord pierces the external abdominal oblique at the *superficial inguinal ring* (Figs. 3.6 and 3.7).

As the testes migrate through the anterior wall down towards the scrotum, they form the inguinal canal running from the deep ring (an opening in fascia transversalis) to the superficial ring (an opening in the external abdominal oblique). In the male, the inguinal canal contains the spermatic cord, the ilioinguinal nerve and the genital branch of the genitofemoral nerve. In the female, the inguinal canal contains the round ligament and ilioinguinal nerve. Think of the canal as a hallway with a floor, a ceiling, an anterior wall, and a posterior wall. To visualize this, take a parasagittal cut through the inguinal canal between the superficial and deep rings—the cut is not in the midline but is slightly off the midline through the right inguinal canal.

1. The *floor* is the easiest layer to visualize as it is the inguinal ligament.
2. The *anterior wall* is the internal abdominal oblique, and the external abdominal oblique—the rectus abdominus fibers do not make their way in front of the spermatic cord. They are not part of the anterior wall.
3. Clinically, the *posterior wall* is the most important boundary. Furthermore, it is subdivided into medial and lateral divisions. The *lateral* posterior wall is a weak area consisting of the fascia transversalis, while the *medial* posterior wall is the strong conjoint tendon—composed of internal abdominal oblique and transversus abdominus.
4. The *roof* is composed of all three muscles (Figs. 3.7 and 3.8).

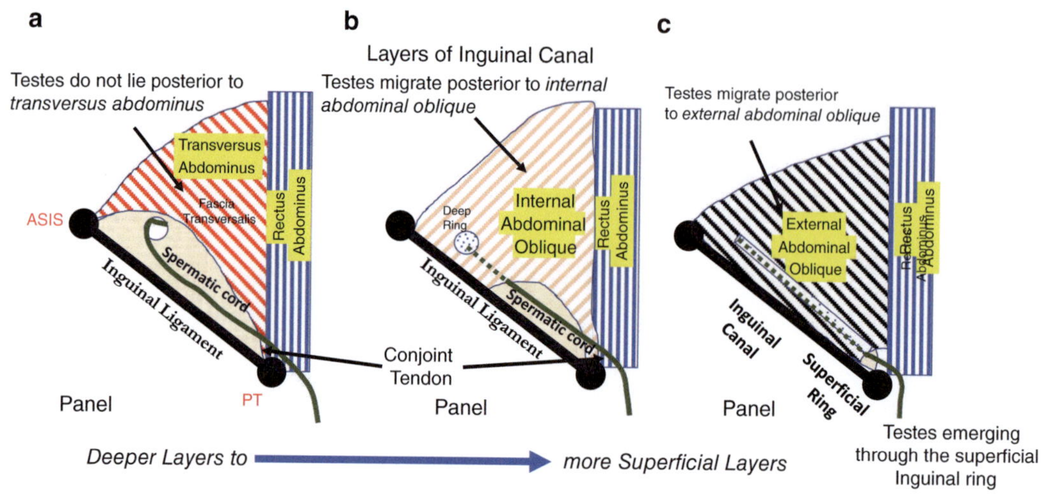

Fig. 3.6 Inguinal Canal. In panel (**a**), the testes have moved through the deep inguinal ring and migrated to scrotum. The internal abdominal oblique arises from the ASIS and arches over the inguinal canal to insert at the pubic tubercle as part of the conjoint tendon. In panel (**b**) the internal abdominal oblique arises from ASIS and portion of the inguinal ligament to arch over and anterior to the spermatic cord, forming part of the anterior wall of the inguinal canal. The ***conjoint tendon*** is made up of the combination of the medial corners of the transversus abdominus and internal abdominal oblique. In panel (**c**) the external abdominal oblique arises from ASIS and inguinal ligament to contribute to the anterior wall of the inguinal canal. The spermatic cord emerges through the external abdominal oblique forming the superficial inguinal ring [10, 11]

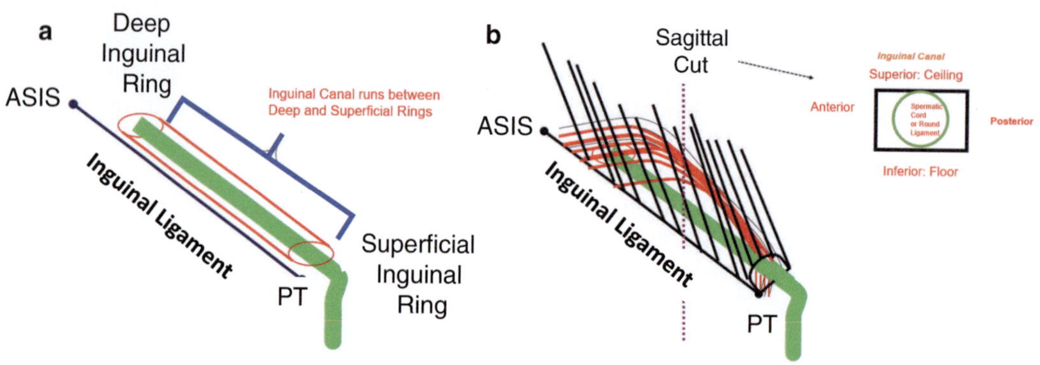

Fig. 3.7 Panel (**a**) shows the path of the spermatic cord through the inguinal canal from deep to superficial ring. Panel (**b**) shows the inguinal canal covered by the external abdominal oblique and the internal abdominal oblique. The sagittal cut through the canal shows the four sides of the canal [10, 11]

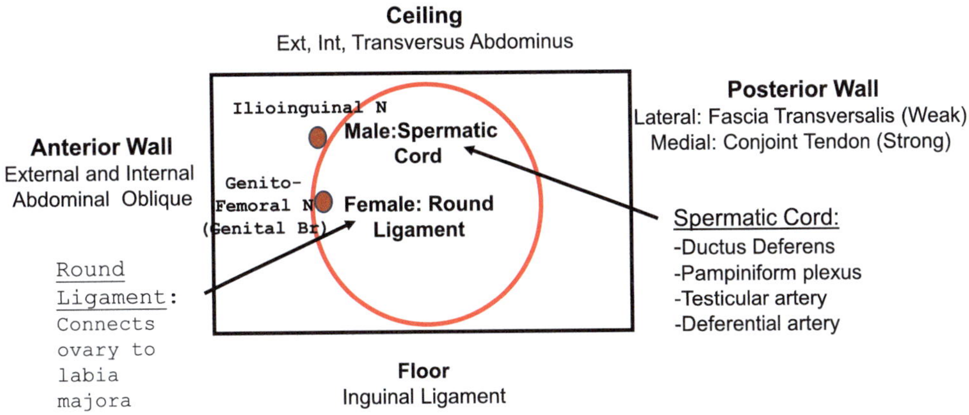

Fig. 3.8 Boundaries of the Inguinal Canal [10, 11]

Inguinal Ligament

The inguinal ligament is the turned under edge of the external abdominal oblique muscle running from the ASIS to the pubic tubercle. It is an important landmark for various clinical scenarios. The external iliac artery passes from the abdominopelvic cavity underneath the inguinal ligament to enter the thigh in the femoral triangle where it turns into the femoral artery. Just before it enters the thigh it gives off the inferior epigastric artery which runs in a superomedial direction. The femoral artery runs with the femoral nerve and femoral vein. This is discussed in detail with the lower limb chapter.

Processes Vaginalis

As the testes descend towards the scrotum during development, they drag a piece of the peritoneal cavity with them. In the adult male, this out pocketing has separated from the peritoneal cavity and has become the *tunica vaginalis*. However, during development, this tunica vaginalis is continuous with the peritoneal cavity via the *processes vaginalis*. This processes vaginalis will eventually degenerate so that the tunica vaginalis is completely separated from the peritoneal cavity. If the communication remains, it is referred to as a *persistent process vaginalis* and is a predisposing factor for a congenital indirect inguinal hernia. A *hydrocele* is a collection of fluid in the tunica vaginalis. The light shown behind it can lead to a red glow. In females, the process vaginalis is referred to as the canal of Nuck.

Indirect Inguinal Hernia

Indirect inguinal hernias start off at the deep inguinal ring. They are more common in males than females. In an elderly male, because of the defect in the anterior abdominal wall, increased pressure on the anterior wall can lead to abdominal contents herniating through the deep inguinal ring. The initial outpocketing of the hernia will be lateral to the pulse of the inferior epigastric artery. Once the hernia is in the deep ring it can then travel down through the canal to eventually exit at the superficial ring to continue onto the scrotum or in a female to the labia majora. If the hernia travels as far as the superficial ring it will be found superior to the pubic tubercle. The indirect inguinal hernia will typically be medial to the pubic tubercle, but it can vary, and it will sometimes be found lateral to it. This is a function of the individual's body weight.

Do not get confused about terminology and geography when referring to these hernias. For instance, the indirect inguinal hernia starts off *lateral to the inferior epigastric artery*; but, given enough time, it can pass through the inguinal canal and then move through the deep inguinal ring where it is now *medial to the artery*.

Direct Inguinal Hernias

In contrast to the pathway of indirect inguinal hernias, a *direct inguinal hernia* will come through the wall at *Hesselbach's triangle*, which is bounded by the inferior epigastric artery, the lateral border of rectus abdominus, and the inguinal ligament. Direct inguinal hernias will be medial to the pulse of the inferior epigastric artery. Direct inguinal hernias will typically spread apart muscle fibers of the anterior abdominal wall and present as a small bulge in Hesselbach's Triangle. However, they can migrate into the end of the inguinal canal or emerge through the deep inguinal ring. They can, although it is not common, migrate all the way to the scrotum or labia majora.

Femoral hernias, which are discussed in more detail with the lower limb, will push through a weakness in the femoral sheath just medial to the femoral vein. The hernia will enter through the femoral ring and enter the femoral canal, which is the medial compartment of the femoral sheath. On examination, femoral hernias will be inferior to the inguinal ligament and, typically, lateral to the pubic tubercle (Fig. 3.9).

Trapezoid of Disaster

If you are inside the pelvic cavity, looking at the posterior wall of the anterior abdominal wall in the region of the inguinal canal there are a considerable number of structures that must be con-

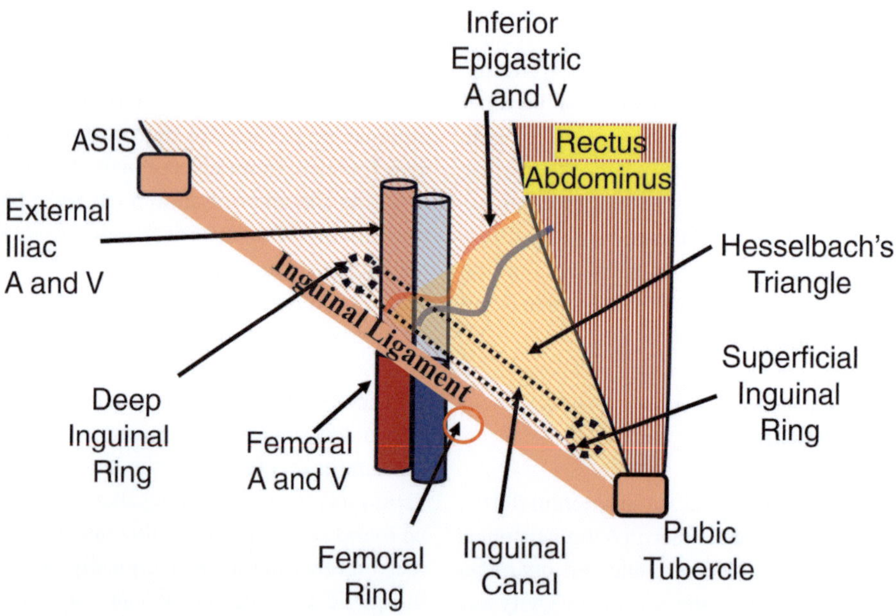

Fig. 3.9 Inguinal Hernias. Indirect inguinal hernias start lateral to the inferior epigastric artery. Direct inguinal hernias start medial to the inferior epigastric artery [10, 11]

sidered during surgery in this region. Surgeons sometimes refer to this region as the trapezoid of disaster *trapezoid of doom*, which is a combination of two triangles:

1. The *triangle of pain* is made up of the iliopubic tract, testicular vessels, and peritoneal fold. It receives its name because there are several nerves in this triangle: femoral, lateral femoral cutaneous, genitofemoral, and ilioinguinal.
2. The *triangle of doom* is bound by the ductus deferens, testicular vessels, and peritoneal fold, and it contains the external iliac artery and vein (Fig. 3.10).

Gubernaculum and Cryptorchidism

During the first six weeks of development there are no outwardly observable differences between a male and female embryo. With the introduction of testosterone at week 7 of development this changes. One major difference is the pathway of the developing gonads. The gubernaculum is a fibrous cord that runs from the gonads, which are now in the abdomen, to either the labia majora in females, or the scrotum in males. The word gubernaculum comes from the Latin word, gubernator, or ship's rudder, or steering. The word governor, the one who steers a state, also comes from the word gubernator. As the gubernaculum shrinks it pulls the gonads downs towards the pelvis—known as the *transabdominal phase*. One idea often seen in textbooks is that it is not really the gonads moving, but that everything else is moving around them, and the gonads are just staying put, held in place by the gubernaculum. However, more recent evidence suggests that the gonads are also moving.

In the male, at about week 25, the testes are located along the inner surface of the anterior abdominal wall. And then on week 26 they start their journey at the deep inguinal ring through the anterior abdominal wall—referred to as the *inguinoscrotal phase*. If the testes do not fully descend into the scrotum this is referred to as *cryptorchidism*—in Greek, crypto = hidden, *Orkhid* = testicle. In these cases, the testes are usually caught in the inguinal canal. Because this can result in reduced sperm counts, surgery is usually called for.

Once the testes arrives in the scrotum, they are thought to be held against the scrotal wall by the *scrotal ligament*. However, the importance of the scrotal ligament has been called into question by recent studies suggesting that in many cases it is not actually attached to the testes or the scrotum

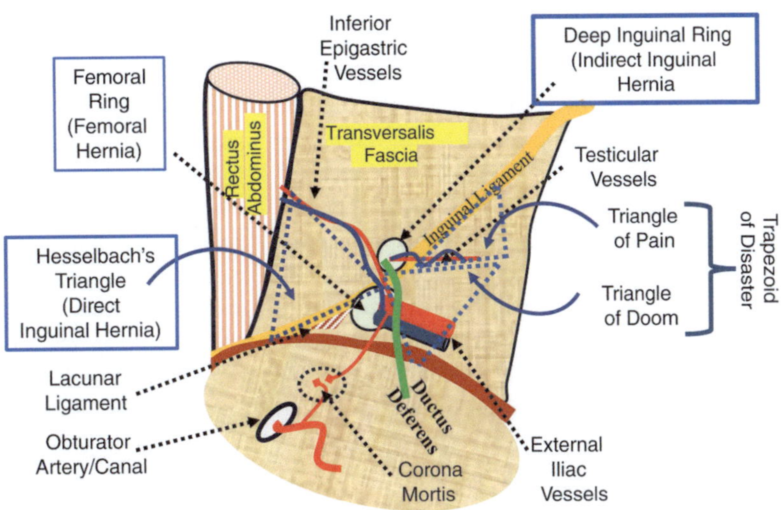

Fig. 3.10 Hernias. This is an internal view. You are in the abdominal pelvic cavity looking at the structures passing from pelvic cavity to the thigh. Indirect inguinal hernias begin lateral to the inferior epigastric artery. Direct inguinal hernias begin medial to the artery. Femoral hernias are inferior to the inguinal ligament [10, 11]

and that it is not really a ligament. It is thought that the scrotum is located outside the abdominal cavity so that the testes with their developing spermatids are kept cooler than the rest of the body. However, birds with a high body temperature have their testes inside their abdominal cavity, and Asian elephants also have abdominal testes.

Layers of Spermatic Cord

As the testes migrate down to the scrotum, they will carry with them the layers that they touch on their journey. The fascia transversalis will become the internal spermatic fascia. Because the testes never touch the transversus abdominus muscle on their way, the transversus abdominus fibers do not get dragged down into the scrotum. The internal abdominal oblique muscle becomes the cremaster muscle and fascia. The external abdominal oblique muscle becomes the external spermatic fascia.

There are three important nerves in the region of the inguinal canal.

1. The *genitofemoral nerve* comes from L1 and as it approaches the inguinal canal it splits into two branches: the femoral branch goes deep to the inguinal ligament and is responsible for cutaneous sensation to the anteromedial thigh. The genital branch innervates the cremaster muscle and joins the inguinal canal near the deep ring. It does not travel through the deep ring, but it does travel through the superficial ring. A test for L1 is the cremaster reflex which is tested by scratching the anteromedial thigh. The sensation travels on the femoral branch of genitofemoral (or in some cases by ilioinguinal nerve since there is considerable overlap), and then the cremaster muscle contracts via efferent signals in the genital branch of genitofemoral.
2. The *ilioinguinal nerve* comes from L1 and enters the spermatic cord. Along with the genitofemoral nerve, it can be damaged during inguinal surgery. It travels through the superficial ring but not the deep ring.
3. The *iliohypogastric nerve* also comes from L1. It runs parallel but superior to the ilioinguinal nerve. The iliohypogastric nerve can be injured during an appendectomy. Both the ilioinguinal and iliohypogastric nerves go to the anterior abdominal wall muscles.

Within the spermatic cord there are several important structures: (1) the *ductus deferens* which carry sperm towards the urethra, (2) the *deferential artery* which supplies blood to the vas deferens, (3) the *testicular artery* carrying blood to the testes, and (4) the *pampiniform plexus* which is the beginning of the testicular vein. On the left, the testicular vein drains into the left renal vein; on the right, it drains into the inferior vena cava. A *varicocele* is a collection of blood pooling in the pampiniform plexus due to a blockage of the testicular vein. When the patient goes from a standing position to lying down, the varicocele will become smaller, as the blood has an easier time draining.

In the female inguinal canal, there is the *round ligament* which connects the labia majora to the uterus. Both the *round ligament* and the *ovarian ligament* are remnants of the *gubernaculum.*

Also in this region is *circle of death*, sometimes referred to as the *corona mortis*. This name comes from a common variation formed by an arterial anastomosis in some individuals. Normally, the obturator artery comes off the anterior division of the internal iliac artery and perforates the obturator foramen to enter the medial thigh. In addition, the external iliac artery usually gives off the inferior epigastric artery which ascends along the anterior abdominal wall. In some individuals, there is a small artery that comes off the inferior epigastric artery and connects to the obturator artery. This small communication is in the vicinity of the lacunar ligament and femoral ring. A surgeon making an anterior approach from the medial thigh to the femoral ring needs to be cognizant of this potential variation. If this artery is nicked during this procedure a significant amount of blood will fill the surgical field. In addition, the blood will collect in the abdominopelvic cavity—the name *"circle of death."*

Abdominal Cavity

The Diaphragm

The abdominal cavity is bounded superiorly by the diaphragm, which is the most important muscle for inspiration. It is a sheet of muscle originating anteriorly from the xiphoid process and ribs 7–12. It runs laterally along rib 12 to insert along the posterior abdominal wall by the crura. The muscle fibers of the diaphragm run from the perimeter towards the center, converging to form the *central tendon*. Along the posterior wall the attachment of the diaphragm forms the *medial and lateral arcuate ligaments* around the anterior portions of the psoas major and quadratus lumborum muscles. When the diaphragm contracts it expands the thoracic space and creates a negative pressure so that air moves into the lungs. There are three major openings in the diaphragm:

1. the *caval hiatus* at the level of T8 with the inferior vena cava, and the right phrenic nerve.
2. the *esophageal hiatus* at the level of T10 with the esophagus and the anterior and posterior vagal trunks, and esophageal branches of the left gastric artery.
3. the *aortic hiatus* at the level of T12 with the aorta, azygous vein, and thoracic duct. The thoracic duct lies just posterior to the esophagus.

A useful saying for the levels and hiatuses is **I** **E**at **A**pples, 8, 10, 12. **I**nferior vena cava, **E**sophagus, and **A**orta at T8, T10, and T12, respectively. Another saying for the hiatus is ***Three gooses And A Duck***, standing for the Esopha*goose*, right va*goose*, and left va*goose* which travel through the esophageal hiatus, and **A**orta, **A**zygous vein, and thoracic **Duck** traveling together through the aortic hiatus.

The diaphragm develops from four different regions, all of which eventually fuse together to from the mature diaphragm.

1. The central portion of the diaphragm starts in the cervical region. This *septum transversum* will eventually migrate inferiorly to form the *central tendon* of the diaphragm. By the end of week 8 it lies near the lumbar vertebrae.
2. Before all the various regions of the diaphragm fuse, the spaces on either side of the septum transversum are referred to as the *pericardioperitoneal canals.* These canals will eventually be closed by the *pleuroperitoneal membranes* which is the original separation between the pleural and peritoneal cavities.
3. The *dorsal esophageal mesentery* surrounds the esophagus and fuses with the pleuroperitoneal membrane. It will eventually become the *crura* of the diaphragm.
4. All these above-named pieces will eventually fuse with outgrowths of the *lateral body wall* that become the edges or peripheral portions of the diaphragm.

The right and left crura arise from the vertebral bodies of L1-L3 and run anterior to encircle the esophageal hiatus. Some of the fibers of the right crus pass to the left side between the aortic and esophageal hiatuses to contribute to the *lower esophageal sphincter. Achalasia* refers to the failure of the sphincter to relax which leads to the bolus backing up in the esophagus. The contracted sphincter leaves a small opening for the bolus to trickle through. On a radiograph it resembles a bird's beak. The thickening of the crura anterior to the aortic hiatus is the *median arcuate ligament.*

The efferent nerve supply to the diaphragm is from the *phrenic nerves* which arise from C 3, 4, and 5. The afferents from the central tendon of the diaphragm travel on the phrenic nerves so pathology of either the superior or inferior surface of the central diaphragm will refer to the neck, or shoulder region, because of the phrenic nerve. However, pathology out on the lateral side of the diaphragm will refer to the body wall because of the intercostal nerves. As mentioned earlier, when the diaphragm contracts the dome of the diaphragm lowers. And when the diaphragm relaxes the dome elevates. So, damage to a phrenic nerve will lead to the dome moving superiorly—it cannot contract. Damage to one phrenic nerve is typically asymptomatic, while bilateral damage can lead to more severe deficits.

The major arteries to the diaphragm are the *superior phrenic arteries*, which are branches of the thoracic aorta, and *inferior phrenic arteries*, which are branches of the abdominal aorta. As the internal thoracic artery descends on the anterior wall near the sternum it eventually divides into two branches: (1) *the musculophrenic artery*, and (2) *the superior epigastric artery*. The musculophrenic branch contributes to the diaphragm. In the neck, the internal thoracic artery gives off a small *pericardiacophrenic* artery which runs with the phrenic nerve to the diaphragm. During heart surgery this artery should be avoided.

A *congenital diaphragmatic hernia* is a malformation that arises because of a failure of the pleuroperitoneal membranes to fuse. This can lead to a defect in the posterolateral portion of the diaphragm, usually found on the left side. In many cases, the intestines will be found in the thorax. If the herniation is large enough it can prevent proper lung development and the lung will be smaller than normal *(pulmonary hypoplasia),* which in turn can lead to pulmonary hypertension. In an infant born with a congenital diaphragmatic hernia the pertinent question for viability concerns the state of lung development.

Abdominal Aorta and Inferior Vena Cava

The abdominal aorta enters the abdomen at the T12 vertebra through the aortic hiatus. Accompanying the aorta are the azygous vein and the thoracic duct. There are unpaired and paired branches coming off the aorta. The three unpaired branches supply the GI tract (Fig. 3.11).

Just as the aorta enters the abdomen it gives two paired branches, *the right and left inferior phrenic arteries* which head towards the diaphragm. Coming off at T12 is the *celiac trunk* supplying the foregut and related structures. Coming off at the superior border of L1 is the *superior mesenteric artery* (SMA) supplying the midgut. Also located at the L1 level, are the paired renal arteries. Moving down the aorta are the *right and left gonadal arteries* to either the testes or ovaries. And coming off at L3 is the *infe-*

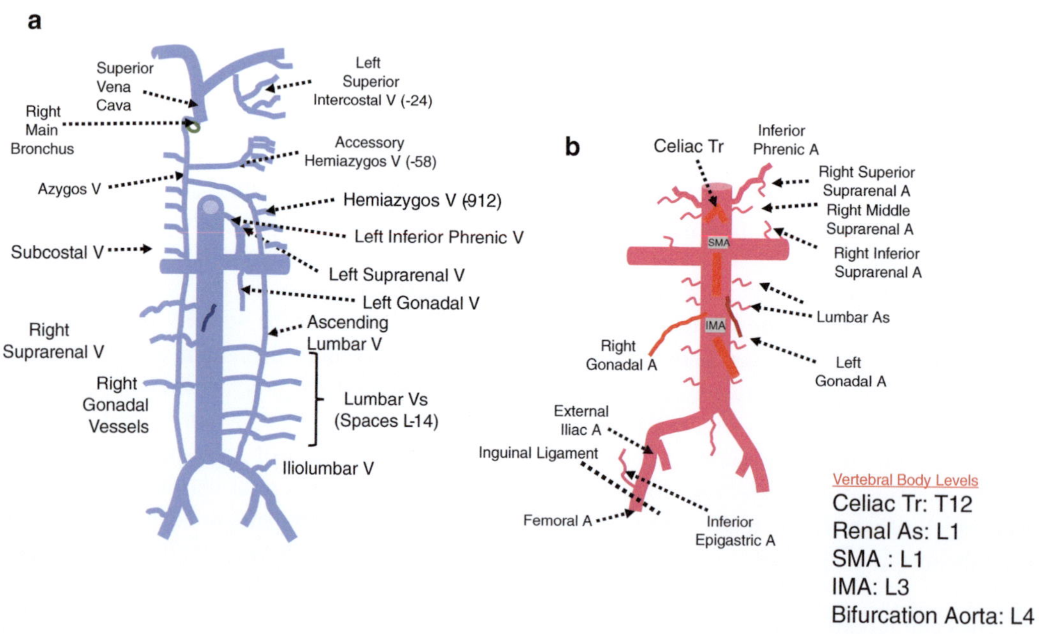

Fig. 3.11 Panel (**a**) shows the inferior vena cava and its branches. Panel (**b**) shows the abdominal aorta and its branches [10, 11]

rior mesenteric artery (IMA) to the hindgut. Coming off the aorta, between the SMA and IMA, in the lumbar region are the four to five lumbar arteries. The aorta ends at the L4 level by bifurcating into the *two common iliac arteries*, which in turn splits into *internal and external iliac arteries*.

Inferior Vena Cava

The inferior vena cava starts at the L5 vertebra where the two common iliac veins merge. Moving up the IVC there are 4–5 *lumbar veins* draining into the IVC and related structures. There is significant variation here. For instance, in some cases, the fifth lumbar vein will drain into the common iliac vein, and in some cases, the second lumbar vein enters the left renal vein. Because of this variation, various books will show slightly different patterns for the lumbar veins. However, regardless of the variations, an important anastomotic channel is formed by the *ascending lumbar veins* which run parallel to the IVC and connect the common iliac and iliolumbar veins in the pelvic region with the azygous, and hemi-azygos veins in the thorax. If the IVC is blocked, these ascending channels provide an alternate path for the return of blood to the heart (Fig. 3.11).

The *right gonadal vein* drains directly into the IVC, while the *left gonadal vein* drains into the left renal vein, which in turn drains into the IVC. Because of this relationship, a mass on the kidney that blocks the left gonadal vein will lead to a varicocele which arises from blood backing up in the gonads. A swollen left testicle could be indicative of a mass on the left renal vein. Each adrenal gland also typically has one vein. On the right side, the adrenal vein drains into the IVC, and on the left it drains into the left renal vein.

Draining into the IVC, near the diaphragm, are the right and *left inferior phrenic veins*. On the right side this vein has a descending branch that connects with the left renal vein in the vicinity of the left suprarenal vein.

As the IVC approaches the liver it forms the posterior wall of the epiploic foramen and then continues posterior to the liver making a groove or tunnel that separates the right and caudate lobes of the liver. As the IVC ascends it is pushed slightly anteriorly by the diaphragm.

Abdominal Contents

Let us start with the GI tract as a simple tube with the mouth at one end and the anal canal at the other end. The entire tract is surrounded by muscle, either smooth or skeletal. At the ends of the tract, the muscles are sphincters formed by a combination of smooth muscle and skeletal muscle. Other than the ends, the rest of the tract is surrounded by smooth muscle. The skeletal muscle at each end is controlled by the somatic nervous system, while the smooth muscle sections are controlled by autonomic nerves, mostly parasympathetic.

The organization of the abdomen is all based on the divisions of endoderm into foregut, midgut, and hindgut. Starting at the beginning of the stomach, the foregut includes the: stomach, the first part of the duodenum, and the top half of the second part of the duodenum. Halfway down the second part of the duodenum, at the greater duodenal papilla, the foregut turns into midgut. The midgut includes the second half of the second part of the duodenum, the third and fourth part of the duodenum, the jejunum, ileum, cecum, ascending colon, and two-thirds of the transverse colon. Close to the splenic flexure, the midgut turns into hindgut. The hindgut then includes the distal one-third of the transverse colon, the descending colon, the sigmoid colon, the rectum, and anal canal. The hindgut ends at the pectinate line. Below the pectinate line we are back to ectoderm, skeletal muscle, and somatic nervous system.

There are three main arteries to the GI tract, *the celiac trunk, the superior mesenteric artery*, and *inferior mesenteric artery*. All three of these arteries are unpaired arteries arising from the abdominal aorta. The celiac artery goes to the foregut, the superior mesenteric to the midgut, and inferior mesenteric to the hindgut. We will see that the organization of the lymphatics and the nerve supply is all based on these three arteries. For instance, the celiac nodes are responsible for lymphatic drainage from the foregut, superior mesenteric nodes from the midgut, and inferior mesenteric nodes from the hindgut (Fig. 3.12).

Peritoneum

The peritoneum is a closed, empty cavity within the abdominopelvic cavity. There is nothing in the peritoneal cavity. The only structure that normally opens into it is the uterine tube. Imagine you have a balloon filled with air, and you make an incision in the anterior abdominal wall and stuff the balloon into the abdomen and then suture the incision closed. The balloon is going to wrap around the abdominal contents. The cavity of the balloon represents the closed peritoneal cavity. You can see in fig. 3.13 that some structures are completely enclosed by the balloon,

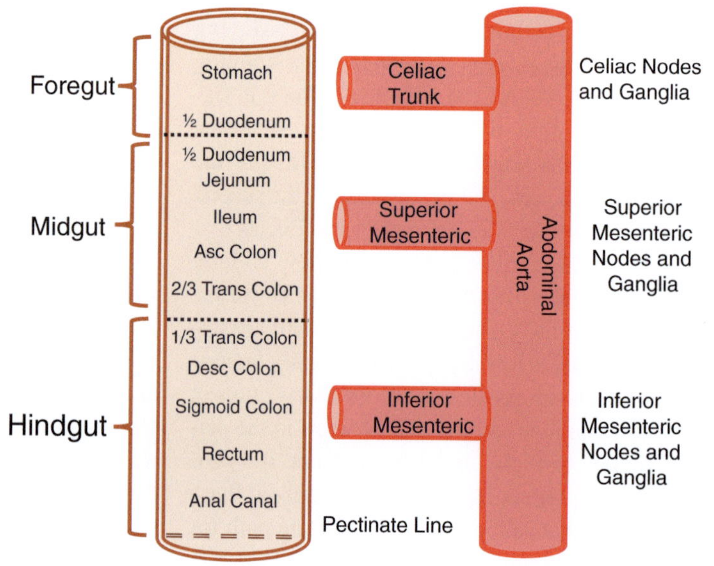

Fig. 3.12 Foregut, Midgut, and Hindgut [10, 11]

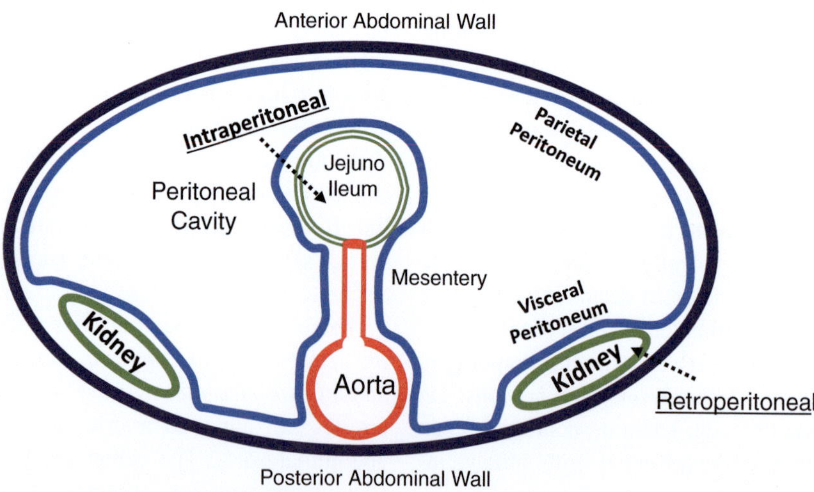

Fig. 3.13 Peritoneal Cavity. The aorta and kidneys are retroperitoneal structures, while the jejunoileum is intraperitoneal. The jejenoileum is connected to the posterior abdominal wall by the dorsal mesentery which contains the superior mesenteric artery [10, 11]

while other structures lie behind the balloon. In the diagram, structures like the aorta and kidneys are behind the balloon and are referred to as *retroperitoneal.* Structures like the jejunoileum are surrounded by peritoneum and are referred to as *intraperitoneal* (Fig. 3.13).

The portion of the peritoneum that abuts the anterior wall is referred to as *parietal peritoneum,* while the layer surrounding organs is referred to as the *visceral peritoneum.* Between these two layers—visceral and parietal—is the peritoneal cavity.

The peritoneum is further divided into several compartments. The major division is into the *greater sac* and *lesser sac (omental bursa).* If you make an incision into the anterior abdominal wall, you are entering the greater sac, which makes up most of the peritoneal cavity. However, behind the stomach is another space—*the lesser sac*. The doorway between the greater and lesser sacs is the *epiploic foramen***.** If you are standing at the right side of a donor and you put your finger in the opening behind the *hepatoduodenal ligament*, part of the lesser omentum, you are moving from the greater sac into the lesser sac. The ceiling of the epiploic foramen is the caudate lobe of the liver (Figs. 3.14 and 3.15).

The *hepatoduodenal* and *hepatogastric ligaments* make up the lesser omentum. Running in the hepatoduodenal ligament are three structures: (1) *the portal vein*, (2) *bile duct,* and (3) *proper hepatic artery*. However, we also need to pay attention to the organization of these three structures in the ligament. The portal vein is the most posterior structure, with the bile duct being anterolateral, and the proper hepatic artery being

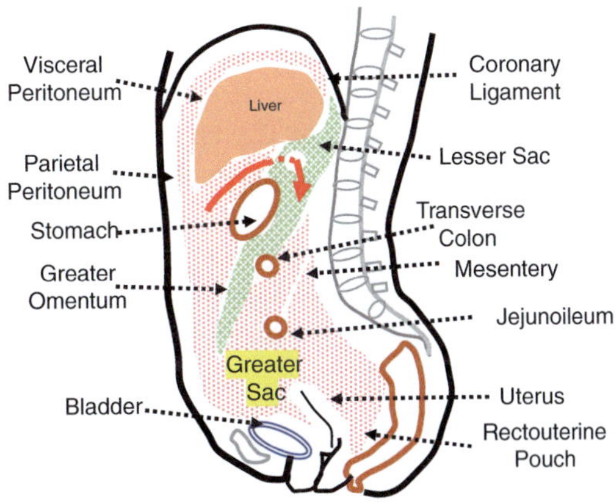

Fig. 3.14 Greater and Lesser Sacs. The red arrow is moving from the greater sac (in red) through the epiploic foramen into the lesser sac (in green) behind the lesser omentum [10, 11]

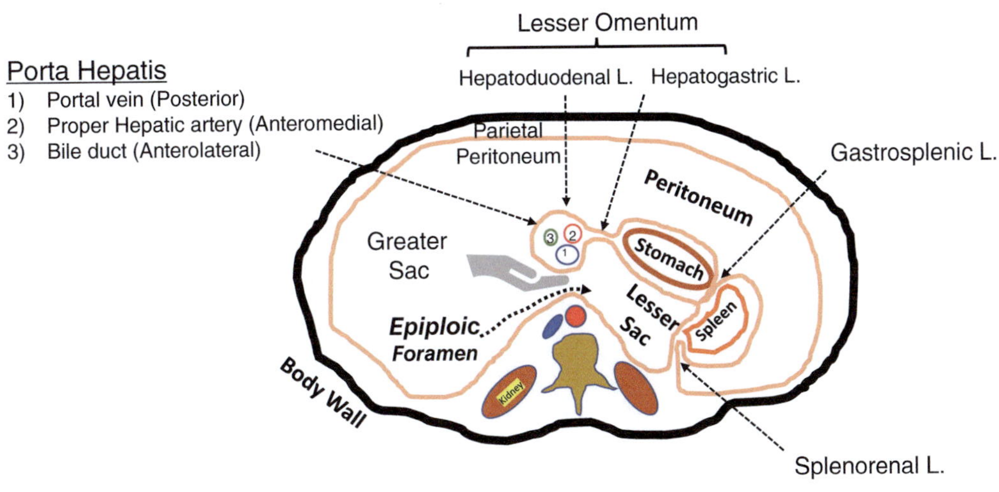

Fig. 3.15 Porta Hepatis. The epiploic foramen is the doorway between the greater sac and the lesser sac of the peritoneal cavity. The finger in the picture is going through the epiploic foramen, posterior to hepatoduodenal ligament. The finger-nail is against the inferior vena cava, and the pad of the finger is against the portal vein. Note the specific location of location of the three structures in the hepatoduodenal ligament making up the porta hepatis [10, 11]

anteromedial. During surgery if you clamp off the hepatoduodenal ligament then you have blocked everything going into and out of the liver. This is called a "pringle maneuver." In Fig. 3.15 the pad of the finger is against the portal vein, and the fingernail is against the inferior vena cava.

Keep in mind that this hepatoduodenal ligament is the anterior wall of the epiploic foramen. If you keep moving your finger towards the midline your finger is now further into the lesser sac, with the lesser omentum and stomach in front of your finger, and the pancreas and posterior abdominal wall behind it. The inferior border of the lesser sac is the transverse mesocolon. An ulcer of the stomach that burrows through the posterior stomach wall will lead to contents collecting in the lesser sac with subsequent back pain because of aggravation of the pancreas (Figs. 3.14, 3.15, and 3.16).

The greater sac is further subdivided into the *supracolic* and *infracolic* compartments which are separated by the transverse mesocolon and greater omentum. The supracolic compartment contains the stomach, liver, and spleen. The infracolic compartment contains the small intestine, ascending colon, and descending colon.

The supracolic and infracolic compartments are connected by two gutters, (1) the *right paracolic gutter,* which is to the right of ascending colon, and (2) *left paracolic gutter*, which is to the left of the descending colon. The paracolic gutter on each side connects with the respective right and left anterior subphrenic spaces found on each side between the diaphragm and the liver. Think of the paracolic gutters as hallways connecting one room to another (Fig. 3.17).

The infracolic compartment is in turn divided into the *right and left infracolic spaces* which are separated by the dorsal mesentery.

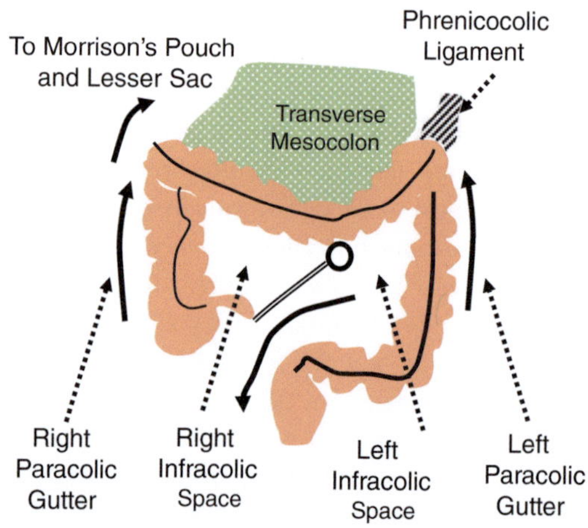

Fig. 3.17 Peritoneal Divisions. On the right side the Phrenicocolic ligament impedes movement from the left gutter to the supracolic space [10, 11]

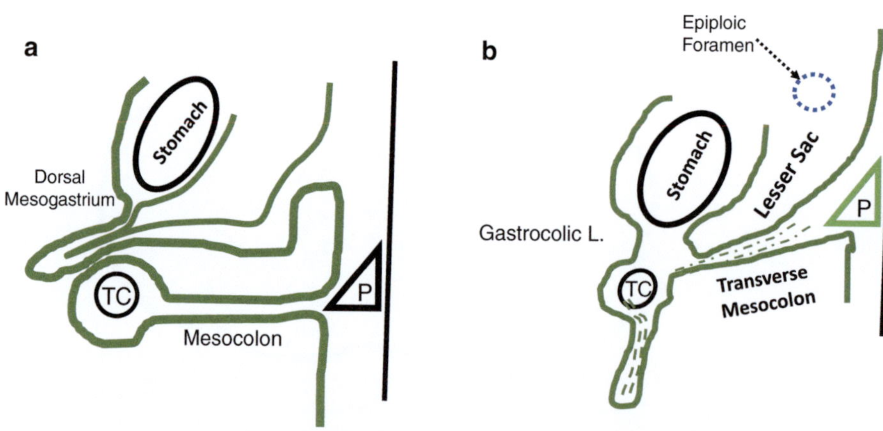

Fig. 3.16 Panel (**a**) The pancreas becomes a retroperitoneal organ during developmental and is considered a secondary retroperitoneal organ. Panel (**b**) The transverse mesocolon is a derivative of dorsal mesentery formed by the fusion of the posterior leaf of the dorsal mesogastrium with the mesentery of the midgut. Posterior to the stomach is the lesser sac. An ulcer in the posterior wall of the stomach that perforates the wall can drain into the lesser sac [10, 11]

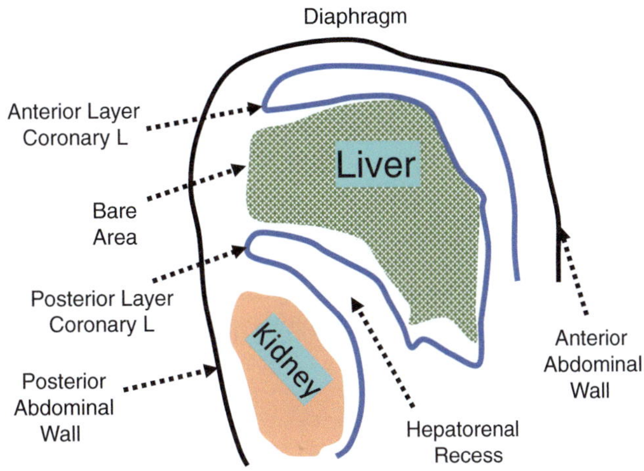

Fig. 3.18 Peritoneum and the Liver. The visceral peritoneum comes up on the diaphragmatic surface of the liver and is reflected onto the undersurface of the diaphragm as the anterior layer of the coronary ligament. On the visceral surface of the liver the reflection creates the hepatorenal recess between the liver and the kidney [10, 11]

On the right side, between the liver and the kidney is the *hepatorenal recess* (Morrison's pouch) which is a subdivision of the peritoneal cavity. The posterosuperior edge of this recess is the posterior layer of the coronary ligament. When a patient is lying down, excess fluid in the peritoneal cavity will typically collect here. As the patient sits up, the fluid will tend to drain into *the rectouterine pouch* in the female or the rectovesical pouch in the male (Fig. 3.17).

Two subdivisions of the peritoneal cavity also surround the liver. On the superior surface of the liver, between the liver and the diaphragm are the right and left *subphrenic spaces* (or suprahepatic spaces) bounded by the coronary ligaments, triangular ligaments, and falciform ligaments. Fluid collecting in the subphrenic space can aggravate the diaphragm leading to pain sensations felt in the neck and shoulder region.

Below the liver the *subhepatic space* (AKA: hepatorenal space or Morrison's Pouch) is a potential space that is normally closed but can open in the presence of excess fluid. The subhepatic space is between the liver and the right kidney (Fig. 3.18).

Retroperitoneal Versus Intraperitoneal

The details will follow but it is useful to look at the big picture first when talking about abdominal structures that are intraperitoneal versus those that are retroperitoneal. Think of a bolus moving down the tract from top to bottom and you will see that we alternate between intraperitoneal and retroperitoneal. Starting with the stomach and the first part of the duodenum, they are intraperitoneal structures. And intraperitoneal structures have a mesentery. In this case, the greater and lesser omentum. Moving down the tract, the 2nd, 3rd, and 4th part of the duodenum are retroperitoneal. Then the jejunoileum is intraperitoneal (dorsal mesentery). Then the ascending colon is retroperitoneal; the transverse colon is intraperitoneal (transverse mesocolon); the descending colon is retroperitoneal; and the sigmoid colon is intraperitoneal (sigmoid mesocolon); and finally, the rectum and anal canal are retroperitoneal (or sub peritoneal) (Fig. 3.19).

Peritoneal Dialysis

Waste products can be removed from the blood via peritoneal dialysis by using the peritoneum as a filter. A tube is inserted into the peritoneal cavity and then fluid (the dialysate) is passed into the peritoneal cavity. There are several types of peritoneal dialysis, but they are all based on the idea that the dialysate will remain in the peritoneum for a set amount of time (the dwell) to absorb waste products from the blood stream. This dialysate containing the waste products is then removed and discarded.

Fig. 3.19 Intraperitoneal versus Retroperitoneal [10, 11]

	Intra or Retro	Peritoneal Folds
Stomach, 1st part Duodenum	Intra	Greater and Lesser Omentum
2, 3, 4th parts Duodenum	Retro	
Jejuno-ileum	Intra	Dorsal Mesentery "The Mesentery"
Ascending Colon	Retro	
Transverse Colon	Intra	Transverse Mesocolon
Descending Colon	Retro	
Sigmoid Colon	Intra	Sigmoid Mesocolon
Rectum	Sub	

Foregut

Stomach

The esophagus turns into the stomach at the diaphragm. This region of the stomach is referred to as the *cardia*. The lower esophageal sphincter, which is a physiological sphincter, is present at this junction. Its job is to open when a bolus of food comes down the esophagus to enter the stomach, and to then close after food enters the stomach. The *phrenoesophageal ligament* attaches the diaphragm to the esophagus to help the two structures operate together. The *fundus* is the top of the stomach and is often filled with air on a barium swallow test. As the stomach approaches the duodenum, it looks like a funnel as it narrows. The large part of the funnel is the antrum, which in turn narrows down to the pyloric region. The *lesser curvature* is towards the right and facing superior. Attached to the lesser curvature is the *lesser omentum,* made up of the hepatoduodenal and hepatogastric ligaments. The *greater curvature* is facing inferior, and it is attached to the greater omentum which is made up of the gastro-phrenic, gastro-splenic, and gastro-omental ligaments.

There are several features that help to keep food in the stomach and prevent backflow into the esophagus. The *angle of His* is the angle between the stomach fundus and the esophagus. In this region, there is also a loose flap of tissue referred to as the *gastroesophageal flap valve* that serves as a flap to prevent contents regurgitating back into the esophagus. When contents move into the stomach, air will push up on the fundus which in turn puts pressure on the gastroesophageal flap valve at the angle of His making it harder for stomach contents to move into the esophagus.

There are two related pathologies in the region of the gastroesophageal junction.

1. A *sliding hiatal hernia* occurs when the gastroesophageal junction herniates into the thorax. Its main characteristic is that the junction moves back and forth between the stomach and the thorax. During swallowing, the gastroesophageal junction can move into the tho-

rax but can then move back to the stomach—it slides.
2. A *paraesophageal hernia* refers to the stomach herniating into the thorax alongside the esophagus. The herniated stomach becomes lodged in the thorax and stays there. It does not move back and forth like a sliding hiatal hernia. The gastroesophageal junction is fixed.

After eating a meal, food will remain in the stomach for several hours. The stomach has three layers of muscle, which are involved in the mechanical aspect of digestion: (1) an outer longitudinal, (2) a circular layer, and (3) and an inner oblique layer. These muscles allow for strong movements of the stomach to break down food into smaller parts. For the chemical component of digestion, the stomach has several important cell types:

1. *Chief cells* secrete both pepsinogen, which in an acidic environment is converted to pepsin, and gastric lipase.
2. *Parietal cells* secrete both HCL to create an acidic environment, and intrinsic factor which is necessary for the absorption of B12 in the duodenum. Intrinsic factor binds to B12 in the duodenum and is then shuttled across the walls of the ileum to enter the bloodstream. In a patient who has had their stomach removed they need an outside source of intrinsic factor.
3. *G Cells* produce gastrin which increases motility.
4. *D Cells* or somatostatin producing cells produce somatostatin which has inhibitory effects on parietal cells and G cells, and they reduce the production of HCL and gastrin. D cells are also located in the duodenum and pancreatic islets.
5. *Enterochromaffin cells* produce serotonin which increases peristalsis.
6. *Enterochromaffin-like cells* in the fundus produce histamine which stimulates parietal cells via the H2 receptor to release HCL. Medications such as ranitidine block the H2 receptor.

During this initial phase of digestion, the pyloric sphincter will remain closed. After two or three hours it will open to allow the chyme to move into the duodenum.

Peptic ulcers are found in the stomach and duodenum. Stomach ulcers will typically lead to pain right after eating while duodenal ulcers will cause pain several hours after eating. *Helicobacter pylori* bacteria in the gastrointestinal tract is a predisposing factor for peptic ulcers. Long term use of non-steroidal anti-inflammatory medications (NSAIDs) can cause peptic ulcers.

Greater and Lesser Omentum

The *lesser omentum* is attached to the lesser curvature. And the greater omentum is attached to the greater curvature. However, there are important subdivisions and details to both structures. The lesser omentum is made up of two parts (Fig. 3.20):

1. the *hepatoduodenal ligament* runs from the liver to the first part of the duodenum and forms the anterior wall of the epiploic foramen.
2. the *hepatogastric ligament* runs from the liver to the stomach and forms most of the lesser omentum. It makes up the anterior wall of the lesser sac.

The greater omentum is attached to greater curvature and the fundus of the stomach and is made up of three subdivisions:

1. the *gastrophrenic ligament* runs from the fundus to the diaphragm.
2. The *gastrosplenic ligament* runs from the left side of the greater curvature to the spleen and contains the short gastric arteries.
3. The *gastrocolic ligament* connects the stomach to the transverse colon and contains as the major portion of the greater omentum. It is also the lateral wall of the lesser sac on the left side.

Duodenum

A prominent characteristic of the duodenum is the presence of circular folds which are easily

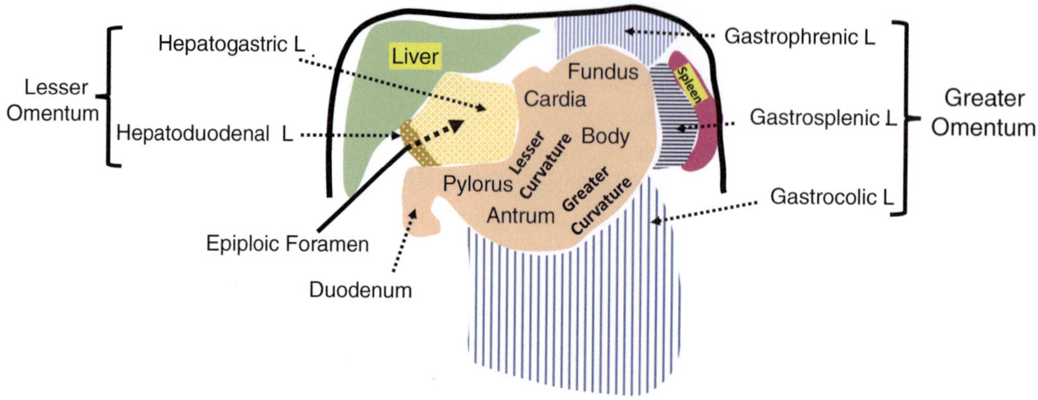

Fig. 3.20 The stomach is suspended in the abdomen by the lesser and greater omentums. The greater omentum is attached to the greater curvature and is made up of the gastrophrenic, gastrosplenic, and gastrocolic ligaments. The lesser omentum is attached to the lesser curvature and is made up of the hepatogastric and hepatoduodenal ligaments [10, 11]

seen on a barium swallow test. However, the first part of duodenum does not have these folds and its surface is smooth. This smooth first part of the duodenum is a radiological landmark sometimes referred to as the duodenal cap. There are four parts to the duodenum. The first part of the duodenum is intraperitoneal, but the second, third, and fourth parts are retroperitoneal. The first part crosses the L1 vertebra, the second part runs parallel to L2, and the third part crosses L3.

1. The first part of the duodenum starts at the pyloric sphincter. Posterior to the first part is the gastroduodenal artery and the common bile duct. This first part of the duodenum is the most common site for duodenal ulcers. An ulcer that destroys the posterior wall of the first part of the duodenum can attack the gastroduodenal artery and common bile duct. The hepatoduodenal ligament runs from the liver to the first part of the duodenum. This ligament forms the anterior wall of the *epiploic foramen* and running in it is the portal vein, and branches of the bile duct, and proper hepatic artery. The first part of the duodenum is anterior to the hilum of the right kidney.
2. The second part of the duodenum has two prominent landmarks on the medial wall. The superior landmark is the *minor duodenal papilla* which is the opening of the accessory pancreatic duct. Moving inferior, the second landmark is the *greater duodenal papilla* which is the opening of the pancreatic duct. On a laparoscopic view, differentiating one papilla from the other can be difficult. One clue, or aid, is that the greater duodenal papilla has a piece of tissue or fold that descends from its inferior portion called the *longitudinal fold.* If you see the longitudinal fold then you are looking at the greater duodenal papilla. If you do not see the extra fold, then you are looking at the minor duodenal papilla. The anterior wall of the second part of the duodenum is crossed by the transverse colon. And the body of the gallbladder rests on top of the second part of the duodenum.
3. The third part of the duodenum crosses anterior to the aorta and posterior to the superior mesenteric artery. See below for a more detailed discussion.
4. The fourth and final portion of the duodenum is pulled superiorly by a ligament which is an extension of the right crus of the diaphragm. This ligament is called the *ligament of Treitz*, or the suspensory muscle of the duodenum, and is the dividing line between the end of the duodenum and the beginning of the jejunum.

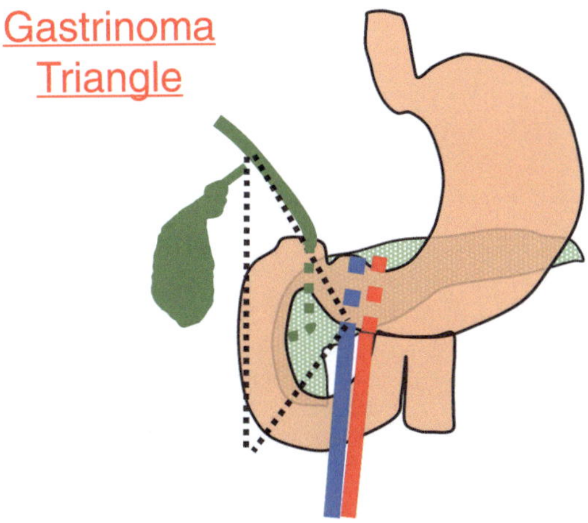

Fig. 3.21 Gastrinoma Triangle. The most common site of tumors arising from the gastrin secreting cells [10, 11]

At the ligament of Treitz, part of which is an extension of the right crus of the diaphragm, the retroperitoneal duodenum turns into the intraperitoneal jejunum. The ligament, which is made up of folded peritoneum, pulls up on the duodenum at this point. It is here where the retroperitoneal duodenum turns into the intraperitoneal jejunum. Near this ligament, the jejunoileum can become twisted and herniated.

Gastrinoma Triangle

The *gastrinoma triangle* is bounded by the cystic duct, the lateral side of the second part of the duodenum and part of the head of the pancreas. It is here in this triangle where many gastric tumors are found (Fig. 3.21).

Celiac Trunk

The celiac trunk is the artery of the foregut. It comes off the abdominal aorta at approximately T12. Right at its origin it has three branches.

1. The *splenic artery* runs behind the pancreas to the spleen where it is found in the *lienorenal ligament.* As it courses along the top of the pancreas it gives off several branches to the pancreas including the *dorsal pancreatic*, and *greater pancreatic* (pancreatica magna). Just before the pancreatic artery enters the spleen, it gives off several branches.
   - (ii) The *short gastric* branches ascend to the fundus of the stomach in the gastrosplenic ligament.
   - (iii) The *left gastroepiploic artery* travels along the greater curvature of the stomach to eventually anastomose with the right gastroepiploic coming from the gastroduodenal artery.
2. The left gastric artery gives off *esophageal branches* to the esophagus and *gastric branches* to the lesser curvature of the stomach.
3. The *common hepatic artery* travels towards the right-side heading towards the liver. It gives off the gastroduodenal artery. Distal to the branching of the gastroduodenal artery the common hepatic artery now becomes the proper hepatic artery.

The gastroduodenal artery terminates into the *anterior and posterior superior pancreaticoduodenal arteries* that perfuse the superior head of the pancreas and the top half of the second part of the duodenum. These two arteries anastomose with their counterparts from the superior mesenteric artery. These anterior and posterior pancreaticoduodenal arteries wrap around the common bile duct.

The *right gastric artery* heads towards the left side of the body and runs along the lesser curvature of the stomach and anastomoses with the left gastric artery (Fig. 3.22).

Midgut

The midgut starts halfway down the second part of the duodenum at the major duodenal papilla. The duodenal jejunal flexure is just below the transpyloric plane. The jejunoileum is approximately 20 feet long when uncoiled. Some portion of the jejunoileum is necessary for life because it is responsible for the absorption of nutrients. Its surface area is about the size of a football field when spread out. There is no sharp dividing line between the jejunum and ileum, instead there is a transition from one to the other. The walls of the jejunum are thicker and wider than the ileum and

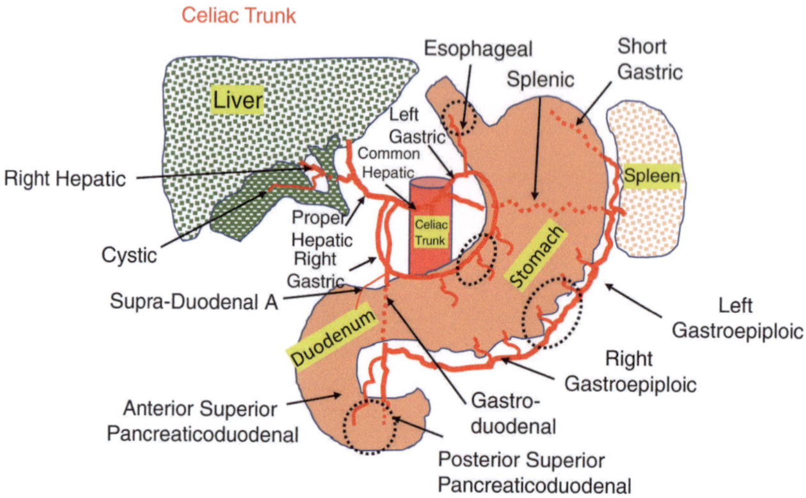

Fig. 3.22 There are three branches of the celiac trunk: (1) common hepatic, (2) splenic, and (3) the left gastric. Coming off the common hepatic is the gastroduodenal artery going posterior to the first part of duodenum. Various anastomoses are shown as black circles [10, 11]

because the jejunum also gets more blood flow it is redder than the ileum.

In the lower right quadrant, the ileum turns into the cecum, which is the beginning of the large intestine. The ileocecal valve separates the ileum from the cecum. The valve is normally closed.

The cecum is a bulbous sac-like structure which marks the beginning of the ascending colon. Instead of the outer longitudinal layer of muscle wrapping around the entire tube of large intestine, the muscle is consolidated into three longitudinal bands referred to as *tenia coli.* More specifically, the three tenia coli are the: tenia libra, tenia mesocolic, and tenia omental, which all originate or come to a point, at the appendix. The effect of the tenia coli on the large intestine is to cause the intestine to bunch up into a series of sac like structures called *haustra*. Hanging off the tenia coli are *epiploic appendages* which are small fat filled packets.

The *ileocecal valve* is a sphincter that normally stays closed. The *ileocecal reflex* is initiated during eating. As an example, take an individual who has just woken up and is now eating breakfast. During the night, fecal material travelled down the ileum and became lodged in the terminal ileum. At breakfast, when food enters the stomach, gastrin is released by the G-cells in the stomach, duodenum, and pancreas. Gastrin has several effects, one of which is to simulate the ileum to contract. The parasympathetic efferent fibers traveling on the vagus nerve will also stimulate the ileocecal valve to open. The combination of the valve opening, plus the contractions will move material from the ileum to the cecum through the valve.

The cecum is a transition zone for where the GI tract moves from peritoneal to retroperitoneal, but there is significant variation between individuals of where exactly this transition occurs. There is typically a *superior ileocecal fold* and an *inferior cecal fold* at the junction where the ileum meets the cecum. These folds form the basis for the *superior* and *inferior ileocecal recesses*. In this region one can also see the appendicular artery, traveling behind the ileum to the appendix. The cecum gives rise to the ascending colon which is a retroperitoneal structure.

At the hepatic flexure, the ascending colon turns into the transverse colon which is an intraperitoneal structure. Its mesentery is the *transverse mesocolon*, whose two layers run towards the pancreas and then split to go either superior or inferior to the pancreas. The attachment of the mesocolon can then be seen anterior to the pancreas which is a retroperitoneal structure. The tail of the pancreas is intraperitoneal and is bounded by the lienorenal ligament. Paralleling the ascending colon, and lateral to the colon, is the right paracolic gutter.

The artery of the midgut is the *superior mesenteric artery,* and its first branch is the *inferior pancreatic duodenal artery*. It heads superiorly to contribute blood to the inferior portions of the head of the pancreas and the second part of the duodenum. It meets and forms an anastomosis with the superior pancreatic duodenal artery from the gastroduodenal artery. This anastomosis occurs on the head of the pancreas and represents the meeting of the artery of the foregut—celiac trunk- with the artery of the midgut—superior mesenteric artery. Blockage of the aorta just above the celiac trunk would lead to enlarged arteries on the head of the pancreas.

As the superior mesenteric continues, its branches can be divided into those on the left and those on the right. On the left are *10–12 intestinal branches*, some of which are *jejunal branches*, and some of which are *ileal branches*. These *jejunoileal branches* head towards the small intestine with several differences between the two groups. In general, the jejunal branches are straighter, thicker, wider, and more vascular (redder). As each branch approaches its target, it divides in two and meets up with the branches from the neighboring artery which is also branching. Where the branches meet there is an arcade, and there can be several levels of arcades: primary, secondary, or tertiary. And all the arcades are connected—like a spider web. From the jejunal branches there is typically just one level of arcades, but from the ileal branches it is common to see secondary and tertiary levels. Coming off the arcades are straight branches or vasa recta which eventually pierce the intestinal wall. At the point where the vasa recta pierce the abdominal wall this leads to a weakness in the wall. This weakness predisposes the intestinal wall to *diverticulosis*, which are small outpocketings of the lining. They are typically asymptomatic and can appear anywhere along the GI tract but are most common along the large intestine. If an infection develops in these outpocketings, this is referred to as *diverticulitis*.

Coming off the right side of the superior mesenteric artery are branches going to the large intestine. There is significant variation in the pattern of these branches, but regardless of the variation they are named for the portion of the large intestine for which they are heading. The *ileocolic artery* heads towards the point where the distal ileum meets the cecum. And coming off the ileocolic artery are the *anterior and posterior cecal arteries*, and the *appendicular artery* which heads posterior to the ileum to travel to the appendix.

The *right colic artery* travels to the ascending colon, while the *middle colic artery* heads towards the transverse colon. Like the intestinal arteries and their arcades, the main arterial branches to the large intestine also branch to meet up with their neighbors, which also branched. This branching forms a continuous channel called the *marginal artery (marginal artery of Drummond)*, which will eventually in turn meet up with the arching branches coming from the inferior mesenteric artery (Figs. 3.22 and 3.23).

Intestinal Villi

The most important job of the small intestine is to absorb the nutrients, such as amino acids and carbohydrates, and water. The surface area of the small intestine is about 250 square meters, or 2700 square feet or about 100 times the surface area of your skin. To increase the surface area of the small intestine there are numerous layers of folds. The first layer of folding involves the plicae circulares which starts about 2 cm from the pyloric sphincter and continues to the ileum. The plicae circular increases the surface area by about six-fold. The next layer of folding is the villi which are finger like extensions into the lumen of the GI tract and which increase the surface area by about ten-fold. The microvilli increase the surface area by about 20-fold. The wall of the small intestine has five layers: mucosa, submucosa, circular muscle, longitudinal muscle, and serosa. The mucosa layer in turn has three layers: epithelium, lamina propria, and muscularis mucosae. The villi are extensions of the mucosa into the lumen of the jejunoileum and are the main site of

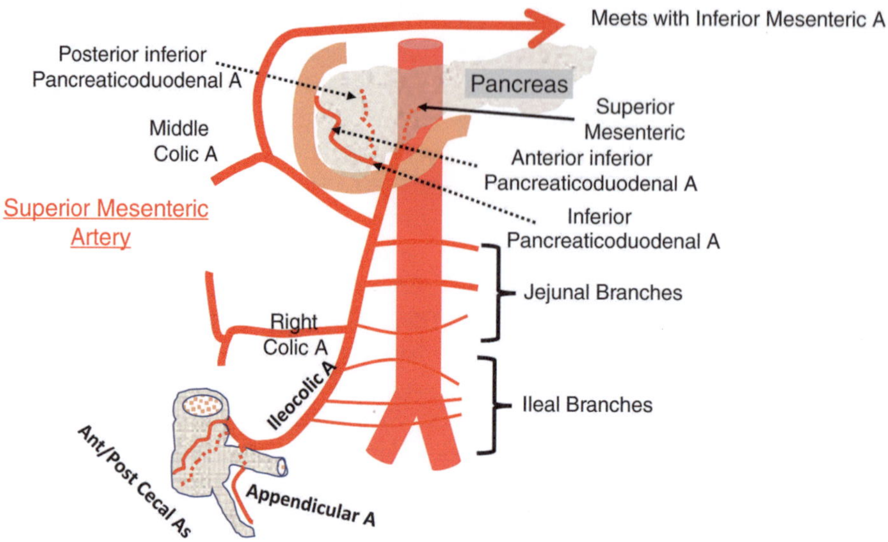

Fig. 3.23 The superior mesenteric artery arises from the abdominal aorta posterior to the neck of the pancreas. It passes anterior to the duodenum. Its first branch is the inferior pancreaticoduodenal artery which divides into anterior and posterior inferior pancreaticoduodenal arteries. These anastomose with branches from the celiac trunk. To the left side, the superior mesenteric artery gives of 10–12 branches to the small intestine, either jejunal or ileal. On the right side it gives off the middle colic, right colic, and ileocolic. The ileocolic gives off cecal branches and an appendicular artery [10, 11]

absorption. The core of the intestinal villi is the lamina propria, a loose connective tissue layer that houses blood vessels and lacteals.

The epithelial layer of the mucosa is made up of several cell types:

1. Absorptive Enterocytes (Columnar Epithelial Cells). These are the most numerous cells. Along their apical border is a ciliated brush border that projects into the lumen of the GI tract to increase the surface area. It is here where nutrients are absorbed by the GI tract.
2. Goblet Cells. These cells are scattered throughout the columnar epithelial layer and release mucous into the GI tract to lubricate it.

   At the base of the villi are the crypts of Lieberkühn which are invaginations from the surface deep into the tissue. At the base of the crypts there are several types of cells (Fig. 3.24).
3. The Paneth cells contain lysozyme and a characterized by large eosinophil cytoplasmic granules.

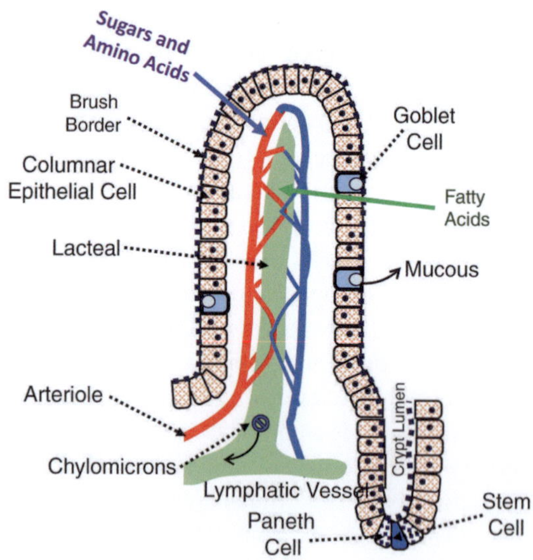

Fig. 3.24 Crypts of Lieberkühn. The most numerous cells in the mucosa layer are the absorptive enterocytes. There are also mucosa secreting goblet cells. In the crypts are the Paneth cells and the stem cells. These stem cells migrate up the villi. It takes about 136 days from the first division to the point where they are sloughed off into the GI tract

4. The stem cells are the cells that give rise to the other cells in the mucosa such as Paneth cells and enterocytes. These enterocytes start at the base of the crypts but then move forward onto the It takes about 142 days for a cell to go from the base of the crypt to eventually be sloughed off.

Hind Gut

The beginning of the hindgut starts with the last one-third of the transverse colon, close to the splenic flexure, and continues into the descending colon, which then turns into the sigmoid colon, and then the rectum. Paralleling the descending colon is the left paracolic gutter. The sigmoid colon is the S-shaped end of the hindgut and is attached to the sigmoid mesocolon. It has a thick muscular layer and is responsible for the movement of fecal material into the rectum.

Inferior Mesenteric Artery

The artery of the hindgut is the inferior mesenteric artery. The inferior mesenteric artery comes off the aorta just behind the horizontal third part of the duodenum. The first branch is the *left colic artery* which has two branches, an *ascending branch* heading towards the splenic flexure and a *descending branch* to the descending colon. The ascending branch runs with the inferior mesenteric vein in the *paraduodenal fold.* It is here where *paraduodenal hernias* can migrate behind these two vessels.

The next group of arteries are the 3–5 *sigmoidal arteries* headed towards the sigmoid colon. The terminal branch of the inferior mesenteric artery is the *superior rectal artery,* traveling down along the sacrum towards the rectum.

Running parallel to the large intestine is the marginal artery which forms an anastomotic network to supply blood to the colon. There are two regions of the descending colon where there are anastomoses between two different arterial systems. These *watershed zones* are susceptible to *ischemic colitis.*

1. *Splenic flexure.* The superior mesenteric artery supplies the proximal two-thirds of the transverse colon. The distal one-third of the transverse colon is supplied by the inferior mesenteric artery. Where these two systems meet is called *Griffith's Point.*
2. *Rectosigmoid junction.* The sigmoidal arteries supply the sigmoid colon. The rectum is supplied by the superior rectal arteries. Where these two systems meet is a potential weak point in the blood supply. This region is referred to as *Sudek's Point* (Figs. 3.25 and 3.26).

Watershed Regions

The arteries to the GI tract cover a wide territory, and some of the cells in the associated structures live close to the arteries while others are located at the periphery. There are advantages and disadvantages for the cells at the periphery which is referred to as a watershed zone. On one hand, cells at the periphery can receive blood from several arteries, but, on the other hand, when blood pressure decreases across the whole territory, then these cells are the first to suffer. These cells are like houses situated at the periphery of the territory supplied by a city water supply—they can get water from two sources, but if pressure in the water system goes down then these are the houses that suffer. Or in the case of hypotension, this affects the cells at the splenic flexure (Fig. 3.25).

Clinical Scenarios

A *volvulus* is a twisting of the small or large intestine and the mesentery that can lead to blockage of the GI tract. It is rare but it is more common in children than adults. In the large intestine it can happen at the cecum, transverse colon, and sigmoid colon. Air will often collect in the twisted section and on radiographs will resemble a coffee bean shape. It is considered an emergency.

Intussusception occurs when one portion of the intestine slips into the neighboring section, like one section of a telescope sliding into the adjacent section. This will lead to blockage of the

Fig. 3.25 Inferior Mesenteric Artery [10, 11]

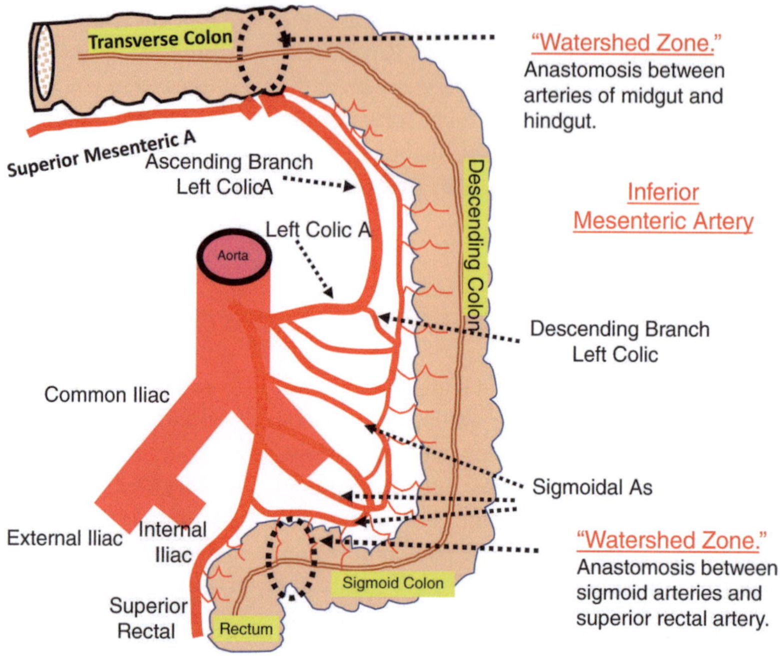

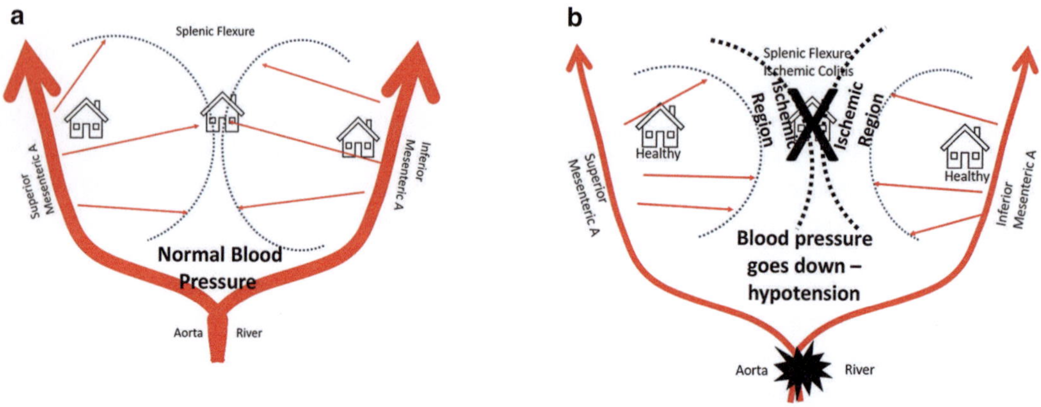

Fig. 3.26 Watershed Zones. As an analogy, compare cells to houses, and arteries to the water supply going to the houses. The aorta gives off the superior and inferior mesenteric arteries, each of which has a perfusion territory. The two territories meet at the splenic flexure. The cells living at this territory can potentially receive blood from both arteries. If we compare these two arterial branches to rivers coming off a main trunk—the aorta—then houses like cells, living at this territory can receive water or blood from both arteries or rivers. However, when there is a drought and water pressure goes down across the system. Then the houses or cells at the periphery of the perfusion ranges will be the first to suffer. Therefore, ischemic colitis usually is evident at the splenic flexure. The houses or cells, living in closer to the arteries or rivers will be spared. These watershed areas are found in several areas of the body—besides the GI tract they are also found in the brain, namely between the middle and anterior cerebral arteries [10, 11]

intestine and often cuts off the blood supply to the affected section. It is considered an emergency.

Mesenteric Adenitis can occur following bacterial or viral infections which leads to inflammation of abdominal lymph nodes in the region of the appendix which can cause pain in the region of the lower right quadrant which can often be mistaken for appendicitis. However, it is only temporary and does not require surgery. It is rare and most often found in preteens.

The Liver

The liver has two surfaces, the *visceral* and *diaphragmatic surfaces*, and is divided anatomically into the *right* and *left lobes* by the *falciform ligament*. The falciform ligament was chosen by early anatomists as the dividing line because of its obvious visual landmark. We will see later that the functional division based on blood flow is slightly different. But for now, sticking with the anatomical divisions, the caudate and quadrate lobes are in the anatomical right lobe of the liver. Starting at the inferior border of the liver, the visceral layer of peritoneal membrane is adherent to the diaphragmatic surface, but near the top of the liver it is reflected onto the inferior surface of the diaphragm. This U-turn of the peritoneum back onto itself creates a fold called the *coronary ligament*. There are two coronary ligaments, one on each side. As you follow either coronary ligament laterally, each one comes to a point called the triangular ligament - either the *right triangular* or *left triangular ligament*. On the opposite side of each coronary ligament, the surface of the liver does not have a peritoneal covering, which is called the *bare area of the liver*. The peritoneum also travels up the posterior surface creating a space which is a continuation of the lesser sac. *Glisson's Capsule* is the connective tissue on the external surface of the liver (Fig. 3.27).

The *porta hepatis* is the doorway to the liver. Several structures pass through the doorway. There are the right and left hepatic arteries and right and left hepatic portal veins going into the liver. And coming out of the liver are the right and left hepatic ducts. Thus, two systems, the artery and vein, are entering the liver at the porta hepatis, and one, the biliary system, is exiting the liver. On the visceral surface of the liver is the *ligamentum venosum* which is the remanent of the ductus venosus which allowed blood to bypass the liver during development. During fetal development, it ran from the portal vein to the inferior vena cava.

Based on the blood flow patterns, we now have a more in-depth understanding of the internal architecture of the liver. Using the perfusion territories of the right and left hepatic arteries and veins, the true dividing line between right and left lobes is a line drawn between the gallbladder fossa and the inferior vena cava, which is slightly to the right of the falciform ligament. The *quadrate lobe* and *caudate lobes* are in the functional left lobe of the liver. However, the caudate lobe receives a dual blood supply from both the right and left hepatic arteries, because it has a small extension called the *caudate process* which is found between the porta hepatis and the inferior vena cava, and it extends over to the right side.

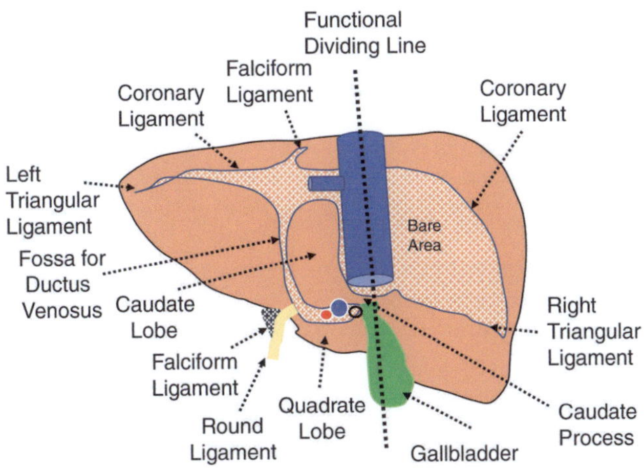

Fig. 3.27 Visceral Surface of Liver. The bare area is not covered by peritoneum. The peritoneal folds make up the coronary ligaments. At the corner of thecoronary ligaments are the triangular ligaments. The porta hepatis contains branches of the portal vein, bile duct and hepatic arteries. A line running from the Inferior vena cava through the gallbladder divides the liver into the functional right and left lobes [10, 11]

Most of the caudate lobe is in the left lobe but the caudate process is in the right lobe.

Liver Architecture

The liver is the chemical processing plant of the body and is involved with several different functions such as: (1) gluconeogenesis which turns amino acids into glucose, (2) the storage of glucose as glycogen which can then be used when energy is low, (3) detoxification of drugs, (4) the production of urea, (5) storage of vitamin A in Ito cells, (6) metabolism of ethanol by alcohol dehydrogenase, and (6) the removal of old red blood cells. The most prominent cells in the liver are the hepatocytes that are lined up in single-file formation forming plate-like structures radiating outward from the portal triad to the central vein (Fig. 3.27).

Blood from both the hepatic artery and portal vein enters the hepatic lobule at the corners and then travels to the central vein. On the way, the blood mixes in the sinusoids which are lined by discontinuous and fenestrated endothelium. Outside the sinusoids are the hepatocytes with their basolateral surface facing the sinusoids. However, there is a small space between the hepatocytes and the sinusoids called the *space of Disse* (perisinusoidal space). In the space of Disse are the *Ito cells* which contain lipid droplets containing vitamin A. Ito cells are also referred to as stellate cells, because of their star-like shape with processes extending from the cell body to enwrap the sinusoids. When the liver is damaged, these Ito cells become activated and are involved in the formation of scar tissue or fibrosis. Sitting inside the sinusoids are the *Kupfer cells* which are phagocytic cells responsible for phagocytosing bacteria, and for destroying old red blood cells to release both iron and bilirubin. The Kupfer cells patrol the sinusoids and remove foreign substances that travel into the liver with the blood from the portal vein (Fig. 3.28).

The apical surfaces of the hepatocytes house the bile canaliculi, which in turn come together to form the *canals of Hering*, which turn into the *bile ductules*, and then the hepatic ducts. While blood is moving from the corners to the center, the bile is moving from the center towards the corners of the lobule. Bile is made up of bile acids, bile salts, and bilirubin. Bile will eventually be secreted into the duodenum, where it plays a role in emulsification of fats. By breaking down larger lipid droplets into smaller droplets, this allows more surface area for the pancreatic lipases to act upon.

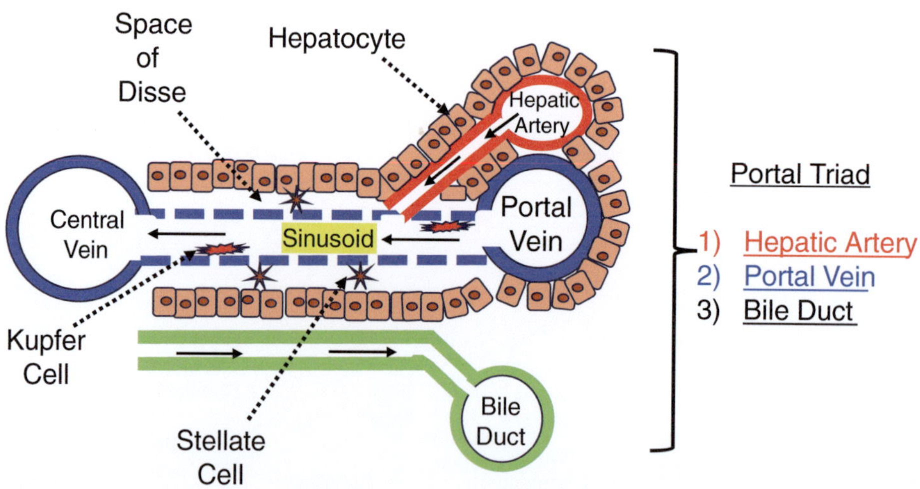

Fig. 3.28 Portal Triad. At the triad are branches of the hepatic artery, portal vein, and bile duct. Blood from the hepatic artery and portal vein comingle at the sinusoid and drain towards the central vein. In the sinusoids are the Kupfer cells. Between the sinusoids and the hepatocytes are the stellate cells. Bile is flowing in the opposite direction to exit the liver

Gallbladder and Bile Ducts

The *gallbladder* is divided into *fundus, body, and neck*. The fundus is at the tip of the ninth costal cartilage in the mid-clavicular line and rests on top of the second part of the duodenum and is pointed inferior and anterior. The fundus is encircled by peritoneum. The body is adherent to the visceral surface of the liver and sits in the gallbladder fossa. Its inferior surface is covered by peritoneum. Bile is made in the liver and transported from the liver to gallbladder to be stored until it is needed. Coming out of the liver are the *right* and *left hepatic* ducts which merge to form the *common hepatic duct*, which in turn merges with the *cystic duct* coming out of the gallbladder, to make up the *common bile duct*. The common bile duct heads inferior, going behind (posterior) the first part of duodenum, to enter the second part of the duodenum at the *greater duodenal papilla* along with the main pancreatic duct. The accessory pancreatic duct comes off the pancreatic duct and enters the duodenum at the *minor duodenal papilla*.

At the greater duodenal papilla, the common bile duct is joined by the *pancreatic duct* which sends digestive enzymes into the duodenum. Bile stones that block the great duodenal papilla will block the pancreatic secretions to the duodenum (Fig. 3.29).

The *proper hepatic artery* branches into the *right and left hepatic arteries*, and the right hepatic artery goes behind (posterior) the common hepatic duct and the gives off the *cystic artery* to the gallbladder in the *cystohepatic triangle* (triangle of calot) which is bounded by the liver, cystic duct, and common hepatic duct. The *cystic artery* lies within the triangle. There is significant variation in the origin of the cystic artery, but it is usually from the *right hepatic artery* (Fig. 3.30).

Liver and Portal System

Blood flow to the limbs involves a single-in-line capillary bed. Oxygen leaves the heart on an artery and travels to the capillary bed where it perfuses across the capillary wall to deliver oxygen to a muscle. The veins then return the oxygen poor blood to the heart. However, the portal system has two capillary beds in-line. There are portal systems in several organs, such as the gastrointestinal tract, the kidney, and the pituitary system. When we talk about the gastrointestinal tract and the hepatic portal system, the first capillary bed is in the wall of the jejunoileum. While the gastrointestinal tract runs from mouth to anus, contents inside the tract are not in the body, per se. Contents that come in through the mouth and leave through the anus have never crossed the body wall. However, within the wall of the jejunoileum are capillary beds so that nutrients such as amino acids, and triglycerides that have been broken down in the gastrointestinal tract are absorbed through the walls of the jejunoileum into veins. These substances along with toxins, such as alcohol and drugs, whether licit or illicit, need to be processed by the liver, and they travel

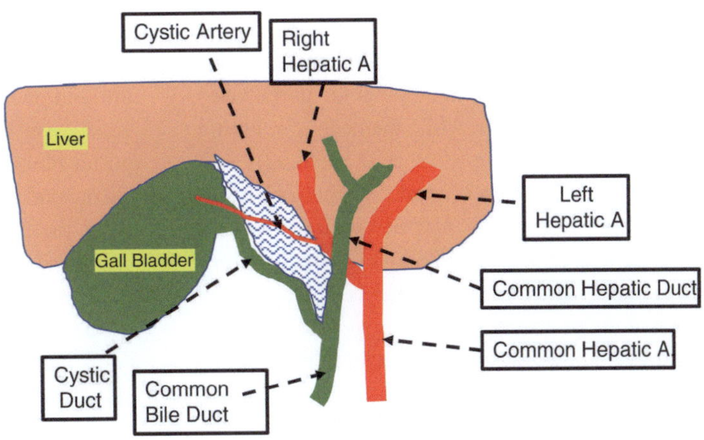

Fig. 3.29 Cystohepatic Triangle (Calot). The triangle is the shaded blue region bounded by visceral surface of liver, cystic duct, and common hepatic duct. (Note the cystic artery coming off the right hepatic artery. The right hepatic artery goes behind the bile duct [10, 11]

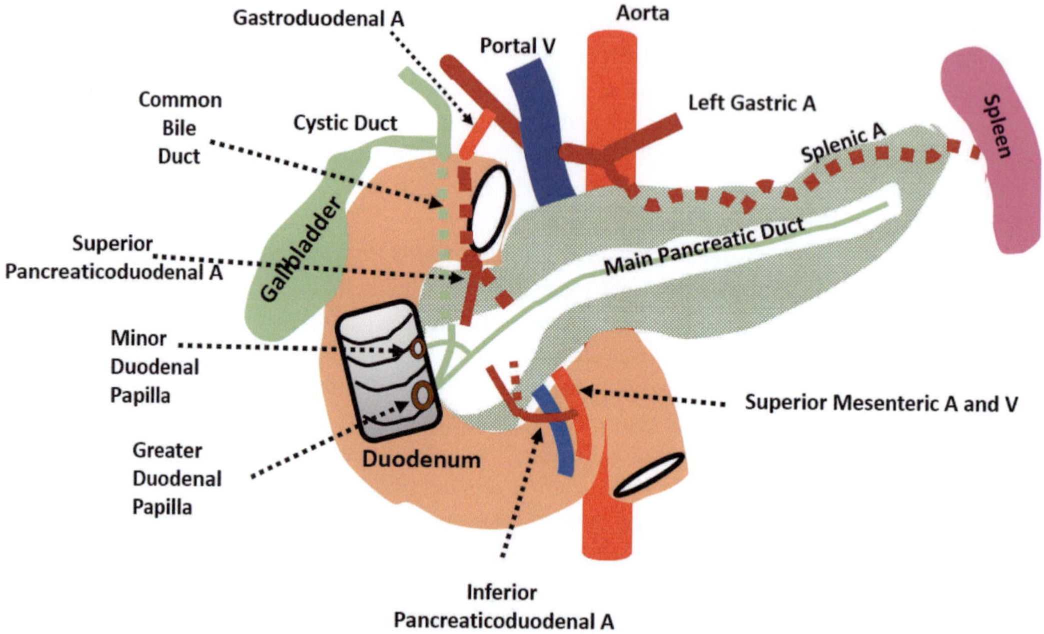

Fig. 3.30 Pancreas, Duodenum, and Gallbladder. Note that the gastroduodenal artery and the common bile duct travel posterior to the first part of the duodenum. The common bile duct joins the main pancreatic duct to enter the duodenum at the greater duodenal papilla. The accessory pancreatic duct enters at the minor duodenal papilla [10, 11]

from that first capillary bed in the jejunoileum to a second capillary bed in the liver via the hepatic portal system.

Pathology in the portal system, such as cirrhosis of the liver, will lead to portal hypertension. This is analogous to putting a dam in the middle of a stream. The water, or in this case the blood, will look for an alternate route around the liver. The blood will now attempt to travel back along the caval system. When blood pressure in the portal veins increases, then pressure in the hepatic veins will typically decrease. Remember the portal veins are going into the liver, while the hepatic veins are coming out of the liver (Figs. 3.31 and 3.32).

The portal system is made by the joining of three large veins. The *inferior mesenteric vein* ascends and joins the *splenic vein* which in turn meets the *superior mesenteric vein* behind the neck of the pancreas, to form the *portal vein*. The portal vein now ascends to the liver in the *hepatoduodenal ligament* (part of the lesser omentum) to enter at the porta hepatis.

The portal system forms several anastomoses with the caval system, and it is at these sites where pathologies will develop in cases of portal hypertension (Fig. 3.31).

1. *Hemorrhoids.* The dividing line in the rectum is the *pectinate line*. Above the pectinate line, normally blood drains to the superior rectal vein, to the inferior mesenteric vein, to the portal vein. While blood below the pectinate line, drains to the inferior rectal vein, to the internal pudendal vein, and then to the inferior vena cava. In the case of liver pathology, the portal blood pressure rises. At the anastomosis around the pectinate line, blood will now cross the line to drain into the inferior rectal vein, and eventually the inferior vena cava. The veins in this region, which are very superficial, can become dilated creating an outpocketing of tissue—referred to as hemorrhoids, which can be classified as internal or external. Internal hemorrhoids are

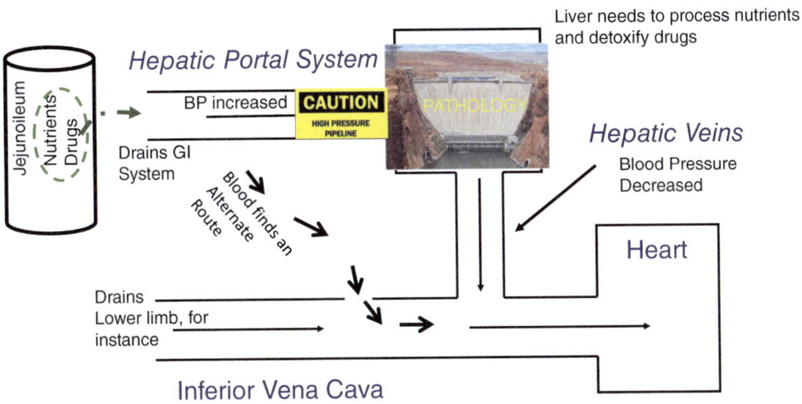

Fig. 3.31 Hepatic Portal versus Inferior Vena Cava. Blood draining the jejunoileum follows the hepatic portal system back to the liver to be processed. Meanwhile, blood from the limbs does not need to go through the liver so it drains via the inferior vena cava back to the heart [10, 11]

Fig. 3.32 Hepatic Portal System [10, 11]

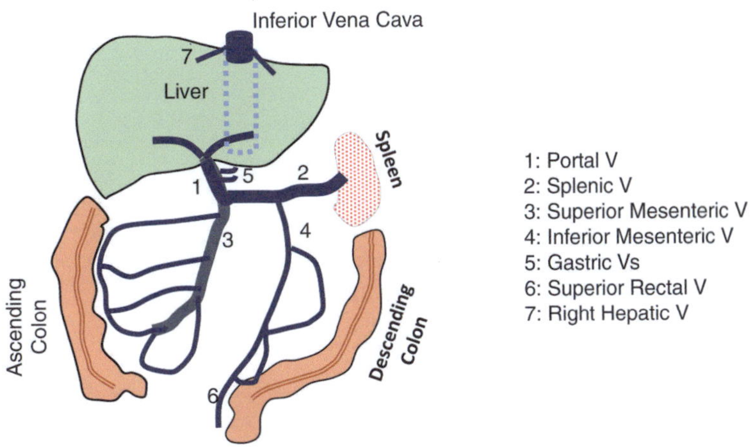

above the pectinate line, while external hemorrhoids are below the pectinate line (Fig. 3.33).

2. *Esophageal Varices.* The terminal esophagus is another site of anastomoses. The esophageal veins in the most distal part of the esophagus drain to the gastric veins and then to the portal vein. Just above this region, the esophagus drains to the caval system, via the azygos veins. With portal hypertension, the veins in this region become dilated and enlarged. The danger is that they can rupture with copious loss of blood and a subsequent emergency.
3. *Caput Medusa.* In the region of the umbilicus, paraumbilical veins follow the round ligament to drain into the left branch of the portal vein. Around the umbilicus are also numerous superficial epigastric veins which drain into the femoral vein. With liver pathology, the anastomoses also lead to dilated veins which radiate out from the umbilicus. These dilated veins are thought to resemble the snakes coming out of Medusa's head.
4. *Splenomegaly.* The splenic vein which drains the spleen can also be backed up because of the increased pressure which can lead to an enlarged spleen (Fig. 3.33).
5. *Ascites.* Normally there is only a small amount of fluid (5-20mls) in the peritoneal cavity. Portal hypertension can lead to excess fluid in the cavity, referred to ascites. The fluid can be removed with paracentesis—placement of a small drainage tube in the peritoneal cavity. Besides portal hypertension, other conditions such as hepatitis or excessive alcohol intake can lead to ascites (Fig. 3.34).

Fig. 3.33 Portal Hypertension. Liver pathology leads to portal hypertension. Venous blood then drains into the inferior rectal vein and back to the inferior vena cava [10, 11]

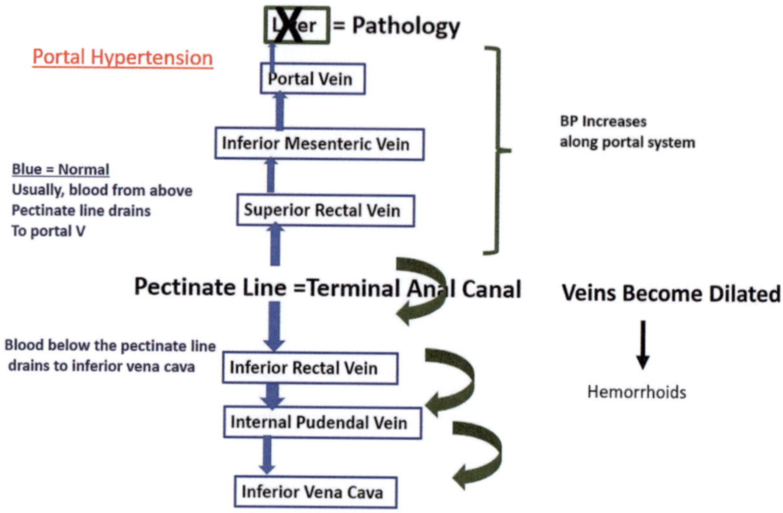

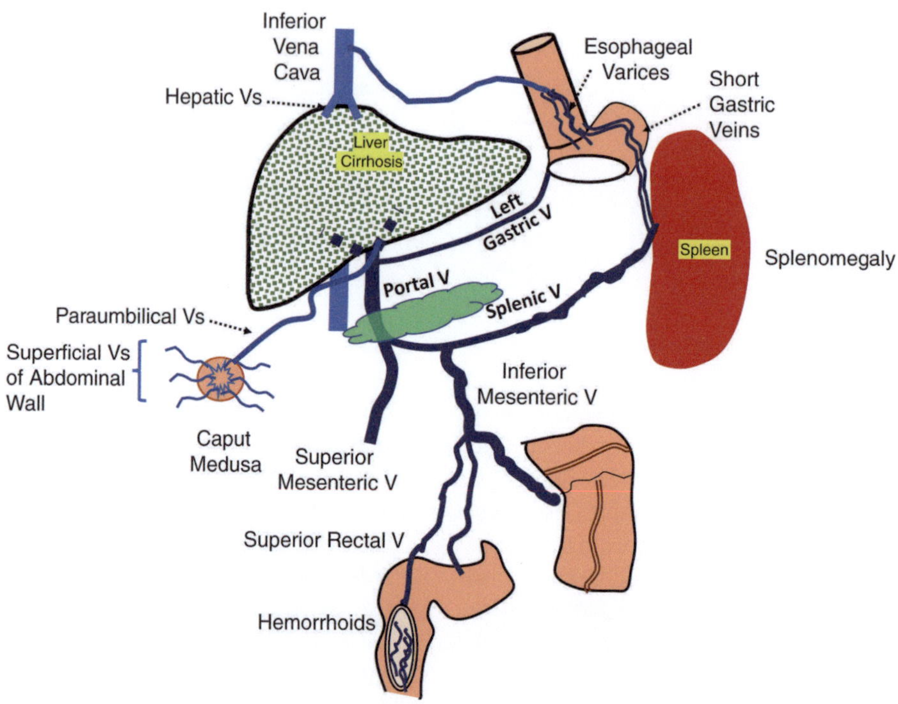

Fig. 3.34 Portal Venous System. Note the inferior mesenteric vein draining into the splenic vein, which then joins the superior mesenteric vein to form the portal vein. Portal hypertension results in esophageal varices, caput medusa, and hemorrhoids. Pancreas pathology will also lead to portal hypertension but the patient will not have esophageal varices or a caput medusa because the veins drain into the portal system above the blockage [10, 11]

Pancreatitis and Portal Hypertension

Pancreatitis can impede blood running in the splenic vein which is referred to as left-sided or sinistral portal hypertension. This may lead to some but not all the same signs as liver induced portal hypertension. For instance, it may lead to splenomegaly, gastric varices or esophageal varices blood backing up in the rectum, the spleen, and the fundus of the stomach. But it will not lead to caput medusa. Liver function will be normal with blockage of the splenic vein (Fig. 3.31).

Liver Subdivisions

There are three ways to divide up the internal architecture of the liver (Fig. 3.35).

1. The most common division is the *classic hepatic lobule* which is a hexagon. As the three structures come into the liver at the porta hepatis. From here they all branch but the branches stay together and are found at the corner of each side of a hexagon. This portal triad has a branch of the hepatic artery carrying oxygen into the liver, a branch of the portal vein carrying nutrients and toxins ready to be metabolized or detoxified into the liver, and a branch of the bile duct carrying bile out of the liver and on towards the biliary tract.

   Blood from the hepatic artery and hepatic portal vein then travels from the corners or periphery of the lobule towards the center to eventually drain into the central vein, which in turn will drain into the hepatic vein and finally the inferior vena cava.
2. The *portal lobule*, a triangle, is simply another way to divide up the liver. Rather than the central vein at the center, the center is one of the portal triads, and the central veins are at the three corners. The blood moves from the center, where one finds a branch of hepatic artery and portal vein, to the periphery.
3. The *liver acinus* is a four-sided trapezoid with four points. The center piece is a line drawn between two portal triads. Blood is moving bilaterally from this midline structure to the central veins at the other two points. As the blood moves from the center towards the periphery, pathologists have divided the regions up into three zones. *Zone 1* is closest to the midline structure and will have the highest concentration of oxygen, so it will be the last of the three regions affected by ischemia. *Zone 3* on the other hand is the farthest away from the center, making it the least oxygenated and most susceptible to ischemia. Zone 3 also has the highest concentration of

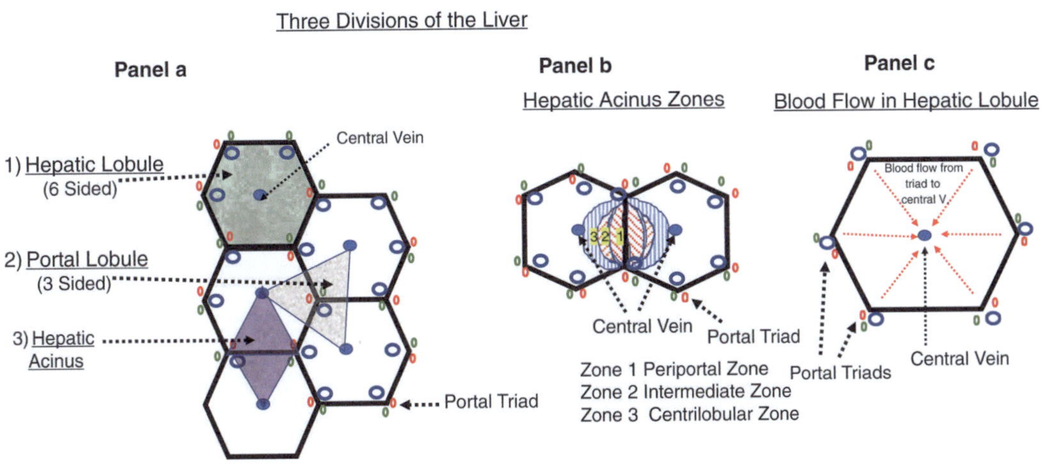

Fig. 3.35 Three Divisions of the Liver. Panel (**a**) shows the three different ways to divide up the liver into segments. Panel (**b**) shows the organization of the hepatic acinus. Panel (**c**) shows the blood flow in the hepatic lobule from the triads at each corner to the central vein [10, 11]

cytochrome P450 leading to the breakdown of metabolic processes building up here (Fig. 3.34).

Pancreas

The pancreas is both an exocrine and endocrine gland. Its exocrine portion involves the production and secretion of pancreatic enzymes. The enzymes travel on the main pancreatic duct to enter the second part of the duodenum at the greater duodenal papilla and minor duodenal papilla. The endocrine portion of the pancreas is handled in physiology textbooks (Fig. 3.36).

Spleen

The spleen lies against ribs 9, 10, and 11 on the left side in the mid-axillary line. In a patient with trauma to this region the spleen can easily be damaged. There are two ligaments associated with the spleen. The *lienorenal ligament* connects the spleen to the kidney. The tail of the pancreas and the splenic artery enter the lienorenal ligament. The *gastrosplenic ligament* connects the stomach and spleen and is part of the greater omentum. Just before the splenic artery enters the spleen, it gives off the *short gastric arteries* that head to the fundus of the stomach.

In some cases, the ligaments do not form properly, and the spleen is able to move within the cavity resulting in a "wandering spleen." Accessory spleens can also be found within the ligaments.

Internal Architecture of the Spleen

The spleen is made up of two different compartments:

1. The red pulp (80% of the spleen) consists of splenic cords and splenic sinusoids and is responsible for removing damaged and aged-red blood cells from circulation.
2. The white pulp (20% of the spleen) is responsible for initiating a primary immune response. The white pulp houses up to one-fourth of the body's lymphocytes and is further divided into three compartments: *the peri arteriole lymphatic sheath* (PALS) which is a collection of T-cells surrounding the central arteriole, the *marginal zone*, and the *follicles* (Fig. 3.37).

The splenic artery enters the hilum and splits into trabecular arteries known as central arterioles which are surrounded by the PALS. Blood percolating out of these arterioles has two different options: (1) The "fast option" involves the blood moving quickly into the venous channels in the

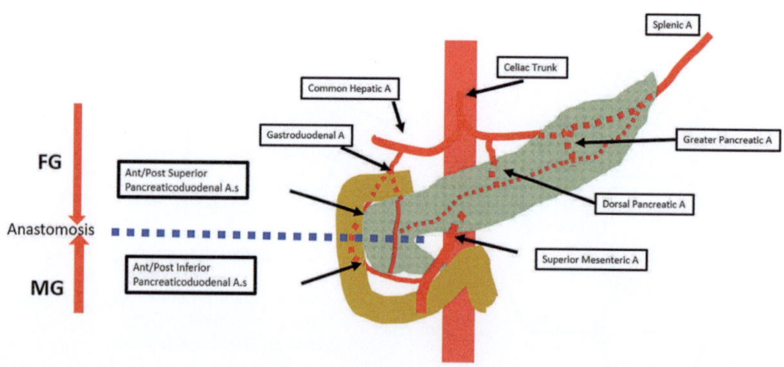

Fig. 3.36 Blood Supply to Pancreas. The gastroduodenal comes from celiac trunk and gives off the anterior and posterior superior pancreaticoduodenal arteries which supply the superior portion of the pancreas and duodenum. The superior mesenteric artery gives of the anterior and posterior inferior pancreaticoduodenal arteries which supply the inferior portion of the pancreas and duodenum [10, 11]

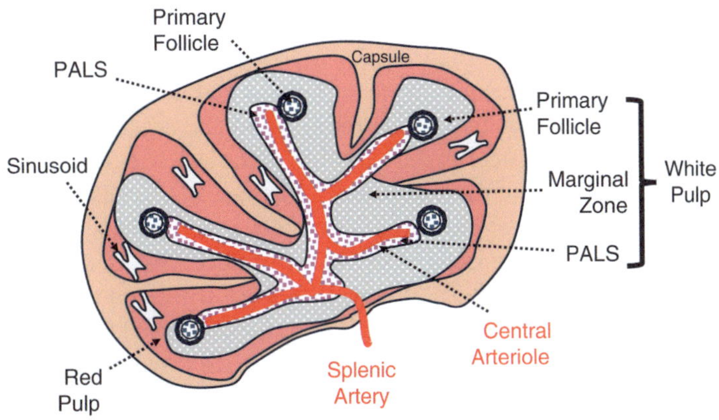

Fig. 3.37 The Spleen. The white pulp consists of the primary follicle, the marginal zone, and the PALS. The central arteriole travels down the PALS towards a primary follicle. The white pulp is surrounded by red pulp. Within the red pulp are sinuses [10, 11]

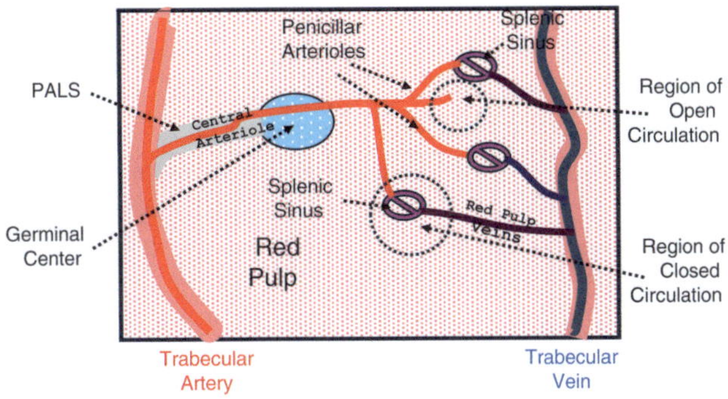

Fig. 3.38 Spleen, Open and Closed Circulation. Blood travelling along the Penicillar arteries has two options: (1) *Open Circulation,* where blood dumps directly into the red pulp to percolate among the cells, (2) *Closed Circulation* where blood empties into a splenic sinus and then travels along the veins

marginal zone. In this scenario, the blood is bypassing the red pulp. Most of the blood uses this pathway. (2) the slow option involves a smaller portion of the blood volume moving out to the red pulp via penicillar arteries (Fig. 3.38).

From the penicillar arteries, the blood can then move to the sinusoids. In this case the blood is always surrounded by endothelium, forming a *closed loop*. But the blood from the penicillar arteries can also move into the stroma of the cords. This is an example of an *open loop* and in this scenario, blood must reenter the system, which occurs between small slits between the cells. It is here where swollen or damaged RBCs are kept from reentry to the blood stream. The RBCs that are denied entry are destroyed by macrophages.

The White Pulp

1. The PALS region surrounding the central arteriole is a T cell rich collection containing mostly CD4+ T cells. The outer portion of the PALS includes T and B cells. It is here where plasma cell formation starts.
2. The marginal zone is located between the PALS and the red pulp and plays a role in antigen processing.
3. The follicles are continuous with the PALS and are filled mostly with B cells. In the presence of antigens, the follicles will typically contain germinal centers, which are less dense and stain lighter than the surrounding tissue.

Referred Pain

The afferent nerve innervation to the GI tract and the visceral peritoneum comes from the autonomic nervous system, which are the thoracic and lumbar splanchnic nerves. The thoracic splanchnic nerves originate in the thorax, descend through the diaphragm, and innervate the GI tract and abdominal organs. These fibers sense pressure and distension from the various portions of the tract. They do not sense pain. In the initial stages of pathology the patient is unable to precisely localize the source of pain. Instead of pointing to the exact source of the pain, they tend to point to regions. Pain from any foregut structure will refer to the epigastric region. Pain from any midgut structure will refer to the umbilical region. Pain from any hindgut structure will refer to the hypogastric region.

Once the pathology has become large enough it will aggravate the parietal perineum which will trigger pain sensations along the somatic nervous system, and the patient will now be able to precisely localize the pain (Fig. 3.39).

Take appendicitis as an example. In the initial stages, when the inflamed appendix is in the initial stages and the appendix is not large, it will aggravate the visceral peritoneum. At this point, the patient will complain of pain around the hypogastric region—they will point to their umbilicus. However, as time goes on, say 4–6 h, and the appendix has gotten larger, it will now aggravate the parietal peritoneum and the pain will be felt in the right lower quadrant. The appendix lies close to the right iliopsoas and an inflamed appendix can also lead to a positive psoas test, meaning that with the thigh placed against the abdomen, extension of the thigh will lead to pain as the inflamed appendix aggravates the psoas muscle. *Rebound tenderness* occurs with cases of peritonitis. When the examiner compresses the affected area there is minimal pain, however when the examiner releases pressure, the patient complains of sudden sharp pain. This is due to pressure on the parietal peritoneum.

Rovsing's sign is a rare finding that sometimes occurs with appendicitis. When pressure is applied to the left lower flank, the patient feels pain in the right lower abdomen. It is not entirely clear why this happens but the pressure on the left side is thought to be caused by gas or intestinal loops pushing towards the right which leads to the appendix rubbing on the anterior wall.

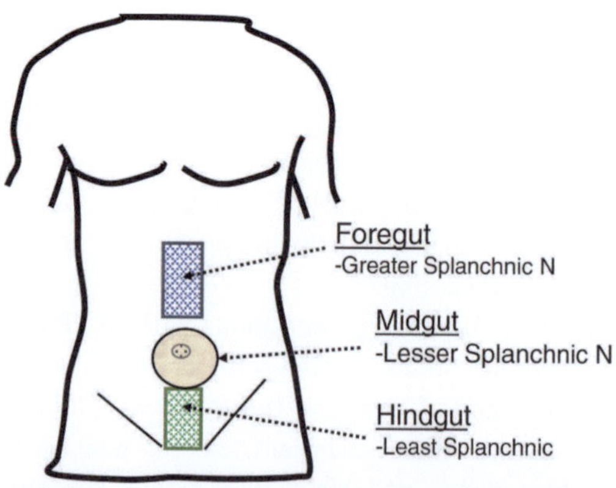

Fig. 3.39 Visceral Sensation. Pain sensation from foregut travels on greater splanchnic nerves and is referred to epigastric region. From midgut on lesser splanchnic nerves and is referred to umbilical region. From hindgut on least splanchnic nerves and is referred to hypogastric region [10, 11]

Greater, Lesser, and Least Splanchnic Nerves

In the section above we used the term thoracic splanchnic nerves and pointed out that these are the sympathetic nerves carrying afferent and efferent fibers to and from the viscera. But we can also be more specific. The thoracic splanchnic nerves include the *greater splanchnic nerve* from T5–9, the *lesser splanchnic nerve* from T10–11, and the *least splanchnic nerve* from T12. These nerves all contain preganglionic sympathetic efferent fibers, and visceral afferent fibers from the GI tract.

The preganglionic sympathetic fibers in the greater splanchnic nerves synapse in the celiac ganglion. The post ganglionic fibers then travel on branches of the celiac trunk to innervate the foregut and related structures. Visceral pain fibers from foregut structures travel on the greater splanchnic nerves back to the spinal cord.

The preganglionic sympathetic fibers in the lesser and least splanchnic nerves travel to the superior mesenteric ganglion and the aorticorenal ganglion, and then travel out on branches of the superior mesenteric artery to reach the midgut structures. Visceral afferents from the midgut structures pass back along these nerves to the spinal cord.

Preganglionic fibers of the lumbar splanchnic nerves travel to the inferior mesenteric ganglion. After synapsing, the fibers pass on branches of the inferior mesenteric artery to the hindgut structures. Visceral afferents also pass on these fibers back to the spinal cord.

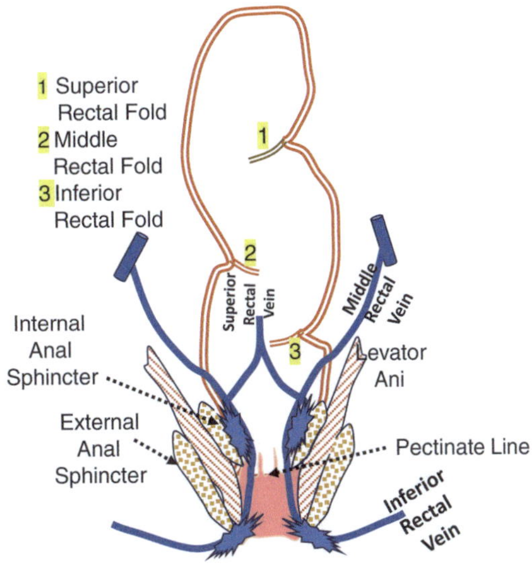

Fig. 3.40 Rectum and Anal Canal. There are three transverse rectal folds, superior, middle, and inferior, projecting into the rectum. The venous drainage below the pectinate line goes to the inferior rectal vein to the internal iliac vein. The venous drainage above the pectinate line drains to the middle and superior rectal veins. The superior rectal veins eventually drain into the portal system [10, 11]

The Rectum and Anal Canal

The rectum is retroperitoneal, or sub peritoneal, because it is inferior to the peritoneal cavity. There are three *transverse rectal folds* also known as the valves of Houston, resembling three shelves stacked on top of each other that serve to slow down the movement of feces through the rectum. The most prominent rectal fold is the middle one, which is referred to as *Kohlrausch's valve*. The space between this middle fold and the anal canal can be expanded to serve as a reservoir for fecal contents. The rectum turns into the short anal canal which ends just above the pectinate line (Fig. 3.40).

The pectinate line is where the hindgut endoderm meets the skin, or ectoderm. It gets its name from the organization of anal valves, anal sinuses, and anal columns, all of which give the pectinate line the appearance of a comb. The anal columns are outpocketings of tissue housing the terminal branches of the superior rectal artery and veins. On the side of each column is a space called the anal sinus. Running from the terminal end of each anal column is a valve which is a thin piece of tissue connecting each column to its neighboring column. The pectinate line is a line of demarcation for the region. The nerve innervation, the arterial blood supply, the venous drainage pattern, the lymphatic flow, and classification of hemorrhoids are all based on the pectinate line (Table 3.1).

Venous Drainage of Anal Canal

The venous drainage above the pectinate line is from the *superior rectal vein*, which drains to the inferior mesenteric vein, and then to the portal vein. The drainage below the pectinate line is from the *inferior rectal vein*, then to the *internal pudendal vein*, the internal iliac vein, and finally to the inferior vena cava. Thus, at the pectinate line there is an anastomosis between the portal vein and the inferior vena cava. With liver pathology, blood pressure in the portal vein will rise which in turn leads to increased pressure in the superior rectal vein. The blood in the anal canal will now look for an alternate route around the liver and will travel from the superior rectal vein to the inferior rectal vein, which will lead to dilated veins, or hemorrhoids in this area. *Internal hemorrhoids* are outpocketings *above* the pectinate line, while *external hemorrhoids* are outpocketings *below* the pectinate line.

The afferent nerve supply above the pectinate line comes from the autonomic nervous system,

Table 3.1 Differences Above and Below the Pectinate Line

	Tissue	Venous Drainage	Arterial Supply	Hemorrhoids	Afferent Nerve	Efferent Nerve	Lymphatic Drainage
Above pectinate line	Hindgut endoderm	Superior rectal V to portal V	Sup rectal A	Internal	Autonomics	Pelvic splanchnic	Abdominal nodes
Below pectinate line	Ectoderm	Inferior rectal V to IVC	Inf rectal A	External	Pudendal	Pudendal	Superficial inguinal nodes

the parasympathetic pelvic splanchnic nerves. These nerves are responsible for sensing pressure and have very few pain fibers. The afferent nerve supply below the pectinate line comes from the pudendal nerve which does carry pain sensation. Most patients will typically not feel internal hemorrhoids; however they will feel the paint from external hemorrhoid and complain of pain and itching.

The lymphatic drainage above the pectinate line is to internal iliac nodes, while the lymphatic drainage below the line will drain to the superficial inguinal nodes. See the anteromedial thigh section for specifics on the superficial inguinal nodes.

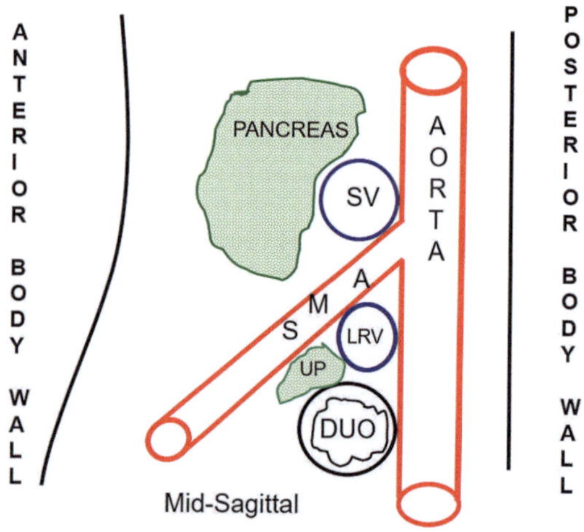

Fig. 3.41 Superior Mesenteric Artery. This midsagittal section shows the superior mesenteric artery emerging from the aorta and passing anterior to the left renal vein, uncinate process of pancreas, and the duodenum [10, 11]

Superior Mesenteric Artery and Nutcracker Syndrome

The superior mesenteric artery (SMA) comes off the aorta at the L1 vertebral body level. The SMA immediately passes the anterior to the left renal vein, which is crossing the aorta to enter the inferior vena cava. Because the inferior vena cava lies to the right of the aorta, the left renal vein passes in front of the aorta to enter the inferior vena cava. Just inferior to the left renal vein where it crosses the aorta is the third part of the duodenum. In front of the SMA is the neck of the pancreas. An analogy to these relationships is that the pancreas is like a fist grabbing the superior mesenteric artery. The pancreas is pushing off from the spleen on the left side and pushing into the duodenum on the right side. The fist, or head of the pancreas is now surrounded by the duodenum. As the hand grabs the SMA, the fingertips extend behind the SMA. The fingertips are analogous to the uncinate process. While most of the hand, or the pancreas, is anterior to the SMA, the tiny uncinate process can slip behind the SMA. The *vascular groove* is the indentation on the uncinate process of the SMA and SMV.

Remember that the pancreas and aorta are retroperitoneal structures, while the superior mesenteric artery is running in the dorsal mesentery. Anterior to the pancreas is the lesser sac, and in front of the lesser sac is the stomach and transverse colon (Fig. 3.41).

Looking anteriorly, as the SMA emerges from the aorta it is surrounded by three veins, like the borders of a window (Figs. 3.42 and 3.43).

1. The *splenic vein* is the top rim of the window, or above the superior mesenteric artery, The splenic vein is coursing from the tail of the

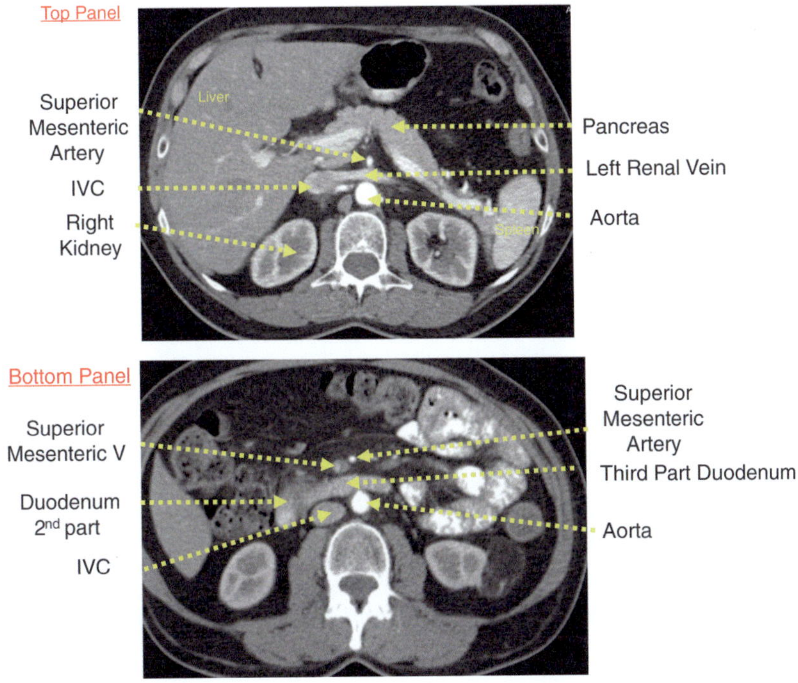

Fig. 3.42 Focus on Superior Mesenteric Artery (SMA). In the top panel we can see the left renal vein (LRV) Between the SMA and the aorta. The LRV is draining into the IVC. We can also see the pancreas in front of the SMA. In the bottom panel we have moved inferiorly, and we now see the duodenum crossing the aorta behind the SMA. The superior mesenteric vein is to the right of the SMA. At this point, the third part of the duodenum is turning into the fourth part [10, 11]

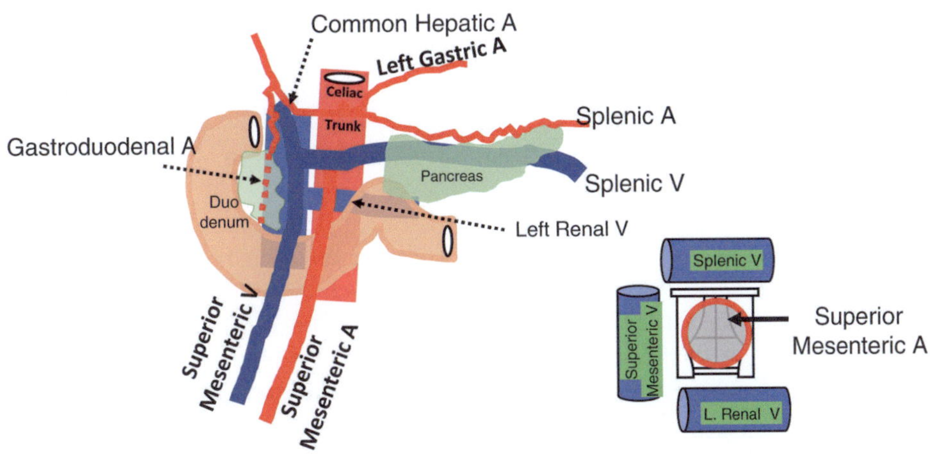

Fig. 3.43 Superior Mesenteric Artery. The emergence of the superior mesenteric artery from the aorta is surrounded on three sides by veins. A section of the pancreas has been removed to see the SMA. Think of the SMA as coming through a window. Above the window is the splenic vein. Below the window is the left renal vein. To the right of the window is the superior mesenteric vein. Note the gastroduodenal artery is passing behind the first part of the duodenum. The celiac trunk has three branches: (1) left gastric, (2) splenic, and (3) the common hepatic [10, 11]

pancreas along the pancreas towards the midline. Along the way it is joined by the inferior mesenteric vein, and then behind the neck of the pancreas it meets the superior mesenteric vein to form the portal vein.

2. the *superior mesenteric vein* forms the right side of the window. Keep in mind that the superior mesenteric vein and artery run together. It makes sense the SMA is found more to left which is same side as aorta, while the superior mesenteric vein is found on right heading towards the liver, also on right.
3. The *left renal vein* forms the windowsill and lies inferior. As mentioned earlier, it crosses from the left kidney, goes across the aorta, and enters the IVC on the right.

Duodenal Fossae and Folds

Near the duodenojejunal flexure where various structures are transitioning from retroperitoneal to intraperitoneal, there is a complicated series of folds and fossae that can lead to weaknesses that in turn can lead to congenital intestinal hernias, classified as either right-sided or left-sided.

Of the two hernias in this region, left-sided are more common. These left-sided hernias are migrations of the intestine into the paraduodenal fossa. The ascending branch of the inferior mesenteric artery and the inferior mesenteric vein run parallel and to the left of the fourth part of the duodenum near the duodenojejunal flexure. At this point, the peritoneum has several folds forming a four-sided window. On the top and bottom of the window are the *superior and inferior duodenal folds* which form the superior and inferior fossae. On the right side of the window is the *paraduodenal fossa* (Landzert's fossa) and on the left side of the window is the *retroduodenal fossa*. The most important fossa in this region is the paraduodenal fossa, or the left side of this window. *Paraduodenal hernias* are herniations of the small intestine into the paraduodenal fossa and are considered left-sided hernias (Fig. 3.44).

Right-sided hernias are associated with the superior mesenteric artery and vein. As the SMA travels over (anterior to) the duodenum, the dorsal mesentery is attached to the superior mesenteric artery. A potential defect at this point can lead to an opening referred to as Waldayer's fossa which can be a site of intestinal herniation. A hernia through Waldayer's fossa is a right-sided hernia going behind the superior mesenteric artery (Fig. 3.43).

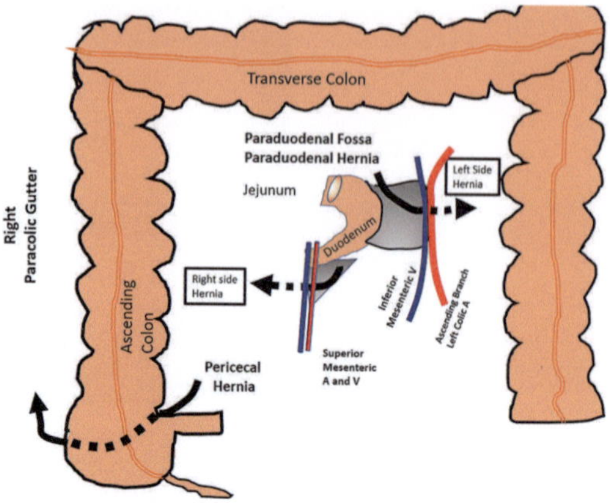

Fig. 3.44 Three internal Hernias. Just lateral to the duodenum is the paraduodenal fold encasing the inferior mesenteric vein and ascending branch of the middle colic artery. (1) Paraduodenal hernias (left-sided) occur just medial to the fold and move into the paraduodenal fossa. (2) Right-sided hernias move behind the superior mesenteric artery and vein. (3) Pericecal hernias move from right to left behind the cecum and can move into the right paracolic gutter [10, 11]

Transpyloric Line

The transpyloric plane or transpyloric line runs across the abdomen through the pyloric region of the stomach at the L1 vertebral body level. It is significant for the structures that it crosses. Rather than just memorizing a list, lets first think about what structures we already know that intersect the transpyloric plane. We will start with the superior mesenteric artery (SMA). We saw earlier that the SMA emerges from the abdominal aorta at L1. As it emerges, it is crossing the left renal vein. Just inferior to the left renal vein is the horizontal part (third part) of the duodenum which is turning into the ascending portion (fourth part) of the duodenum about to join the jejunum. So, the SMA, the left renal vein, the L1 vertebra, and the conus medullaris all lie in the transpyloric plane—remember the spinal cord ends at L1. Likewise, the first part of the duodenum also lies in the plane, as does the pyloric region of the stomach.

Anterior to the SMA, is the neck of the pancreas. To the right of the SMA is the superior mesenteric vein, so you can think about the SMA emerging through the window, mentioned earlier, bounded by three veins; the superior mesenteric vein to the right, the splenic vein is above, and the left renal vein is below. All these veins lie in the transpyloric plane.

The pancreas, except for its tail, is a retroperitoneal structure. Anterior to the pancreas, the visceral peritoneum both from above and below the pancreas merge to form the transverse mesocolon. So, the transverse mesocolon is also in the transpyloric plane. As the pancreas pushes off the spleen and into the duodenum, it comes to lie on top of the hilum of the right kidney. The hilum of the right and left kidneys, pancreas, and the spleen (lower border) all lie in the transpyloric plane.

And as we already discussed, the neck of the gallbladder rests on the first part of the duodenum, so the neck of the gallbladder is also on the transpyloric plane.

A gallstone ileus occurs when an adhesion forms between the gallbladder neck and the first part of the duodenum. The adhesion leads to a fistula between the two with the gallstones migrating into the duodenum. They can eventually become lodged in the ileocecal valve leading to a bowel obstruction.

Internal Pancreas

The exocrine portion of the pancreas is made up of *serous acini* which drain into intercalated ducts. The acini produce pancreatic juice containing digestive enzymes such as lipases, nucleases, and α-amylase, plus bicarbonate (HCO_3^-). The pancreatic digestive enzymes are highly reactive and while their ability to break down various products is beneficial in the duodenum; these enzymes pose a potential problem for pancreatic tissue. Fortunately, there are several biological mechanisms in place to protect pancreatic tissue, such as,

1. Pancreatic acini secrete trypsinogen which is the inactive form of trypsin. The conversion of inactive trypsinogen to active trypsin occurs in the duodenum. In addition, the pancreas secretes a trypsin inhibitor.
2. The presence of HCO_3^- in the pancreatic acini ensures that the enzymes will not be active.

The pancreas also has an endocrine function. Scattered throughout the organ there are small islets of Langerhans (pancreatic islets) containing three types of secretory cells: (1) A cells secrete glucagon, (2) B cells secrete insulin, and the D cells secrete somatostatin, and (4) PP cells secrete pancreatic polypeptide.

After a meal, glucose levels will be high, which leads to secretion of insulin by the B cells. Insulin binds to receptors on the membrane of muscle and adipose cells which leads to an increase in the number of glucose transporters on the cell membrane. This increases the movement of glucose from the blood stream into the cells—blood glucose is lowered making insulin a hypoglycemic hormone.

In a fasting state, the glucose levels will be low, and the A cells will secrete glucagon which will lead to:

1. *Glycogenolysis* is the breakdown of glycogen into glucose. This leads to the liver very quickly releasing glucose into the blood stream, making glucagon a hyperglycemic hormone.
2. *Gluconeogenesis* is the production of new glucose molecules in the liver. This process takes longer and will occur between meals. These glucose molecules also enter the blood stream.

Kidneys

The kidneys lie on the posterior abdominal wall running from the T12 to the L3 vertebrae. Because of the liver's location on the right side of

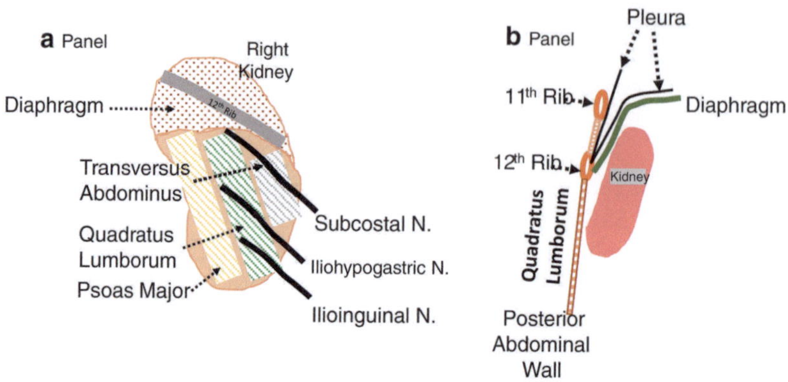

Fig. 3.45 Panel (**a**) is a posterior view of kidney. Note the top part of the kidney that comes up above rib 12 is covered by the diaphragm. Three nerves of the posterior abdominal wall lie posterior to the kidney. Panel (**b**) shows a view from the side. Note that the pleura adherent to the diaphragm comes down between the kidney and posterior abdominal wall [10, 11]

the body, the right kidney is slightly lower than the left kidney. The posterior surface of the right kidney is crossed by the 12th rib, and the posterior surface of the left kidney by the 11th and 12th ribs. The diaphragm is attached to the 12th rib on each side, so the diaphragm and its accompanying parietal pleura, on the medial side, come down between the posterior abdominal wall and the kidneys. This relationship needs to be accounted for when performing procedures in this area. For instance, a needle biopsy of the kidney that approached the kidney above the 12th rib could potentially transfer an infection from the liver to the pleural cavity. An approach below the 12th rib would not go through the pleura (Fig. 3.45).

The inferior posterior surface of each kidney is about three muscles. Moving from medial to lateral:

1. The *iliopsoas* is the chief flexor of the hip. The psoas major originates from the transverse processes of T12-L4 and descends on the posterior wall. Meanwhile, the iliacus arises from the superior pelvic brim. The two muscles come together to make up the iliopsoas to reach the lesser trochanter. Both muscles are innervated by direct branches from L1-L3 (not the femoral nerve). The *genitofemoral nerve* pierces the psoas on its course to the inguinal region. *The Thomas Test* is used to test tightness of the iliopsoas. In brief, with the patient lying on the exam table in the supine position they lift their lower limb off the table and are asked to resist the examiner's downward force on the lower limb. The psoas can be aggravated in patients who spend much of their day sitting in a chair all day at a desk. NASCAR accidents have been blamed on psoas strain.
2. The *quadratus lumborum* runs from rib 12 to the iliac crest. When the muscle is active on one side it is a lateral flexor. When both are active it is an extensor. It also assists with stabilizing the 12th rib.
3. The *transversus abdominus* also forms part of the posterior abdominal wall.

The hilum of the kidney, at the L1 vertebra level, is the opening at the medial border of the kidney. Starting anteriorly and moving posteriorly, the hilum transmits the renal **V**ein, renal **A**rtery, and the renal **P**elvis (VAP). The renal arteries arise at the level of L1, just inferior to the superior mesenteric artery. The origin of the left renal artery is slightly higher than the right renal artery. The

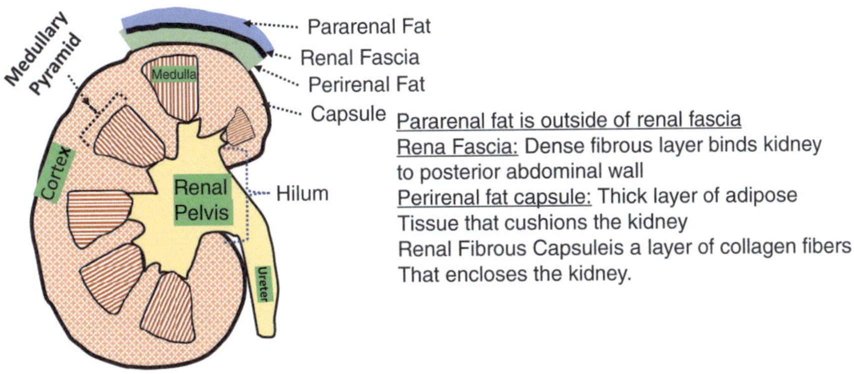

Fig. 3.46 Internal Kidney. Urine formed in the medulla will drain to the renal papilla, which drains into the minor calyx. Several minor calyces will form a major calyx, which in turn will form the renal pelvis [10, 11]

right artery is longer because it needs to go posterior to the IVC. On the other hand, the left renal vein is longer because of its longer route to the IVC over (anterior to) the aorta. The left kidney is usually used for transplants because of its longer renal vein. Because the kidneys ascend during development, it is not uncommon to see accessory renal veins.

Lloyd's test involves a soft punch, either directly or indirectly, on the posterior abdominal wall just behind the kidney. Pain indicates a kidney stone or infection.

Renal Fascia

The kidney has a strong fibrous capsule made of dense irregular connective tissue surrounding it. Outside of the capsule is a loose layer of adipose tissue—the perirenal fat, which serves as a shock absorber. And then outside of the perirenal fat is the renal capsule—also known as Gerota's fascia. On the anterior surface, the renal fascia on the right and left sides fuse in front of the aorta and inferior vena cava. Outside of the renal fascia is the pararenal fat. The kidneys are retroperitoneal. The adrenal glands are in the perirenal space and are also surrounded by perirenal fascia (Fig. 3.46).

Renal Blood Supply

The blood supply to the kidneys comes from the *right and left renal arteries*, each of which then split into 4–5 *segmental arteries*. The segmental arteries give off *interlobar arteries* which ascend in the renal columns alongside the edges of the renal medulla. The interlobar arteries then make a 90° turn to run along the top of the medullary pyramids as the *arcuate arteries*. The arcuate arteries then give off the *interlobular arteries* which give off *afferent arterioles* which then enter the glomerulus. Coming out of the glomerulus are the *efferent arterioles* that then wind around the proximal and distal convoluted tubules. Coming out of this network are the *peritubular capillaries* that turn into the *interlobular veins* and then drain back along a similar pattern as the arterial side (Fig. 3.47).

The blood flow of the kidney is a portal system. Remember that the portal systems have two capillary beds in line. In the kidneys, the first capillary bed is the glomerulus, and the second capillary bed is the peritubular capillary network. One thing to note is that in the kidneys the connection between the glomerulus and the peritubular capillary network is the *efferent arteriole*, which contrasts with the portal vein where the first and second capillary beds are connected by a vein (the portal vein).

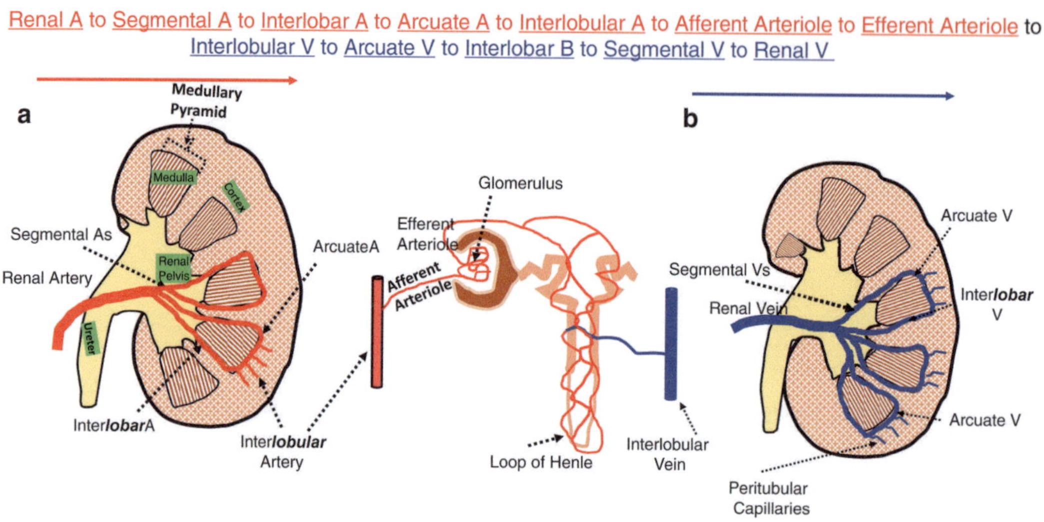

Fig. 3.47 Panel (**a**) shows the blood coming into the kidney from the renal artery. Panel (**b**) shows the blood leaving the kidney and eventually draining into the renal vein [10, 11]

Adrenal Glands

The adrenal glands, or suprarenal glands, are triangular and sit on top of the kidneys nestled between the great vessels. The right adrenal gland abuts the inferior vena cava. The adrenal cortex has three zones (think salt, sugar, and sex):

1. *Zona Glomerulosa* produces aldosterone which causes the distal convoluted tubule and the collecting tubule to reabsorb sodium.
2. *Zona Fasciculata* releases cortisol.
3. *Zona Reticulata* produces androgens.

Although there are variations, the arterial pattern is similar on both the right and left sides. Both the *right and left superior suprarenal arteries* come off the *inferior phrenic arteries*. The *middle suprarenal arteries* come off the abdominal aorta. The *inferior suprarenal arteries* come off the renal arteries. The venous drainage for the adrenals is not symmetrical and is different on the right versus left sides. On the right side, the suprarenal vein drains into inferior vena cava, while on the left the suprarenal vein drains into the left renal vein. At this point an extension of the left inferior phrenic vein sends a branch down to the left renal vein. Given the proximity of the inferior phrenic vein and the left suprarenal vein to each other where they drain into the left renal vein, it is not uncommon to see a common trunk for these two branches (Fig. 3.48).

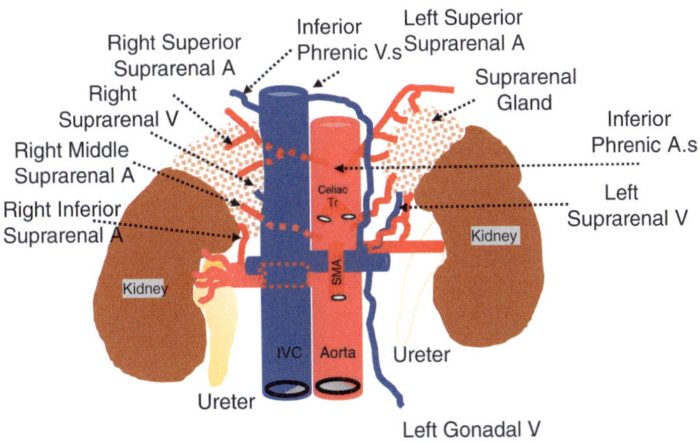

Fig. 3.48 Blood supply to suprarenal glands. There are three arteries to the adrenal gland: (1) superior suprarenal artery from the inferior phrenic artery, (2) middle suprarenal arteries from the abdominal aorta, and (3) inferior suprarenal arteries from the renal arteries. There is typically only one vein. On the right side the vein drains into the IVC, and on the left it drains into the left renal vein. Note that on the left side, the left inferior phrenic vein sends a branch to the left renal vein [10, 11]

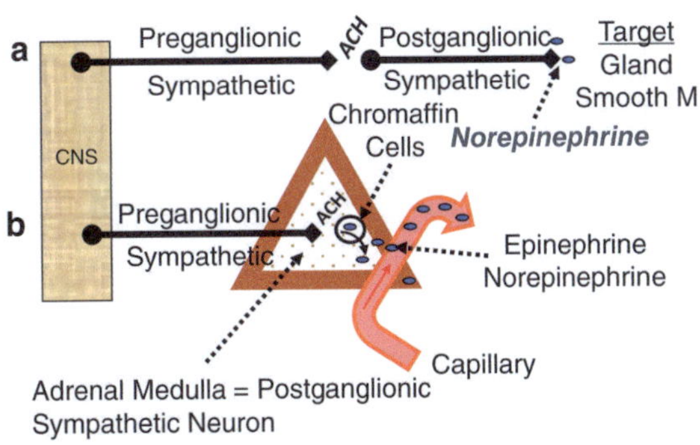

Fig. 3.49 Adrenal Medulla. Panel **(a)** shows the typical scenario with pre- and post ganglionic sympathetic neurons The preganglionic sympathetic nerve releases acetylcholine at the synapse with a postganglionic nerve which in turn releases epinephrine and norepinephrine to act on a target. Panel **(b)** shows how the adrenal medulla is equivalent to a post ganglionic sympathetic neuron. A preganglionic cholinergic neuron comes out of the CNS and travels to the adrenal medulla where it stimulates the chromaffin cells to secrete epinephrine and norepinephrine into the capillaries to have a systemic affect [10, 11]

Adrenal Medulla

The adrenal medulla is equivalent to a post ganglionic sympathetic neuron. It is innervated by prganglionic sympathetic neurons. When stimulted, the chromaffin cells in the adrenal medulla secrete norepinephrine and epinephrine into the systemic blood stream (Fig. 3.49).

Ureters

The *ureters* descend from the renal pelvis down to the bladder. As they travel down the posterior abdominal wall, they lie on top of the psoas major muscle. They enter the pelvis crossing the pelvic brim anterior to the bifurcation of the common iliac artery. As the ureters descend, they are crossed by several structures: either the right or left colic artery traveling to the large intestines; either the ileocolic artery on the left or the sigmoidal arteries on the right; and then the left or right gonadal arteries. And at the pelvic brim, lateral to the ureters, are the ovarian vessels entering the pelvis.

In females, just lateral to the cervix, the ureter crosses inferior to the uterine artery—"water under the bridge." During a hysterectomy or other pelvic surgeries this relationship is important. In males, just before the ureter enters the bladder it is crossed by the ductus deferens (Fig. 3.45).

Kidney stones can get caught up at either the: (1) the renal pelvis, (2) the pelvic brim (the most common site), or (3) at the entrance to the bladder. As the stones move down the ureter, the patient will first complain of pain in the epigastric region. As the stone descends it will aggravate the psoas major leading to pain which causes the patient to flex at the hip. By assuming the fetal position, the patient is trying to relieve the pressure of the stone on the psoas major. Extension of the patient's lower limb will lead to significant pain because of increased aggravation of the psoas. As the stone enters the bladder the patient will complain of pain in the inguinal canal region—the L1 dermatome (Fig. 3.50).

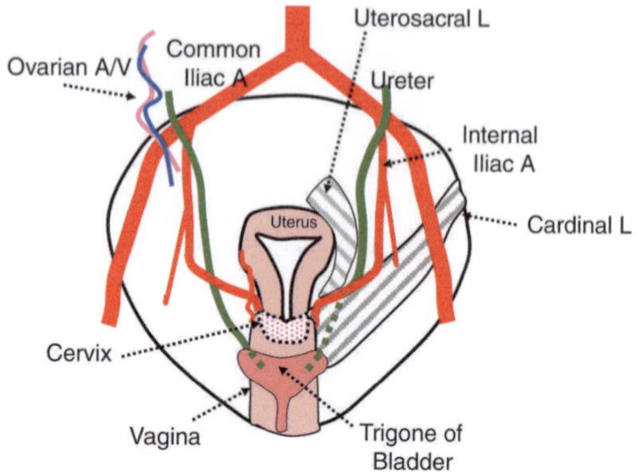

Fig. 3.50 Uterine Artery and Pelvic Ligaments. The cardinal ligament runs medial to lateral, while the uterosacral ligament runs anterior to posterior. The ureter enters the pelvic cavity just lateral to the origin of the common iliac artery. The ureter then passes under the uterine artery. The uterine artery runs in the cardinal ligament towards the cervix [10, 11]

Nerves of Posterior Abdominal Wall

Along the posterior abdominal wall are several nerves:

1. The *subcostal nerve* is found just inferior to the 12th rib.
2. The *iliohypogastric nerve* (L1) winds around the abdominal wall running parallel and superior to the inguinal ligament.
3. The *ilioinguinal nerve* also winds around the abdominal wall to travel through the inguinal canal, exiting at the superficial ring.
4. The *lateral femoral cutaneous nerve* travels medial to the ASIS to enter the thigh.
5. The *genitofemoral nerve* splits into a genital and femoral branch. The genital branch is found in the spermatic cord and it innervates the cremaster muscle. The femoral branch carries sensory fibers coming from the anteromedial thigh.

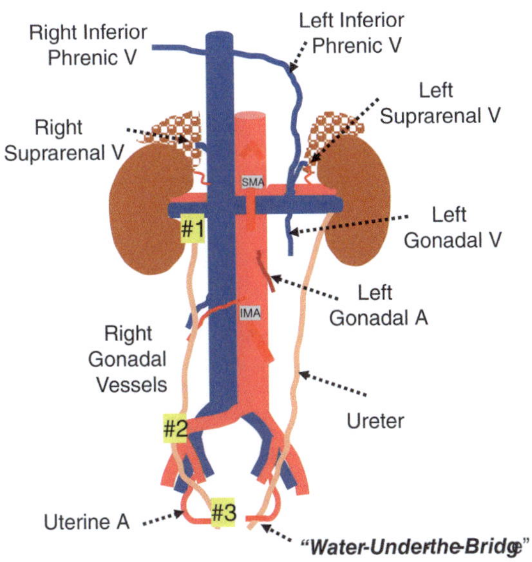

Fig. 3.51 Branches of Aorta and Inferior Vena Cava. On the right side, the adrenal gland and the gonads drain into the IVC. However, on the left side, the gonads and adrenal gland drain into the left renal vein, which then drains into the IVC. The SMA passes anterior to the left renal vein. The ureter enters the pelvis lateral to the common iliac arteries and veins. The ureter then passes under the uterine artery just lateral to the cervix *(Water-under-the-Bridge)*. There are three common locations for kidney stone blockage (1) at the renal pelvis, (2) where the ureter crosses the pelvic brim and (3) where the ureter enters the bladder [10, 11]

Branches of the Abdominal Aorta

As a summary of the abdominal aorta. Consider a stick figure drawing of a person standing up with a hat. Their hat is the diaphragm, their eyes are the inferior phrenic arteries, the nose is the celiac trunk, the mouth is the superior mesenteric artery, and the goatee just underneath the mouth is the left renal vein. The upper limbs are the renal arteries with the fingers representing the segmental arteries of the kidneys. The nipples are the gonadal arteries (either testicular or ovarian), the chest hair represents the lumbar arteries, the belly button the inferior mesenteric and the common iliac arteries are the lower limbs (Figs. 3.51 and 3.52).

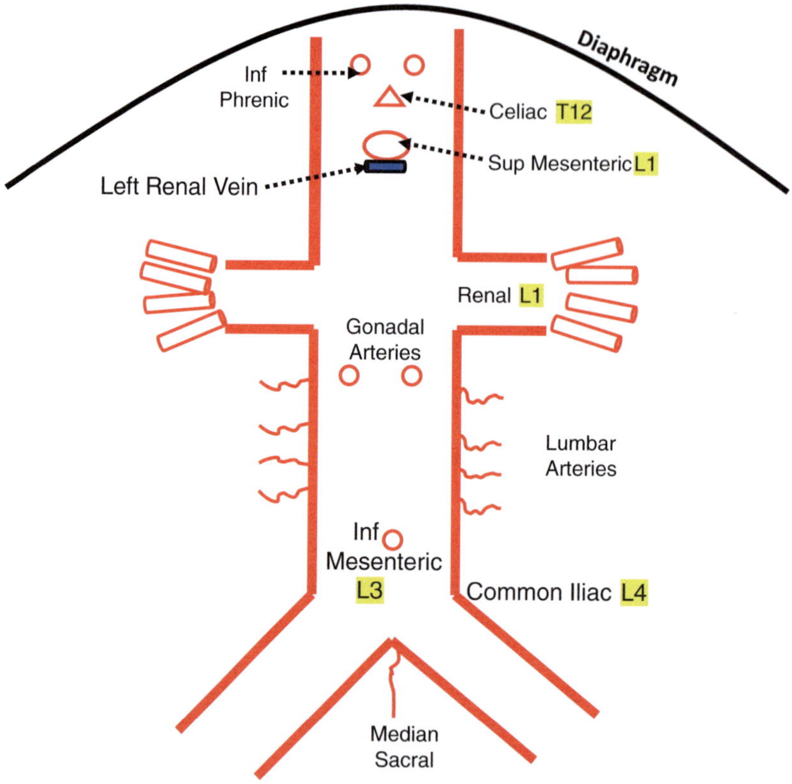

Fig. 3.52 Abdominal Aorta

Historical Snippet: The Pernkopf Atlas

Edward Pernkopf (1888–1955) was the lead illustrator of a four-volume anatomical atlas, known originally for the superb quality of its illustration, and used by countless numbers of medical students. However, in the 1990's, due to the immense work of several scholars, the history behind the illustrations emerged. For their models, Pernkopf and his team of assistants used political prisoners executed by the Nazis during WW II. It would be comforting to think of these illustrators as noble artists and scientists who unwittingly used the bodies of murdered people delivered to the University's morgue, but it is more complicated.

Rather than hide from their association with the Nazis, several of the artists proudly broadcasted their allegiances by weaving images, such as the Nazi Cross and the Waffen SS lightning-bolt, into their signatures.

But it is not just the atlas that has drawn attention to Pernkopf. After the Nazis entered Austria, Pernkopf became the Dean of the medical school and one of his first official actions was to purge 153 of the 197 faculty members from the University. The overwhelming majority of the exiled member were Jewish, three of them were Nobel laureates, and several were Department Chairs. Following their expulsion, many were sent to concentration camps, and several committed suicide.

On April 26, 1938, just a month after Hitler's troops entered Austria, Pernkopf presided over a medical school faculty meeting. He gave his speech that day from the lectern in the Anatomical Theatre at the University of Vienna, flanked by guards. The backdrop consisted of Nazi flags and Adolf Hitler's portrait. We know something about that day because the speech was subsequently published in the academic journal, the *Viennese Medical Weekly*, a well-respected medical journal and there is also a picture of the event.

In his speech, Pernkopf stressed the need for "the exclusion of the genetically inferior from future generations by sterilization and other means," and he ended his speech with his arm raised and a rousing shout out for Hitler, "we as doctors will gladly place at his service our lives and our souls. So shall our cry express what we wish with all our hearts: Adolph Hitler, Sieg heil, Sieg Heil, Sieg Heil."

The above description is just a brief overview of Pernkopf and his atlas. Whether the Pernkopf atlas should still be used is a matter of debate.

Further Reading

1. Carstens P. Revisiting the infamous Pernkopf anatomy atlas: historical lessons for medical law and ethics. Fundamina. 2012;18(2):23–49.
2. Cavale G, Bellier A, Marnas G, Boisson B, Robert Y, Rabattu PY, Chaffanjon P. Anatomy and histology of the scrotal ligament in adults: inconsistency and variability of the gubernaculum tests. Surg Radiol Anat. 2018;40(4):35–370.
3. Cesta MF. Normal structure, function, and histology of the spleen. Toxicol Pathol. 2006;34:455–65.
4. Darda DM. The gubernaculum and the evolution of testicular descent. J Human Anat Physiol Soc. 2017;12(3):12–9.
5. Davey WW. Rovsing's sign. BMJ. 1956;2(4983):28–30.
6. Hanzalova I, Schafer M, Demartines N, Clerc D. Spigelian hernias: current approaches to surgical treatment. Hernia. 2021. Available at: https://dpo.org/10.1007/s10029-021-02511-8;26:1427–33.
7. Hartsock JA, Beckman ES. A human paradox: the Nazi legacy of Pernkopf's atlas. Conatus. 2019;4(2):317–39. https://doi.org/10.12681/cjp.21076.
8. Hutson J, Nation AB, Southwell BR. The role of the gubernaculum in the descent and undescent of the testis. Ther Adv Urol. 2009;1(2):115–21.
9. Izbicki JR, Yekebas EF, et al. Extrahepatic portal hypertension in chronic pancreatitis: an old problem revisited. Annal Surg. 2002;236(1):82–9.
10. Leo J. Medical neuroanatomy for the boards and clinic: finding the lesion. 2nd ed. Switzerland: Springer; 2024a.
11. Leo J. Clinical anatomy and embryology: A guide for the classroom, clinic, and clinic. 2nd ed. Springer; 2024b.
12. Moore K, Dalley AF, Agur A. Clinically oriented anatomy. 7th ed. Baltimore: Lippincott Williams and Wilkin; 2014.
13. Norton SA. On first looking into Pernkopf's atlas. Archives Dermatology. 2001;137(5):549–51.
14. Leo JV. Was this the worst faculty meeting ever? Times Higher Educations. 1938;23:2023.
15. Peters M, Syed RK, Katz M, Moscona J, Press C, Niijar V, Bisharat M, Baldwin D. May-Thurner syndrome: a not so uncommon cause of a common condition. Proc (Baylor University Medical Center). 2012;25(3):231–3.
16. Rosse C, Gaddum-Rosse P. Hollinshead's textbook of anatomy. Lippincott-Raven; 1997.
17. Snell R. Clinical anatomy by region. 9th ed. Lippincott Williams and Wilkins; 2012.
18. Thompson JT, Taylor MA, McKie LD, Diamond T. Sinistral portal hypertension. Ulster Med J. 2006;75(3):175–7.
19. Weismann G. Springtime for Pernkopf. Hosp Pract. 1985;15:142–68.
20. Williams DJ. The history of Eduard Pernkopf's Topographische Anatomie des menschen. J Biocommun. 1988;45(1):19–29.

Kidney Function 4

A Sodium Ion's Journey Through the Nephron and Collecting Duct: An Autobiography

As an introduction to kidney function, consider this short travel diary from the point of view of a single sodium molecule – written in the first person.

I am a single sodium molecule on a long, tortuous journey through the nephron and the collecting duct. Just a moment ago, I was in the blood stream, specifically a specialized capillary tuft, called the glomerulus. The capillary wall of the glomerulus has a fenestrated wall, and combined with its high pressure, I was able to slip through the capillary wall. Then I crossed the visceral layer of Bowman's capsule and entered the urinary space.

And I am not alone. I am traveling with 249 of my closest friends—other sodium molecules. Unfortunately, only several of us, possibly just one of us, will make it to the finish line, where we will be released into the urine. Most of us will not complete the journey because we will work our way out of the tube by passing through various doorways to reenter the host organism's blood stream. There are three doorways that we will encounter on this journey, each of which has a very specific requirement about who can pass through.

The reason only several of us will make it to the end has to do with our host organism's regulation of blood pressure, and the fact that we like to drag water molecules with us. The amount of fluid in the blood stream has a large effect on blood pressure, and one way to control whether water is excreted or absorbed is to control the movement of us—sodium. One of the roadblocks we will encounter are different medications prescribed by a clinician, to prevent our movement through these doorways—think of these medications as security guards that are specific to one of the three doors. If the organism wants to retain more water, then more of us will move through the doorways. Conversely, if the organism wants to excrete more water, then the doorways will be blocked.

Proximal Tubule

We sodium molecules are not alone on this journey. When we crossed the urinary space, besides water, we also took with us many other molecules such as glucose, K^+, Cl^- and other ions. The first part of our journey is through the proximal tubule, the interior wall of which is an interdigitated surface of projections called the brush border. As we move through the lumen along the brush border, we sense that there are fewer of us on the other side of the brush border, and this exerts a force on us. In the spirit of equality, 168 of my colleagues now cross the brush border and enter the cells of the proximal tubule—they also drag with them water and other molecules. The driving force

J. Leo, *Gross Anatomy, Neuroanatomy, and Embryology for Medical Students*,
https://doi.org/10.1007/978-3-031-87151-1_4

here is the low concentration of sodium on the other side of the brush border, in the cells of the proximal tubule, which in turn is created by the NaK^+Atpase pump (active transport) on the basolateral surface of the cells, where the pump moves 3 Na^+ molecules out of the cell and 2 K^+ molecules into the cell. At the end of this segment there are only 82 of us left inside the tubular lumen.

Loop of Henle Descending Limb

The tube we are now traveling through is starting to become narrower and will eventually form a loop. There is the descending part of the loop, the bend in the loop, and the subsequent ascending limb. And most importantly, the ascending and descending limbs have different doorways along their apical membranes. The descending limb does not have any doors for us to move into the blood stream (some of us slip through, but not many), but it does allow water to move across into the bloodstream. With the water leaving the tube, and us staying behind, we are all now crowded in closer together so that at the bottom of the tube the congestion is now elbow-to-elbow.

Loop of Henle Ascending Limb

After the bend, the tube starts to ascend. There is a short, thin segment of this ascending limb but it quickly starts to widen and is now called the thick ascending limb or TAL. Along this segment there are doorways marked NKCC2 which we can travel through to get back to the blood stream, and 62 of my Na^+ friends go through this door. And furthermore, each of them carries one K^+ and 2 Cl^- ions through the doorway. Some of the K^+ ions that got carried into the cell realize the error of their ways and slip back into the tubule through a doorway marked renal outer medullary potassium channel (ROMK).

A unique feature of the TAL is that the cells are impermeable to water. The Na^+ molecules moving from the tubular lumen to the blood stream do not carry water molecules with them. This leads to the concentration of sodium in the TAL decreasing as we move up the ascending limb. In other words we are not so crowded as we ascend the TAL.

There is a potential pitfall we may encounter at this point, namely furosemide. This drug blocks the NKCC2 doorway and slows down our movement from the tubular lumen to the bloodstream.

Distal Convoluted Tubule

Our journey continues into a short but wide convoluted pathway. The first part of this segment has a doorway marked NaCL, and 10 more of our Na^+ colleagues disappear though this doorway. Each Na^+ molecule takes a Cl^- ion with it. However, if thiazide is present, it blocks the doorway preventing many of us from moving through the doorway.

Macula Densa

As we move along this thick ascending limb, we must pass through the macula densa, a sensor tasked with getting a head count. If there are not enough of us in the tube then this sensor will tell the juxtaglomerular cells (JG) to slow us down, by constricting the afferent arteriole of the glomerulus. The JG cells also release renin to tell the liver to secrete angiotensinogen which will then convert it to angiotensin to tell the adrenal gland to secrete aldosterone. The aldosterone will then open doorways to allow more of us to cross over into the blood stream.

Collecting Duct

As we move along the tubule, another 10–20 of us will move from the tubular lumen into the blood stream through a doorway marked ENaC. Since only Na^+ moves through this channel, the positive charge inside the cell tends to build up. This leads to K^+ moving into the tubular lumen to be excreted in the urine.

A potential problem for us in this segment is the presence of potassium sparing blockers (such as amiloride) which allows fewer of my colleagues to move into the blood stream, which in turn leads to not as many K^+ ions being secreted. On the other hand, if aldosterone is present then there will be more ENaC channels in the membrane allowing more of us to enter the bloodstream.

As we move through the collecting duct, the amount of crowding in the duct is related to the water content in the tubular lumen. If there is an abundance of water in the tubular lumen then we will have lots of room to move around (we are less concentrated) and if the amount of water in the tubular lumen goes down, then we will be overcrowded (more concentrated). The degree of crowding in the lumen is under control by ADH. If our host organism senses low blood pressure, then it will want to retain water. In this case the posterior pituitary will release ADH which signals the collecting duct cells to insert aquaporin channels in the membrane. These channels move water from the tubular lumen to the cell and raise blood pressure. If blood pressure is too high, then ADH levels will decrease and more water will stay in the tubular lumen (diluted urine).

As I complete my journey to the renal papilla and enter the urine, I am the only one of the original 249 molecules of sodium to make it this far. At any given time, this number can vary a bit (from 1–10) depending on the host organism's internal environment. My colleagues that reentered the bloodstream will repeat this whole journey many times a day and have the same fate as me (Fig. 4.1).

And now for the specifics. As you study kidney function, with its ions, channels, medications, and pathologies, everything relates, one way or another, to sodium. When you study the various aspects of the kidney, whether it is pharmacology, physiology, histology, genetics, or pathology and you want to test yourself, ask yourself: How does it relate to sodium?

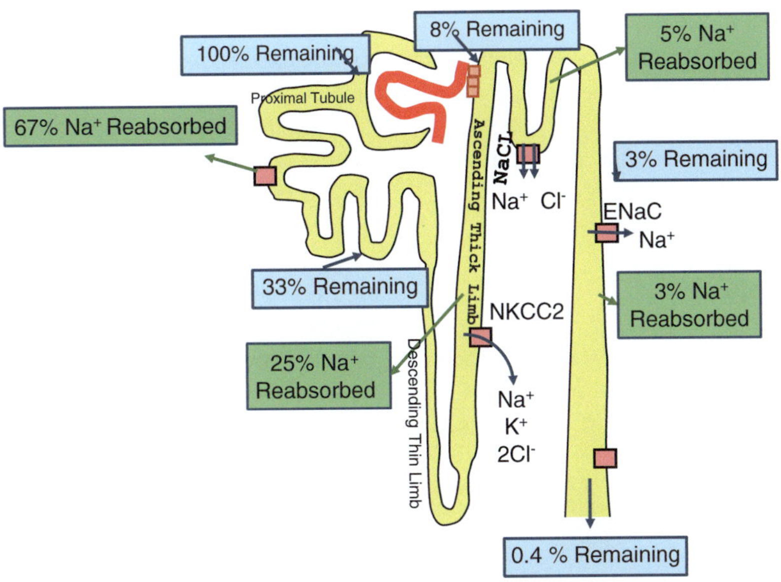

Fig. 4.1 Sodium Reabsorption along the Nephron. In the proximal convoluted tubule, almost 67% of the Na^+ is reabsorbed. The ascending thick limb of the loop of Henle absorbs another 25%. Thus, by the time the fluid has reached the macula densa almost 92% of the sodium has been reabsorbed. The distal tubule then absorbs another 5% of filtered sodium. The collecting duct only absorbs about 3 to 5% of the total Na^+ but this fine tuning is extremely important

The Kidney

At Bowman's capsule a large amount of water, sodium, and other ions enter this tubular network. A major job of the kidney is to reabsorb most of the water and ions that have moved into this tubular network. How the kidney handles the reabsorption of sodium chloride is a major determinate of blood pressure, and a failure of the kidney to appropriately handle the flow of Na^+ can lead to hypertension. Besides reabsorption of Na^+, the flow of the fluid through the tubule network accomplishes several other functions, including the secretion of metabolic waste products such as urea and potassium, the absorption of ions other than Na^+, and maintaining the body's proper acid/base balance.

When looking at the movement of a given molecule through the kidney's tubular network consider the following terms:

1. Filtration is the amount of a given molecule moving from the glomerulus into the urinary space.
2. Absorption is the amount of that molecule that is taken back up during its path through the tubular network.
3. Secretion is the amount of the molecule that is secreted into the tubular network during the fluid's path.
4. Excretion is the amount of the molecule finally released via urine.

Bowmans Capsule

Bowman's capsule resembles a hand reaching out and grabbing a ball—the glomerulus. The glomerulus is a round tuft of capillaries that receives blood from an afferent arteriole and sends blood out via an efferent arteriole. The layer of Bowman's capsule adjacent to the fenestrated endothelium of the glomerulus is the visceral layer and it has interdigitations or extensions called podocytes that reach out to cover the capillaries. Between the podocytes are filtration slits that allow substances from the capillary lumen to cross over and enter the urinary space. This visceral layer of Bowman's capsule turns back on itself to become the parietal layer and between the visceral and parietal layers is the urinary space. Along with water, other molecules such as glucose, bicarbonate, and amino acids move from the blood and cross the visceral layer of Bowman's capsule to enter the urinary space. From here the fluid continues its trip through the tubular network. The amount of fluid and solute moving across Bowman's capsule into the urinary space is referred to as the glomerular filtration rate (GFR).

The blood pressure in the glomerulus is high and it can be fine-tuned by controlling the width of the arterioles. For instance, substances such as angiotensin that constrict the efferent arteriole, or substances that dilate the afferent arteriole such as prostaglandins, will increase the pressure (Fig. 4.2).

Keep in mind that once all this fluid enters this tubular system is now out of the body and is on its way to being excreted in the urine. Fortunately, not all this fluid will be excreted, because the cells of this tubular system have various specialized transport mechanisms on their apical membranes so that as the fluid moves through the tubular network the body reabsorbs most of the water, sodium chloride (Na^+Cl^-), other ions, glucose, and amino acids.

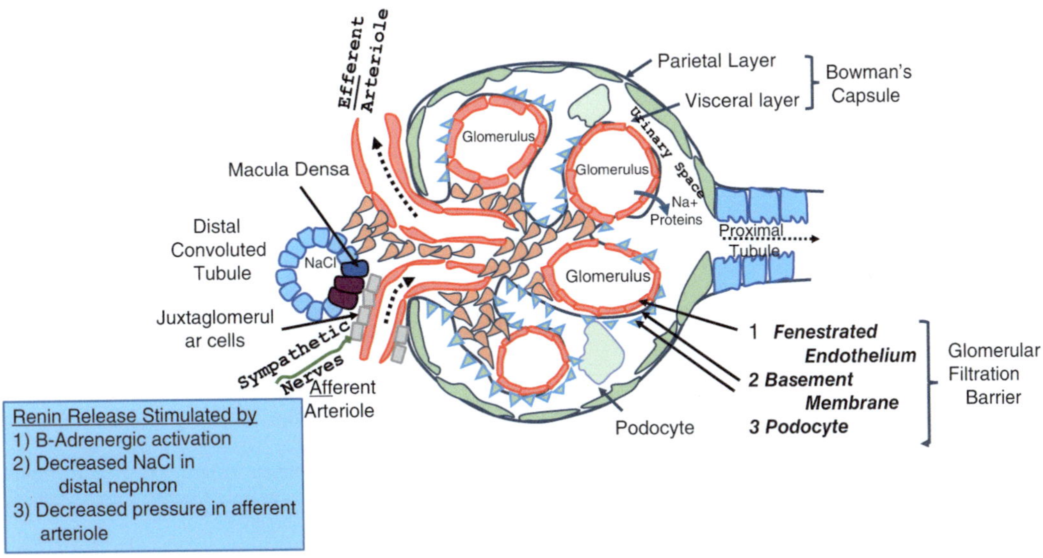

Fig. 4.2 Bowman's Capsule . The glomerular filtration barrier includes the fenestrated endothelium, the basement membrane, and the podocyte with their foot processes. Between the foot processes are the filtration slits

Water and Na⁺ Reabsorption

Proximal Tubule

The proximal tubule is the site of between 60–70% (typically 67%) of the reabsorption of water and Na^+. The cells lining the proximal tube are cuboidal epithelium with microvilli extending from the apical membrane into the lumen. Along the basolateral membranes of the proximal tubes are Na^+/K^+-ATPases moving Na^+ out of the cell and K^+ into the cell. This creates a sodium gradient so that Na^+ moves from the lumen into the cells, then to the interstitium, and finally the blood stream. The sodium moves across the apical membranes through various co-transporters. The sodium takes with it: glucose, amino acids, and various vitamins (Fig. 4.3).

As an example of cotransport, take Na^+ and Cl^-. The movement of Na^+ across the membrane brings Cl^- with it because of its negative charge. And the movement of the Na^+ ion across the membrane also takes H_2O with it—the so-called "obligatory" water reabsorption. The fluid that remains in the proximal tubule continues into the loop of Henle.

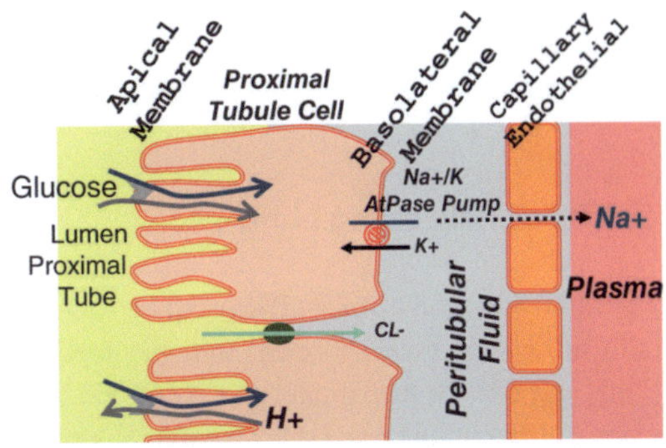

Fig. 4.3 Proximal Tubule and Sodium Retention . The Na^+/K^+ ATPase on the basolateral surface drives the sodium gradient. Na^+ then moves from the lumen of the proximal tube into the cell and then into the blood stream. On the apical membrane are co transporters where certain molecules such as glucose that follow Na^+ across the membrane

Loop of Henle

The *loop of Henle* consists of a thin descending limb, a thin ascending limb, and a thick ascending limb. There are both short-looped nephrons which begin in glomeruli located in the outer and mid regions of the cortex called *cortical nephrons* (7/8 of all the nephrons) and long-looped nephrons which begin at the junction of the cortex and medulla, appropriately called *juxtamedullary nephrons* (1/8 of all nephrons). A single loop of Henle is formed by a descending limb entering the medulla, doing a U-turn, and heading back towards the cortex as an ascending limb which then turns into the distal tubule. The reabsorption of water is made possible because *the ascending thin limb is impermeable to H_2O.*

Descending Thin Limb

The simple squamous cells of the descending thin limbs are freely permeable to water because of the presence of permanent aquaporin-1 channels. While most segments of the nephron are involved with Na^+ and Cl^- reabsorption, the descending limb is an exception, as it is not involved in significant movement of Na^+Cl^-. Moving down the descending limb, the osmolarity of the interstitium increases from about 300 to 1200 mOsmol/kg which draws the water from the lumen into the surrounding interstitium.

The Thick Ascending Limb

The thick ascending limbs (TAL) can be found in both the cortex (short-looped) and the medulla (long-looped). Approximately 30% of the total reabsorption of Na^+ and Cl^- occurs along the thick ascending limb. Most importantly, *these cells of the TAL are impermeable to water*. As the Na^+ and Cl^- move from the lumen to the interstitial fluid, with no accompanying water movement, the concentrations of these ions increase in the interstitium surrounding the tube.

The cells of the TAL contain a Na^+ K^+ 2 Cl^- transporter (NKCC2) that cotransports these ions from the TAL cells into the lumen. The loop diuretics act by inhibiting the movement of CL^- across this channel. And because the movement of Na^+ and K^+ is dependent on the movement of Cl^-, these other two ions are also inhibited (Fig. 4.4).

In addition to the three ions moving across the membrane from the lumen into the cell at the NKCC2 channel, K^+ also moves back across at

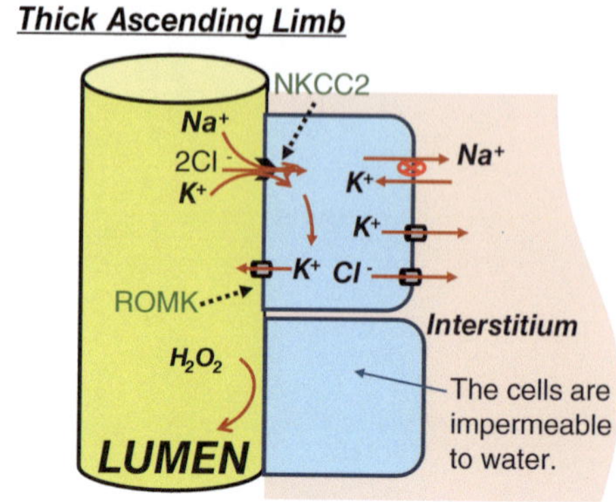

Fig. 4.4 Thick Ascending Limb. The cells lining the lumen are impermeable to water. Na^+ and K^+ are Cotransporters on the lumen surface. The NKCC2 transports Na^+, K^+, and 2 Cl^- ions into the cell. Some of the K^+ leaks out at the ROMK channel

the apical K^+ (ROMK) channels from the interior of the cell to the lumen. The thick ascending limb ends as the macula densa.

Distal Convoluted Tubule

The distal convoluted tubule is a short segment that runs from the macula densa to the collecting duct. It does not absorb significant amounts of water. But it does absorb 5–10% of filtered sodium. The cells are cuboidal epithelium with an apical membrane facing the lumen and a basolateral membrane facing the interstitium. The DCT is divided into two segments: an early segment, and a late segment. The cells of both these segments contain Na^+/K^+ ATPase pumps along their basolateral membranes. But their apical segments are different.

The apical membrane of the early segment is characterized by the presence of the NaCl cotransporter. Note that this Na^+Cl^- cotransporter has replaced the NKCC2 transporter present in the loop of Henle. For every Na^+ molecule that moves across the membrane, a molecule of Cl^- follows it, so there is no change in the membrane electrical potential of these cells in the early segment of the distal convoluted tube. The Na^+ Cl^- cotransporter is the site of the inhibition by the thiazide diuretics, which are given for patients with hypertension. These drugs decrease the movement of NA and CL from the lumen into the cells and blood stream.

The late stage of the DCT however is characterized by a higher concentration of epithelial sodium channels (ENaC). In this case the movement of just Na^+ into the cell leaves the lumen with a slightly negative charge, which in turn drives the movement of other ions. For instance, to offset the inward Na^+ movement, K^+ ions are now moving from inside the cell to the lumen through the renal outer medullary potassium secretory channel (ROMK) channels. In the DCT, the term for this movement of K^+ is *potassium recycling*. This is because some potassium is brought from the lumen into cell through the NaCl channel, and some potassium is moved from the cell into the lumen through the ROMK channel. Keep in mind that as more Na^+ is reabsorbed, then more potassium will be secreted.

In addition, Ca^{2+} also passes from the lumen to the cell via calcium channels on the apical surface which are regulated by parathyroid hormone. Calcium then moves from the cell into the interstitial fluid via Ca^{2+} ATPase or a $3Na^+/Ca^{2+}$ antiporter.

These cells of the distal convoluted tubule are impermeable to water so the interstitial tissue with its increased ion concentration is now hyperosmotic. The fluid in the lumen has fewer ions but more water. In other words, the interstitial tissue fluid in the renal medulla is now saltier than the fluid in the tubule.

Collecting Duct—Fine Tuning Sodium Chloride Reabsorption

The ends of the distal convoluted tubules turn into collecting tubules, and several collecting tubules merge to form a collecting duct. The collecting ducts pass through the cortex and medulla. Near their ends, they merge and terminate at the renal papilla which empties into the renal calyx. There are two types of cells in the collecting ducts: (1) Principal cells which are involved with Na^+ retention, and (2) Intercalated cells which have elevated levels of carbonic anhydrase and are involved with acid-base regulation.

In birds and mammals, it is the collecting ducts that create concentrated urine—hypertonic urine. At one point in time, it was thought that this was the job of the loops of Henle, but we now know that the fluid delivered to the start of the collecting duct is less concentrated than the surrounding interstitial fluid making it evident that it is the collecting duct's job to concentrate the urine. As the collecting ducts pass through this hypertonic interstitial fluid in the medulla created by the loop of Henle and the countercurrent multiplier water is drawn out of the tubular lumen (Figs. 4.5 and 4.6).

It is also the job of the collecting duct to fine-tune the concentration of the final products of molecules such as Na^+, K^+, H^+ and water, to determine what is excreted by the body. While the collecting duct only controls a small percentage of what is reabsorbed, this fine-tuning ability is critical.

By the time the fluid reaches the collecting duct, approximately 80% of the water and 90% of the Na^+ has been reabsorbed.

On the apical membrane of the principal cells are the epithelial sodium channels (ENaC). As the Na^+ moves into the cell, the cell becomes slightly positively charged. This positive charge drives K^+ out of the cell via ROMK channels. In this case, the term is *potassium secretion*.

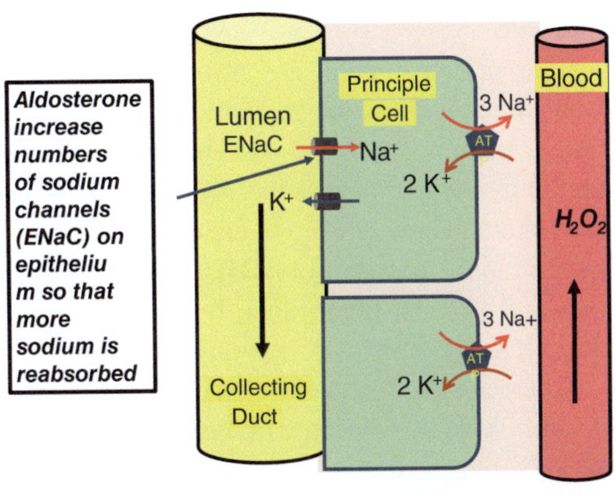

Fig. 4.5 The Principal Cell of the Collecting Duct and Sodium Reabsorption. Sodium moves from the lumen through the EaNC channels. At the same time, K^+ is moving into the lumen

Fig. 4.6 The Principal Cell of the Collecting Duct and Water Retention. Aquaporins 3 and 4 are present in the basolateral membrane. Aquaporin 2s are held in reserve within the cell. In the presence of ADH the pores are released from their reservoir and migrate to the apical cell membrane

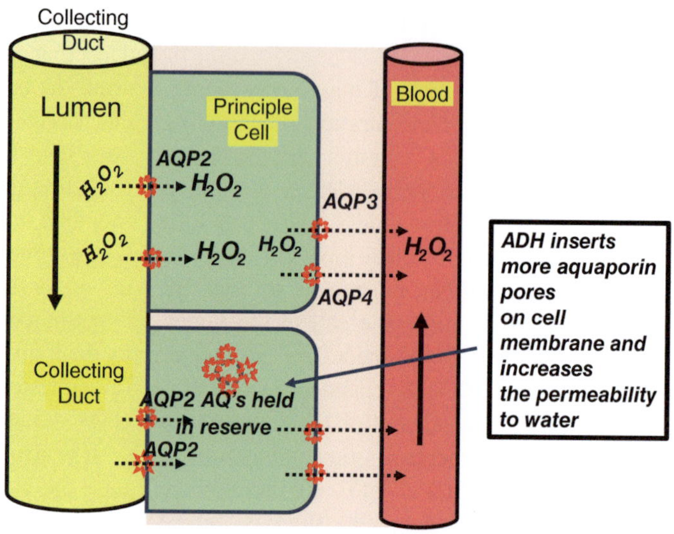

Conversely, the potassium sparing diuretics get their name because when they block the ENaC channels they prevent the movement of Na^+ from the tubular lumen into the cells and then into the blood stream. By blocking the movement of sodium into the blood stream they also slow down the movement of K^+ into the urine—*potassium sparing*.

In addition, as the Na^+ concentration increases in the cell, this positive charge leads to an influx of Cl^- ions into the cell. The principal cells are connected to each other via tight junctions. Cl^- ions are transported from the lumen into the cell paracellularly via channels within these tight junctions.

The principal cells are also involved with water retention via the regulation of aquaporin (AQ) channels. AQ 3 and 4 channels are located on the basolateral membrane. AQ 2 channels are sequestered together deep in the cell in a holding pattern. In the presence of ADH, these AQ 2 s are moved from their intracellular holding pattern to the cell membrane.

There are two forms of intercalated cells: Type A and Type B. The type A cells have H^+/K^+-ATPase pumps on their apical membranes so that H^+ is secreted into the tubular fluid. This also returns bicarbonate to blood stream via an anion exchanger. Type B cells have an apical anion chloride-bicarbonate exchanger (pendrin) that releases bicarbonate into the tubular fluid, and a H^+-ATPase pump on the basolateral surface that releases H^+ into the blood stream. Think Type A for "acid" (acidosis)—in acidosis, H^+ is released into urine, and Type B for "basic" (alkalosis) -in alkalosis, bicarbonate is released into urine (Fig. 4.7).

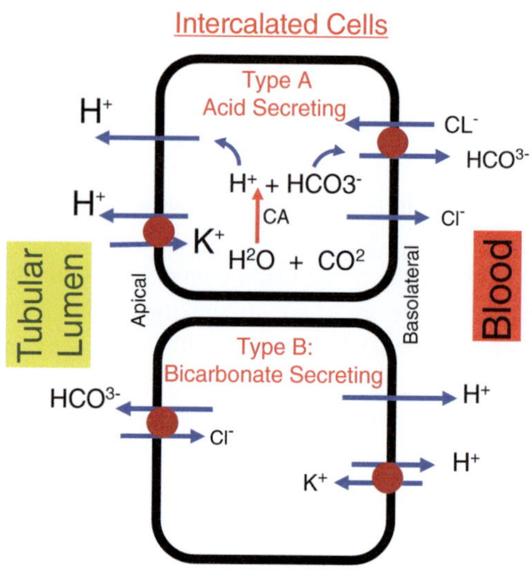

Fig. 4.7 Intercalated Cells. Type A are acid secreting cells. In response to acidotic conditions they secrete H^+. Type B are Base secreting cells and in response to basic conditions, they secrete HCO_3^-

Antidiuretic Hormone (ADH) and Water Retention

Antidiuretic hormone controls the collecting duct's ability to absorb water. In cases of dehydration, ADH will signal the collecting ducts to reabsorb the water passing through them, or conversely if the body does not need water, then ADH levels will drop so that the collecting ducts allow most of the fluid to remain in the lumen to be excreted in the urine. In other words, in the absence of antidiuretic hormone (ADH), the collecting duct cells are impermeable to water. In the presence of ADH, the principal cells increase the amount of water absorbed by the collecting ducts.

ADH is under control by higher centers and is intimately tied to blood pressure. When the baroreceptors in the neck sense low blood pressure, they signal the hypothalamus and posterior pituitary to release ADH which increases water retention. ADH acts on the principal cells in collecting ducts and distal convoluted tubule by inserting aquaporin channels in the membrane. With an upregulation of the aquaporin channels, more water is absorbed by the body, leading to less urine output. With the increased volume of fluid retained by the body, blood pressure increases. In addition, ADH moves urea channels to the distal regions of the convoluted tubule to increase the movement of urea from the lumen of the duct to the interstitial tissue.

Whether the urine is concentrated or not is a clue to the concentration of ions in the blood. In an individual who retains water, the urine will become more concentrated. Conversely, if they are excreting water the urine is less concentrated.

One way to alter the concentration of Na^+ in the blood is to increase or decrease the amount of water that the body either retains or excretes. Normal sodium levels are between 135 and 145 mEq/L. Hypernatremia, which is too much NA^+ in the blood stream ($Na > 145$ mEq/L), is typically the result of dehydration, vomiting, diarrhea, or diuretics. Hyponatremia, which is too little Na^+ in the blood stream, can result from drinking too much, congestive heart failure with fluid retention, or the Syndrome of Inappropriate Antidiuretic Hormone (SIADH).

A normal response to elevated levels of Na^+ in the blood (hypernatremia) would be for the posterior pituitary to release ADH which then increases water retention by the collecting duct. This leads to concentrated urine because the body is reabsorbing water—urine osmolality will be higher than in the serum. It should make sense that ADH is trying to counteract the hypernatremia by absorbing water. But what to make of the at odds scenario of hypernatremia with low urine osmolality? In this case the body is not responding appropriately by absorbing water. Most likely the ADH pathway has gone awry, and there are two possible culprits. Either there is a deficit in the kidney's ability to respond to ADH, or there is a deficit in the body's ability to make ADH.

On the other hand, take hyponatremia. Normally, when an organism is taking in enough fluid, ADH secretion will decrease so that urine output increases. If Na^+ in the plasma is low (hyponatremia) then the body will want low levels of ADH so that water is excreted in the urine, to raise the concentration of Na^+ in the blood. In contrast, the syndrome of inappropriate ADH secretion (SIADH) results in an excess of ADH, and more water retention which can lead to seizures, nausea, and vomiting.

Urea, ADH, and Urea Recycling

Deep in the medulla, near the loop of Henle, the concentration of solutes is approximately 1200 mm. About half of this amount—600 mm–comes from NaCl, and the other half comes from urea. At the start of the collecting duct, the concentration of urea in the lumen is high. As the body needs to absorb water from the collecting duct at this point, the high concentration of urea in the collecting duct would seem to be fighting against the water's ability to move from the collecting duct. Fortunately, there is a mechanism in place to account for this—urea recycling (Fig. 4.8).

As the fluid travels down the collecting duct there is a difference between the proximal (top

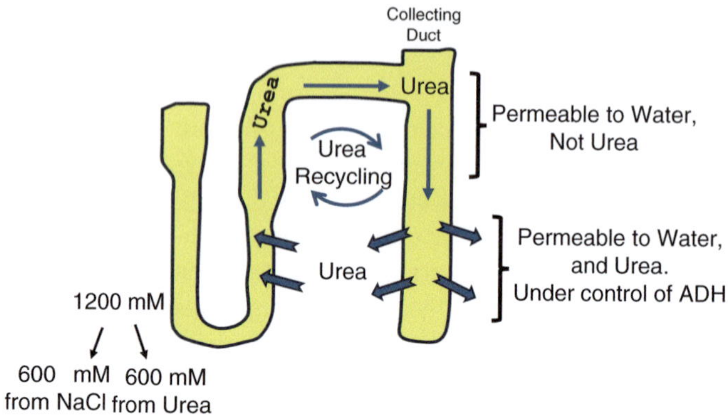

Fig. 4.8 Urea Recycling. The top of the collecting duct is permeable to water but not urea. The bottom of the collecting duct is permeable to water and urea. The urea travels from collecting duct, to interstitium, to thin ascending limb, to go back to collecting duct

of) and the distal (bottom) portions of the collecting duct. The top of the collecting duct is impermeable to urea, but permeable to water, so the water can freely move from the tube to the interstitium. As the fluid moves down the collecting duct, urea becomes more concentrated. However, the bottom of the collecting duct is permeable to urea. Towards the bottom of the collecting duct, the urine is very concentrated which leads to urea, along with water, diffusing out of the tubule and into the interstitium. The urea build-up in the deep medullary region contributes to the region's high osmolarity outside of the distal collecting duct. As the urea builds up in the interstitium, some of it will diffuse into the thin ascending limb which in turn adds to the concentration gradient as the fluid comes out of the loop and starts its ascent up the ascending limb—the recycling. It will also diffuse into the ascending limb of the vasa recta. This circular movement of urea from the lumen of the collecting duct to the interstitial tissue, to the thin ascending limb, and then back to the collecting duct is like a roundabout along a road, with the car getting caught in the roundabout doing several turns before finally getting back on the road.

Diabetes Insipidus

Due to a deficit with ADH, Patients with diabetes insipidus excrete copious amounts of urine and in turn drink a lot of water. The shortage of ADH in diabetes insipidus can be caused by a deficit in the brain (central) or the kidney (nephrogenic). Central diabetes insipidus results from a tumor, surgery or trauma to the pituitary or hypothalamus. Nephrogenic diabetes insipidus results from a failure of the kidney to respond to ADH due to a kidney infection, medication side effect (lithium for instance), elevated levels of calcium, low levels of potassium, or a blockage of the urinary tract. This leads to a loss of the collecting duct to reabsorb water. With the patient losing water, they will become hypernatremic.

Potassium

At Bowman's capsule, a significant amount of K^+ enters the proximal tubule. Most of it is absorbed by the proximal tubule, but by the time the fluid reaches the distal tubule, about 5 to 10% of the filtered potassium remains. Because of the Na^+/K^+ ATPase on the basolateral membrane, K^+ levels rise in the cells of the collecting duct. The membrane potential at the apical membrane is negatively charged and this electrical gradient drives K^+ from the cell into the tubular lumen—excretion. Under most conditions, K^+ is excreted at the collecting duct but under conditions of K^+ depletion, it will be reabsorbed.

Juxtaglomerular Apparatus

The juxtaglomerular apparatus consists of three cell types: (1) the macula densa cells, (2) the mesangial cells, and (3) the juxtaglomerular cells (JG cells).

The macula densa is a salt sensor which detects the concentration of Na^+ ions in the thick ascending limb. It resembles a plaque and consists of 20–30 cells that are larger and thicker than the rest of the TAL. The apical membranes of the macula densa cells face the lumen of the TAL, while their basal membranes face the afferent arteriole. Along the apical border of these cells, the presence of the NKCC2 cotransporters allows Na^+ and Cl^- to move into the cell. The Na^+ levels then activate the second messenger system adenosine, which leads to constriction of the afferent arterioles by the juxtaglomerular cells to slow the glomerular filtration rate (GMR). This signaling pathway is known as tubuloglomerular feedback.

The juxtaglomerular cells also release renin which activates the renin-angiotensin-aldosterone system to increase Na^+ reabsorption. There are three triggers that lead to an increase in renin: (1) Decreased perfusion pressure in the kidneys, (2) an increase in sympathetic nerve activity and (3) reduced concentration of Na^+Cl^- in the macula densa (Fig. 4.9).

Renin converts the inactive plasma enzyme angiotensinogen to angiotensin1. Angiotensin 1 is then catabolized to angiotensin 2 by angiotensin converting enzyme (ACE). One effect of angiotensin 2 is to stimulate the zona glomerulosa in the adrenal cortex to release aldosterone. Aldosterone then increases the absorption of Na^+ and the secretion of K^+ in the collecting duct by increasing the activity of ENaC along the apical cell membrane and by increasing the activity of the Na^+/K^+ -ATPase along the basolateral cell membrane. Because of ACE's ability to regulate the amount of angiotensin I, it sits in the catbird seat when it comes to controlling blood pressure. By constricting blood vessels, ACE increases blood pressure, which is why ACE inhibitors such as lisinopril are given to patients with hypertension. The ACE inhibitors lead to vasodilation of blood vessels.

Segmental Differences in Sodium Transport Mechanisms

In summary, Na^+ reabsorption along the tubular network varies from one region to another depending on what type of transporter is found in each segment. The first three listed below are on the apical membrane. The fourth one, the Na^+K^+ ATPase pump, is on the basolateral membrane.

1. $Na^+K^+2Cl^-$ transporter (NKCC2) is found on the apical membrane of the thick ascending limb and transfers these three ions into the lumen of the tubule. Because two positive charges (Na^+ and K^+) move along with two

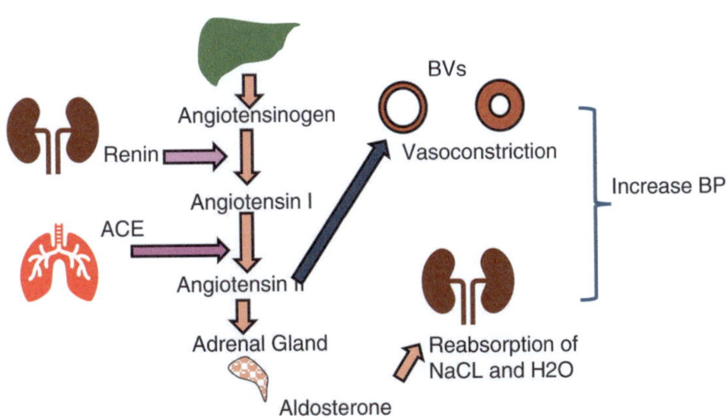

Fig. 4.9 Renin/Aldosterone. In response to low blood pressure, the liver secretes angiotensinogen, which is converted into angiotensin I by Renin. Angiotensin I is then converted into angiotensin II by ACE. Angiotensin II stimulates the adrenal gland to produce aldosterone which leads to reabsorption by kidney of NaCL and H20. Angiotensin II also leads to vasoconstriction

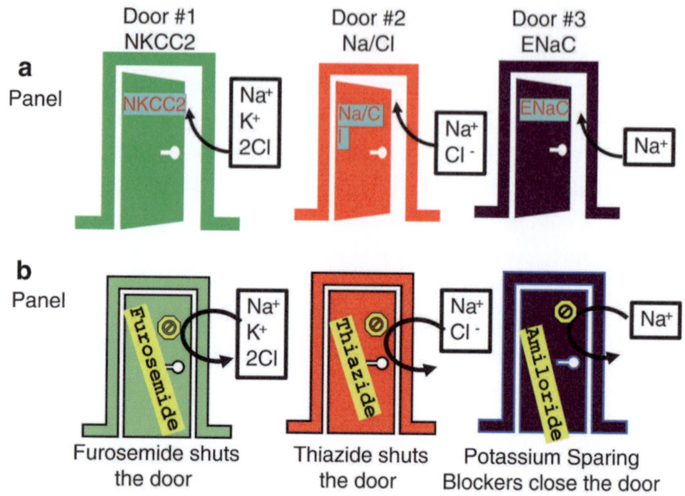

Fig. 4.10 Sodium Channels along Kidney Tubule. There are three doorways: #1 is the NKCC2 channel along the thick ascending limb. #2 is the Na/Cl channel along the distal convoluted tubule. #3 is the ENaC channel along the collecting duct. Each channel can be blocked by a specific medication [4]

negative charges (2 Cl^-) there is no change in membrane potential with ion movement. Furosemide (Lasix) blocks the NK2CC pump and is given for edema and hypertension. With blockage of the NKCC2 pump, more sodium remains in the tubular network, which in turn leads to more K^+ leaking back into the lumen (hypokalemia). When the NKCC2 is inhibited, more of these ions are excreted which leads to a decrease in blood pressure. Conversely, aldosterone increases the activity of NKCC2 so blood pressure will increase. Because it is an anti-vasoconstrictor it can be used in patients with COPD.

2. *Na^+Cl^- Cotransporter.* Located in the apical membrane this pump moves Na^+ and Cl- together in the same direction. Its principal location is on the apical membrane of the cells of the distal convoluted tubule. These channels are thiazide sensitive. Thiazides are used for the treatment of hypertension because they block the reabsorption of N^+ and CL^- and H_2O.
3. *ENaC.* The epithelial sodium channel. Located on the apical membrane this channel moves sodium from outside the cell to inside. It is found on the principal cells of the collecting ducts and on the cells towards the ends of the distal convoluted tubule. Amiloride acts on these channels. Because blockage of these channels does not affect K^+, they are known as *potassium-sparing diuretics.*
4. *Na^+K^+ -ATPase Pump.* This channel is located on the basolateral membrane, in contrast to the channels below which are on the apical membrane. As fluid moves along the tubule it encounters a sodium gradient that tends to drive sodium from the lumen of the tube into the cells. This Na^+ gradient is established by the Na^+K^+ -ATPase pumps located on the basolateral membrane. These channels use ATP to move 3 Na^+ out of the cell, and 2 K^+ ions into the cell. With a decrease of Na^+ in the cell, this drives sodium from the tubular lumen across the apical border of the tubular cells, then into the interstitial fluid, and from there then into the blood (Fig. 4.10).

Counter Current Multiplier

The focus of this section is the countercurrent multiplier. To examine this system, we are first going to look at the benefits of a countercurrent multiplier on a simpler system—not the kidney, but a simple heat exchange system. Then we will look at the countercurrent multiplier in the kidney with its descending and ascending limbs, then we will add in the vasa recta, and then focus on the collecting duct. After we have looked at the movement of the major players, we will then focus on more details of each type of cell and the role that each one plays.

Heat Exchange and the Benefits of a Counter Current Multiplier

Imagine a simple straight tube with water running through it. As the water enters the tube, the temperature is 40°. About halfway down the tube we now add a jolt of heat to increase the temperature of the water to 50°. The water exiting the tube is now at 50°. But, if we take the tube and bend it back on itself (a 180° bend), such that we have the water in each half of the tube running in different directions, we have now created a counter current exchange system. If we add the same jolt of energy to increase the heat right at the tube's bend to 50°, the water coming out of the bend is still at 50°, however there is now a temperature gradient in the system and the water at the bend, and just past the bend, deep down in the structure will heat up to a point much hotter than 50°. While we have added the same jolt of energy that we added to the straight tube, with the folded tube we have both increased the heat and trapped it. How does this happen?

Looking at the details we can see how the architecture of the 180° bend contributes to much hotter fluid in the tube. Right as the water comes out of the bend it will be 50°, but this is where the counter current multiplier benefit kicks in. Some of this heat will dissipate to the water in the parallel tube which is about to enter the bend. This water entering the bend could now be bumped up to 45°, and as this water now enters the bend and gets its jolt of heat it will heat up to 55°. As this water enters the tube some of its heat will dissipate to the other side so that the water about to enter the bend is at 50°, which is then heated to 65° - and the loop continues. The result is that with each successive turn, the water heats up to where the water entering the bend is much hotter. In other words, just by bending the tube back on itself the water is heated up to a point much hotter than a straight tube (Fig. 4.11).

This type of system is extremely important in animals that inhabit cold environments where heat conservation is essential. Besides its importance in heat exchange it is also important in gas exchange. For instance, in the swim bladders of fish where O_2 levels in the swim bladders are extremely high. Rather than the O_2 diffusing out of the bladder it is captured by the arteries. But heat and gas aside, let us move onto the kidney's countercurrent multiplier.

The Single Pass

Within the kidney, there is a horizontal osmotic pressure gradient, such that in the cortical region (outer region) the pressure is low—in the 300 MM range, but deep in the medulla (deeper region) the osmotic pressure is high—in the 1200 mM range. In other words, there are a lot of

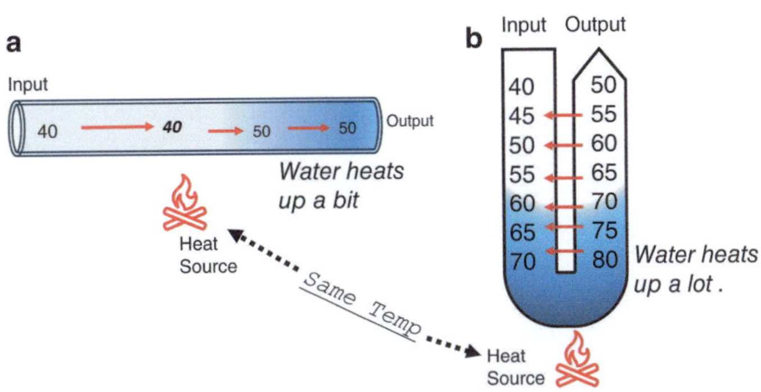

Fig. 4.11 Counter Current and Counter Exchange. In panel (**a**) the heat applied to the straight tube is very straightforward. In panel (**b**) with the tube bent back on itself, the heated water in the ascending limb dissipates some of its heat to the descending limb, so the fluid delivered to the bend keeps getting hotter and hotter. In both the straight and curved tubes, the inputs and outputs are the same, but in the system with the curved tube, the water in the bend and the lower tube is hotter [4]

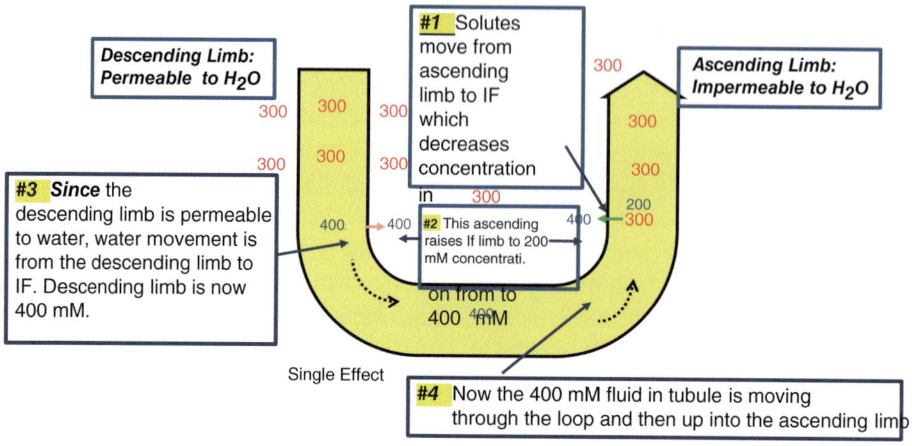

Fig. 4.12 Single Effect: The system starts at 300mM. At the end of one cycle the fluid delivered to the beginning of the ascending limb is at 400 Mm. Since this is a loop, with each subsequent pass the concentration being delivered to the ascending limb increases [4]

solutes in the deep medullary tissue—the interstitial tissue is very salty (Fig. 4.12).

Before looking at the details, we are going to look at the big picture view. As a starting point, imagine that the entire system is at 300 mM. This includes the contents of descending limb and ascending limbs which are running parallel to each other, and the surrounding interstitial fluid in both the cortex and medulla. There are two important properties that form the basis for the counter current multiplier. On one hand, the *descending limb is permeable to water but not solutes* (Na^+ and K^+ for instance), and, on the other hand, the *ascending limb is permeable to solutes but not water*. Or put another way, the *ascending limb is impermeable to water*.

Step #1 Starting with the ascending limb, which is sometime referred to as the diluting segment, there are channels in the cell membrane that allow solutes to perfuse out of the cell into the IF. (More to come on the specifics of the cell membranes in the next section). This movement of solute from the lumen of the tube to the surrounding tissue raises the IF pressure to 400, This in turn will lower the fluid in the ascending limb to 200 mM. Note that the difference in osmolality between the fluid in the ascending limb and the IF will be 200 mM, with it being higher in the IF. Keep that 200 mM difference in mind as we follow on.

Step #2 The descending limb, with its pressure at 300 mM, is now traveling through this milieu of 400 mM. And as it travels through here, there is osmotic reabsorption of water—remember the neat trick of the kidney is that while the ascending limb is *impermeable* to water, the descending limb is *permeable* to water.

Step #3 As this fluid at 400 mM moves down through the descending tube, it enters the bend, and then continues up into the ascending limb. As it approaches the beginning of the ascending limb, the pumps are still moving solute out of the fluid, so that the fluid drops to 300 mM. The IF will now be at 500 mm—remember a 200 difference between the lumen of the ascending limb and the IF. Note that with this one turn of the exchange, we have increased the osmotic pressure in the ascending limb and the IF, granted it is not by a huge amount, but it is a start. This is referred to as the *Single Effect* (or Single Pass)–we have just focused on one turn of the countercurrent exchange. We started with an osmotic pressure in the IF outside of the ascending limb of 300 mM and at the end of one turn of the loop we are at 500 mM.

Multiple Passes

With each exchange, as the fluid in the tubule travels down towards the loop it becomes more concentrated. As it makes a U-turn at the loop and now travels up the ascending limb, we are back to solute moving out of the limb into the interstitial fluid. This solute extraction from the ascending limb results in water extraction from the descending limb (Fig. 4.13).

Just as in the example of the water temperature we looked at above, with each turn of the loop, the pressure in the tubule keeps rising. With each successive turn of the loop there is an increase in pressure until we reach an equilibrium state. The result is a horizontal gradient of pressure that increases as we move from the superficial region of the medulla to the deeper regions. After one turn of the loop the pressure in the ascending limb is 300 mM but in the IF it is 500 mM. The fluid in the descending limb moving into the bend is at 500 mM also. As it enters the bend it will drop to 400 mM which gives 600 in the IF. At the next turn the ascending limb will be 500 and the IF 700, and on and on until equilibrium is reached where the osmolality values in the loop of Henle (in mOsm/kg) are: Descending limb = 800, the bend 1200, Ascending limb: 800. And then in the interstitial fluid are: Cortex –300, Outer medulla –800, and inner medulla –1200.

The Vasa Recta: Countercurrent Exchange

If we look at the interstitial fluid in the lower regions of the medulla, it seems problematic because the fluid leaking out of the descending limb into the surrounding tissue needs to go somewhere. Fortunately, passing through this region are the blood vessels in the form of another loop called the vasa recta.

Imagine for a moment what would happen if the blood vessels just passed straight through the kidney from cortex to medulla. All the fluid

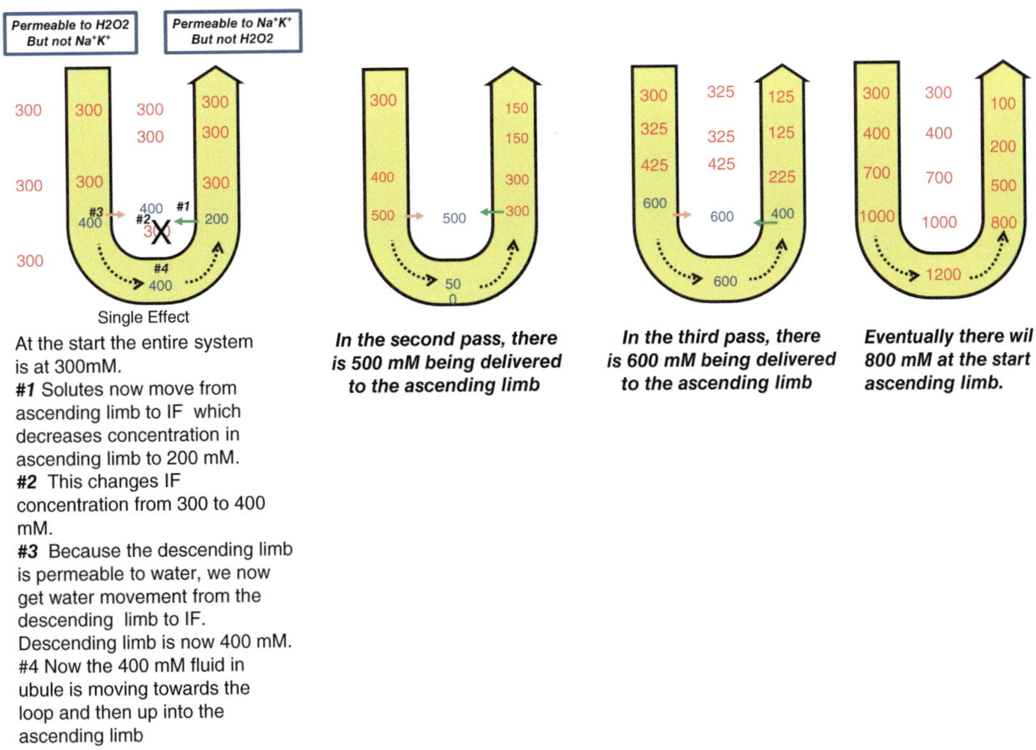

Fig. 4.13 The Countercurrent Multiplier [4]

would leak out of the interstitial fluid and the all-important countercurrent multiplier that we just described would be destroyed. Again, another fortunate feature is that the blood vessels form the vasa recta with an ascending and descending limb. The vasa recta do not *create* the hypertonic renal medulla, but they *preserve* it.

Because the vasa recta loop parallels the loop of Henle, it allows solutes to enter the descending limb of the vasa recta—solutes are entering, and water is leaving. But as the vasa recta ascends, it all reverses and the solutes flow back out of the vasa recta, and the water flows into the ascending vasa recta (Fig. 4.14).

It might be tempting to think that the blood going into the vasa recta is the same as the blood coming out, but there is a crucial difference. The blood in the ascending limb of the vasa recta is losing some water, so the fluid in the ascending vasa recta is slightly more diluted. In other words, in the vasa recta there is a net loss of water. Fortunately, the blood in the vasa recta moves very slowly so that there is less removal of solutes. Conversely, if the blood moved quickly through the vasa recta, then more solutes would be removed from the surrounding interstitial tissue.

The vasa recta emerge from the efferent arterioles of the juxtamedullary nephrons. They are equivalent to the peritubular capillaries that also emerge from the efferent arterioles of the glomeruli.

Old "Recycled" Bicarbonate

In the proximal tubule, the bicarbonate molecule cannot move directly across the apical membrane from the tubular lumen into the cells. Instead, it dissociates into smaller molecules which can cross the apical membrane, then reforms into bicarbonate, which can now move across the basolateral membrane into the blood stream. How does it do this? Carbonic anhydrase (CA) is in both the tubular lumen and the inside of the cell. In the tubular lumen, the CA splits H_2CO_3 into H_2O and CO_2. The CO_2 then crosses from the lumen into the cells of the proximal tubule where CO_2 and H_2O combines to form H_2CO_3 to then dissociate via CA to form HCO_3^- (bicarbonate) and H^+. The HCO_3^- then moves across the basolateral membrane into the blood stream. In addition, on the apical membrane of these cells there is a Na^+ H^+ antiport channel that is moving Na^+ into the cell and H^+ out of the cell. The Na^+ then moves across the cell to exit at the basolateral membrane and following the Na^+ is the HCO_3^- ion back into the blood stream. And at the same time, as the H^+ ions build up in the cell they are

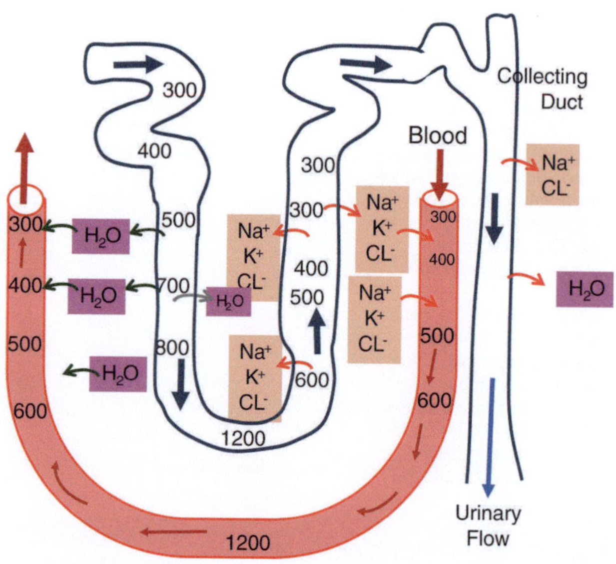

Fig. 4.14 Vasa Recta. As the vasa recta travels down into the medulla solutes are moving from the lumen into the vasa recta, but as the vasa recta travels up the medulla, water is moving from lumen to interstitium to blood

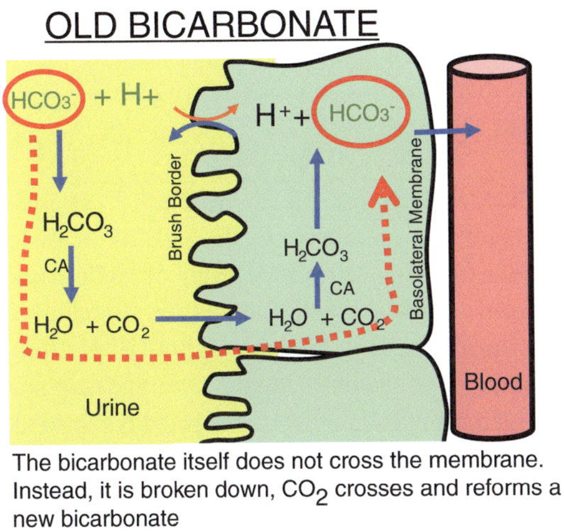

Fig. 4.15 Recycling of Bicarbonate ("Old" Bicarbonate) In the proximal tubule H^2CO_3 is broken down to H^+ and HCO_3^-. The HCO_3^- crosses the basolateral membrane and ends up in the blood stream. The H^+ ion crosses the apical membrane and combines with HCO_3^- to form H_2CO_3 which then divides into CO_2 and H_2O. It is the CO_2 which crosses the apical membrane to enter the cell [4]

moved across the apical membrane into the tubular fluid which maintains the H^+ gradient which brings Na^+ into the cell (Fig. 4.15).

Note that the Na^+ gradient is driving Na^+ from the tubular lumen to the cell and then to the interstitial fluid, while the H^+ ion is moving the opposite direction, and this movement of the H^+ ion leads to the HCO_3^- being absorbed. About 90% of the bicarbonate is reabsorbed by the proximal tubule. Note that the body has not generated bicarbonate in the proximal tubule in this process, it has just reabsorbed what was already originally present but filtered at the glomerulus, thus the term "old" or "recycled" bicarbonate. Drugs that inhibit carbonic anhydrase reduce the reabsorption of bicarbonate and the activity of the Na^+/H^+ exchanger.

Also note that with the H^+ ions there is an even trade with the bicarbonate. For each H^+ ion that moves from the proximal tubule cell into the tubular lumen, there is a molecule of HCO_3^- that is moved from the lumen to the blood stream. The more H^+ is secreted, the more HCO_3^- is retained, and vice versa, the more H^+ ion that is retained the more HCO_3^- that is excreted.

New Bicarbonate

Besides the recycling of bicarbonate in the above explanation, the kidneys are sometimes required to produce new bicarbonate. There are two major pathways involved in producing new bicarbonate.

In the cells of the distal nephron, carbonic acid is broken down into H^+ and HCO_3^- These two products then go in different directions. H^+ moves across the apical membrane to enter the tubular fluid, while HCO_3^- moves across the basolateral membrane to enter the interstitial fluid. At the apical membrane, the movement of H^+ out of the cell does not move a molecule of HCO_3^- across into the cell. This movement of HCO_3^- to the interstitial fluid has created a "new" bicarbonate in this step—as opposed to the "old" bicarbonate. The H^+ ion moves across the apical membrane to the tubular fluid because of the presence of an H^+/K^+ ATPase on the apical cell membrane. This pump is moving H^+ out of the cell and K^+ into the cell.

Since there is no bicarbonate buffer for the H^+ to bind to, instead these H^+ ions join the phosphate and ammonia buffer systems to be excreted in the urine:

$$H^+ + HPO_4^{2} \leftrightarrow H_2PO_4^-$$

$$H^+ + NH_3^+ \leftrightarrow NH_4^+$$

$H_2PO_4^-$ cannot be reabsorbed from the lumen so once an H^+ binds to HPO_4^{2-} then the H^+ is on its way to being excreted.

Calcium Reabsorption

Calcium leaves the blood stream at Bowman's capsule and enters the proximal tubule. About two-thirds of the calcium will be reabsorbed via a paracellular pathway, mostly due to positive luminal forces generated by the NKCC2 channels. One-third of the calcium will be reabsorbed via a transcellular pathway using an apical Ca^{2+} (ENaC) in the apical cell membrane. Once in the cell, sodium will cross the basolateral cell membrane via a $3Na^+/1\ Ca^{2+}$ exchanger. Most of the calcium—60–70%—will be reabsorbed along the proximal tubule, approximately 35% will be absorbed along the TAL, and the rest along the collecting duct.

Calcium sensors (CaSR) are located on the basolateral surface of the TAL cells that are the basis for a negative feedback loop. This mechanism involves elevated levels of calcium leading to less activity of the NKCC2 channel via a G-protein pathway. With less activity of the NKCC2 channel, there is less K^+ coming into the cell and subsequently less K^+ going back through the ROMK channels to the tubular lumen. With the reduction in luminal potential there is now less Ca^{2+} movement from the tubular lumen into the cell and the blood stream.

Four Commonly Used Medications

Although these medications and genetic syndromes are mentioned in various places within this chapter, here they are discussed together and summarized. Understanding these three medications and the three genetic syndromes aides in understanding the movement of sodium along the nephron.

Carbonic Anhydrase Inhibitors reduce the movement of sodium from the tubular lumen into the bloodstream. The inhibition of CA in the proximal tubule cells leads to a decrease of H^+ into the lumen via the Na^+/H^+ antiporter. This in turn reduces the movement of Na^+ from the lumen into the cell. The Na^+ is released into the urine, and the Na^+ takes water with it, leading to diuresis.

Furosemide one of the loop diuretics, (Lasix) blocks the NKCC2 channel along the TAL which leads to less movement of Na^+. However it will also lead to less movement of K^+ into the cell—the patient will be hypokalemic. The urine will be diluted. In addition, with less movement of K^+ into the cells, and now less K^+ moving back through the ROMK channel (the inward rectifier) this leads to a reduction in the positive luminal potential. With the lower potential, this leads to less movement of Ca^{2+} from the tubular lumen to the blood stream—*lower levels of calcium in the blood -hypocalcemia.*

Thiazide Diuretics block the Na^+/Cl^- channel on the apical membrane of the cells of the distal tubule which leads to low levels of sodium and chloride inside the cell. In addition, if sodium is low inside the cell, then the activity of Na^+/Ca^{2+} exchanger on the basolateral membrane responds by increasing its activity and to bring Na^+ into the cell via the Na^+/Ca^{2+} exchanger, which in turn leads to calcium being excreted by the cell—*higher levels of calcium in the blood (hypercalcemia)*. The main side effect of the thiazides is the potassium loss resulting in hypokalemia. Due to an increase of Na^+ delivery to the late nephron segments (Fig. 4.16).

As a side bar, the thiazides are often used to treat diabetes insipidus and this seems paradoxical. Why would we treat a condition with polyuria by administering a diuretic? While they are several proposed mechanisms, the most likely is that by blocking the Na^+/Cl^- co-exchanger this leads to a less sodium reabsorption in the distal tubule, more sodium secretion, and a reduction of extracellular fluid volume, which leads to a reduction in GFR sodium, and increased water reabsorption. The result is that there is less water in the urine.

Some Potassium Sparing Diuretics act on the ENaC channels which normally allow Na^+ to move from the lumen to the cell and then to the blood stream. When the concentration of Na^+ increases inside the cell this leads to movement of K^+ from the cell to the lumen. When this ENaC channel is blocked, there is now less movement of K^+ into the lumen and less excretion of potassium, hence the name potassium sparing (Fig. 4.17).

Other potassium sparing diuretics act by blocking aldosterone receptors or the production of aldosterone. Remember, aldosterone usually increases the activity of the ENaC channel.

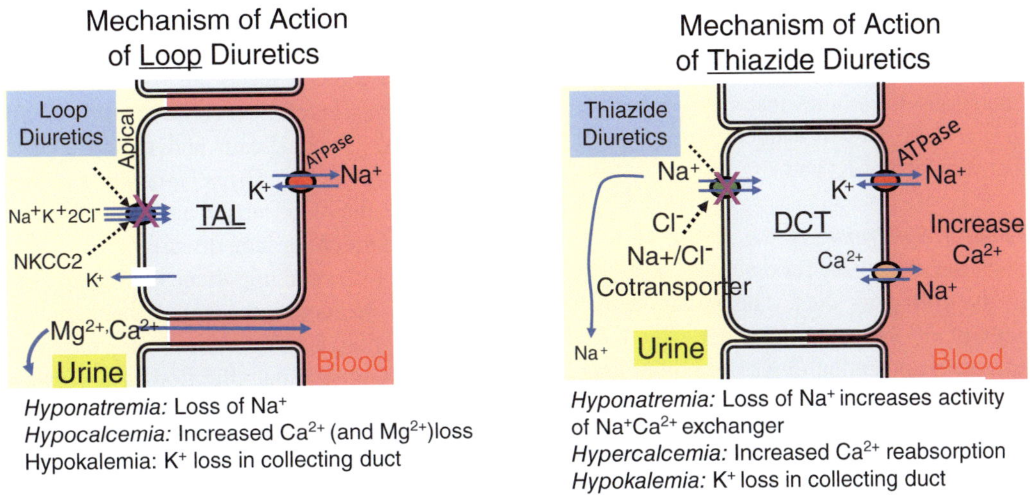

Fig. 4.16 Mechanism of Action of Diuretics. Panel (**a**) the loop diuretics block the NKCC2 receptor along the apical membrane of the thick ascending limb (TAL). The Thiazide diuretics block the Na^+/Cl^- coexchanger, also located on the apical membrane. With the sodium levels inside the cell dropping, this leads to increased activity of the Na^+/Ca^{2+} exchanger, thus calcium levels inside the blood are increased [4]

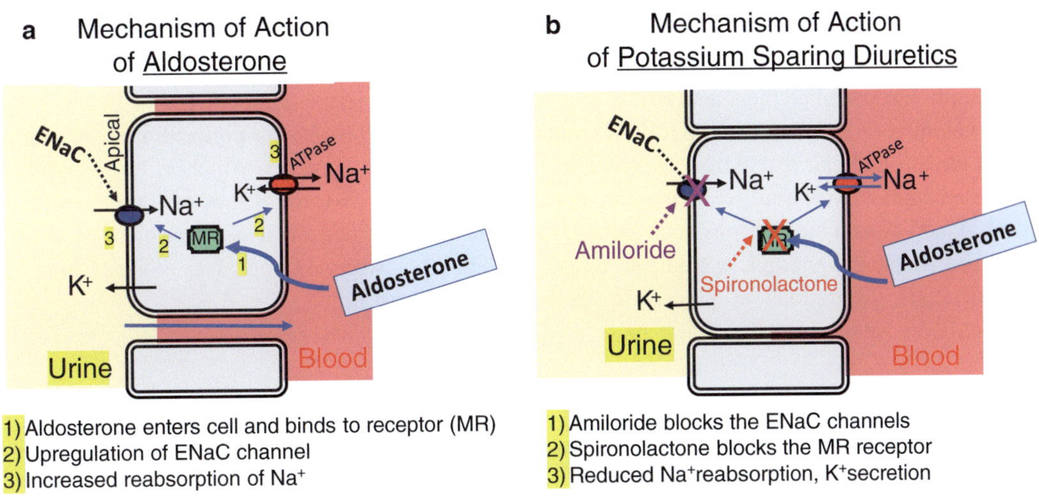

Fig. 4.17 Mechanism of Action of Potassium Sparing Diuretics. Panel (**a**) aldosterone binds to intracellular receptor which upregulates the ENaC channels and the Na^+/K^+AtPase leading to increased absorption of Na^+ and water. Panel (**b**) Spironolactone blocks the MR receptor (aldosterone antagonist) and Amiloride blocks the ENaC channel. Sodium reabsorption is decreased, and potassium is not affected [4]

Three Genetic Disorders

Just like the medications above, there are three genetic mutations, each of which affects one of the three sodium channels along the tubular network. While they are very rare, they aide in our understanding of kidney function.

Bartter's Syndrome is a defect in the gene for the NKCC2 transporter. These patients will have low levels of serum calcium—elevated levels of calcium in the urine.

Gitelman's Syndrome is a genetic condition that results in a mutation (loss of function) of the thiazide sensitive NaCl cotransporter in the distal convoluted tubule leading to hypertension and hypokalemia. The hypokalemia comes from alterations in volume that lead to increases in aldosterone, with subsequent absorption of NA^+ and secretion of K^+ and H^+.

Liddle's Syndrome is the result of a genetic mutation in the gene for the ENaC channel found in the collecting duct. The mutation increases activity of the ENaC channel which leads to increased absorption of Na^+ and other ions leading to hypertension (Fig. 4.18).

Altered Ion Levels

Normal potassium levels are between 3.6 to 5.2 mmols/L. *Hyperkalemia* is too much K^+ and can result from ingesting too much K^+ in the diet. Elevated levels of K^+ are found in orange juice, melons, and bananas. It can also result from a deficit in the ability of the kidney to excrete potassium. Uncontrolled diabetes can also lead to hyperkalemia. *Hypokalemia* is too little K^+ in the blood stream and can result from diarrhea, certain medications, vomiting, drinking too much alcohol, and certain medications. Low potassium can lead to muscle cramps, weakness, fatigue, and twitches. Alterations in potassium levels, whether they are too high or too low, affect nerve conduction.

Normal chloride levels are 96 to 106 mEq/L. *Hyperchloremia* refers to elevated levels of chloride in the blood stream and typically results from kidney deficits. *Hypochloremia* is too little chloride in the blood stream and typically results from heart failure or lung disease.

There are several important values that can be examined to determine renal function. The amount of fluid moving across at Bowman's capsule is the glomerular filtration rate. However, what comes out in the urine does not equate to the GFR, because as the fluid moves through the tubular system, some will be reabsorbed and some will be secreted. Fortunately, inulin is a molecule that comes across at Bowman's capsule and is not subject to secretion or absorption as it moves through tube. If one knows the starting and ending values of inulin, one can determine GFP. Inulin is not produced in the body but can be injected into the blood stream and then monitored in the blood stream and urine to determine GFR. The volume of inulin in the urine divided by the plasma concentration of inulin equals inulin clearance which in turn is equivalent to GFR. Normal values of inulin clearance for young women are in the range of 110 ± 15 mL/min for women and for young men is 125 ± 15 mL/min.

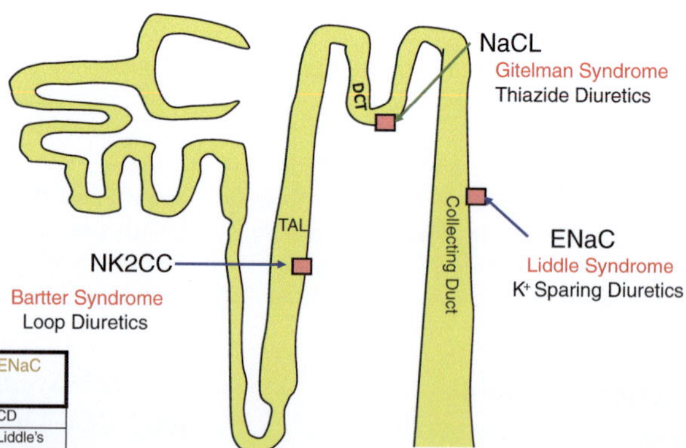

	NKCC2	Na^+Cl^-	ENaC
Location	TAL	DCT	CD
Genetics	Bartter's	Gitelman's	Liddle's
Drug	Furosemide	Thiazide	Amiloride

Fig. 4.18 Three Medications and Three Genetic Syndromes. The loop diuretics and Bartter's syndrome affect the NAKCC2 transporter in the thick ascending limb (TAL), the thiazide diuretics and Gitelman syndrome affect the Na^+/Cl^- Co-exchanger in the distal convoluted tubule (DCT). and the K^+ sparing diuretics and Liddle syndrome affects the ENaC channel in the collecting duct [4]

Creatinine, produced by the muscles, can also be used to measure GFR, and, like inulin, is filtered at Bowman's capsule and then excreted. Like the formula above for inulin, creatinine clearance is determined by the volume of creatinine in the urine divided by the creatinine in the plasma which equals the creatinine clearance rate which in turn equals GFR. There are two errors or complications with measuring creatinine clearance but fortunately these errors cancel each other out. On one hand, the kidneys do secrete some creatinine into the tubular fluid. About 20% of the creatinine excreted in the urine comes from secretion. However, on the other hand, the common test for measuring creatinine in the plasma overestimates the amount by 20%. While one complication affects the numerator of the equation, and another complication affects the denominator of the equation—both by 20%, they cancel each other out. For a healthy individual creatinine can be a good estimate of GFR but in pathological states the errors can be problematic when it comes to using creatinine as a measure of GFR.

Acid Base Maintenance

Consuming foods produces a net amount of acids. The body has three mechanisms in place to handle this production of H^+ ions: (1) Chemical buffering, (2) a Respiratory Response, and (3) a Renal Response.

1. Chemical buffers can either absorb H^+ ions or give up H^+ ions as needed to maintain the optimal pH for the body, and they act very quickly—think of them as the first line of defense. There are several chemical buffers such as the phosphate buffer and protein buffers. In addition, an essential buffer in the body which involves both the lungs and the kidneys is:

   The HCO_3^- (base) can absorb H^+ ions, while the H_2CO_3 (carbonic acid) can give up H^+ ions. In water this reaction can take up to a minute but in the presence of the enzyme carbonic anhydrase, it takes milliseconds. In addition to the chemical buffers, the lungs and kidneys also play a role in maintaining the proper pH (Fig. 4.19).

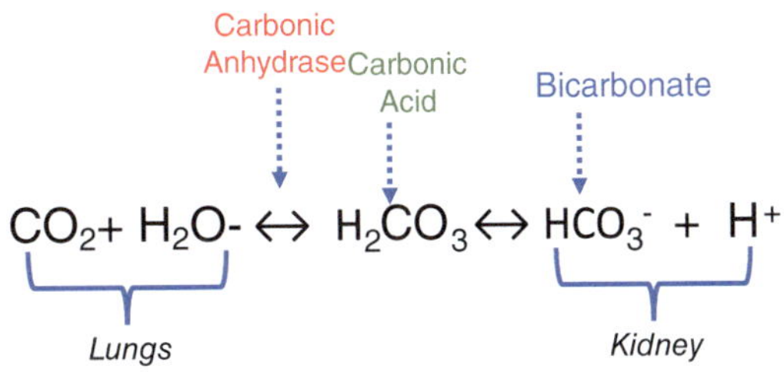

Fig. 4.19 The Bicarbonate Buffer

2. The lungs act quickly by changing the pCO_2 which changes H_2CO_3.
3. The kidneys take longer by removing either H^+ or HCO_3^-.

In the lungs, respiration controls the amount of CO_2, so that increases or decreases in CO_2 will drive the reaction either to the right or the left. In the kidneys, increases or decreases of HCO_3^- will drive the reaction one way or the other. To counteract the H^+ we ingest daily, the distal tubule of the healthy kidney is excreting H^+. As we saw earlier, as H^+ is excreted, a new molecule of HCO_3^- is being produced and absorbed into the bloodstream.

Respiratory Acidosis and Alkalosis

A respiratory acidosis or alkalosis comes from increasing or decreasing the partial pressure of CO_2. The optimal pH of the blood is 7.40. Adding or subtracting components from the above equation will alter the direction of the reaction one way or the other. Fig. 4.20 focuses on what moves the reaction towards either the right or the left and the subsequent pH levels. We can see the effects of either holding one's breath or increasing the breathing rate. If the patient is holding their breath this increases the CO_2 levels in the blood stream which drives the reaction towards the right and increases the H^+ concentration leading to respiratory acidosis.

On the other hand, by increasing the breathing rate, the patient is expelling CO_2 which leads to a reduction of CO_2 in the blood stream which

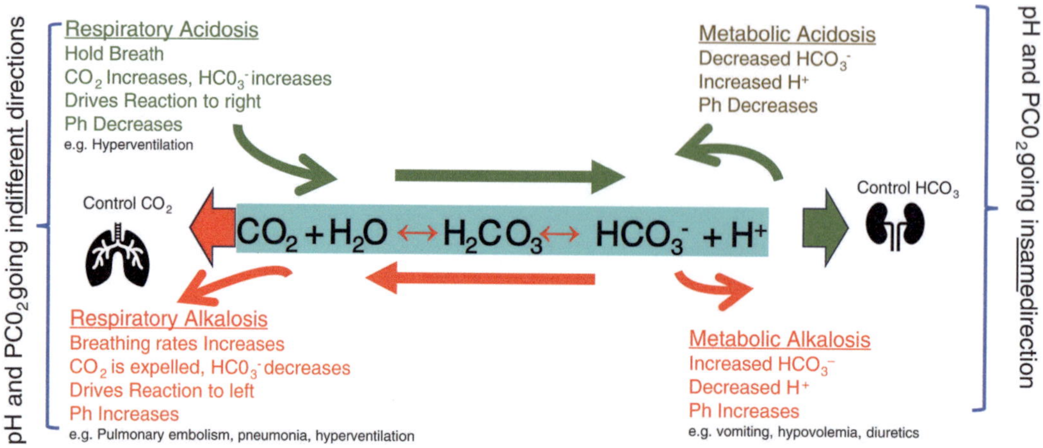

Fig. 4.20 Acidotic versus Alkalotic Patient And Direction of Reaction. This figure starts with the pH of the patient, either acidotic or alkalotic, and then looks at the direction of the reaction. Holding one's breath drives the reaction to the right and increases H^+. Excessive breathing drives the reaction to the left and decreases H^+. If the kidneys are secreting HCO_3^- this increases H^+, while retaining HCO_3^- secretes H^+ [4]

drives the reaction to the left. This reduces the H^+ concentration and leads to a respiratory alkalosis (Fig. 4.20).

Metabolic Acidosis and Alkalosis

A metabolic acidosis or alkalosis comes from lowering or raising HCO_3^- levels in the blood. With a metabolic acidosis, there is secretion of HCO_3^- and retention of H^+. Metabolic acidosis can result from diabetes mellitus or diarrhea.

On the other hand, with a metabolic alkalosis, there is retention of HCO_3^- which leads to excretion of H^+. Metabolic acidosis can be caused by antacids, vomiting, and increased renal H^+ secretion.

Once you understand the equation and the movement of the various ions, a straightforward way to remember all of this when you are looking at arterial blood gases (ABGs), is that *when pH and pCO2 levels are going in opposite directions then it is a respiratory problem.* If you are a Star Wars fan, think CPO, – CO_2 and **pH O**pposite and CPO is a **R**obot.

Conversely, *when pH and CO_2 levels are going in the same direction then the source of the problem is metabolic.*

One way to look at the balancing act between CO_2 and HCO_3^- is by thinking of them as opposite weights on the two ends of a teeter-totter—as the concentration of a substance on one end of the teeter-totter goes up, that end goes down, while the other end goes up. Looking at Fig. 4.21 we can see CO_2 on one end and HCO_3^- on the other end. On either end of the teeter totter we can increase or decrease the concentration of that substance. This results in two scenarios at each end for a total of four scenarios (Fig. 4.21).

1. Increasing the amount of CO_2 leads to *respiratory acidosis.*
2. Decreasing the amount of HCO_3^- leads to *metabolic acidosis.*
3. Decreasing the amount of CO_2 leads to *respiratory alkalosis.*
4. Increasing the amount of HCO_3^- leads to *metabolic alkalosis.*

Compensation

We can also see that when the body finds itself in one of these scenarios it will respond and try to correct it. If the problem comes from the respiratory system, the kidneys will try and compensate; vice versa, if the initial problem is with the kidneys, the lungs will try and compensate. The lungs can respond very quickly, the kidneys take

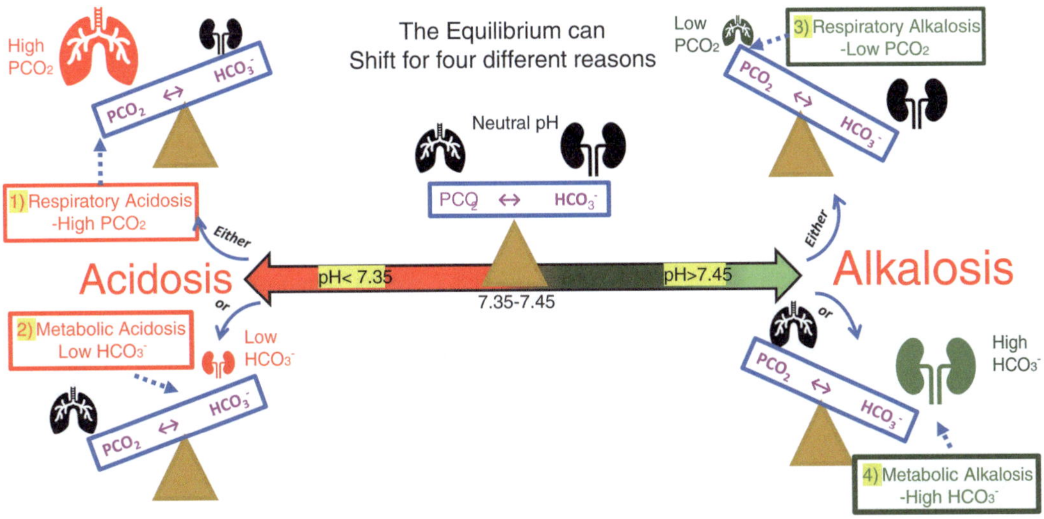

Fig. 4.21 Causes of Acidosis and Alkalosis. Acidosis can be caused by (1) high levels of CO_2 (respiratory) or (2) low levels of HCO_3^- (metabolic). Alkalosis can be caused by either (3) low PCO_2 (respiratory) or 4) high HCO_3^- (metabolic) [4]

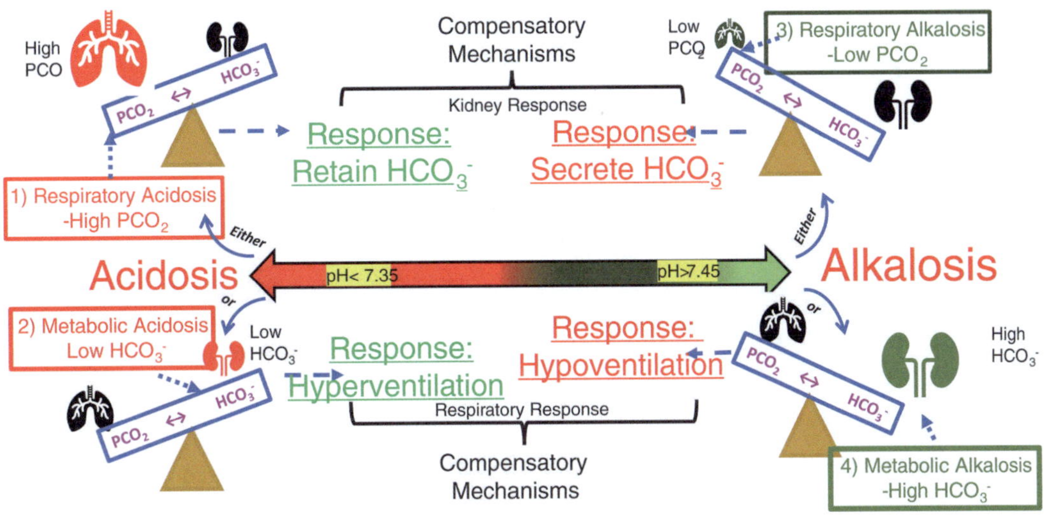

Fig. 4.22 Causes of Acidosis and Alkalosis Plus Compensatory Responses. With metabolic issues, the body will have a respiratory response. With respiratory issues, the body will have a metabolic response [4]

days to respond. When the compensatory response brings the pH back within the normal range this is considered a *full compensation*, when the response only brings the pH back in the right direction but not all the way, it is considered a *partial compensation* (Fig. 4.22).

1. With a respiratory acidosis, caused by elevated levels of CO_2, the kidneys will retain HCO_3^- and secrete H^+.
2. With a metabolic acidosis, caused by low levels of HCO_3^-, the patient will hyperventilate to blow off CO_2.

3. With a respiratory alkalosis, caused by low CO_2 levels, the kidneys will secrete HCO_3^- and retain H^+.
4. With a metabolic alkalosis, caused by elevated levels of HCO_3^-, the patient will hypoventilate to retain CO_2.

Keep in mind that an individual with a normal pH could still have a problem, but it is because of the compensation that the pH is normal. Both metabolic alkalosis and acidosis are due to alterations in bicarbonate. The kidneys can recycle bicarbonate "old bicarbonate" or they can make new bicarbonate.

The Anion Gap

If you determine that a patient has a metabolic acidosis, there is one more step: You need to calculate the anion gap to determine the cause of the metabolic acidosis. The anion gap is the *measurable* difference between the cations and anions. Note the adjective, *measurable*, which is important, because if you could measure all the cations and anions in the extracellular space, you find that they are equal—there would be no difference. However, we cannot measure all the anions. Thus because we take the measurable ions, we come up short with the anions. The formula for this is the cations minus the anions, or

$$\left[Na^+\right]\text{minus}\left[Cl\right]\text{minus}\left[HCO_3\right] \\ = \text{The Anion Gap.}$$

The measurable cations are Na^+ and K^+ but the K^+ is so minimal that we can ignore it. The two anions are Cl^- and HCO_3^-. The healthy anion gap is 11 mmol/L, but measurements can vary from one lab to another. Either below 10 mmol/L or above 14 mmol/L is considered problematic. A low anion gap is rarely found. Using normal laboratory values we can see the calculation: 136–100 – 25 = 11.

In the case of a high anion gap, the extracellular space is losing bicarbonate which binds with H^+. A high anion gap (greater than 10 mmol/L) can be caused by several conditions and remembered with the Mnemonic KARMEL: standing for Ketoacidosis, Aspirin, Renal failure, Methanol, Ethylene Glycol, and Lactic acidosis (Figs. 4.23 and 4.24).

In a patient with metabolic acidosis and normal anion gap, they are losing bicarbonate, so something else must be compensating to maintain the normal anion gap. In this scenario of the bicarbonate loss, Cl^- is moving from the cells into the extracellular space to make up for the lost bicarbonate. Normal anion gap metabolic acidosis can be caused by losses of bicarbonate via the GI tract, renal tubular acidosis, carbonic anhydrase inhibitors, and excess administration of saline (Fig. 4.25).

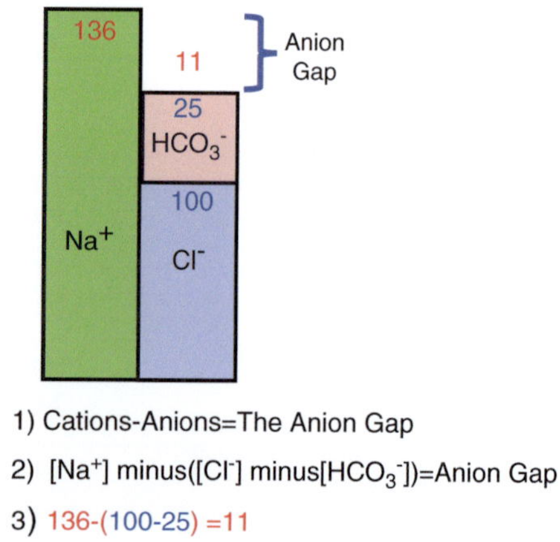

Fig. 4.23 The Anion Gap. Various ways of showing the anion gap

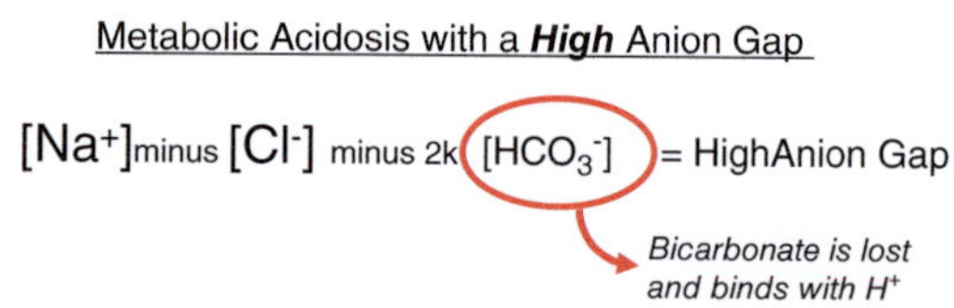

Fig. 4.24 Metabolic Acidosis with a High Anion Gap. In this case the bicarbonate is being lost and binding with the H+

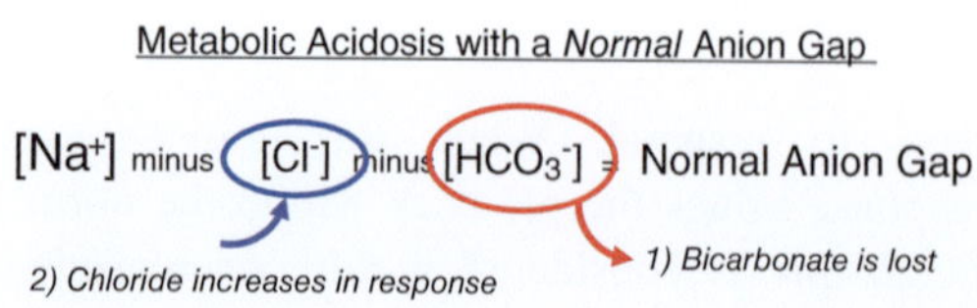

Fig. 4.25 Metabolic Acidosis with a Normal Anion Gap. In this case the bicarbonate is being lost and binding with the H^+ however to counteract this, the cells are releasing chloride into the extracellular space

Acidosis or Alkalosis? Metabolic or Respiratory?

When you are looking at lab values, there are several steps to determine the source of an acid base disturbance:

1. Start by looking at the pH to determine if the patient is acidotic (pH below 7.35) or alkalotic (pH above 7.45). The question then becomes is it a metabolic or respiratory issue.
2. The next step is to look at their bicarbonate and pCO_2 levels to determine whether the primary cause if metabolic or respiratory (Fig. 4.26).
   (a) Acidotic: Low Bicarbonate = Metabolic. High PCO_2 = Respiratory
   (b) Alkalotic: Low pCO_2 = Respiratory. High Bicarbonate = Metabolic
3. The last step is to determine the anion gap.

Another way to think about this is imagine if the patient is alkalotic, and has low CO_2 levels, then it is a respiratory alkalosis. However, if they have high HCO_3^- levels, then they have metabolic alkalosis. With kidney failure, the kidney is unable to make and absorb HCO_3. With this reduction in plasma levels of HCO_3^- there is an increase of H^+ leading to metabolic acidosis. The lungs will compensate by increased respiration.

Arterial Blood Gas Questions

Remember CPO—R For when **C**O_2 and **p**H are going in **O**pposite directions this a **R**espiratory matter. It is the reverse for Metabolic issues.

Ion	Normal Level (In mmol/L)
pH	7.35–7.45
Sodium	135–145
Potassium	3.6–5.2
Bicarbonate	22–26 mEq/L
Chloride	96–106
pCO_2	35–45mmol/Hg

Fig. 4.26 Normal levels of ions in serum

Patient One

$$pH = 7.6 \quad pCO2 = 20 \; HCO_3^- = 20$$

Patient Two

$$pH = 7.2 \quad pCO2 = 80 \; HCO_3^- = 30$$

Patient Three

$$pH = 7.3 \quad pCO_2 = 33 \; HCO_3^- = 15$$

$$Na+ = 136 \; Cl- = 109$$

Patient Four

$$pH = 7.33 \; pCO_2 = 54 \; HCO_3^- = 41$$

Patient Five

$$pH = 7.32 \; pCO_2 = 53 \; HCO_3^- = 31$$

Patient Six

$$pH = 7.51 \; pCO_2 = 50 \; HCO_3^- = 34$$

Patient Seven

$$pH = 7.42 \; pCO_2 = 44 \; HCO_3^- = 33$$

Patient Eight

$$pH = 7.19 \; pCO_2 = 15 \; HCO_3^- = 7$$

$$Na^+ = 138 \; Cl^- = 95$$

Answers

Patient (1) pH and pCO_2 going in opposite direction = Respiratory alkalosis. pH still out of normal range = Uncompensated.

Patient (2) pH and pCO_2 going in opposite directions = Respiratory acidosis. pH still out of normal range—Uncompensated.

Patient (3) pH and pCO_2 going in same direction = Metabolic acidosis. HCO_3^- is low - partial compensation. Plus, anion gap = 136–109-15 = 12. Normal anion gap (NAGMA)

Patient (4) pH and pCO_2 going in opposite directions = Respiratory acidosis. HCO_3^- – is high—partial compensation.

Patient (5) pH and pCO_2 going in opposite directions = Respiratory acidosis, pH is on low side but in normal range - fully compensated.

Patient (6) pH and pCO_2 going in same directions = metabolic alkalosis. Lungs are trying to bring pH back in range, but still not in normal range—partial compensation.

Patient (7) pH and pCO_2 going in same direction—metabolic alkalosis. pCO_2 is high and is bringing pH back into normal range- fully compensated.

Patient (8) pH and pCO_2 going in same direction—metabolic acidosis. Anion Gap 138–95—7 = 36. High anion gap metabolic acidosis (HAGMA)

Further Reading

1. Hamilton PK, Morgan NA, Connoly GM, Maxwell AP. Understanding Acid-Base Disorders. Ulster Med J Grand Rounds. 2017;86(3):161–6.
2. Kriz W, Kaissling B. Structural organization of the mammalian kidney. In: Seldin and Giebisch's The Kidney. 4th ed; 2008. p. 479–563. Available at: https://doi.org/10.1016/B978-012088488-9.50023-1.
3. Leo J. Medical neuroanatomy for the boards and clinic: finding the lesion. 2nd ed. Switzerland: Springer; 2024.
4. Leo J. Clinical anatomy and embryology: a guide for the classroom, clinic, and clinic. 2nd ed. Springer; 2024.
5. Magaldi A. New insights into the paradoxical effect of thiazides in diabetes insipidus therapy. Nephrology Dialysis Transplant. 2000;15:1903–5.
6. Moor MB, Bonny O. Ways of calcium reabsorption in the kidney. Amer J Physiol: Ren Physiol. 2016;310:F1337–G1350.
7. Pallone TL, Turner MR, Edwards A, Jamison RL. Countercurrent exchange in the renal medulla. Amer J Physiol Integr Compare Physiol. 2003;284:R1153–75.
8. Roy A, Al-bataineh MM, Pastor-Soler N. Collecting duct intercalated cell function and regulation. Clin J Amer Soc of Nephrol. 2015;10(2):305–24.
9. Sato K, Hall C, Glaser S, Francis H, Meng F, Alpini G. Pathogenesis of Kupffer cells in cholestatic liver injury. Amer. J Pathol. 2016;186(9):2238–47.

5 The Pelvis and Perineum

Introduction

As an introduction to the pelvic region, imagine the bony pelvis like a bucket, and into this bucket we drop a funnel. But then underneath the funnel, we are going to add an extra layer of support. The sides of the bucket are the bony pelvis and the obturator internus muscle. The funnel is the muscular *pelvic diaphragm*. And the extra layer of support under the pelvic diaphragm is the *urogenital diaphragm*. The space between the pelvic diaphragm and the urogenital diaphragm is the *ischiorectal fossa*. And within this fossa, on the medial wall of the obturator internus is the *pudendal canal*, housing the pudendal nerve and internal pudendal artery and vein (Fig. 5.1). Now for the details.

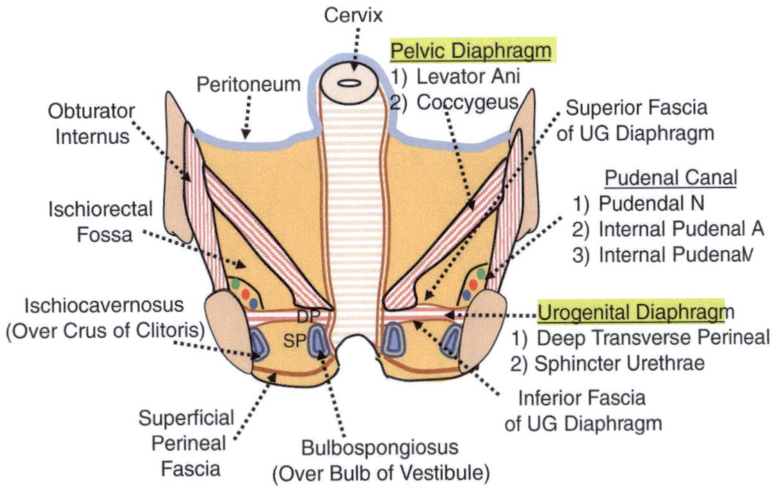

Fig. 5.1 Pelvic diaphragm. The bony pelvis resembles a bucket, whose walls are the obturator internus. Dropped into the bucket is a funnel, the pelvic diaphragm. Inferiorly is the urogenital diaphragm. The pudendal canal is found in the ischiorectal fossa. *SP* superficial space, *DP* Deep Space [3, 4]

J. Leo, *Gross Anatomy, Neuroanatomy, and Embryology for Medical Students*,
https://doi.org/10.1007/978-3-031-87151-1_5

Pelvic Diaphragm

The pelvic diaphragm is made up of two muscles: (1) *coccygeus*, and (2) *levator ani,* and the levator ani in turn has three divisions (Fig. 5.2).

1. The fibers of the *pubococcygeus* run from the pubic bone to the coccyx in an anterior to posterior direction.
2. The most medial portion of the pubococcygeus is the *puborectalis*. Starting at the pubic bone, the fibers run posterior towards the rectum, but unlike the pubococcygeus which attaches to the coccyx, the fibers of puborectalis make a 180° turn around the rectum and head towards the contralateral pubic bone. They form a sling around the rectum to keep fecal material inside the rectum.
3. The *iliococcygeus* runs from the ischium to the coccyx with the fibers running in a mediolateral direction, as compared to the anteroposterior running fibers of pubococcygeus. The iliococcygeus also attaches to the tendinous arch of levator ani. In four-legged animals the muscle is attached along the bony rim of the pelvis, but as humans stood up, gravity and the weight of the internal muscles pushed down on the iliococcygeus to push it away from the bone.

The *coccygeus muscle* is fused with the *sacrospinous ligament*.

The pelvic diaphragm muscles—*levator ani* and *coccygeus*—are innervated by direct branches from S3 and 4 (sometimes S2 contributes). During deliveries, the pelvic diaphragm is stretched. Kegel exercises help to strengthen the pelvic diaphragm. In some instances, a weak pelvic diaphragm can lead to prolapse of the internal organs. Prolapses are categorized by where in the perineum the organ emerges. Anterior prolapses typically involve the bladder emerging anterior to the vagina—*cystocele.* Posterior prolapses involve the rectum or intestines emerging posterior to the vagina—*rectocele*. And apical pro-

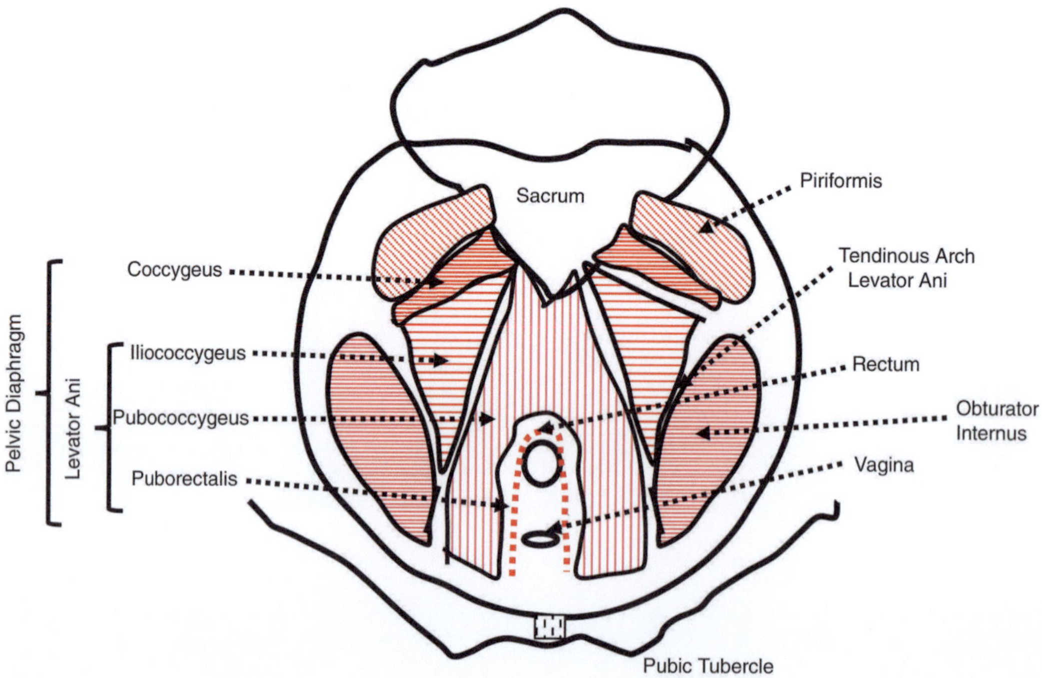

Fig. 5.2 Pelvic diaphragm. The pelvic diaphragm is made up of levator ani and coccygeus. The levator ani is made up of the iliococcygeus, pubococcygeus and puborectalis. The iliococcygeus arises from the tendinous arch of levator ani [3, 4]

lapses involve the uterus emerging though the vagina.

In the lithotomy position, the perineum can be seen as a diamond shaped pelvic outlet with four points to it. On the sides, the two points are the ischial tuberosities, anterior is the pubic symphysis and posterior is the coccyx. By drawing a line between the two ischial tuberosities, the perineum is further subdivided into two smaller triangles:

1. the *anal triangle* is bound superiorly by the pelvic diaphragm and contains the internal and external anal sphincters.
2. the *urogenital triangle* contains the urogenital diaphragm, which is the extra layer of support mentioned earlier. In the lithotomy position the urogenital triangle blocks the view of the pelvic diaphragm.

Internal Iliac Artery

The internal iliac artery arises from the common iliac artery and enters the pelvic cavity anterior to the sacroiliac joint. There is significant variability in its branching pattern, but it has anterior and posterior divisions. The posterior division gives off three branches (Fig. 5.3):

1. The *iliolumbar artery* divides into an *iliac* branch descending towards the ileum and a *lumbar* branch ascending towards the lumbar vertebrae.
2. The *superior gluteal artery* heads inferior and typically runs between the lumbosacral trunk and the S1 ventral root. It then leaves the pelvis through the greater sciatic foramen and enters the gluteal region superior to piriformis (supra piriform recess). As it approaches the gluteal muscles it travels between the gluteus medius and gluteus minimus. In cases of pelvic fractures, the superior gluteal artery is the most often injured vessel.
3. The *lateral sacral artery* heads down along the sacrum lateral to the ventral sacral foramina.

The anterior division of the internal iliac artery sends branches to the pelvic viscera, the medial thigh, and the gluteal region:

1. The distal portions of the right and left *umbilical arteries*, which transmitted blood to the placenta during development, become obliterated in the adult. Their remnants are found on the posterior surface of the anterior abdominal wall as the *medial umbilical ligaments*. But

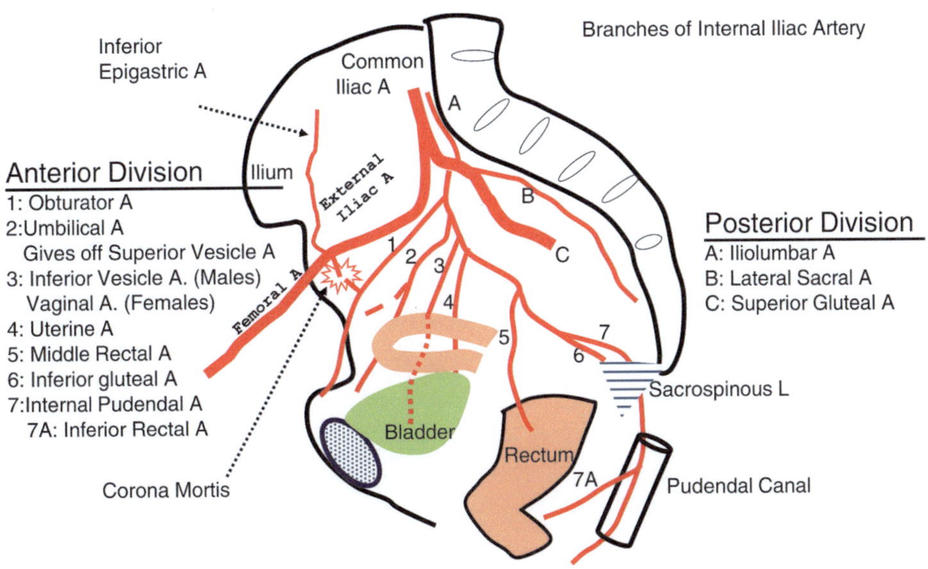

Fig. 5.3 Branches of the internal iliac artery [3, 4]

the proximal portion remains as the *superior vesicle artery* which goes to the bladder.

2. The *obturator artery* leaves the pelvis through the obturator foramen to reach the medial thigh.
3. The *middle rectal artery* supplies the rectum.
4. The *uterine artery* supplies the uterus. The uterine artery heads towards the cervix in the cardinal ligament traveling over the ureter. As it reaches the uterus it divides into an ascending branch heading towards the uterus, and a descending branch heading towards the vagina. The ascending branch of the uterine artery has a curvy, twisted path so that in a pregnant woman the artery can stretch as the uterus expands.
5. The *inferior gluteal artery* leaves the pelvis through the greater sciatic foramen inferior to the piriformis to enter the gluteal region.
6. The *internal pudendal artery* leaves the pelvis through the greater sciatic foramen, but then reenters the pelvis through the lesser sciatic foramen. It does a 100° turn around the sacrospinous ligament to enter the pudendal canal which is made up of the fascia of obturator internus.
7. *Sampson's Artery,* also known as the artery of the round ligament, runs under the round ligament and is the anastomosis between the uterine artery and the ovarian artery. Most sources list it as a branch of the uterine artery. Sampson's artery is a bit of minutia for future OB-GYN physicians.
8. The *inferior vesical artery* is present in males, in females there is a *vaginal artery*.

The visceral peritoneum in the abdominal cavity extends down into the pelvic area and overlays the various organs. The lowest point in the peritoneal cavity is the *rectouterine pouch* in females and *rectovesical pouch* in males. In the supine position, excess fluid in the peritoneal cavity can collect in the rectouterine pouch and drain via the paracolic gutters to the hepatorenal recess. In the sitting position, the fluid will drain out of the hepatorenal recess and collect in the rectouterine pouch.

Internal Pudendal Artery

Traveling with the pudendal nerve is the internal pudendal artery. Its branching pattern is like the nerve branches (Fig. 5.4):

1. The *inferior rectal artery* comes off at the beginning of the pudendal canal and crosses the ischiorectal fossa with the inferior rectal nerve.
2. The *perineal artery* supplies the superficial perineum.
3. The *artery to the bulb* supplies the bulb of the vestibule or penis.
4. The *dorsal artery of the penis or clitoris* supplies these two structures.

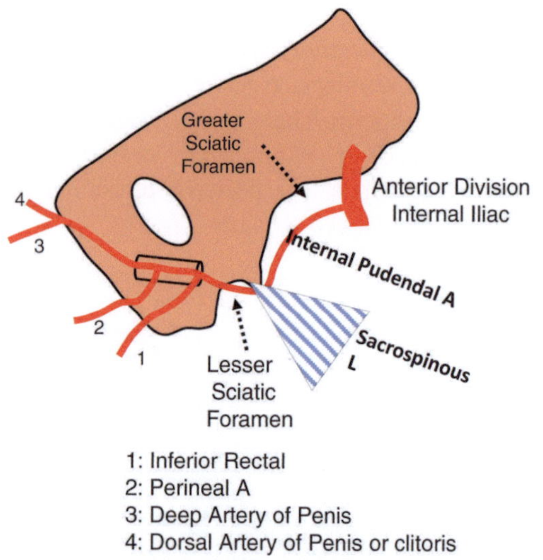

Fig. 5.4 Branches of internal pudendal artery. The internal pudendal artery comes off the anterior division of the internal iliac and leaves the pelvis through the greater sciatic foramen. It then wraps around the sacrospinous ligament and renters the pelvis through the lesser sciatic foramen. It continues into the pudendal canal. At the entrance to the canal, it gives off an inferior rectal artery. In the canal it then gives off a perineal artery. At the end, the artery divides into the deep artery of the penis and the dorsal artery of the penis or clitoris [3, 4]

Pudendal Nerve

The *pudendal nerve* comes from S 2, 3, and 4 and enters the pudendal canal and travels to the perineum. The pudendal canal lies against the obturator internus muscle and is made up of the fascia of obturator internus. There are some autonomic fibers that travel on the pudendal nerve but it is primarily a somatic nerve carrying voluntary nerve fibers. On the way it has several branches (Fig. 5.5).

1. The *inferior rectal nerve* is the first branch and arises right at the beginning of the pudendal canal. It crosses the ischiorectal fossa, heading medially, to supply the anal region. It has a motor and sensory component. The motor component supplies the external anal sphincter. The sensory component is to the skin around the anus. The anal wink is a test for the inferior rectal nerve. In a healthy individual, when the skin around the anus is scratched, the external anal sphincter contracts confirming that the inferior rectal nerve, the pudendal nerve, and S 2, 3, and 4 are all intact. During a delivery, if there is a tear through the perineal body and into the external anal sphincter, the nerve at risk is the inferior rectal nerve.
2. The *perineal nerve* also has motor and sensory branches. The motor nerve supplies all the muscles of the deep and superficial spaces except for the internal urethral sphincter. The sensory branch is either the posterior scrotal or posterior labial branch. In addition, in females this nerve is responsible for sensation from the terminal one-third of the vagina.
3. The *dorsal nerve of the clitoris or penis* is the terminal branch of the pudendal nerve and is responsible for sensation from the penis or clitoris.

A pudendal nerve block can be used for episiotomies or other surgeries in this region to block pain sensation. The nerve can be anesthetized at the ischial spine.

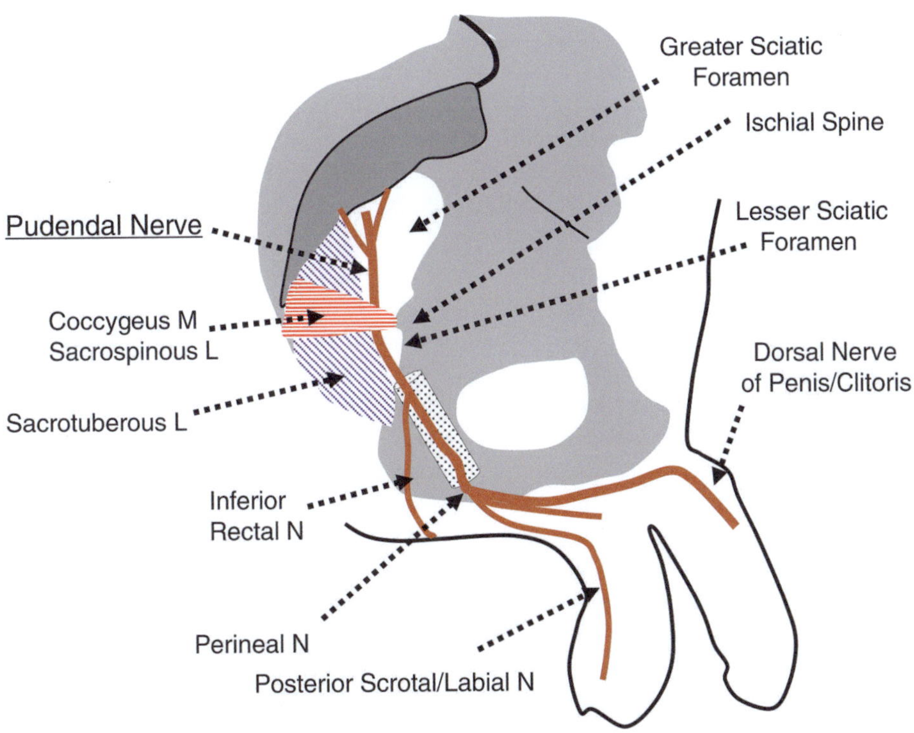

Fig. 5.5 Pudendal nerve and its branches [3, 4]

The pudendal nerve, a somatic nerve, should not be confused with the pelvic splanchnic nerves which are made up of parasympathetic fibers. The pelvic splanchnic nerves travel along the walls of the pelvic organs such as the bladder and the prostate. They approach the pelvic diaphragm from above. As they travel through the pelvic diaphragm they are called cavernous nerves. Again, these nerves pierce the pelvic diaphragm reaching the erectile tissue from above. The pudendal nerve is reaching the pelvic region by approaching from below.

Erectile Tissue

There is erectile tissue in both males and females. In females the bulb of the vestibule and the crus of the clitoris come together to form the clitoris. In males the bulb of the penis and crus of the penis come together to form the penis. Both the clitoris and the penis receive parasympathetic nerve innervation from the cavernous nerves, and sensory innervation from the pudendal nerves.

Semen Production

Semen is the medium for sperm transport, it nourishes the sperm, and it maintains the pH between 7 and 8. It originates from four structures:

1. The *seminiferous tubules* in the testes produce about 10% of the seminal fluid.
2. The *bulbourethral glands* produce pre-ejaculatory fluid which acts as a lubricant and neutralizes uric acids. They make a small contribution to semen (1%)
3. The *prostate* produces a thin milky-white fluid that combines with the seminal fluid in the prostatic urethra via 20–30 small prostatic ducts draining into the prostatic sinuses. It contains the clotting enzyme PSA which breaks down semen clots. It produces about 30% of semen.
4. The *seminal vesicles* (AKA, seminal glands) are sub-peritoneal and lie between the rectum and the prostate where they can be palpated via the rectum. They produce most of the semen (60%).

The Bladder

The bladder sits just posterior to the pubic bone. The space between the bladder and the pubic bone is the retropubic space which is not part of the peritoneal cavity. Most of the bladder consists of smooth muscle referred to as the *detrusor muscle*. The interior of the bladder has a triangular shaped trigone with three points. Two of the points are made by the ureters entering the bladder. At the center point, the lumen of the bladder turns into the neck of the bladder, which in turn forms the beginning of the urethra. Surrounding the urethra just as it enters the prostate is the *internal urethral sphincter*.

When the bladder is full, it rises above the pubic bone. Bladder injuries can result in urine draining into the peritoneal cavity (intraperitoneal) or around the peritoneal cavity (extraperitoneal). For instance, in an automobile accident, if the driver has a full bladder, the dome of the bladder can rupture, which in turn tears the visceral peritoneum over the dome. This leads to urine draining into the peritoneal cavity. Pelvic fractures tend to damage the anterior surface of the bladder right behind the pelvic bone. In this case, urine can drain into the retropubic space which is separated from the peritoneal cavity.

At the base of the bladder is the internal urethral sphincter which is also smooth muscle. The detrusor and the internal sphincter work together for voiding and filing of the bladder. When the bladder is filling up, the detrusor relaxes and the internal urethral sphincter contracts. When the bladder is filled and needs to empty, the detrusor will contract, and the internal urethral sphincter will relax. This coordinated activity is under control of the pelvic splanchnic nerves (Fig. 5.6).

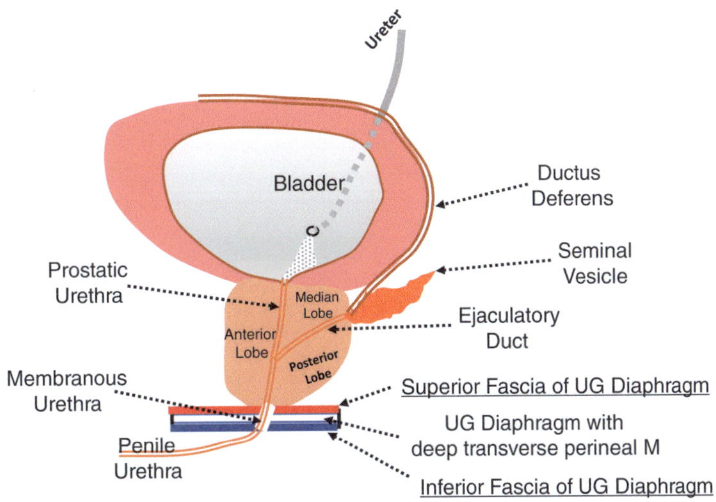

Fig. 5.6 Urogenital diaphragm. The urogenital diaphragm is located between the superior fascia and inferior fascia of the urogenital diaphragm. Emerging from the bladder is the prostatic urethra, which then travels through the urogenital diaphragm as the membranous urethra, which becomes the penile urethra

The internal urethral sphincter is related to the superior surface of the prostate. On the inferior surface of the prostate is the external urethral sphincter which is skeletal muscle under control of the pudendal nerve.

Prostate

The prostate sits between the bladder and the urogenital diaphragm. The prostatic urethra leaves the bladder and travels through the prostate. Along the way, the ejaculatory ducts join the prostatic urethra. The prostatic urethra and the ejaculatory ducts divide the prostate up into five lobes. In a mid-sagittal cut one can see: the *anterior lobe* in front of the prostatic urethra; the *median lobe* between the prostatic urethra and the ejaculatory duct; and the *posterior lobe* posterior to the ejaculatory duct. Moving laterally on either side are the *lateral lobes* of the prostate. The median lobe is the site of begin prostatic hypertrophy, while the posterior lobe is the site of prostatic carcinoma. The prostate is surrounded by a fine network of nerve fibers, the prostatic plexus, which in turn gives rise to the cavernous nerves which travel through the urogenital diaphragm to reach the erectile tissue in the superficial perineal space (Fig. 5.6).

The interior of the prostatic urethra is not a simple round tube but is instead shaped like an oval in cross section. On the posterior wall of the prostatic urethra is a protuberance called the *seminal colliculus*. And on the seminal colliculus are three small openings:

1. The *prostatic utricle* is a blind ended sac.
2. On each side of the utricle are the paired *openings of the ejaculatory ducts.*

At the edges of the seminal colliculus are the *prostatic sinuses* where the glands of the prostate open. In the retropubic space is a venous network—the prostatic plexus—which is responsible for the venous drainage of the prostate. This network communicates with the venous networks higher up and can be the cause of prostatic carcinoma spreading to the lungs.

Uterus

The uterus typically rests on top of the bladder with the cervix pointing posteroinferiorly. It is usually in an anteverted and anteflexed position. There are three layers to the uterus.

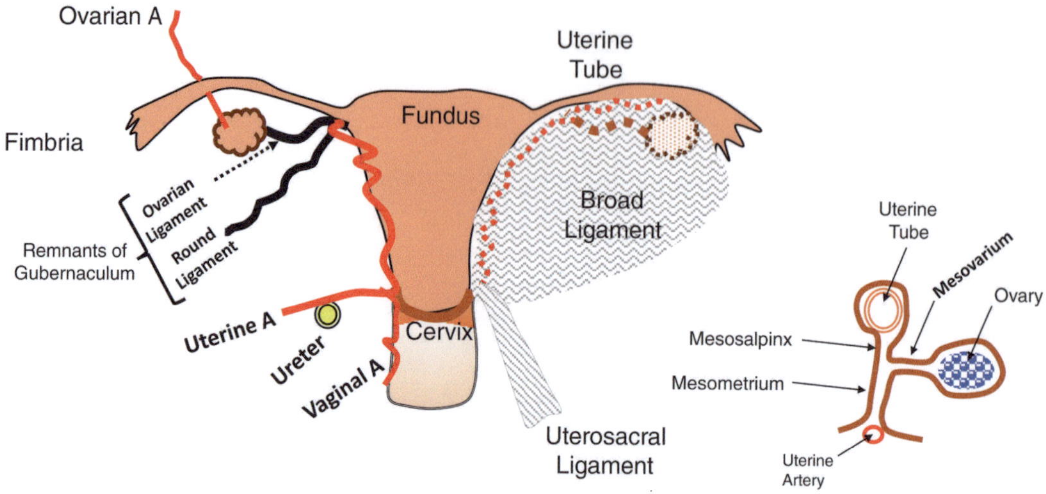

Fig. 5.7 Broad Ligament. The broad ligament is made up of the mesosalpinx, mesometrium, and mesovarium. The ovarian ligament and the round ligament are remnants of the gubernaculum. The ureter runs inferior to the uterine artery

1. *Endometrium* is the inner lining with abundant glandular tissue.
2. *Myometrium* is the middle muscular layer.
3. *Perimetrium* is the thin serous layer of peritoneum covering the uterus.

The fundus of the uterus is the superior rounded section. The horns (cornu) are located at each corner Coming into the cornu are the uterine tubes. The cervix is bounded by the superior portion of the vagina. Around the cervix is a continuous space referred to as the *fornix* which can be divided into anterior, lateral, or posterior fornix.

The peritoneum descends along the posterior wall and is reflected onto the superior surface of the uterus at the rectum. This gives rise to the lowest point in the female peritoneal cavity: the rectouterine pouch. Fluid either from an ectopic pregnancy or an infection in the peritoneal cavity, can be aspirated via the posterior fornix (Fig. 5.7).

Ovary, Uterine Tube, and Broad Ligament

At ovulation, the egg leaves the ovary and crosses the peritoneal cavity and is picked up by the fimbria to enter the uterine tube. From here the ova moves into the ampulla. If sperm are present, fertilization will occur in the ampulla of the uterine tube. It takes approximately seven days for the developing embryo to move into the uterus. Implantation typically occurs along the posterior surface of the uterus.

The ovary is attached to the cornu of the uterus by the *ovarian ligament*. Also, attached to the cornu is the *round ligament* running from the cornu through the deep inguinal ring, through the inguinal canal to connect to the labia majora. The round ligament and the ovarian ligament are both remnants of the *gubernaculum*. At one point the ligaments are continuous and do not touch the uterus, but during development, the gubernacu-

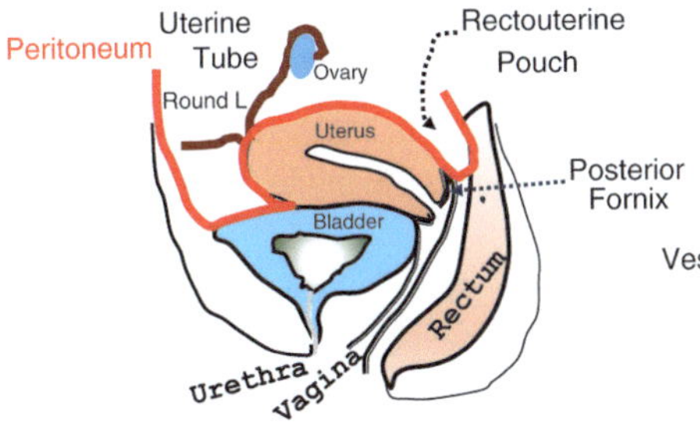

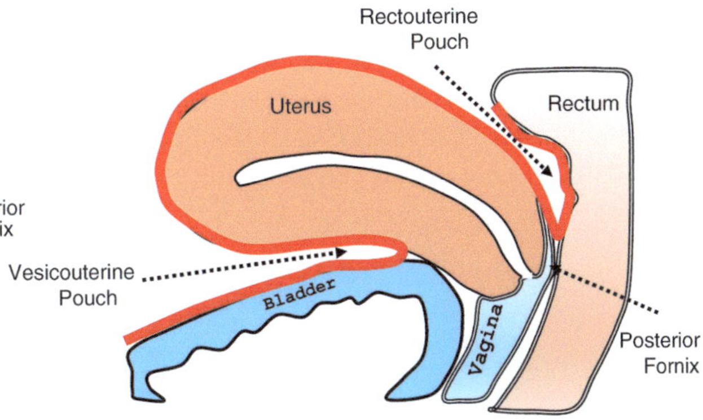

Fig. 5.8 Peritoneum in the pelvis. Starting on the posterior abdominal wall, the peritoneum, shown in red, descends and is reflected from the rectum to lie on top of the uterus and bladder. Note the proximity of the rectouterine pouch and the posterior fornix [3, 4]

lum shortens, it comes to touch the cornu of the uterus, giving rise to the two different sections: the round ligament and the ovarian ligament (Fig. 5.8).

Broad Ligament

The peritoneum is like a sheet draped over the internal female organs, and as such, it can be divided into three subdivisions:

1. The *mesosalpinx* is the mesentery folded around the uterine tube (salpinx = tube).
2. The *mesovarium* is the mesentery folded around the ovary.
3. The *mesometrium* is the mesentery along the sides of the uterus. Running along the base of the mesometrium is the cardinal ligament.

The blood supply to the uterus comes from the uterine artery which approaches the uterus and divides into an ascending branch which travels up along the edge of the uterus to anastomose with branches of the ovarian artery which came from the descending aorta. The descending branch of the uterine artery descends towards the vagina to anastomose with the vaginal artery. As the uterine artery approaches the uterus it travels superior to the ureter (*water under the bridge*).

Cardinal and Uterosacral Ligaments

The *cardinal ligament* (Mackenrodt's Ligament) runs transversally from the cervix and vagina to the lateral pelvic wall. It sits at the base of the broad ligament and the uterine artery runs in it on its way to the uterus. The two *uterosacral ligaments* are U-shaped, with each one running from the posterior cervix and vagina towards the sacrum (Fig. 5.8).

Superficial Space and Deep Perineal Spaces

In the perineal region there are three layers of fascia and two layers of muscle. To talk about these layers, we are going to use a Big Mac as an analogy. Remember, a Big Mac, has three layers of bun and two hamburger patties. The bottom layer or bun is the *superficial perineal fascia*, the middle layer of bun is the *inferior fascia of the UG diaphragm* (perineal membrane), and the top layer of the bun is the *superior fascia of the UG diaphragm*. Between the bottom bun and middle bun is the *superficial perineal space*. Starting from superficial and moving deep we are going to discuss each layer.

The bottom layer of the bun is the superficial perineal fascia, also known as Colle's fascia.

Colle's fascia is continuous with Scarpa's fascia on the anterior abdominal wall, and with the fascia lata on the thigh. At the line between the urogenital and anal triangles, Colle's fascia is attached to the perineal body (Figs. 5.9, 5.10 and 5.11).

In the superficial perineal space, the space between the bottom and middle buns, there are three muscles:

1. The *ischiocavernosus* runs from the inferior pubic rami towards the penis or clitoris.

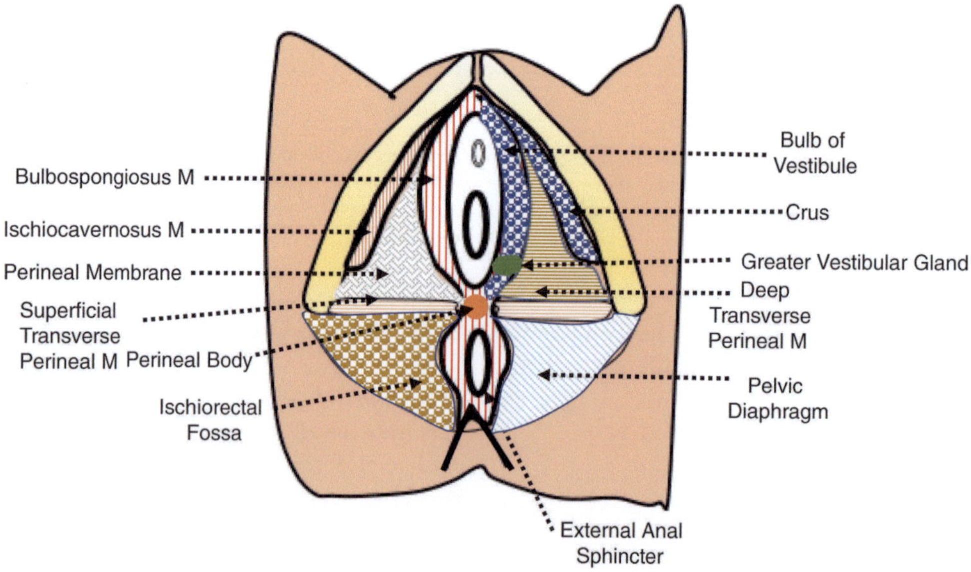

Fig. 5.9 Perineum. On the patient's right are the muscles of the superficial space and the fat filled ischiorectal fossa. On the patient's left are the structures of the deep perineal space and the pelvic diaphragm [3, 4]

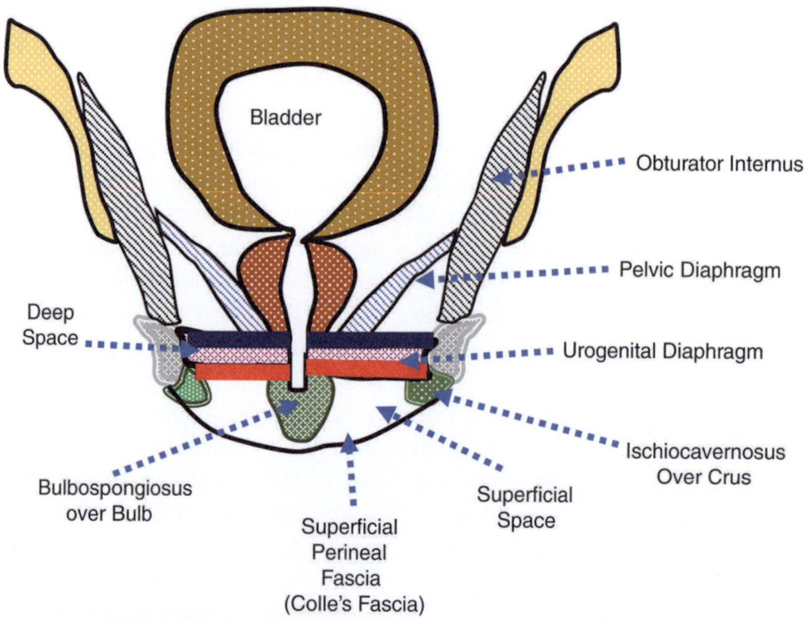

Fig. 5.10 The urogenital diaphragm is bounded by the superior and inferior fascia of the urogenital diaphragm. In the superficial space are the ischiocavernosus and bulbospongiosus muscles over the crus and bulb, respectively [3, 4]

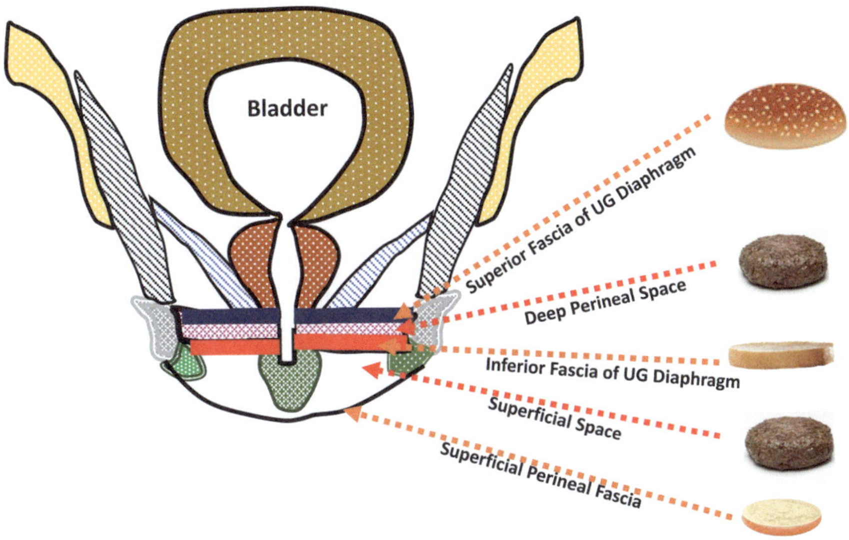

Fig. 5.11 The perineum. The layers of the perineum are compared to the layers of a big mac [3, 4]

2. In females the *bulbospongiosus* is found on the sides of the vestibule. In males the bulbospongiosus is fused in the midline on the bulb of the penis.
3. The two *superficial transverse perineal* muscles run from the ischial tuberosities towards the midline and meet at the perineal body. The bulbospongiosus muscle and the external anal sphincter muscle also meet at the perineal body.

These muscles of the superficial space are sitting on top of the erectile tissue which is also in the superficial space:

1. The *crura* of the penis or clitoris are deep to the ischiocavernosus muscle.
2. The *bulb of the vestibule* (females) or the *bulb of the penis* sit just under the bulbospongiosus.

And in females, the *greater vestibular glands* are found in the superficial space located in the posterior one-third of the vestibule.

The middle layer of the bun is the *inferior fascia of the urogenital triangle*, also known as the perineal membrane. This is a thick dense layer that serves as an anchoring point for the erectile tissue (bulbs and crura).

If we peel this layer away, we are now looking at the muscles and structures in the deep space. There are two muscles (Fig. 5.11):

1. The *deep transverse perineal* muscle is a very thin sheet running across the urogenital triangle from one inferior pubic ramus to the other.
2. Within the deep transverse perineal muscle is a small sphincter—the *sphincter urethrae* with the *membranous urethrae* running through it. This sphincter is skeletal muscle which is innervated by the perineal branch of the pudendal nerve.

Also in this deep space, in males are the *bulbourethral glands*. However, while the glands are in the deep space, their ducts drain into the urethra in the superficial space. Of note, remember that in females the greater vestibular glands are in the superficial space.

Dartos and Cremaster Muscles

The *dartos muscle* (sometimes referred to as the dartos fascia) is smooth muscle that is continuous with Scarpa's fascia. It wrinkles the scrotum to alter the surface area for heat exchange. In chilly weather it will contract to pull the testes closer to the body and to decrease the surface area, and in warm weather it relaxes to increase the surface area of the scrotum. It is innervated by sympathetic fibers.

The *cremaster muscle* is an extension of the internal abdominal oblique muscle and travels in the inguinal canal to the testes. It is innervated by the somatic nervous system. Muscle fibers are usually visible running along the spermatic cord. In females there are some rudimentary fibers on the round ligament.

The Testes

The tunica albuginea surrounds the testes. It is a thick white-colored layer with septa that divides the testes into lobules, which contain the *seminiferous tubules*. Sperm start their development in the seminiferous tubules. The developing spermatogonia travel through the seminiferous tubules and then into the straight tubules. The straight tubules then merge into the rete testes, which in turn drain into the efferent ductules. The efferent ductus then connects to the head of the epididymis. The three parts of the epididymis are the head, body, and tail. From the tail, the sperm then enters the ductus deferens (Fig. 5.12). *Orchitis* is an inflammation of the testes from an infection. It sometimes goes along with mumps.

Penis

The penis is composed of three tubes that resemble a tripod. The three tubes are flared out at the base, but then come together to make up the penis. The base is composed of a single bulb of the penis and two crus of the penis. Where these

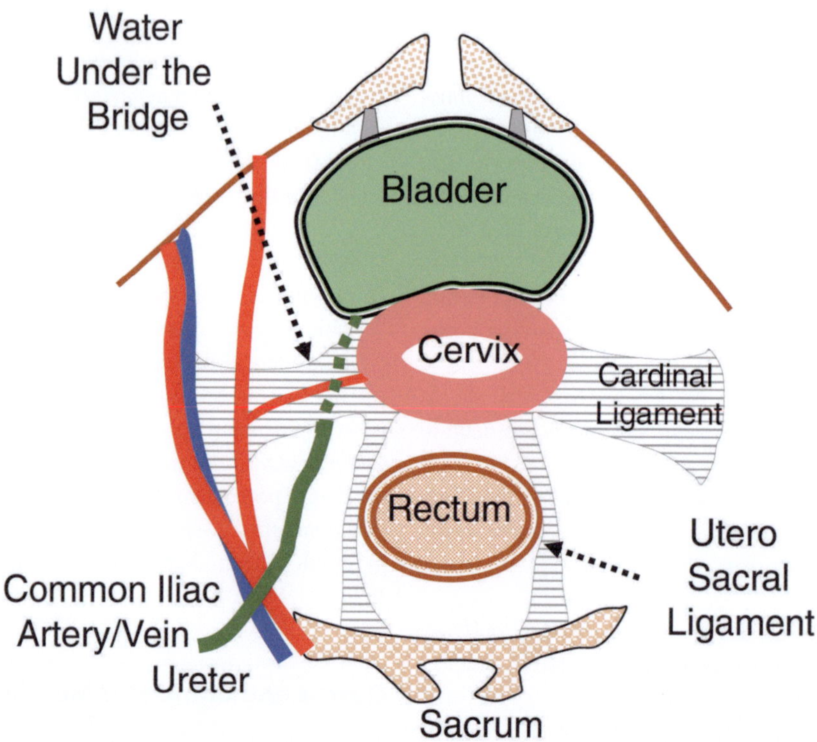

Fig. 5.12 "Water under the bridge." The uterine artery comes off the internal iliac artery and travels to the uterus in the cardinal ligament. Going under the uterine artery is the ureter heading to the bladder. The uterosacral ligament runs from the sacrum to the uterus and cervix [3, 4]

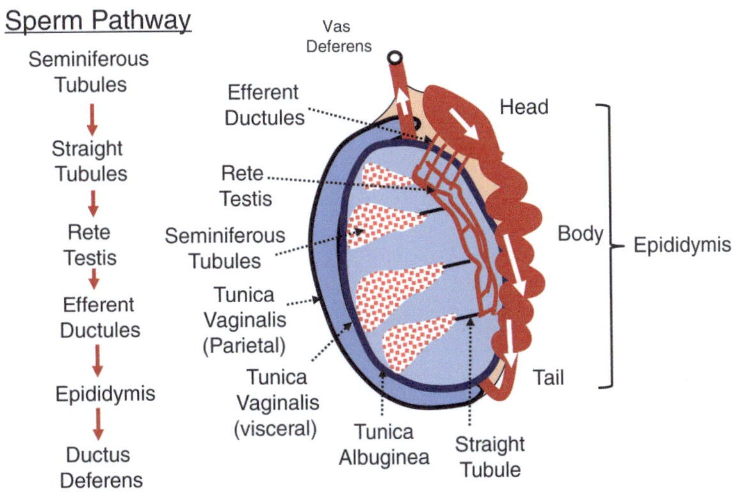

Fig. 5.13 Testes and sperm production. Sperm is made in the testes and then follows the tract depicted in the image above. The white arrows show the pathway of sperm [3, 4]

three pieces come together, the bulb becomes the corpora spongiosum, and each crus forms a corpora cavernosa. At the end of the penis is the glans of the penis which is covered by the foreskin or prepuce. Traveling through the corpus spongiosum is the spongy or penile urethra (Fig. 5.13).

The penis is encircled by a thick tough membrane referred to as *Buck's fascia*, also known as the deep perineal fascia, that holds the three tubes together. Deep to the fascia is the single *deep dorsal vein* of the penis which drains to the prostatic plexus. This deep dorsal vein of the penis is surrounded on each side by a *dorsal artery of the penis* and then two *dorsal nerves of the penis*. The two dorsal arteries of the penis come from the internal pudendal arteries. The dorsal nerves of the penis come from the pudendal nerve and there are carrying sensory information from the penis. They do not carry parasympathetic fibers. Outside of this collection of veins, arteries, and nerves is the superficial penile fascia, and outside this layer is the *superficial dorsal vein of the penis*. Within each corpus cavernosum is a deep artery of the penis.

The Clitoris

The clitoris is homologous to the penis and is similar structurally. However instead of three tubes, it is composed of two tubes—the two corpora cavernosum arising from the crura. The bulb of the vestibule does not have an extension that merges onto the clitoris like it does in the penis. Surrounding the clitoris is the tunica albuginea, and then more superficially is the clitoral fascia. Outside of the tunica albuginea is the deep vein of the clitoris, the two dorsal arteries of the clitoris, and the two dorsal nerves of the clitoris. Outside of the clitoral fascia is the superficial dorsal vein of the clitoris. Sensation from the clitoris travels on the dorsal nerves of the clitoris. The two cavernous nerves carry parasympathetic information for erection (Fig. 5.14).

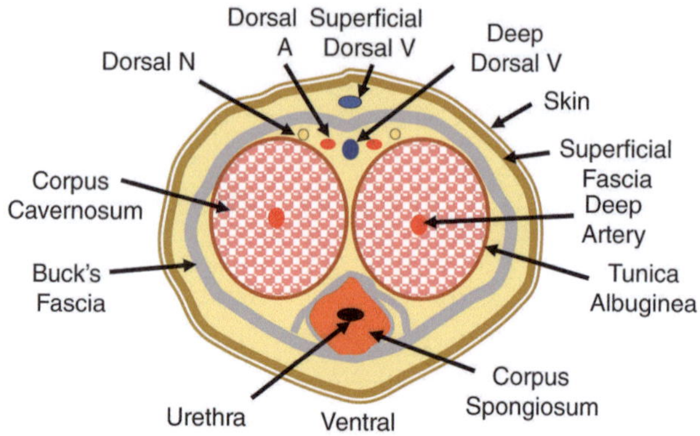

Fig. 5.14 Cross section of penis [3, 4]

Episiotomies and Caesarean Sections

During difficult deliveries, when the clinician believes that the perineum might tear, episiotomies can be performed. They are typically made in either a mediolateral or midline direction. There are advantages and disadvantages to either one. Mediolateral cuts avoid the anal canal, and even if the tear continues it will move laterally and avoid the anal canal region. Midline cuts avoid the nerves and arteries located laterally, but they can continue tearing posteriorly into the anal canal. And while the tough perineal body can prevent the tear from continuing posteriorly, if the tear does go through perineal body, then the tear can move into the anal canal.

There are two main types of C-sections, a high vertical incision, or a low transverse incision. High incisions used to be more common (they are sometimes referred to as a classical incision), but the lower transverse incisions are more common now. The low incision avoids the more vascular superior part of the uterus. In addition, after delivery the upper portion will contract and retract as it moves back towards its pre-pregnancy state. This contraction and retraction will not happen with the lower portion. The lower incision also gives better access to the actual presenting part of the delivery.

Pudendal Versus Pelvic Splanchnic Nerves

Both the pudendal nerve and the pelvic splanchnic nerves come from sacral levels 2, 3, 4. However there are major differences between the two. The pelvic splanchnic nerves emerge from the ventral sacral foramina as multiple thread-like fibers to travel down on the walls of the various organs such as the rectum, bladder, and uterus. As they pass over these organs, they also provide the parasympathetic nerve supply to the organs. As the fibers come out of the sacrum they are first referred to as the inferior hypogastric plexus or one of its subsidiary plexuses such as rectal, vesicle, uterine, or prostatic plexus. These nerves are especially susceptible to trauma during pelvic surgery. Emerging from the prostatic plexus in the male, and the uterovaginal plexus in the female, are the two *cavernous nerves* traveling through the urogenital diaphragm from superior to inferior to reach the erectile tissue of the bulb (penis/vestibule) and the crus (penis/clitoris) (Figs. 5.15 and 5.16).

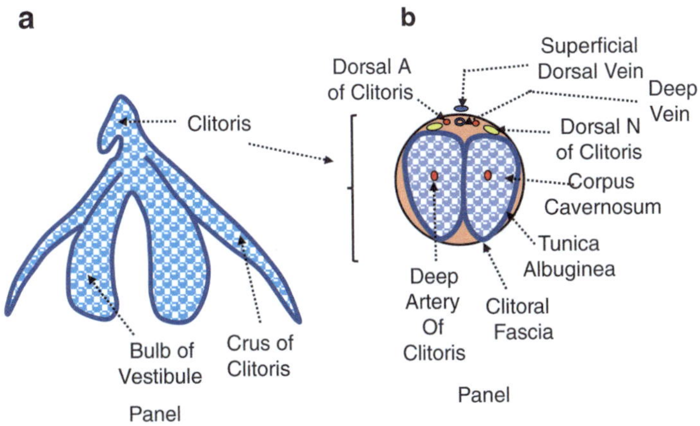

Fig. 5.15 Clitoris. Panel (**a**) Female erectile tissue. Surrounding the vestibule are the bulbs of the vestibule. More laterally, on both sides, is the crus of the clitoris. Panel (**b**) is a close-up of the clitoris. The clitoral fascia surrounds the two corpora cavernosum. Running in the center of the Corpora cavernosum are the deep arteries of the clitoris. The deep vein, the dorsal nerves, and the dorsal arteries of the penis are found deep to the clitoral fascia [3, 4]

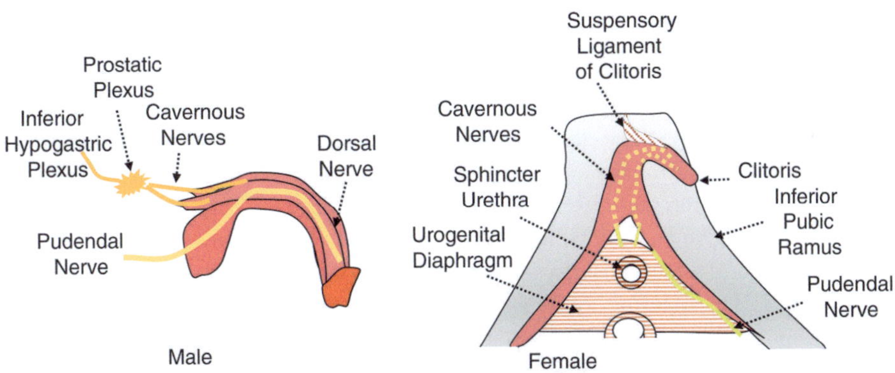

Fig. 5.16 Pelvic splanchnic and pudendal nerves. The inferior hypogastric nerves arise from S 2,3, 4 and form the cavernous nerves that supply the erectile tissue in the male and female. The pudendal nerve, also S 2,3,4, carries somatomotor fibers to the muscles of the deep and superficial spaces, and sensory fibers from the dorsal nerve of penis and clitoris [3, 4]

The pudendal nerve on the other hand travels through the pudendal canal and approaches the urogenital diaphragm from below. An example of trauma that could injure the pudendal nerve is a bike rider who falls forward off the seat and lands with the cross bar beneath their legs. The pudendal nerve is a somatic or voluntary nerve that carries sensory fibers from the perineal region and provides the motor supply to all the muscles of the deep and superficial spaces. It is not responsible for erection (Fig. 5.17).

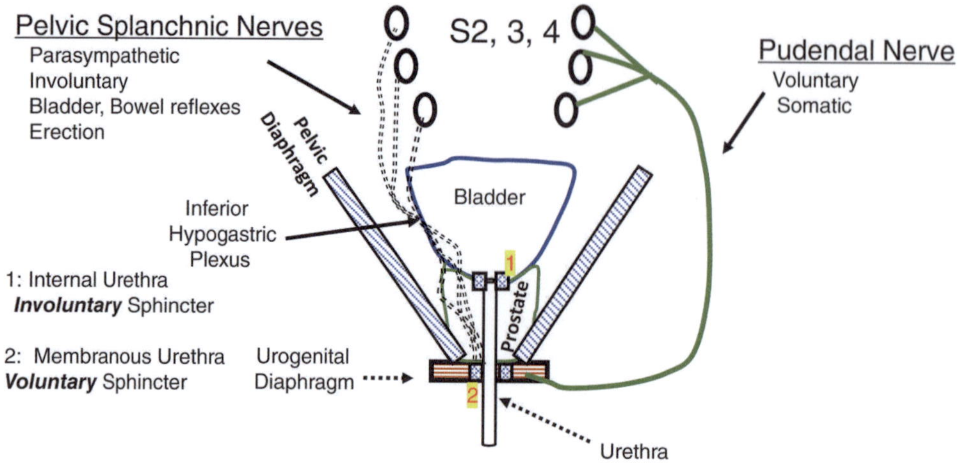

Fig. 5.17 Both the pelvic splanchnic nerves and the pudendal nerves come from S2,3,4. On one side the figure shows the pelvic splanchnic nerves joining the inferior hypogastric plexus and descending along the pelvic organs to approach the perineal structures from above. On the other side the pudendal nerve is shown leaving the pelvis and approaching the UG diaphragm from below [3, 4]

Anal Canal

An important division of the anal canal occurs at the pectinate line. This is where the hindgut endoderm meets the ectoderm. Because of this embryological meeting point, there are important structural differences above and below the pectinate line. For instance, the arterial supply above the pectinate line is the superior rectal artery, which comes from the inferior mesenteric artery; and below the pectinate line the blood supply is from the inferior rectal artery via the internal pudendal artery. Likewise, as discussed with the liver, the venous drainage above the line follows the superior rectal vein, to the inferior mesenteric vein, and eventually to the portal vein. The blood below the pectinate line follows the inferior rectal vein, to the internal pudendal vein, and eventually to the inferior vena cava (Fig. 5.18).

The afferent nerve supply to the anal canal above the pectinate line comes from the pelvic splanchnic nerves which are parasympathetic. Because there are no significant pain fibers associated with these nerves, a needle placed in the anal canal above the pectinate line will not cause severe pain. However, the skin below the pectinate line is innervated by the pudendal nerve, meaning that a needle placed below the pectinate line will cause considerable pain (Fig. 5.17).

Above the pectinate line the mucosal layer of the anal canal is thrown into folds called anal folds. Under each fold is a branch of the venous structures. In a patient with portal hypertension, the venous network here can prolapse into the rectum. Hemorrhoids above the pectinate line are referred to as internal hemorrhoids, while those below the pectinate line are referred to as external hemorrhoids. At the distal end of each fold there is a flap of tissue that extends from one fold to another. This series of anal valves connecting one fold to another ends up forming a ring around the terminal rectum. The space above each valve is an anal sinus.

Tears in the anal canal in the region of the anal valves and pectinate line can lead to infections that spread into the ischioanal fossa. These can lead to abscesses and fistulas developing in this region. In some cases, these fistulas can run from the anal canal, through the ischioanal fossa, and then open through the skin onto the external environment.

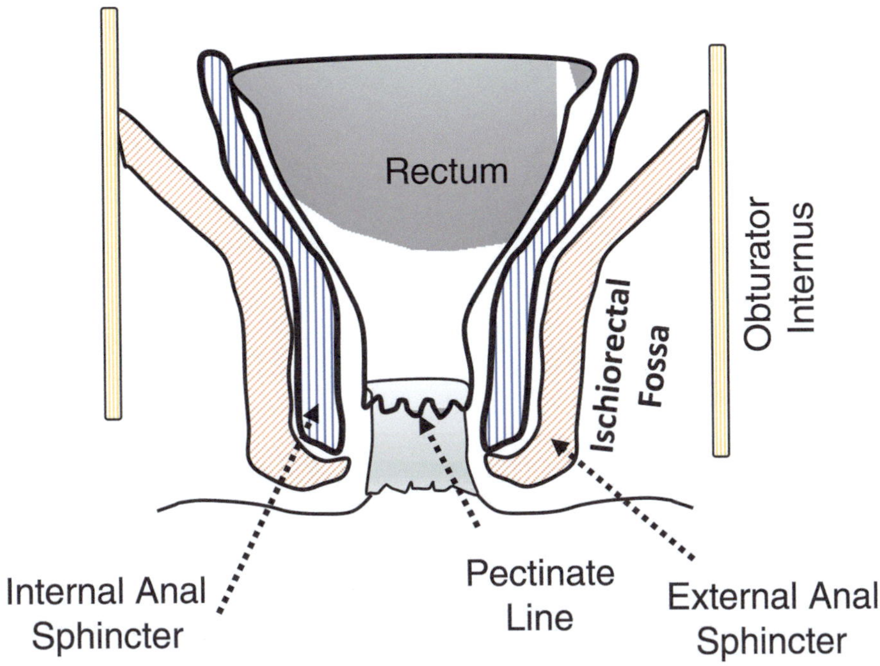

Fig. 5.18 Anal canal. The pectinate line is the transition from endoderm to ectoderm. Surrounding the terminal anal canal are the internal anal and external anal sphincters. Between the sphincters and the obturator internus is the ischiorectal fossa [3, 4]

Bladder and Bowel Control

Bladder and bowel control operate on the same basic mechanisms. The names of the various sphincters change whether you are talking about the bowel or bladder, but the nerve control of the two is similar. We will look at bowel control first. The exchanger bowel has internal and external anal sphincters. The internal anal sphincter is smooth muscle under control of the autonomic system via the pelvic splanchnic nerves coming from S 2, 3, and 4. The external anal sphincter is skeletal muscle under control of the somatic nervous system via the inferior rectal nerve, a branch of the pudendal nerve (Fig. 5.19).

The diagram shows three different states of bowel control (Fig. 5.18). In the first panel, the anal canal is empty. The pudendal nerve and external anal sphincter are relaxed, while the internal anal sphincter is tonically active. In the middle panel, material has moved into the anal canal. This activates the sensory afferent nerves, which travel back to the cord at S2, 3 and 4 and make a connection to the efferent pelvic splanchnic nerves to relax the internal anal sphincter. This is strictly a reflex loop with no conscious or cortical input at this point. If the individual is a six-month-old infant, then the fecal material will come out. The six-month-old's corticospinal tract is not developed enough to send a signal from the cortex down to the cord, and onward to the pudendal nerve, so the infant is strictly operating on the reflex arc.

In an adult, when something moves into the canal and the internal anal sphincter relaxes, the adult can then voluntarily fire their pudendal nerve and contract the external anal sphincter. The adult will then look for the bathroom, sit down, relax, pick up a magazine or a board review book, and release their external anal sphincter to void. This entire process is sometimes referred to as the Urge-to-Purge.

When it comes to the bladder, instead of an internal and external anal sphincter, there are the internal and external urethral sphincters, plus the

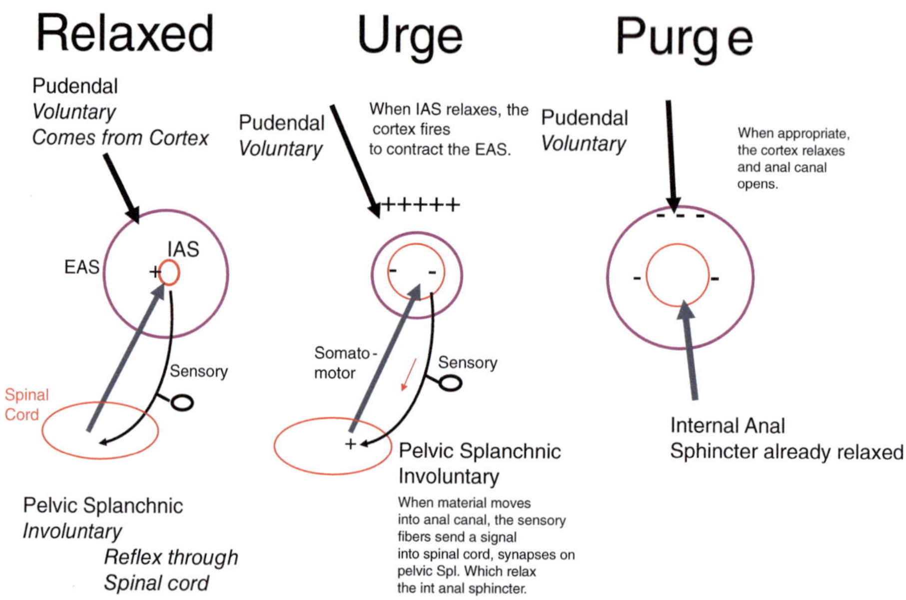

Fig. 5.19 Autonomic projections to the internal and external anal sphincters

detrusor muscle. During the filling stage, the internal urethral sphincter is contracted, and the detrusor is relaxed. During voiding the detrusor contracts, and the internal and external urethral sphincters relax. With this in mind, we have two lesions to discuss.

Superior Hypogastric Plexus

The superior hypogastric plexus is a collection of fibers resting on top of the sacral promontory. Coming out of it, on both sides are the right and left hypogastric nerves, which are sympathetic fibers descending along the sacrum. Along the way they are joined by the pelvic splanchnic nerves to make up the inferior hypogastric plexus. The most important function of the superior hypogastric plexus is that it receives the pain fibers from the pelvic viscera such as uterus and ovary. A superior hypogastric nerve block is used to block painful sensations from these organs.

Pelvis

The *innominate bone* or *os coxae* is made up of three bones that fuse together. Together these three bones form the lateral sides of the pelvis.

1. the *pubis* has both a superior and an inferior pubic ramus projecting out of its body.
2. the *ischium* has two important landmarks. One is the *ischial spine* where the sacrospinous ligament attaches. The second is the *ischial tuberosity* where the sacrotuberous ligament and hamstring muscles attach. Projecting anteriorly is the ischial ramus which meets the inferior pubic ramus.
3. the *ilium* is the largest of the three bones and has a fan-shaped look to it. The *iliac crest* runs from the *anterior superior iliac spine* to the *posterior superior iliac spine*. Along the lateral wall, are three lines: the posterior, anterior, and inferior gluteal lines, for the attachment of the gluteus maximus, gluteus medius, and gluteus minimus, respectively.

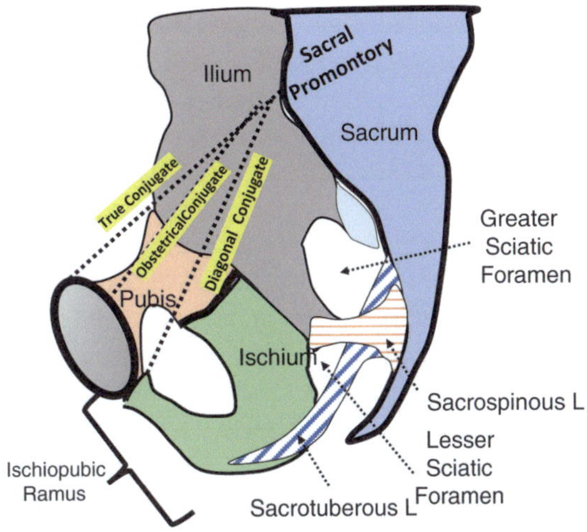

Fig. 5.20 Innominate bone. The three bones that make up the innominate bone are the pubis, ischium and Ilium. Note the pubis and ischium meet to form the ischiopubic ramus. The true conjugate runs from the top of the pubic symphysis to the sacral promontory. The obstetrical conjugate runs from the pubic bone to sacral promontory. The diagonal conjugate runs from the inferior level of the pubic symphysis to the sacral promontory. During a vaginal exam, the diagonal conjugate can be measured. Taking 2 cm off the diagonal conjugate gives a rough estimation of the obstetrical conjugate

All three of the bones that comprise the innominate bone: the pubis, ischium, and ilium meet at the *triradiate cartilage* to form the acetabulum of the hip joint. The *obturator foramen is* the large round opening whose boundary is made up of pubis, ischium, and ilium.

The two innominate bones (right and left) meet in the anterior midline at the *pubic symphysis.* Posteriorly, they meet at the sacrum. There are major differences between the male and female innominate bones due to the fact that in females the fetal head moves through the canal during delivery.

The *pelvic inlet* is a line from the superior pubic symphysis to the sacral promontory. It is widest in the transverse section. The pelvic outlet is taken from a line drawn from the lower border of the pubic bone to the coccyx. The widest diameter of the outlet is in the anterior posterior direction. During delivery, because the fetal head diameter is largest in the anterior to posterior section, as the fetus moves though the pelvic inlet it will be looking off to the side, but as it moves through the pelvic outlet it will be facing posterior as it passes through the pelvic outlet (Fig. 5.20).

Some Differences Between Apes and Humans

I am only pointing out the differences between humans and apes because it provides some insight into human pelvic anatomy. It is interesting to note that in chimpanzees, the fetal head does not have to rotate as it moves through the pelvic canal. As it comes through the pelvic inlet, the fetal chimp is facing forward, and as it comes through the outlet it is still facing forward. The much larger human brain makes the entire delivery process more complicated and has necessitated changes to the human pelvis. The human baby comes through the pelvic inlet facing the side and then rotates so that when it comes through the outlet it is facing posteriorly. Much of the human pelvis can be seen considering this need for this enlarged human brain plus the need for bipedalism. Keep in mind that the human brain goes through its brain growth spurt postnatally.

1. The secondary ossification centers in the pubic rami do not fuse until the third decade which allows these pubic rami to lengthen

after the rest of the skeleton has stopped growing, which leads to a larger pelvic outlet. The pubic symphysis remains malleable.

2. The ischial spines in humans assume a more lateral position which allows more room for the fetal head.
3. Because the fetal chimpanzee is facing anterior when it emerges from the pelvic outlet, the mother can easily see the face of the fetus and she can clean it as it emerges from the inlet. This allows her to be alone during the delivery. With the human fetal head facing posteriorly, it is hypothesized that this leads to the need for members of the community to assist the mother.
4. In chimpanzees, the gluteus medius and minimus are extensors at the hip which leads to chimps having a natural Trendelenburg gait -their hips and knees are in flexed positions. The organization of these muscles allows for more hip mobility, which results in improved tree climbing but a reduced ability to walk long distances. In addition, the hands in chimpanzees are used for walking so they cannot be used for working. Compared to chimpanzees, in humans the gluteus medius and minimus are positioned more laterally, allowing these muscles to serve as abductors. These abductors at the hip along with the lordotic curve in humans allows for extension at the hip and the subsequent upward stance that allows humans to free up their hands. Besides being able to walk long distances with their hands free, they can now use tools. A downside for humans is that we have more lumbar vertebrae and they are also larger which can lead to spondylolysis and spondylolisthesis, something which is unheard of in chimpanzees.

There are also differences between the male and female human pelvis. The female pelvis tends to be lighter and thinner than the male pelvis. The pelvic inlet in females is oval shaped with the long axis of the oval running from side to side. The pelvic inlet in males, because of the jutting out of the sacral promontory, is shaped like a heart. The pelvic outlet in females is rounder and wider, while in males it is thinner and smaller. The pelvic cavity in females is cylindrical with short parallel sides, while in males it is cone shaped with long sides projecting medially. The pubic arch in females is wider and has a circular shape and is about the size of the angle between your second and third fingers when spread. In females, the ischial tuberosities are everted, while in males they are inverted. The subpubic arch in males is narrow and triangular shaped and can be represented by the angle between your first and second fingers when spread.

Sacrum

The sacrum is a wedge-shaped bone made up of the five fused vertebrae of S1-S5. Superiorly it articulates with the L5 vertebra, and inferiorly it articulates with the coccyx. Posterior to the fused vertebrae is the sacral canal with the cauda equina running in it. At the end of the sacral canal is the sacral hiatus where a sacral epidural nerve block can be administered. On the anterior surface are the anterior sacral foramina, and posterior are the posterior sacral foramina. On the lateral sides are the two sacral ala (wings) which each form one side of the sacroiliac joint. On the lateral surface of the ala are the *auricular surfaces* (not articular but auricular, because they look like an ear) that form one half of the sacroiliac joints.

The *sacroiliac joint* has a small amount of movement in children, but in adults it is fused. Sacroiliac joint disease is characterized by small movements at the joint which lead to chronic pain. The *Faber test* is used to evaluate the hip. The patient is in a supine position and places one ankle on the opposite knee—like the tailor's position. In this position, the lower limb is now abducted, flexed, and externally rotated (the FABER test). The examiner now pushes down on the flexed knee. Pain is thought to be indicative of either sacroiliac joint or hip joint pathology.

On the anterior and posterior surface of the sacrum are the four anterior and posterior sacral foramina, through which emerge the ventral and dorsal rami of the sacral nerves. Medial to the anterior sacral foramina are the sympathetic trunks and the lateral sacral arteries. On the posterior surface, one can see the *iliac crest* turning into the *posterior superior iliac spine* which is an important landmark. It marks the middle of the SI joint, the S2 vertebra, and the end of the dural Superficially, the dimple just above the buttocks is directly over the posterior superior iliac spine.

Lymph Nodes

The lymph nodes are kidney shaped in-line filters that transport proteins, lipids, lymphocytes, and other substances back to the blood stream. An afferent lymphatic duct brings lymph into the node at the convex surface. The lymph then travels through the node to exit at the hilum as the efferent lymphatic duct. The afferent and efferent lymphatic ducts are found on opposite sides of the lymph node (Fig. 5.21).

Lymph nodes can initiate a primary immune response because they are the site where antigen-presenting cells carrying antigens in the lymph meet naïve lymphocytes coming from the blood stream. This interaction triggers this primary immune response. To understand how these interactions occur, it is important to understand the architecture of the lymph nodes. There are three zones to a lymph node, and each zone merges into its neighboring zone with no sharp demarcation, or epithelial layer between them:

1. the *medulla* is the site of a reticular meshwork housing plasma cells which are mature B lymphocytes. The medullary sinus is the site of the macrophages.
2. the *paracortex* (deep cortex) is the site where T lymphocytes meet antigen presenting cells.
3. the superficial cortex (sometimes referred to as just the cortex) is the site of primary and secondary germinal centers. Secondary follicles are characterized by the presence of a germinal center with B lymphocytes.

Primary follicles (or nodules) are immature follicles. As they mature into secondary follicles and the germinal center expands, the cells in the center are pushed outward towards the periphery forming a mantle and a margin. These germinal centers are made of follicular dendritic cells (FDCs) that are arranged in rows. Secondary follicles have a more lightly stained germinal center because they are made up of large lymphoblasts that are dividing. Within 2–3 weeks the cells have been dispersed and the germinal center is gone.

The nodes are surrounded by a connective tissue capsule that sends trabeculae into the node's parenchyma. The endothelium of the afferent lymphatics is continuous with the subscapular sinus, the cortical sinus, and the efferent lymphatics. As the lymph passes through the node it bathes the germinal centers with plasma and contacts the immune fighting cells. As the sinuses

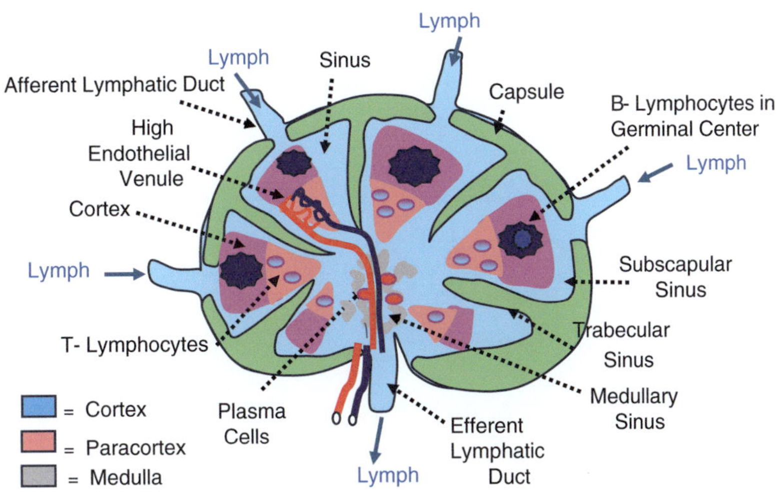

Fig. 5.21 Lymph node. There are three regions. (1) Superficial cortex with the lymphatic follicles. (2) Paracortex with T-Cells. (3) Medulla with plasma cells. The artery enters at the hilum and travels to the paracortex where it forms a capillary bed. On the venous side of the capillary bed are the high endothelial venules (HEVs)

pass through the node, the lymph can pass through discontinuous epithelium to percolate through the lymphocytes.

High Endothelial Venules

Each node has an artery entering the hilum that passes into the paracortex where it breaks up into a capillary bed. On the venous side of the capillary bed are the high endothelial venules, which get their name because of the presence of tall cuboidal endothelial cells. These cells have receptors that bind to the lymphocytes in the blood stream. These receptors facilitate the transfer of the lymphocytes into the reticular meshwork. The B lymphocytes enter the surrounding area and if the B cell meets its antigen on a follicular dendritic cell, it starts clonal expansion. Within 3–4 days of this interaction, there will be a visible germinal center which will remain like this for 2–3 weeks. The mitotic activity will eventually stop, and the germinal center will disappear (Fig. 5.22).

Unlike the blood system, which has a central pump to move blood along, there is no central pump to move the lymph along. In addition, compared to the high-pressure blood circulatory system, the lymphatic system is a low-pressure system. This creates a problem that must be overcome. The problem being that this low-pressure lymph system needs to drain into the high-pressure system at some point. Consider the various pressures in the network of pipes involved in the lymph's return to the circulatory system. At the aorta, right after coming out of the heart, the blood pressure is at its highest point (120 mmHg). As you travel along the system, the pressure drops. Right before entering the heart, the pressure is at its lowest (5 mmHg). The lymphatics wisely enter the venous system close to this point. On the left side, the thoracic duct enters at the junction of the internal jugular vein and the subclavian vein, and on the right side the right lymphatic duct also enters at the same junction. The other mechanism involved in moving lymph along this low-pressure system is that there is an extensive system of one-way valves that keep moving the lymph towards the neck without allowing it to move in a retrograde direction.

Lymphatic Bulbs

Another difference between the blood and lymphatic circulations is that the heart and its vessels are a closed continuous loop with no beginning or end, while the lymphatic system is an open system that starts as a blind-ended-sacs. The start of a lymphatic channel is a small dilated bulbous structure which drains into ever larger tubular structures. The endothelial cells of the bulb overlap in this region and are shaped like an oak leaf. The cells have a discontinuous basement membrane, no smooth muscle around them, and their tips are anchored to the extracellular matrix by fibers composed of fibrillin. Because of these specializations they form *button-like junctions* creating one-way valves. When pressure in the surrounding tissue rises, these overlapping cells act to allow fluid to enter the lymphatic channel. These same valves prevent the fluid from leaving

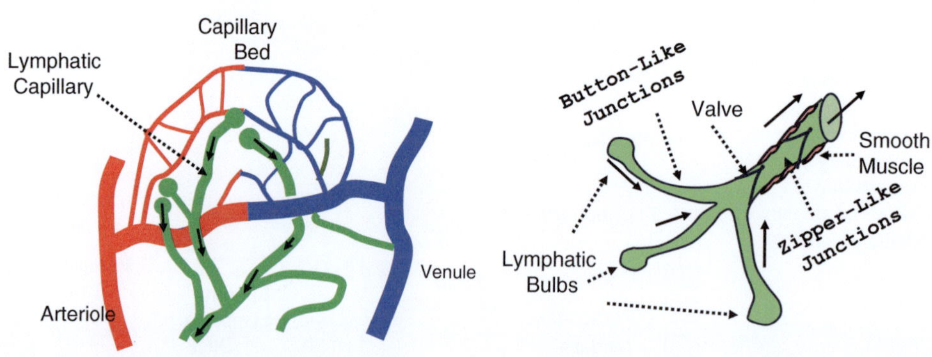

Fig. 5.22 Start of lymphatic circulation

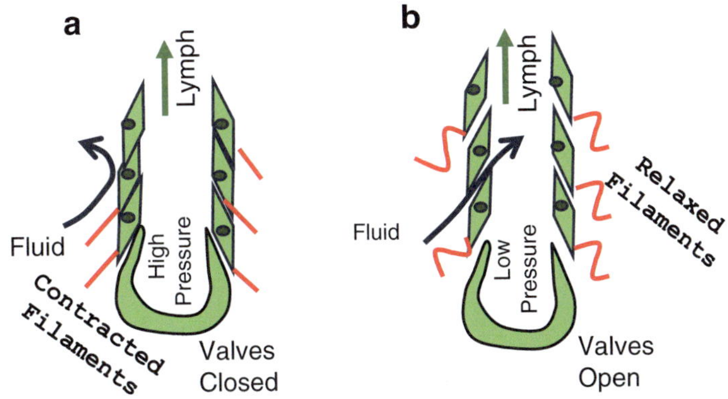

Fig. 5.23 Lymphatic capillaries. Panel (**a**) When pressure is high inside the lymphatic bulb, the channels between the leaf like cells are closed. Panel (**b**) When pressure is low inside the lymphatic bulb, the valves are open, and lymph can enter the bulb

the bulb. Once this interstitial fluid enters the bulb it is now referred to as *lymph* (Fig. 5.23).

From the lymphatic capillaries the lymph then enters the collecting vessels which have an endothelial layer that forms *zipper-like junctions* which are less permeable than the button-like junctions. These vessels are also surrounded by a layer of smooth muscle. The muscle cells in the walls of the lymphatic channels play a role in propelling lymph along the network.

The forces pushing lymph along the network come from the passive action of the surrounding musculature. When the bulb is compressed, the lymph is forced along the network. The pressure is the bulbs is extremely low—in the 1–3 mm Hg range. As the lymph moves along the system, the pressure rises—in the larger lymph vessels it is in the range of 10–20 mm Hg.

Historical Snippet: Ignaz Semmelweis, The Savior of Mothers

The idea that health care workers should wash their hands between seeing patients came from Ignaz Semmelweis, a Hungarian physician. In 1847. Semmelweis was working at a hospital in Vienna where there were two maternity wards. One of the clinics was staffed by medical students and it had a 10% maternal mortality rate due to puerperal fever; the second clinic which was run by midwives only had a 4% rate. After careful observation, Semmelweis concluded that the cause of the increased rate in the clinic run by medical students was that the students were coming from the anatomy lab after dissecting the cadavers. And, while it is hard to imagine today, they were not washing their hands and transferring the bacteria to the pregnant women. Semmelweis suggested that handwashing would reduce the rate of infection. Unfortunately, his advice was ignored. The medical community did not pay attention to him, and he died in 1865. It was not for another 20 years that his ideas were accepted. His simple but once ridiculed idea is now a mainstay of medical practice. In Budapest, Semmelweis University is named after him; the house he was born in, and grew up in, is now the Semmelweis Museum (Fig. 5.24).

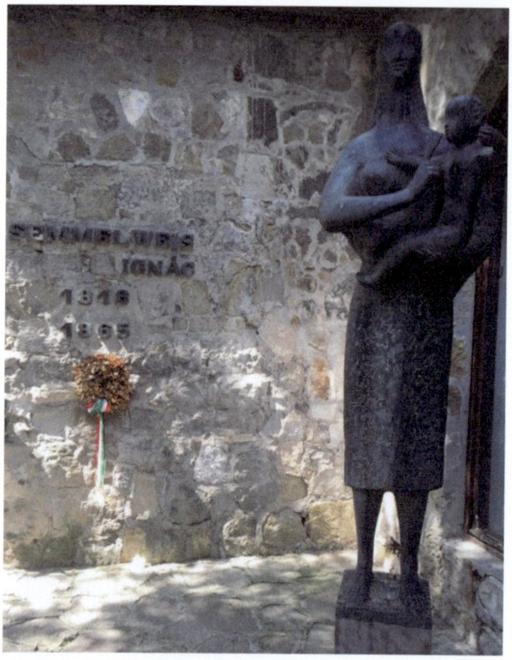

Fig. 5.24 Tomb of Ignaz Semmelweis. Semmelweis is buried in the garden of the house where he was born and grew up in. It is now the Semmelweis Museum, Library, and Archive of the History of Medicine, in Budapest Hungary. The statue, *Motherhood* by Miklos Borsos, honors Semmelweis as the "Savior of Mothers"

Further Reading

1. Boutefnouchet T, Bassett J, Patil S. Anatomy and clinical relevance of the "Corona Mortis": a review of the literature and current aspects of management. J Orthop Rheumatol. 2016;3:2.
2. Iskra, T, Balawender K, Przybycien W, RUtowicz B, Mazur M, Solewski W. Pelvic cavity and its space-anatomical overview. Folia Med Cracov. 2024;63(4):89-98.
3. Leo J. Medical Neuroanatomy for the boards and clinic: finding the Lesion. 2nd ed. Cham: Springer; 2024.
4. Leo J. Clinical anatomy and embryology: a guide for the classroom, clinic, and clinic. 2nd ed. Springer; 2024.
5. Moore K, Dalley AF, Agur A. Clinically oriented anatomy. 7th ed. Baltimore: Lippincott Williams and Wilkin; 2014.
6. Razak L. Pathophysiology of pelvic organ prolapse, pelvic floor disorders, Raheela M. Rizvi. IntechOpen; 2018. https://doi.org/10.5772/intechopen.76629. Available from: https://www.intechopen.com/chapters/60935
7. Ross JA, Davison AZ, Sana Y, Appiah A, Johns J, Lee CT. Ovum transmigration after salpingectomy for ectopic pregnancy. Hum Rep. 2013;28(4):937–941.
8. Rosse C, Gaddum-Rosse P. Hollinshead's textbook of anatomy. 5th ed. New York: Lippincott-Raven; 1997.
9. Said H. Endoscopic anatomy of the groin: implications for transabdominal preperitoneal herniorrhaphy. Anat J Afr. 2012;1(1):2–10.
10. Seif E, Iwanaga J, Oskouian RJ, Loukas M, Tubbs RS. Comprehensive review of the cardinal ligament. Cureus. 2018;10:e2846. https://doi.org/10.7759/cureus.2846.
11. Sharma V, Lehmann T, Stuckas H, Funke L, Hiller M. Loss of *RXFP2* and *INSL3* genes in Afrotheria shows that testicular descent is the ancestral condition in placental mammals. PLoS Biol. 2018;16:e2005293. Available at: www.journals.plos.org/plosbiology/article/file?id=10.371/journal.pbio.2005293&type=printable
12. Simon LV, Sajjad H, Lopez RA, Burns B. Bladder rupture. Stat Pearls; 2020. Available at: https://www.ncbi.nim.nih.gov/books/NBK470226/
13. Snell R. Clinical Anatomy by region. 9th ed. Lippincott Williams and Wilkins; 2012.
14. Standring S. Gray's anatomy: the anatomical basis of clinical practice. London: Elsevier; 2005.
15. Vallabhajosyula R, Mathur M, Kathirvel R, Madan AI, Kang J, Mogali SR. Getting back to the basics: reintroduction of pelvic anatomy concepts for obstetrics and gynecology residents. In: Proceedings of Singapore healthcare; 2020. p. 1–7. https://doi.org/10.1177/2010105820935913.
16. Willard-Mack CL. Normal structure, function, and histology of lymph nodes. Toxicol Pathol. 2006;34:409–24.
17. Winsberg E. We need scientific dissidents now more than ever. Chronicl Higher Educ. August 10, 2023. Available at: We Need Scientific Dissidents Now More Than Ever (chronicle.com)
18. Wong JW, Lai T, Carney M. Sampson's Artery revisited. HSOA J Reprod Med Gynaec Obstet. 2017;2:005. https://doi.org/10.24966/RMGO-2574/100005.

6 The Lower Limb

Gluteal Region

There are three gluteal muscles (Fig. 6.1):

1. *Gluteus Maximus* is the largest muscle of the buttocks. Its origin is a semi-circular line running from the posterior gluteal line of the ilium, along the sacrum, the sacrospinous ligament, and the coccyx. It inserts into the iliotibial tract, the linea aspera and gluteal tuberosity of the femur. In the standing position, the muscle covers the ischial tuberosity, but in the sitting position, it rises over the ischial tuberosity so that you sit on your ischial tuberosity and not the gluteus maximus. The gluteus maximus is a strong extensor at the hip joint. It is most important in going from a sitting to a standing position. Running up and down the stairs will strengthen the muscle. It is innervated by the inferior gluteal nerve. Patients with damage to the nerve will have difficulty standing—getting out of

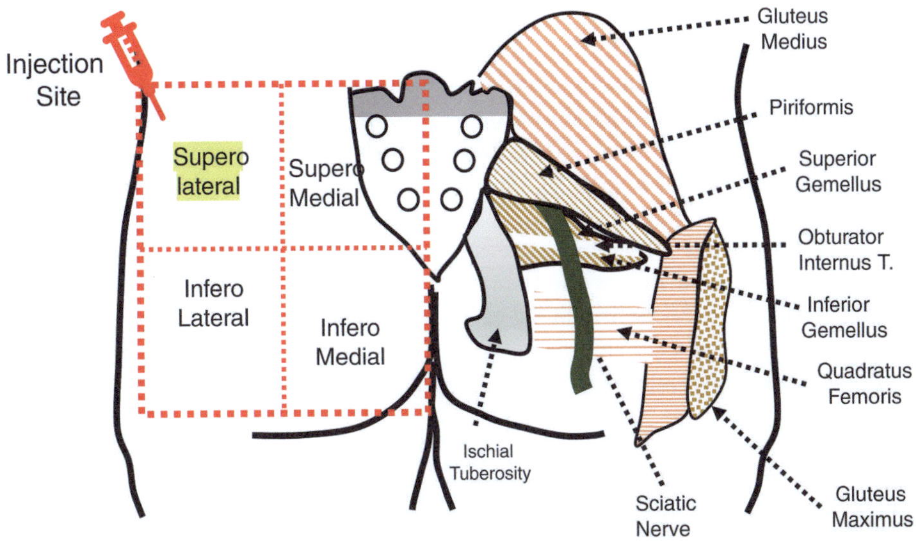

Fig. 6.1 Gluteal region. The piriformis is a landmark for the gluteal region. Emerging inferior to it is the sciatic nerve which in turn is passing over the superior gemellus, obturator internus and the inferior gemellus [13, 14]

J. Leo, *Gross Anatomy, Neuroanatomy, and Embryology for Medical Students*,
https://doi.org/10.1007/978-3-031-87151-1_6

the car for instance. It is also a lateral rotator at the hip.
2. *Gluteus Medius* is deep to gluteus maximus. It arises from the ilium and inserts into the greater trochanter.
3. *Gluteus Minimus* is deep to gluteus medius. It arises from the ilium and inserts into the greater trochanter. Both gluteus medius and minimus are abductors and medial rotators of the hip. But gluteus medius and minimus are more complicated, and their actions should be considered together.

Trendelenburg Sign and Trendelenburg Gait

Gluteus medius and minimus work together to stabilize the pelvis when the contralateral foot is lifted off the ground. For instance, when you are in a standing position, and lift your left foot off the ground, the tendency to fall is to the left. As an analogy, imagine kicking out the leg of a dining room table; the table will fall towards the unsupported side. In a healthy human, lifting the left leg off the ground results in a tendency to fall to the left, but this does not happen because the right gluteus medius and minimus will contract to stabilize the pelvis, and prevent the lean to the left. With damage to the medius and minimus on the right side, if the person lifts their left leg off the ground they will tend to fall to the left. In the same patient, they will not have a deficit when they lift their right leg off the ground.

If you suspect a patient has a weak gluteus medius and minimus on the patient's left side, you ask them to stand and lift their right leg off the ground. If the left muscles are weak, the patient will fall towards the right. This is known as *Trendelenburg's sign*. This patient will also have a "waddling gait" or *Trendelenburg gait*. When this patient is walking, each time they lift their right leg off the ground they will tend to fall to the right, so they will counteract this tendency by excessively leaning to the left.

Deep to the three gluteal muscles are the six deep lateral rotators. All these muscles run from the sacral region laterally to insert along the posterior side of the greater trochanter of the femur (Fig. 6.1).

1. The triangular shaped *piriformis* runs from sacrum to the greater trochanter through the greater sciatic foramen and it is the major landmark in this region. Most of the other muscles and the nerves and arteries in this region are explained based on their relationship to piriformis. They are either superior (supra piriform recess) or inferior (infra piriform recess) to piriformis.
2. Inferior to piriformis are three muscles that form a triangle, sometimes referred to as the triceps coxae (three hip muscles). The middle muscle of the group is the *obturator internus*. If you are dissecting the gluteal region and have removed the three large gluteal muscles, the main muscle belly of the obturator internus is out of view, but you can see its tendon sandwiched between two smaller muscle bellies. The tendon is a sharp white line at this point. On either side of the tendon of obturator internus is the *superior gemellus* or *inferior gemellus*. The two gemelli arise from the ischial spine. The sciatic nerve emerges from the pelvis inferior to piriformis and passes over (posterior to) these three muscles. Obturator internus is also discussed in more detail in the pelvis chapter, as its muscle belly forms the lateral wall of the pelvic cavity. The tendon of obturator internus passes from the pelvis to the gluteal region by traveling through the lesser sciatic foramen (Fig. 6.3).
3. *Obturator externus* is typically not visible in the gluteal region with a posterior approach. It also inserts on the greater trochanter. It is discussed in more detail with the medial thigh.
4. *Quadratus femoris* is inferior to the triceps coxae and is also a deep lateral rotator.

Greater Trochanter

The greater trochanter is a major attachment point on the superior femur for several muscles coming from different regions of the pelvis and the thigh. To aid in the understanding of all these

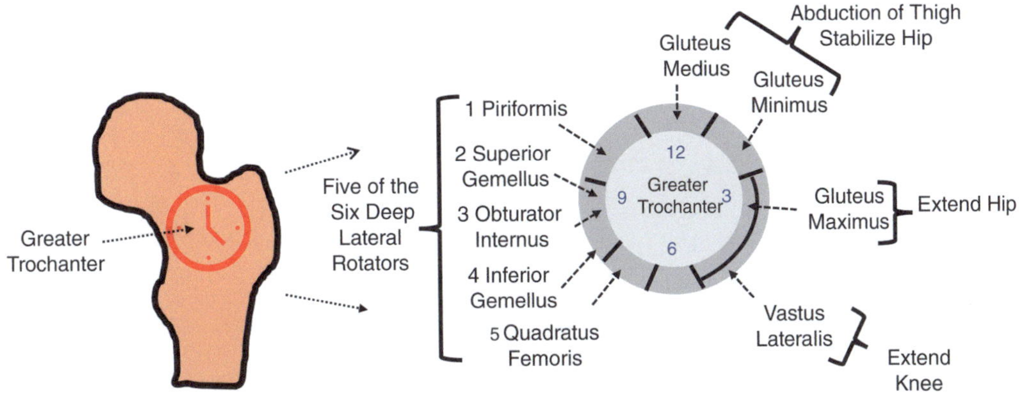

Fig. 6.2 Insertions onto greater trochanter. The greater trochanter is pictured as a clock face with the various muscles attaching to it. The gluteus medius and minimus insert superiorly act to abduct at the hip. While the deep lateral rotators can be seen inserting medially [13, 14]

muscles, it helps to think of these insertions on the greater trochanter as a clock face. If we look at the greater trochanter from a posterior view, we can divide up the muscles and their insertions as the points on the clock. Starting at the 12 o'clock, we see gluteus medius attached to the top of the greater trochanter. And then moving in a clockwise direction to the 2 o'clock position we can see the gluteus minimus. By coming in superiorly and attaching to the top of the greater trochanter, both these muscles, gluteus medius and minimus, are involved in abduction at the hip joint. The gluteus maximus starts posteriorly and comes in at an angle to insert from about the 2 to 5 o'clock positions. Because of the angle that it is coming into the clock, it assists with extension at the hip (Fig. 6.2).

Overlying the gluteus maximus but projecting inferiorly is the origin of vastus lateralis from the gluteal tuberosity, which contributes to knee extension. At the seven o'clock position is the attachment of the quadratus femoris. At the nine o'clock position the triceps coxae, sometimes called the conjoined tendon, can be seen inserting. As mentioned above, this common tendon is made up of the superior gemellus, tendon of obturator internus, and the inferior gemellus. Moving to the 10 o'clock position is the attachment for piriformis. We can see on the medial side of the trochanter, from about the 7 to 10 o'clock position, the group of muscles which are the deep lateral rotators: quadratus femoris, inferior gemellus, obturator internus, superior gemellus, and the piriformis. In addition to the location of the muscles there are several bursae in this region which are designed to facilitate the gliding motion of the muscles. The superficial trochanteric bursa is located superficial to the gluteus medius muscle—in the center of the clock, and deep to gluteus maximus. There is also a small deep trochanteric bursa found deep to the gluteus medius. The bursa can become inflamed which leads to pain in the region of the greater trochanter.

Nerves and Vessels of Gluteal Region

The gluteal region is described as four quadrants. Most of the important nerves and arteries of the gluteal region are in the inferior medial quadrant. An injection in this gluteal region is typically given in the superolateral quadrant to avoid these underlying structures.

1. Emerging from the pelvis, superior to the piriformis is the *superior gluteal nerve*, *artery*, and *vein* which travel between the gluteus medius and minimus. The superior gluteal nerve innervates the gluteus medius and minimus. The superior gluteal vessels are often injured with pelvic fractures (Fig. 6.3).

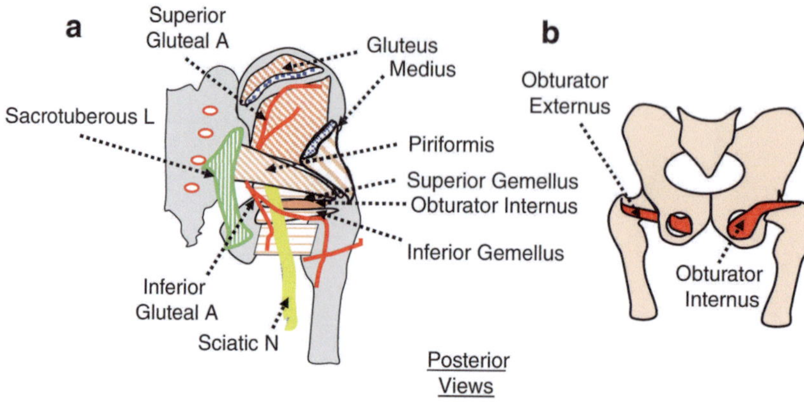

Fig. 6.3 Panel (**a**) Deep, Posterior Gluteal Region. The gluteus maximus is not shown**.** The gluteus medius has been cut to show the superior gluteal A, V, and N passing between gluteus medius and minimus. Inferior to piriform is the sciatic nerve and the triceps coxae made up of three muscles: (1) the superior gemellus, (2) the tendon of obturator internus, and (3) the inferior gemellus. Panel (**b**) highlights the difference between obturator internus and externus [13, 14]

2. Emerging inferior to the piriformis is the *inferior gluteal nerve, artery, and vein***.** The nerve innervates the gluteus maximus.
3. The *pudendal nerve* is the major nerve of the pelvis, but it makes a brief appearance in the gluteal region. It emerges from the pelvis close to the inferior gluteal nerve, but while the inferior gluteal nerve heads posterior to the gluteal region, the pudendal nerve does a quick 90° turn and heads back into the pelvis by traveling between the sacrospinous and sacrotuberous ligaments, and back through the lesser sciatic foramen. Traveling with the pudendal nerve is the internal pudendal artery and vein.
4. The *posterior femoral cutaneous nerve* also emerges inferior to piriformis through the gluteal region to enter the posterior thigh. It gives a branch to the inferior gluteal region (inferior cluneal nerve) and to the perineum (perineal branch) to supply the posterior regions of the labia majora and the scrotum.
5. The *sciatic nerve* is the largest nerve in the body, even larger than the spinal cord, and it emerges inferior to piriformis to travel lateral to the ischial tuberosity on its way to the posterior thigh. The sciatic nerve has two divisions at this point: the *common fibular division*, and the *tibial division*. At this point, the two divisions are typically wrapped together in the same sheath. As they continue traveling towards the knee, they will eventually split as they approach the popliteal fossa. However, in some individuals the split occurs higher up in the pelvis with the common fibular division traveling through the piriformis. In this case, the individual may present with sciatica-like symptoms and complain of weakness in the muscular compartments innervated by the common fibular nerve (Fig. 6.4).

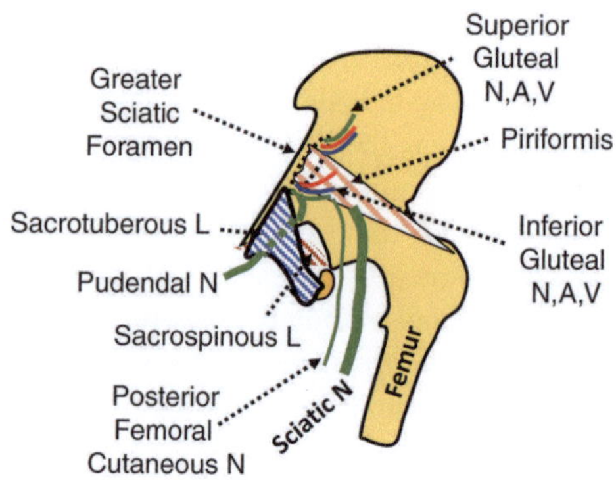

Fig. 6.4 Piriformis Relationships. Emerging above piriformis is the superior gluteal neurovascular bundle. Emerging below the muscle is the inferior neurovascular bundle. The pudendal nerve also emerges inferior to piriformis, but it does a U-turn and re-enters the pelvis between the sacrotuberous and sacrospinous ligaments [13, 14]

Piriformis

Because of the proximity of the sciatic nerve to the piriformis, the nerve can be aggravated by the muscle. Patients with piriformis syndrome will complain of pain in the gluteal region, particularly in the region of the sciatic notch. With the patient starting in the supine position, they will often complain of pain with hip movements, particularly with flexion, abduction, and internal rotation at the hip (the FAIR test).

Trochanteric Bursitis

As the gluteus medius and minimus pass over the *greater trochanter* there is a bursa between the muscles and the bone. This bursa can become inflamed, leading to hip pain. Tendinopathy of the medius and minimus can also lead to pain in this region. In fact, it is hard to tell whether the pain is coming from bursitis or tendinopathy. The tendons of the medius and minimus and the associated bursa can be compressed by the overlying iliotibial band. Exercises to strengthen the medius and minimus are thought to alleviate the pain.

Cutaneous Sensation in Gluteal Region

Cutaneous sensory information from the superolateral quadrant of the gluteal region travels on the *superior cluneal nerves* which are branches of the dorsal rami of L 1, 2, and 3; sensation from the inferolateral quadrant is via the *inferior cluneal nerves* which are branches of the posterior femoral cutaneous nerve; sensation from the superomedial quadrant is via the *medial cluneal nerves* which are branches of the dorsal rami of S 1, 2, and 3; and sensation from the inferomedial quadrant is via the *perforating cutaneous nerve*, from the ventral rami of S, 2 and 3.

Superficial Venous Drainage of the Lower Limb

For all the arteries of the lower limb, there are equivalent veins. For instance, the anterior tibial artery has an equivalent vein—the anterior tibial vein. However, there is a separate pattern of drainage for the skin and superficial fascia. The *great saphenous vein* starts as the dorsal venous arch on the dorsum of the foot and runs anterior to the medial malleolus and continues posteromedial to the knee, and then tracks along the medial thigh to drain into the femoral vein by piercing the fascia at the saphenous opening. The vein is sometimes harvested for coronary bypass procedures. To find the vein, one can look anterior to the medial malleolus, or medial to the femoral artery (Fig. 6.5).

The other significant superficial vein of the lower limb is the *lesser saphenous vein* which starts from the lateral side of the dorsal venous arch and drains the lateral foot and posterior leg. It pierces the fascia in the popliteal fossa to join

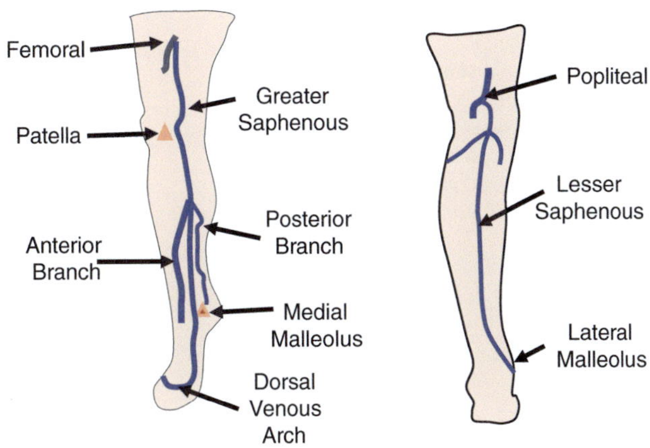

Fig. 6.5 Superficial veins of lower limb [13, 14]

the popliteal vein. These superficial veins have a series of valves that assist in moving the blood against gravity. With aging these valves can be compromised which leads to varicose veins.

A deep vein thrombosis (DVT) can develop in the deep veins, especially in sedentary individuals. Long airplane flights are a predisposing factor. Symptoms include pain and swelling in the calf. In some patients a deep vein thrombosis can lead to pulmonary embolism (venous thromboembolism). To test for a DVT, the patients lies supine, and the foot is dorsiflexed. A subsequent pain in the posterior leg suggests the presence of a DVT (Homan's sign). While not as common, a thrombosis can also develop in the superficial veins. These can usually be seen on a physical exam and will typically resolve with time (Fig. 6.6).

Right before the great saphenous vein enters the femoral vein, it has three branches: (1) superficial external pudendal vein, (2) superficial circumflex iliac vein, and (3) the superficial epigastric vein. All three of these veins drain the regions described by their names. Of note, the corresponding arteries are branches of the femoral artery (Fig. 6.7).

These superficial veins have one-way valves at various points inside the vein which keep the blood moving towards the heart (uphill). As the muscles contract, the veins above the contraction

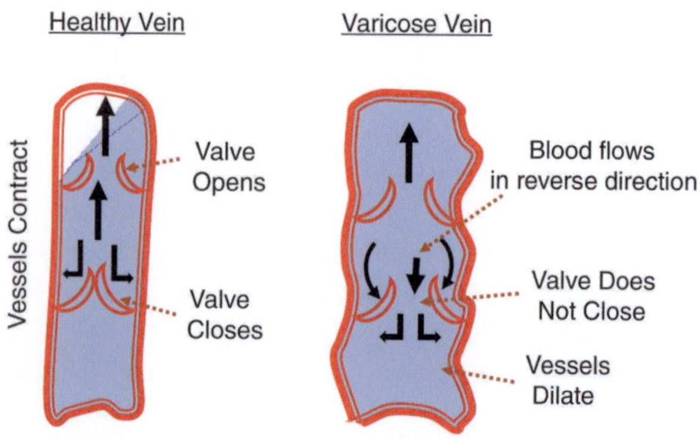

Fig. 6.6 Normal versus varicose veins. In the healthy vein, the valves work in tandem. As the vessel wall contracts, the downstream valves open, while the upstream valves close. This prevents backflow into the veins. In varicose veins the valves do not close, and the blood will pool in the veins leading to dilated veins [13, 14]

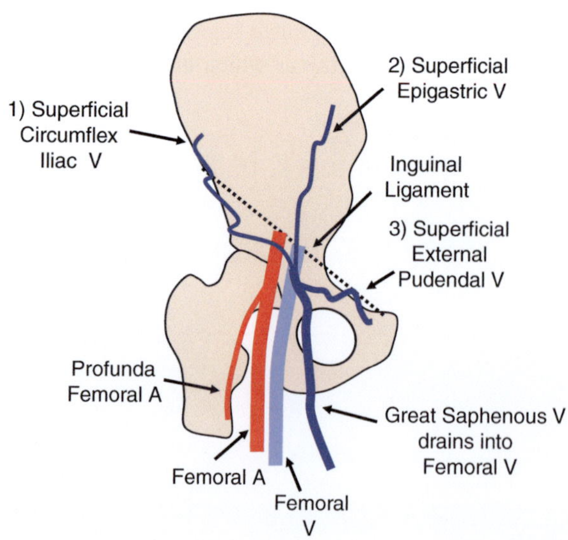

Fig. 6.7 Branches of great saphenous vein. (1) Superficial circumflex iliac, (2) Superficial epigastric, and (3) Superficial external pudendal veins. These are all branches of the great saphenous vein. The corresponding arteries (not shown) are branches of the femoral artery [13, 14]

open, while the veins below the contraction close, so that the blood moves in one direction—superiorly. In elderly individuals, these veins lose their elasticity, and the valves remain open which allows the blood to move inferiorly and pool in the legs. This leads to dilated veins known as varicose veins. Women are more likely to be affected by varicose veins than men. The reason for this is unknown. It can also occur in pregnant women but will usually improve following the delivery.

The Thigh

Both the thigh and the leg each have three compartments. In the thigh there are the anterior, posterior, and medial compartments; and in the leg there are the anterior, posterior, and lateral compartments.

The nerve supply to the thigh is straightforward because the muscles in each compartment are innervated by one nerve, however each compartment has one exception to this rule. The anterior thigh compartment is innervated by the femoral nerve except for pectineus that is innervated by the femoral and obturator nerves. The medial thigh compartment is innervated by the obturator nerve except for the "hamstring" portion of adductor magnus which is innervated by the tibial division of the sciatic nerve. The posterior thigh compartment is innervated by the tibial division of the sciatic except for the short head of the biceps which is innervated by the common fibular division of the sciatic.

Fascia Lata and Iliotibial Band

The *fascia lata* is a thick tough layer of fascia surrounding the thigh. It is connected to the gluteal fascia which in turn is connected to the thoracolumbar fascia superiorly. The *iliotibial tract* is a thickened layer of the fascia lata on the lateral thigh and runs from the superior iliac crest to *Gerdy's tubercle* on the anterolateral side of the proximal tibia. Within the superior portion of the iliotibial tract is the *tensor fascia lata,* which contracts the iliotibial band, leading to extension and lateral rotation of the leg. It is also involved in adduction and medial rotation of the thigh. It is innervated by the superior gluteal nerve.

Iliotibial syndrome occurs when the muscle is overactive which leads to pain from the lateral thigh or knee. It is a common injury in runners. Patients will often complain of pain when standing, getting out of a chair, or getting out of the car. Exercises to develop the gluteus medius, such as running up and down stairs are often recommended.

Anterior Thigh

The bulk of the anterior thigh is made up of the quadriceps, but it also includes the sartorius and the pectineus. The pectineus is confused as it sits right between the anterior and medial compartments, and some authors will group it with the anterior compartment while other authors will group it with the medial compartment. Since it needs to have a home, I will talk about it as being in the anterior compartment (Fig. 6.8).

The *sartorius,* the longest muscle in the body, is sometimes referred to as the "Tailor's muscle" which alludes to the tailor sitting with the leg crossed with the hip flexed, the knee flexed, and the lower limb laterally rotated at the hip. The tailor would then put a sheet over their thighs to catch anything they dropped. The sartorius runs from the anterior superior iliac spine (ASIS) to the medial side of the proximal tibia.

Sitting deep to the sartorius is the quadriceps group of muscles which include the three vasti muscles and the rectus femoris. The vastus medialis, vastus lateralis, and vastus intermedius, all originate from the femur, and come together with the rectus femoris to make up the *quadriceps tendon* which runs over the patella and then continues as the *patellar tendon.* Together with the rectus femoris they are all involved with extension of the knee. In addition, the rectus femoris is a hip flexor.

One might expect all the muscle fibers of vastus medialis to be orientated in a superior to inferior direction. However, if one looks closely at the inferior fibers of vastus medialis, which are

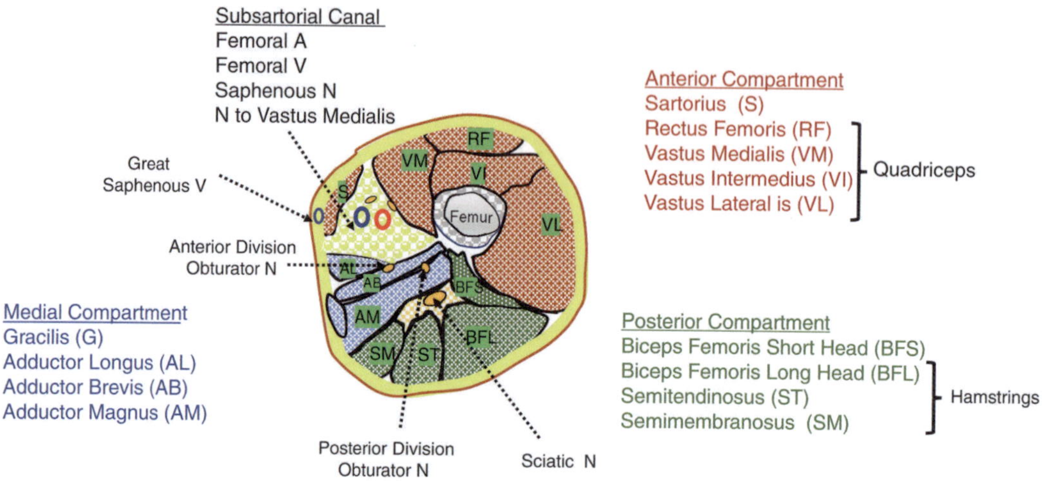

Fig. 6.8 Cross section of thigh. In the medial compartment, gracilis is most medial with adductor longus, brevis, and magnus organized in three planes. The adductor brevis is between the anterior and posterior divisions of obturator nerve. In the posterior compartment are the hamstrings: semitendinosus, semimembranosus, and the long head of biceps femoris. In the anterior compartment are the quadriceps and sartorius. The cross section is below pectineus thus it is not in the image [13, 14]

easily seen medial to the patella, you will see that they are angled so that they enter the patellar tendon from the side. This orientation helps to counteract the patella's tendency to slip laterally. In an individual who exercises a lot the vastus medialis stands out and is shaped like a tear drop.

Of note is that both the sartorius and the rectus femoris span the hip and the knee joint. Both contribute to hip flexion, however their actions at the knee differ. The rectus femoris arises from the *anterior inferior iliac spine* and runs over the front of the knee and joins the patella tendon to insert into the tibial tuberosity, making it a knee extensor. The sartorius on the other hand runs to the medial side of the knee to insert on the medial surface of the tibia, making is a knee flexor.

Osgood-Schlatter disease primarily occurs in adolescents. The patellar tendon attaches to the tibial tuberosity and excessive strain can lead to inflammation of the attachment site.

Myositis Ossificans is a common injury in athletes that arises from repeated trauma or bruising to a muscle that can result in bone forming within the damaged region. It often happens in the quadriceps. Resting after an injury is the best way to prevent bone from forming. With an appropriate amount of rest, the bone tissue will typically be reabsorbed.

Pes Anserinus

The *Pes Anserinus* is a point on the medial tibia where three tendons insert. One mnemonic for remembering this is, "**S**ay **G**race before **T**ea" standing for the **S**artorius, **G**racilis, and semi-**T**endinosus. The three muscles and the Pes Anserinus are like an upside-down tripod, with each muscle, or leg of the tripod coming from a different compartment: sartorius from the anterior compartment, gracilis from the medial compartment, and semitendinosus from the posterior compartment. Deep to the pes anserinus is the *pes anserinus bursa* which can become inflamed (Fig. 6.9).

Medial Thigh

The bulk of the medial thigh compartment is made up of the three adductors—brevis, longus, and magnus. On the medial edge of the medial compartment is the strap-like *gracilis* muscle. At

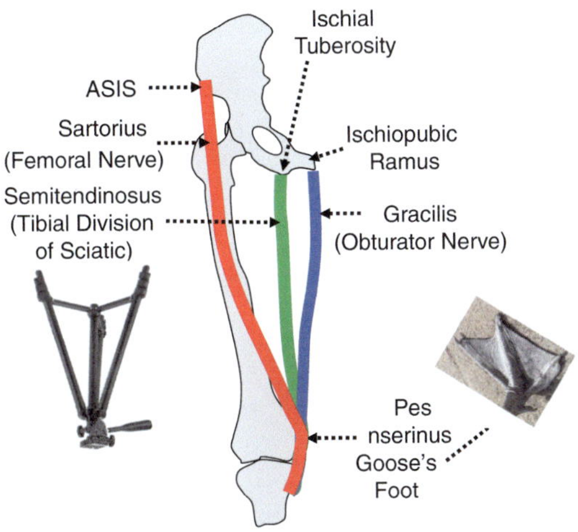

Fig. 6.9 Pes anserinus: There are three muscles that contribute to the pes anserinus (Latin: Goose Foot) and form an *upside-down tripod:* (1) Sartorius arises from ASIS, (2) Semitendinosus from the ischial tuberosity, and (3) Gracilis from the ischiopubic ramus. Each muscle originates from a different compartment and is innervated by the nerve of that compartment [13, 14]

the superior medial corner, the *pectineus* makes a brief appearance in the medial thigh. The muscles of the medial thigh are organized in three planes. The first plane houses the *adductor longus* and the *pectineus*. Deep to the adductor longus and pectineus, in the middle layer, is the *adductor brevis*. And then in the deepest layer is the *adductor magnus*. The entire medial thigh is innervated by the obturator nerve, with one exception. The *obturator nerve* is a branch of the lumbosacral plexus and comes through the obturator foramen and enters the thigh where it splits into *anterior* and *posterior divisions* proximal to the adductor brevis. The anterior division is easily seen passing anterior to the adductor brevis and entering the gracilis. The posterior division of the obturator nerve passes posterior to the adductor brevis.

All the adductors originate from the pubic ramus in the vicinity of the obturator foramen and then fan out to insert along the posterior surface of the femur near the linea aspera.

Like all the thigh compartments, when it comes to the medial thigh, there is one exception to the notion that each compartment is innervated by one nerve. The "hamstring portion" of adductor magnus is innervated by the tibial division of the sciatic nerve. The hamstring portion of adductor magnus is the most medial part of the muscle, it is thin and can be seen attaching to the *adductor tubercle* of the femur. Strain on the adductors is a common injury to horseback riders. Groin strains result from increased pressure on the adductor muscles of the medial thigh. The most common groin strain involves adductor longus.

The obturator nerve innervates both the hip and knee joint leading to a patient complaining of pain in one of these joints when the pathology is in the other joint. In addition, because of the obturator nerve's pathway through the pelvis, a difficult delivery or a pelvic mass can aggravate the obturator nerve (Figs. 6.10 and 6.11).

The obturator externus is located outside the obturator membrane. And runs from the outer surface of the obturator membrane and pubic and ischial rami to the medial surface of the greater trochanter. It is one of the six deep lateral rotators of the hip.

Posterior Thigh

The posterior thigh is composed of the three hamstrings which all arise as a group from the ischial tuberosity. As the hamstrings travel inferiorly, they separate to go in different directions and head for different insertion points. The long head of the *biceps femoris* crosses over the sciatic nerve to head towards the lateral side of the tibia, while the *semitendinosus* and *semimembranosus* travel to the medial side. The long head of the biceps femoris is joined by the short head of the biceps femoris at about the midpoint of the posterior thigh. The biceps femoris then inserts into the fibula and lateral condyle of the tibia, but more specifically its tendon splits to go around the fibular collateral ligament. The semitendinosus inserts at the pes anserinas on the medial tibia, and the semimembranosus has an extensive attachment to the tibia, medial meniscus, and the medial collateral ligament. All the hamstrings are innervated by the *tibial division of sciatic*, except for the short head of the biceps which is innervated by the *common fibular nerve*.

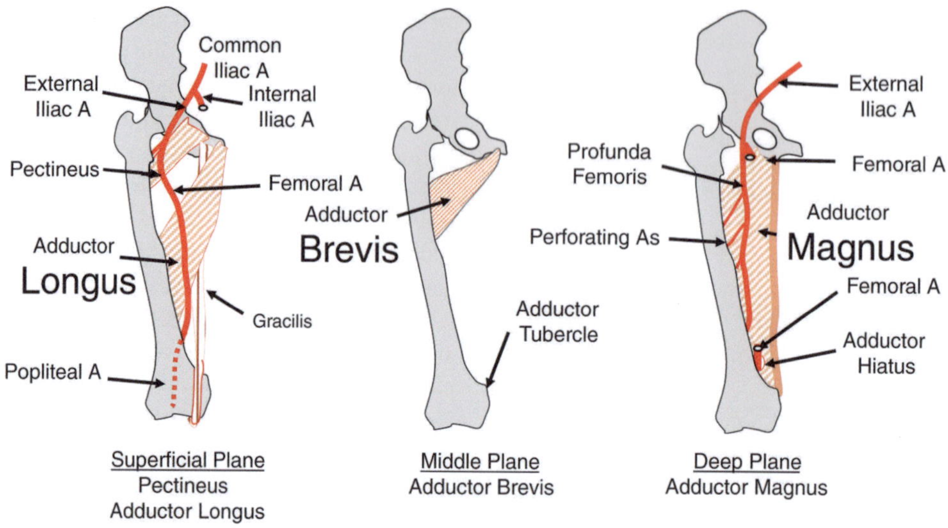

Fig. 6.10 The three adductors. The figure shows the Longus, Brevis, and Magnus and their relationship to each other and the major arteries. The muscles are organized into three planes. The most superficial, or the first plane, includes adductor longus and pectineus. The middle, or second plane, houses the adductor brevis. The deepest, or third plane, houses the adductor magnus. The femoral artery lies superficial to the muscles of the first plane. The profunda femoris artery lies superficial to the adductor magnus [13, 14]

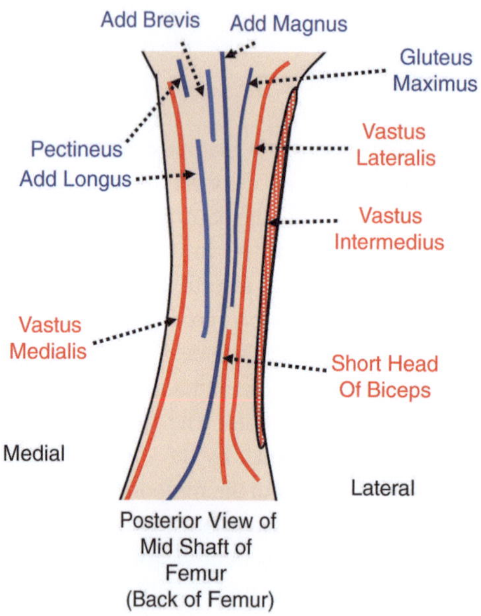

Fig. 6.11 Muscular attachments to the posterior femur

The hamstrings extend at the hip and flex at the knee. Hamstring injuries can occur when the muscle is stretched. A good example of this is a hurdler's injury. When a runner goes over a hurdle, they are putting maximum strain on the hamstrings by flexing at the hip and extending at the knee. If a hurdler goes down in severe pain during a race and grabs their posterior thigh, it is likely that they either tore the hamstrings or avulsed the ischial tuberosity—the origin of the hamstrings. Another common way to injure the hamstrings is in a water-skiing accident. When the skier is first getting pulled by the rope to go from a seated to a standing position their skis are pointed straight up and their upper limb is extended out over their feet. When the engine is first put into gear this motion puts a sudden strain on their hamstrings.

In the femoral triangle, the femoral artery gives off the *profunda femoris artery* (also known as the deep femoral artery) which has several important branches. Close to its origination is the *lateral femoral circumflex artery* which forms a "T."

The profunda femoris artery also gives off the *medial femoral circumflex*. Both the medial and lateral femoral circumflex arteries provide blood to the femoral head, but the medial femoral circumflex is the more important one. To reach the femoral head, the branches of these two arteries travel on the surface of the femoral neck.

It seems counterintuitive, but the profunda femoris artery which is in the medial compartment also supplies blood to the posterior thigh. As the profunda femoris descends in the thigh anterior to the adductor magnus, there are three to four *perforating branches* that pierce the adductor magnus at various points adjacent to the femur to gain access to the posterior thigh muscles. The second perforating branch supplies blood to the femur.

A *slipped capital femoral epiphysis* involves the ball of the femoral head slipping off the femoral neck, typically posterior. The femoral head stays in the joint, but the femur moves—the metaphysis shifts relative to the epiphysis. This is most often seen in teenagers.

Femoral Triangle

The f*emoral triangle* is bound by two muscles and a ligament. The medial border of the triangle is the adductor longus, the lateral border is the sartorius, and the superior border is the inguinal ligament, which runs from the anterior superior iliac spine to the pubic tubercle. The lateral floor is iliopsoas, and the medial floor is pectineus. There are several important structures in the canal. A common mnemonic is NAVL standing for femoral **N**erve, femoral **A**rtery, femoral **V**ein, and **L**ymphatics. Some authors will use the mnemonic NAVEL, where the E stands for empty space, but we will see that both mnemonics mean the same thing. The "L" in the mnemonic stands for Lymphatics and refers to the *deep inguinal nodes.*

Surrounding the femoral artery, femoral vein and lymphatics is the *femoral sheath* which is a continuation of the abdominal sheath. In addition, the sheath can be subdivided into three compartments, appropriately named the: lateral, intermediate, and medial compartments. Furthermore, the medial compartment of the femoral sheath is referred to as the *femoral canal,* and the opening of the femoral canal is the *femoral ring.* Just medial to the femoral ring is the *lacunar ligament* (Figs. 6.12 and 6.13).

When pressure in the abdominal cavity rises, abdominal contents look for a weakness in the anterior wall. The femoral artery and vein act to block contents from herniating through the wall at this point, so the contents will tend to herniate through the femoral ring, which except for some lymph nodes is relatively "empty" and weak.

The NAVL mnemonic will help with numerous scenarios. As a starting point, the femoral artery sits halfway between the ASIS and the pubic tubercle and lies over the femoral head. If you want to block the femoral nerve, one way to find it would be to find the pulse of the femoral artery, and then move laterally. If one wants to find the great saphenous vein, then you could start at the femoral artery, move medially to the femoral vein, and then find the great saphenous vein opening into the femoral vein. And most importantly, femoral hernias which herniate through the femoral ring will be medial to the femoral vein. And the femoral hernia will be lateral to the lacunar ligament.

The femoral nerve sits on top of the medial portion of the iliopsoas. An infection inside the abdominal cavity can lie deep to the fascia of psoas major. The infection can then travel down close to the insertion point of iliopsoas to lie mostly lateral to the femoral nerve. Moving even further laterally is the lateral femoral cutaneous nerve which comes under the inguinal ligament just medial to the ASIS (Fig. 6.14).

Meralgia paresthetica is a loss of cutaneous sensation to the anterolateral thigh from damage to the lateral femoral cutaneous nerve. Either a belt or jeans that are too tight can aggravate the nerve at this point. Likewise, in the later stages of pregnancy, increased pressure from the abdominopelvic cavity can aggravate the nerve (Fig. 6.14).

Superficial Inguinal Lymph Nodes

The *superficial inguinal nodes* are found distal to the inguinal ligament and resemble a "T" shape, with the top part of the "T" running parallel to the inguinal ligament, and the descending part of the "T" running down the anterior thigh. The nodes

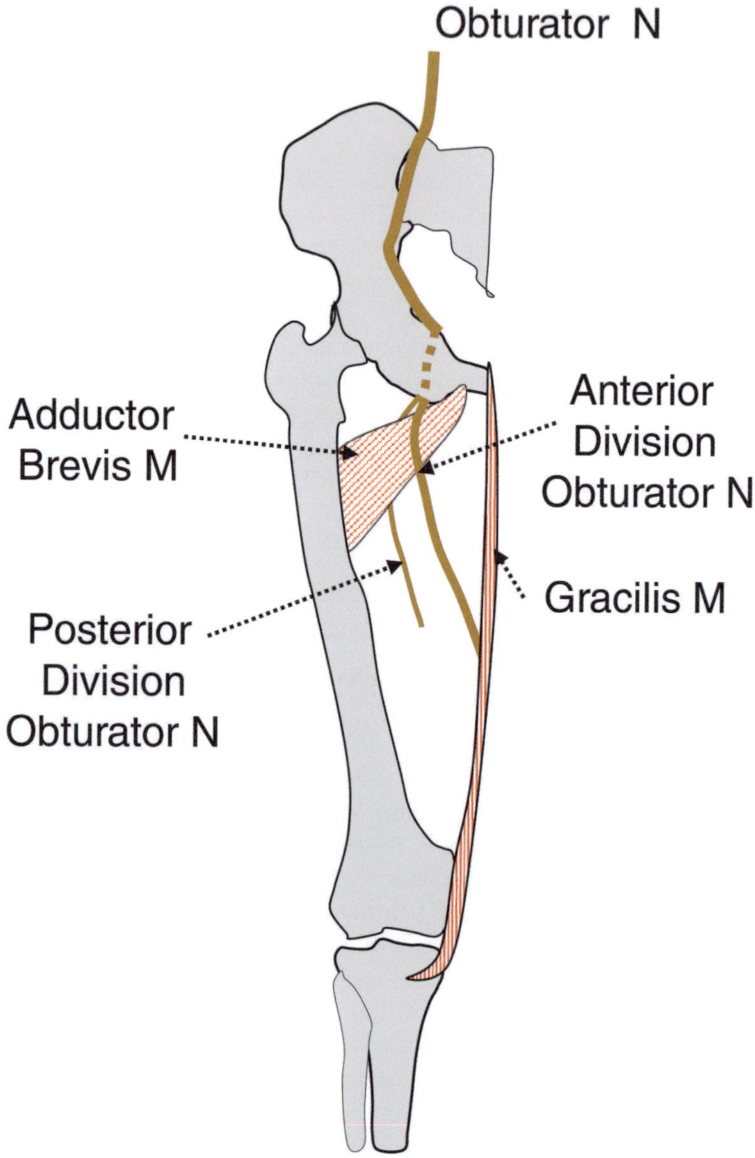

Fig. 6.12 Obturator nerve. The obturator nerve comes from L2, 3, and 4. As it enters the medial thigh it splits into and anterior and posterior divisions that are separated by the adductor brevis muscle [13, 14]

drain the entire superficial lower limb except for the lateral leg and the fifth and lateral side of the fourth toe, which in turn drain into the popliteal nodes. Stepping on a rusty nail with your big toe could lead to swollen superficial inguinal nodes; while stepping on a tack with the little toe could lead to swollen popliteal nodes The superficial nodes also drain the anterior abdominal wall below the umbilicus, the superficial gluteal region, and the superficial perineum. It might seem counterintuitive, but the superficial nodes also drain the cornua of the uterus due to the lymphatics that track along the round ligament which is running from the fundus of the uterus down along the inguinal canal to the labia majora (Fig. 6.15).

Femoral Nerve

The *femoral nerve* arises from L 2, 3, and 4 and descends within the abdominal cavity lateral to the *iliopsoas* muscle. In the abdominal cavity the nerve is large. It enters the thigh by passing

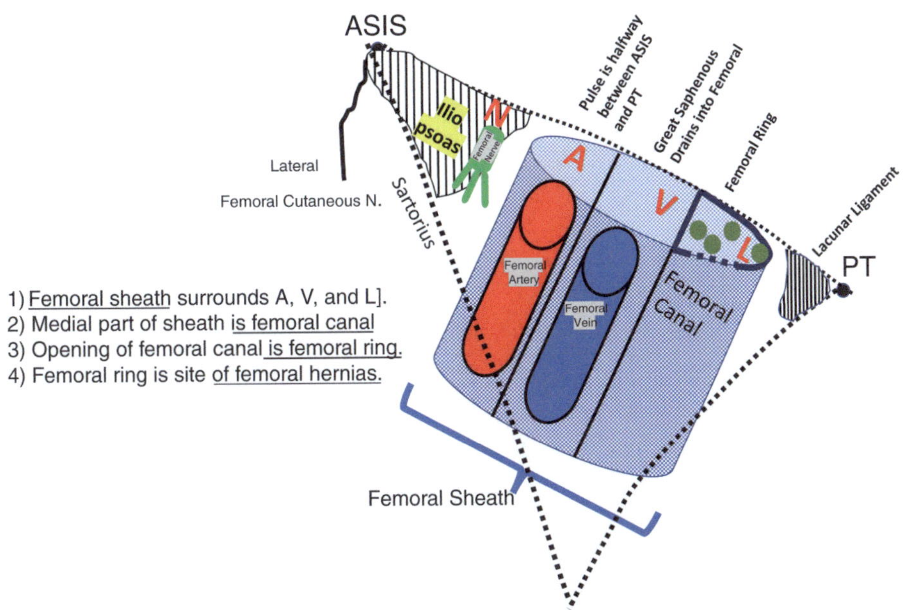

Fig. 6.13 Femoral triangle. The femoral triangle is bounded by the inguinal ligament, adductor longus, and sartorius. Within the canal, from lateral to medial are the femoral nerve, artery, and vein, and the deep inguinal nodes [13, 14]

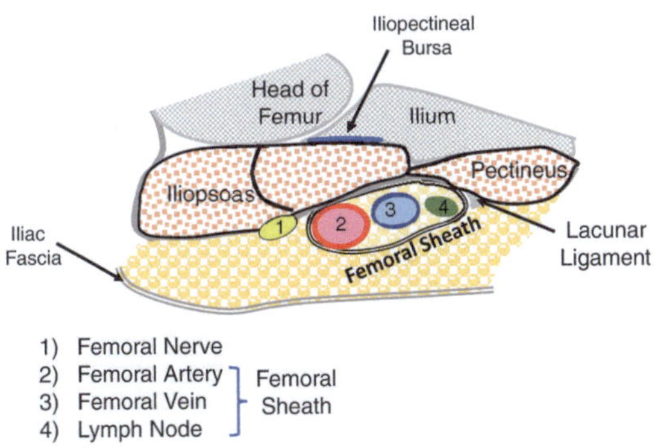

Fig. 6.14 Transverse section through the femoral sheath. The femoral sheath surrounds the femoral artery, femoral vein, and lymphatics (deep inguinal nodes). The femoral nerve is outside of the femoral sheath resting on the iliopsoas. Note the femoral artery located anterior to the head of the femur [13, 14]

deep to the inguinal ligament and enters the femoral triangle just lateral to the femoral artery. It is not housed in the femoral sheath. In the femoral triangle the femoral nerve is medial to the iliopsoas muscle. As soon as the nerve passes deep to the inguinal ligament it immediately divides into many small branches that each travel on to innervate the muscles in the anterior thigh. These branches are named for whichever muscle they are innervating, such as the nerve to vastus medialis, or the nerve to vastus intermedius, or the nerve to rectus femoris (Fig. 6.16).

Subsartorial Canal

At the inferomedial corner of the femoral triangle, the femoral artery, femoral vein, and branches of the femoral nerve continue as a group to dive deep to the sartorius in the appropriately named adductor or *subsartorial canal*. At this point, most of the branches of the femoral nerve have terminated in muscles, however there are typically two nerve branches remaining: the *nerve to vastus medialis*, and the *saphenous nerve*. The nerve to vastus medialis will eventually terminate in its muscle but the *saphenous nerve* will continue past the knee by passing just deep to the tendon of sartorius near its insertion point. The saphenous nerve will then continue down to the foot and is responsible for cutaneous sensation to the medial leg and medial foot as far as the ball of the medial foot (Fig. 6.15).

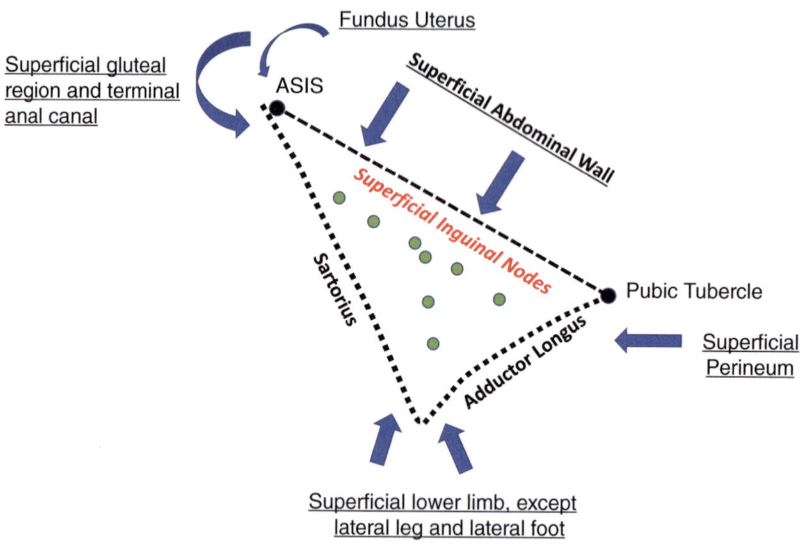

Fig. 6.15 Superficial inguinal nodes. The nodes are shaped like a "T" with one branch running parallel to the inguinal ligament and one branch running down the femoral triangle. The structures draining into the nodes are underlined [13, 14]

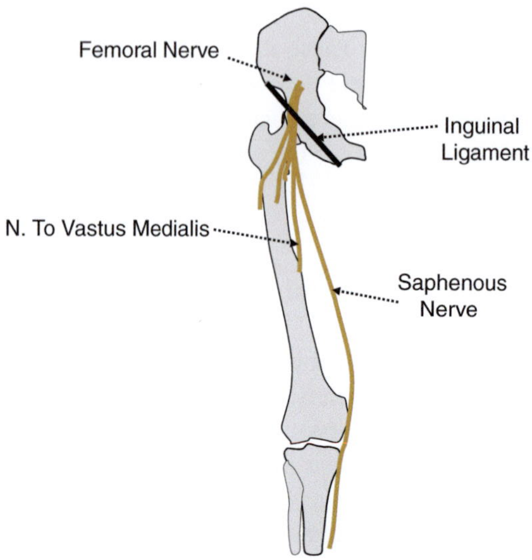

Fig. 6.16 The femoral nerve (L2, 3, and 4). As it passes deep to the inguinal ligament it divides into numerous branches that go to the muscles of the anterior thigh. The only branch to go past the knee joint is the saphenous nerve [13, 14]

Adductor Hiatus

As the femoral artery and vein travel down through the *adductor canal* (subsartorial canal) on top of adductor magnus, they will eventually travel through an opening in adductor magnus called the *adductor hiatus*. They emerge from the hiatus in the popliteal fossa and are now called the popliteal artery and vein.

Femoral Artery

Soon after it comes under the inguinal ligament, the femoral artery gives off the *profunda femoris artery*. Near its origin, there are two important branches. The lateral femoral circumflex artery which proceeds laterally and gives off three appropriately named branches: the *ascending, transverse, and descending branches*. The descending branch can travel as far as the knee joint and anastomose with the genicular arteries to provide collateral circulation in the event of a blocked femoral artery (Figs. 6.16 and 6.17).

The cruciate anastomosis is a point on the posterior hip where four arteries come together: (1) descending branch of inferior gluteal, (2) an ascending branch of the first perforating artery from the profunda femoris, (3) a transverse branch of lateral femoral circumflex, and (4) an ascending branch of the medial femoral circumflex.

The second important branch of profunda femoris is the *medial femoral circumflex* artery which heads to the hip joint and runs between pectineus and obturator externus. Both the lateral and medial femoral circumflex send retinacular branches to the femoral head. Obturator hernias are rare, but they occur when abdominal contents slip through the obturator canal and enter the medial thigh either between adductor longus and brevis or between adductor brevis and magnus—following the same path as either the anterior or posterior division of the obturator nerve (Fig. 6.18).

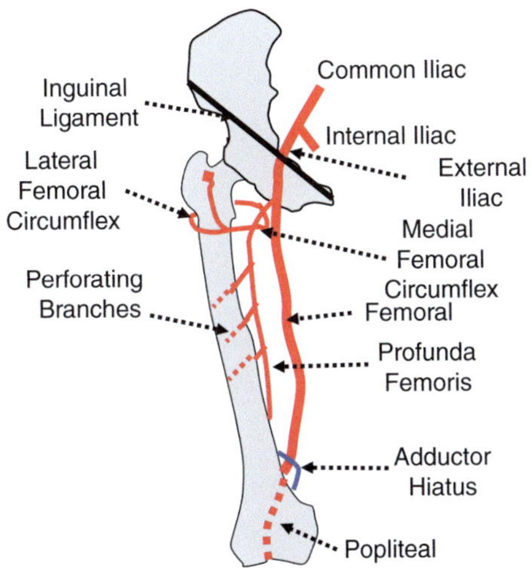

Fig. 6.17 Femoral artery and its branches. Shortly after the femoral artery emerges under the inguinal ligament it gives off the profunda femoris (Deep Femoral) artery [13, 14]

Hip Joint

The hip joint is a ball and socket joint, which is surrounded by three strong, tough ligaments: the *iliofemoral, ischiofemoral, and pubofemoral.* The iliofemoral ligament (Bigelow Ligament) is the strongest ligament in the body and consists of two bands, resembling a Y and provides support during extension of the hip. The ischiofemoral ligament is located on the posterior surface of the hip joint and prevents excessive internal rotation. The pubofemoral ligament runs inferior to the joint and limits external rotation (Fig. 6.19).

While the hip is the strongest joint in the body, it is at its weakest when an individual is in a seated position. A dashboard injury occurs to a rider in the front-seat of a car when the car's front-end

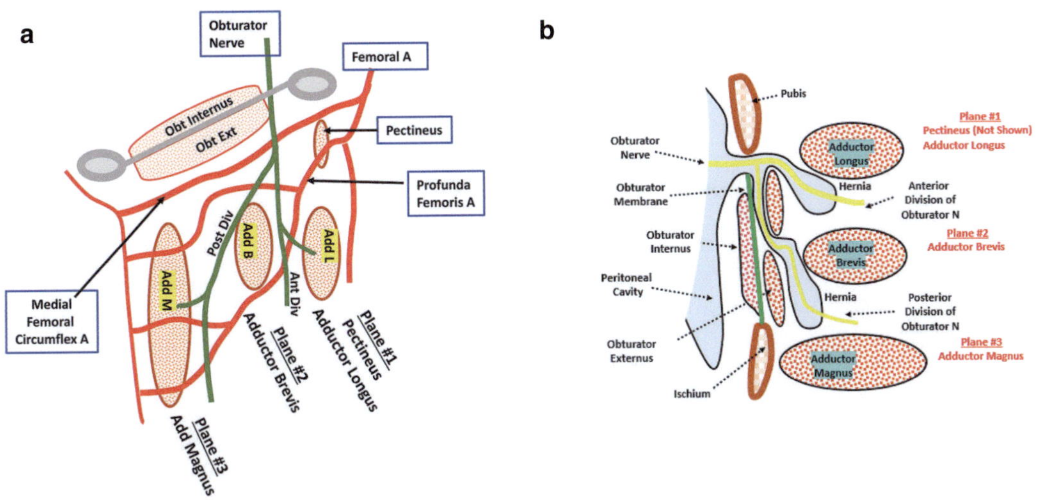

Fig. 6.18 Three planes of muscles in the medial thigh. Panel (**a**) The obturator nerve splits into two branches to go around adductor brevis. Panel (**b**) shows the potential pathways for an obturator hernia [13, 14]

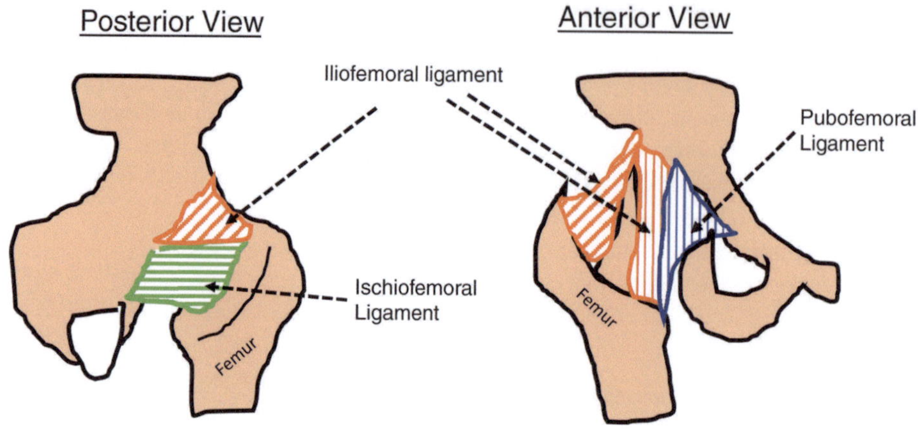

Fig. 6.19 Hip ligaments. From the anterior view, one can see the two bands of the iliofemoral ligament plus the pubofemoral ligament. From the posterior view one can see the top of the iliofemoral plus the whole of the ischiofemoral ligament [13, 14]

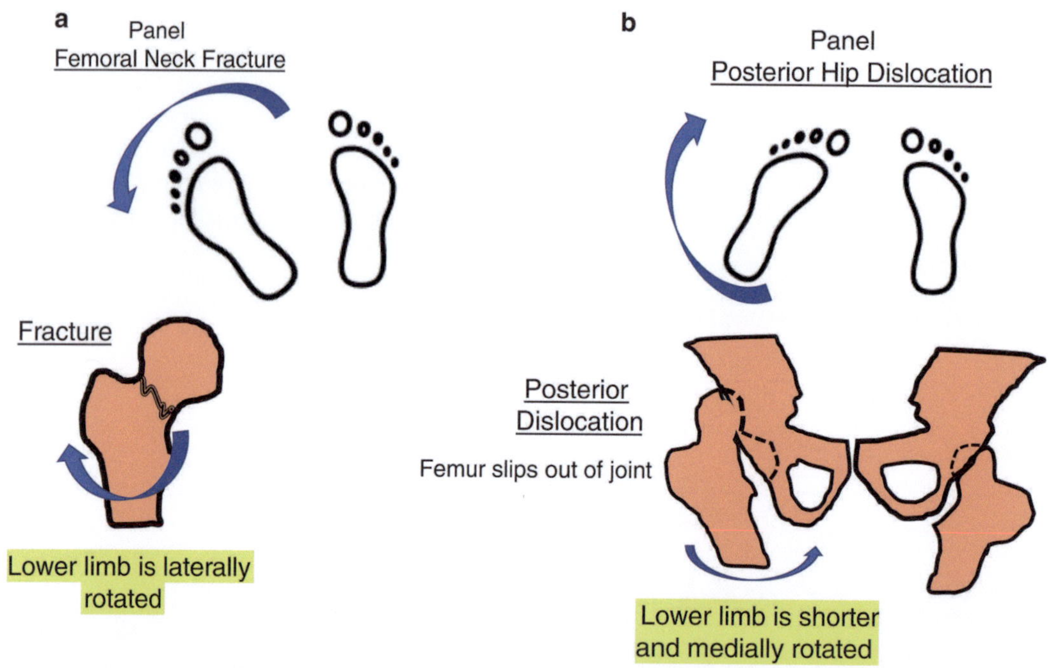

Fig. 6.20 Panel (**a**) With a fracture of the femoral neck the lower limb will be laterally rotated due to the action of iliopsoas. Panel (**b**) In the case of a posterior dislocation, the lower limb will be medially rotated and shorter. The femur has slipped out of the socket and has come to rest on the posterior ischium [13, 14]

slams into an object and their knees hit the dashboard. The force, combined with the seated position, results in a posterior dislocation of the hip joint such that the femoral head pushes through the acetabulum and ischiofemoral ligament. The femoral head then comes to lie posterior to the ischium. This leads to the lower limb being medially rotated and noticeably shorter (Fig. 6.20).

The *angle of inclination* is determined by drawing two lines: one line straight down the femur through the femoral shaft, and another line drawn through the neck of the femur. The range of the normal angle between the two lines is about 105° to 140°. Coxa vara is a decreased angle, which predisposes one to femoral neck fracture. Coxa valga is an increased angle (Fig. 6.21).

As mentioned above, the most important blood supply to the hip and particularly the femoral head comes from the *medial* and *lateral femoral circumflex arteries*, which are typically branches of the profunda femoris artery (the medial is the most important of the two). They form a continuous ring surrounding the femoral head between the lesser and greater trochanters. Emerging from this ring are several retinacular branches traveling on the outer surface of the femoral neck to reach the femoral head. There is also a tiny artery traveling in the ligament of the head of the femur, the *foveal artery* (artery to the head of the femur) which come from the obturator artery. In children the foveal artery plays a significant role, but in adults it is non-existent.

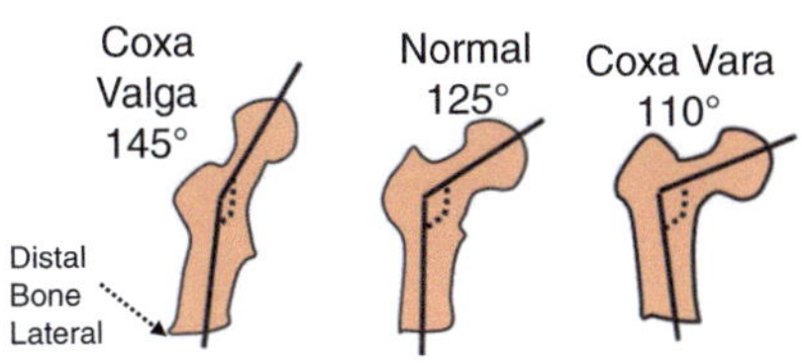

Fig. 6.21 Angle of inclination. Angle between one line drawn down the femoral neck, and a second line drawn down the femur. Normal is 125°. An increased angle is Valga and a decreased angle is Vara [13, 14]

Fractures to the femoral head will result in the lower limb being laterally rotated and shorter. The lateral rotation occurs because of the attachment of iliopsoas to the lesser trochanter. Fractures here, especially in older individuals, will result in avascular necrosis of the femoral head due to disruption of the arteries (Fig. 6.22).

Anastomosis Around Hip

There are two anastomotic networks in the vicinity of the hip joint. The cruciate anastomosis sits near the lesser trochanter and is made up of the transverse branches of medial and lateral femoral circumflex arteries, a descending branch of the inferior gluteal artery, and the ascending branch of the first perforating artery. The trochanteric anastomosis is made up of the medial and lateral femoral circumflex arteries and branches of the superior and inferior gluteal arteries. These networks connect the internal iliac and the femoral arteries and provides blood flow to the head of the femur (Figs. 6.23 and 6.24).

Fractures of the Femoral Neck

While a fracture of the femoral neck will often compromise the blood supply to the femoral head, in contrast an intertrochanteric fracture will

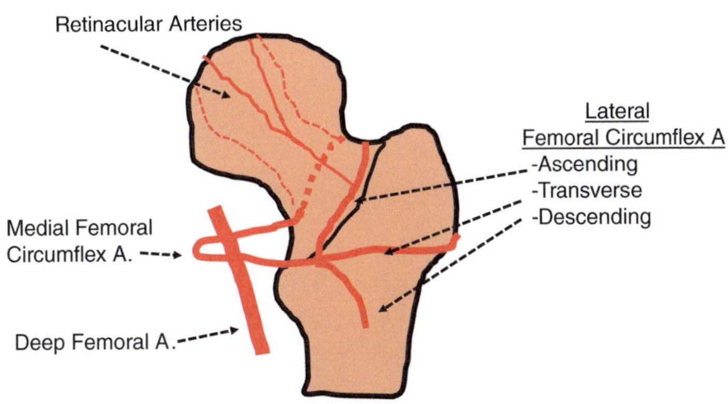

Fig. 6.22 Femoral head. The blood supply to the head of the femur comes mainly from the medial femoral circumflex artery which sends retinacular branches along the external surface of the femoral neck to reach the head. The lateral femoral circumflex has three branches: ascending, descending, and transverse [13, 14]

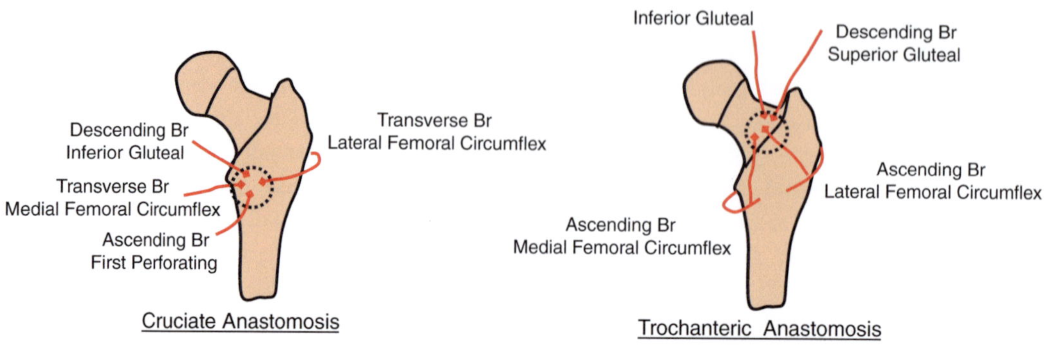

Fig. 6.23 Panel (**a**) Cruciate Anastomosis The four arteries involved meet near the lesser trochanter. Panel (**b**) Trochanteric Anastomosis. Four arteries form a network to supply blood to the femoral head [13, 14]

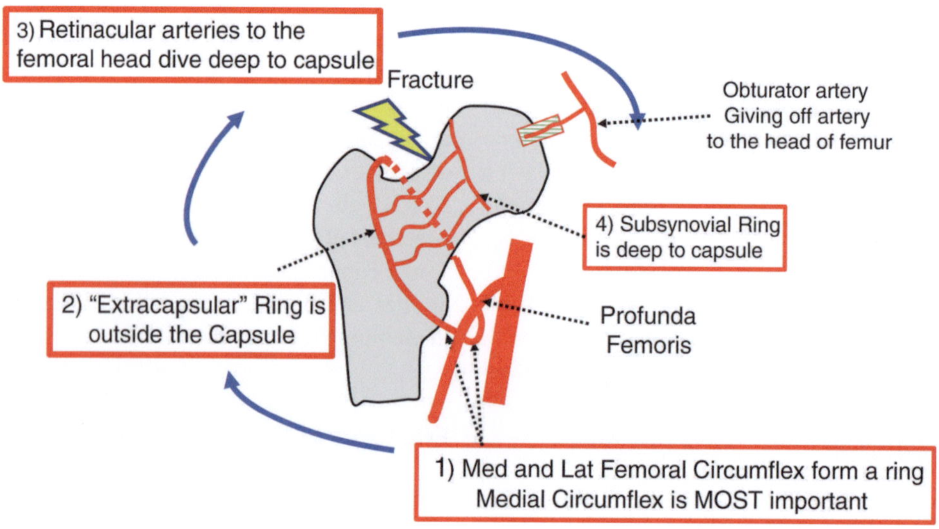

Fig. 6.24 Blood supply to the head of femur. (1) the medial and lateral femoral circumflex arteries form an extracapsular ring near the trochanters. (2) The ring is outside the capsule. (3) The retinacular arteries arise from the ring and travel to the head of the femur. (4) There is a subsynovial ring deep to the capsule. Fractures at the neck will compromise the blood flow to the femoral head. There is a branch of the obturator artery—the artery of the ligament of the head of the femur—that is insignificant in adults [13, 14]

usually spare the blood supply to the femoral head. And with a subtrochanteric fracture, the blood flow to the femoral head should not be in danger. Fractures of the femoral neck are intracapsular while the trochanteric and subtrochanteric fractures are extracapsular. Fractures of the femoral neck in the elderly can lead to increased mortality with some studies showing that in women, death rates within a year after a hip fracture are 4.5 times higher than those without a fracture. And some studies have suggested that a hip fracture has carries a worse prognosis than a cancer diagnosis (Figs. 6.24 and 6.25).

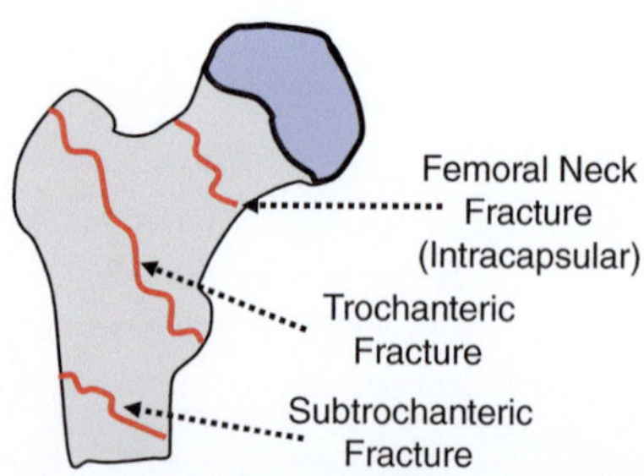

Fig. 6.25 Three femoral fractures. Femoral neck fractures will typically destroy the blood supply to the femoral head. Trochanteric fractures will often spare the blood flow to the femoral head. Subtrochanteric fractures should not disrupt the blood flow to the femoral head [13, 14]

The Knee

The synovial membrane encases the knee joint to make up the synovial joint. There are several important bursae around the joint. Some of these bursae connect with the knee joint and some are separate compartments. The *suprapatellar bursa* is an outpocketing of the synovial membrane that extends superior to the patella, which makes it a suitable location for draining excessive fluid in the knee joint. On the other hand, the *prepatellar bursa* and *infrapatellar bursa* are not continuous with the knee joint. The prepatellar bursa sits directly in front of the patella and patellar tendon, so excessive friction here can lead to bursitis. The term "roofer's knee" refers to a roofer who is on their knees putting pressure on the prepatellar bursa. The infrapatellar bursa on the other hand sits anterior to the knee but lower down on the patellar tendon than the prepatellar bursa. The term "clergyman's knee" refers to the praying person who is aggravating this bursa. A *Baker's cyst* refers to an abnormal outpocketing of the synovial membrane around semitendinosus in the posteromedial popliteal fossa. The cyst will typically appear as a small protuberance in this region. The cysts were first described by William Baker, a surgeon in Fig. 6.26.

In the center of the joint cavity are two important ligaments, the *anterior* and *posterior cruciate ligaments*. These ligaments are named for their attachment to the tibia. In other words, the anterior cruciate starts from the anteromedial tibia and runs posteriorly and laterally to the femur. The posterior cruciate runs from the posteromedial tibia laterally to insert onto the femur. The two ligaments cross each other, making an X, with the anterior cruciate running from anterior to the posterior cruciate. The ligaments are surrounded by the synovial membrane—they are not in the synovial cavity but are extracapsular. The anterior cruciate resists anterior forces. If it is torn, when the patient is sitting on an exam table with the leg free (not touching the floor), the leg can be pulled anteriorly. This anterior drawer sign is indicative of a torn anterior cruciate ligament. Likewise, a posterior drawer sign is indicative of a torn posterior cruciate ligament. The posterior cruciate ligament resists hyperextension.

A variant of the anterior drawer test is the *Lachman test*. In brief, with the patient supine on the exam table and the knee flexed 20°, the examiner then checks for stability by pushing on the tibia. The *Reverse Lachman's test* is used to check for PCL stability (Fig. 6.27).

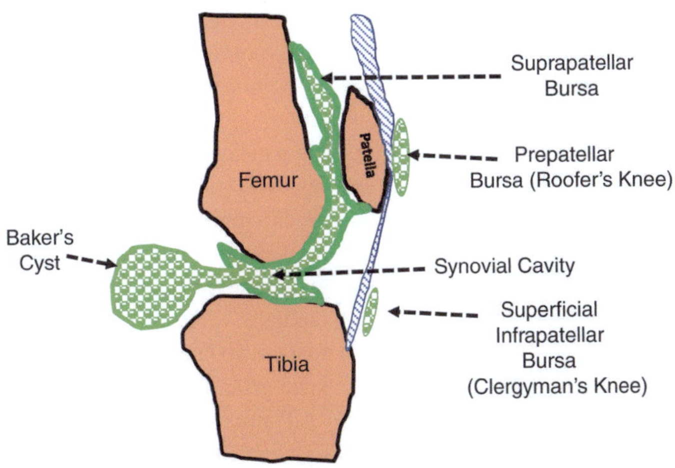

Fig. 6.26 Knee bursa. The synovial cavity comes between the femur and tibia. It extends superiorly as the suprapatellar bursa. The prepatellar and superficial infrapatellar bursa are separated from the synovial joint. Excess fluid can be drained via the suprapatellar bursa. A Baker's cyst is an extension of the synovial cavity posteriorly. It will usually be found in the region of semimembranosus muscle [13, 14]

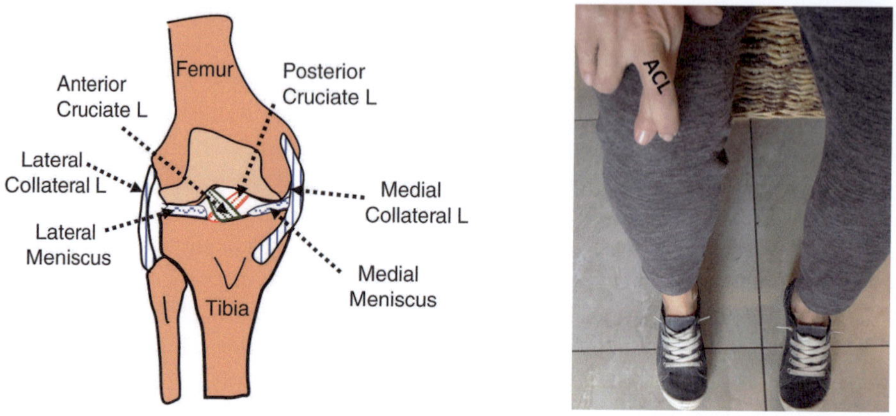

Fig. 6.27 Cruciate ligaments. The cruciate ligaments are named after their attachment to the tibia. The anterior cruciate is attached to the anterior tibia, while the posterior cruciate is attached more posterior on the tibia. If you place your crossed fingers on your knee, they are running in the direction of the cruciates [13, 14]

For a straightforward way to remember the orientation of the ACL and PCL, you can fold your fingers and place your hands on your knee to see the orientation of the ligaments. The ACL is anterior to the PCL. If you are looking at a radiograph of the knee, you can take your crossed fingers and hold them up to the radiograph in the anatomical position to help identify which ligaments on the radiograph (Fig. 6.29).

On the sides of the knee joint are the medial and lateral collateral ligaments. A common injury, often referred to as the *unhappy triad (O'Donoghue's triad),* involves a blow to the lateral posterior knee that damages the anterior cruciate (ACL), the medial collateral ligament (MCL), and the medial meniscus (MM). Just a word of caution here, this is the traditional definition of the unhappy triad, when it is not so clear cut, and the patient does not always present with the textbook scenario. Some authors talk about the triad consisting of the ACL, MCL, and the lateral meniscus—not the medial meniscus *(Shelbourne's triad)* (Figs. 6.28 and 6.15).

Meniscus

The medial and lateral meniscus sit atop the tibial plateau. They are shaped like a "C" with the medial meniscus being larger and more open at the ends. The end of each meniscus is attached to the bone via an anterior and posterior horn. The anterior horns of each meniscus are connected by the transverse ligament. Tears in the meniscus can from injuries that twist the knee joint. There are several common tears each of which has a different shape to it, and they all have very descriptive and appropriate names such as: bucket-handle, longitudinal, tear drop, etc.

Patella

The patella (*small pan* in Latin) is a triangular shaped bone with the base facing superior and the apex pointing inferior. The posterior surface is smooth while the anterior surface is rough. The smooth posterior surface is important for tracking the patellar tendon between the medial and lateral condyles of the femur. The quadriceps tendon tends to pull the patella laterally, but this is resisted by the higher and more vertical surface of the lateral condyle along with the tendons of vastus medialis. The patella sits in the intercondylar fossa (also known as the trochlear groove). During knee extension the patella moves superiorly.

Trauma to the knee can lead to a patellar dislocation, which usually moves in a lateral direction (Fig. 6.30). They are more common in female athletes. *Chondromalacia* of the patella lead to degeneration of the posterior surface of the patella.

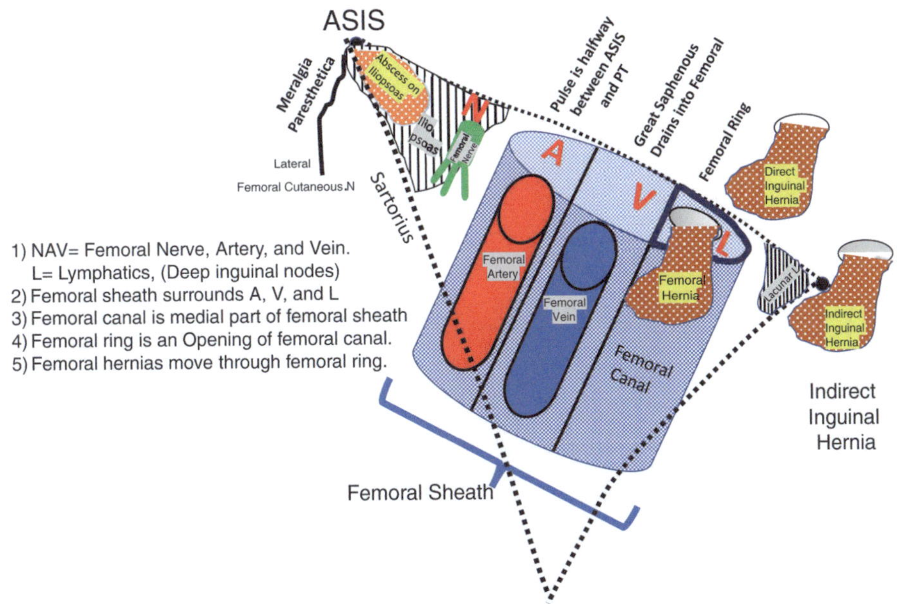

Fig. 6.28 Hernias. Location of the various hernias and their relationship to the pubic tubercle. Note this image is showing where the hernias emerge and that while the indirect inguinal emerges medially, it starts lateral to the inferior epigastric artery [13, 14]

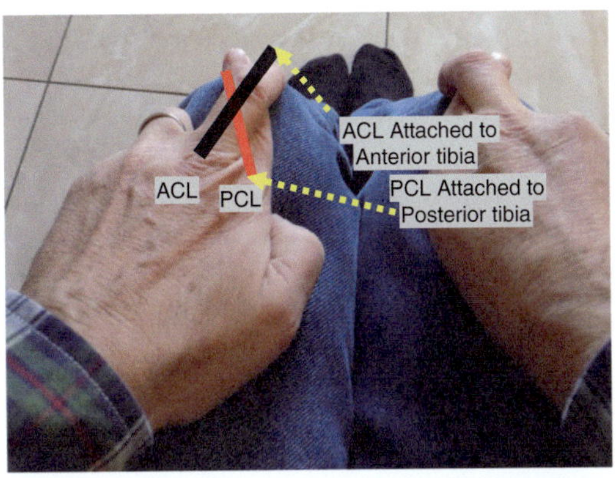

Fig. 6.29 Orientation of ACL and PCL. The anterior cruciate runs anterior to the posterior cruciate ligament. If you cross your fingers and place your hands on top of your knees, you have the orientation of the ligaments [13, 14]

Articularis Genu

The articularis genu is a small muscle that lies deep to the vastus intermedius. During knee extension it pulls the suprapatellar bursa superior to prevent the bursa from getting caught between the femur and tibia. It is innervated by the femoral nerve and is often considered as part of the quadriceps—the littlest quad.

The Popliteal Fossa

The *popliteal fossa* is bounded superomedially by the semitendinosus and the semimembranosus; superolaterally by the biceps femoris; and inferomedially and inferolaterally by the medial and lateral heads of the gastrocnemius. Located superficially in the fossa, is the sciatic nerve splitting into the common fibular and tibial nerves. Moving deeper is the popliteal vein and then the popliteal artery. The floor of the fossa is made up of the popliteus muscle.

The Knee and the Screw-Home Mechanism

If our ability to stand upright for a long time—say standing in line for a sporting event—was entirely based on our thigh muscles, we would

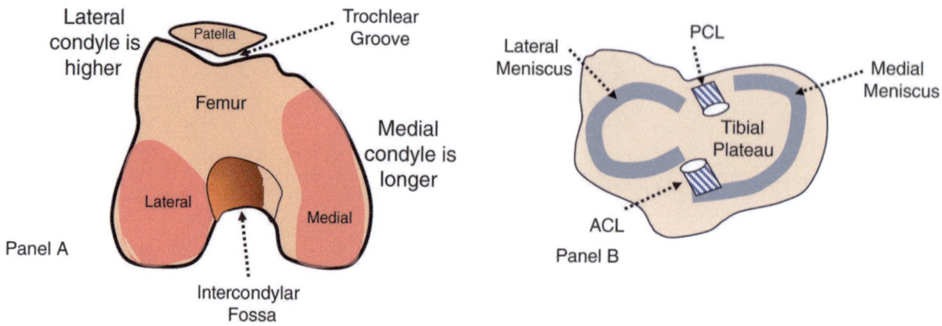

Fig. 6.30 Panel (**a**): Distal Femur. Note that the medial femoral condyle has more surface area than the lateral femoral condyle. This allows the medial side to have more movement during flexion and extension at the knee. For instance, at terminal extension, with the foot off the ground, the tibia will rotate laterally, while with the foot on the ground the femur will rotate medially. The medial and lateral condyles also help to hold the patella in place within the trochlear groove. The quadriceps tendon tends to pull the patella laterally, but this is resisted by the higher and more vertical lateral condyle. Panel (**b**): Tibial plateau with the C-shaped medial and lateral meniscus [13, 14]

expend a significant amount of energy and quickly tire. Fortunately, the knee joint has a unique energy saving feature. To preserve energy when standing our knee locks into place, which is referred to as the screw-home mechanism. When the knee is locked, or screwed home, the integrity of the knee is maintained by the ligaments and the shape of the bones, and not by the muscles.

While the knee is considered a hinge joint, it is not like the simple hinge on a door which allows a door to swing in one plane. The knee joint is more complicated, and besides swinging at the hinge it also has a gliding motion. The tibiofemoral joint is made up of the distal femur and the proximal tibia. The distal end of the femur has two rounded ends called the medial and lateral femoral condyles, which both meet on the flat tibial plateau. However, the medial femoral condyle is about ½ inch longer than the lateral femoral condyle so that during flexion and extension of the knee joint, the medial side has more room to rotate which leads to rotation of the knee joint either medial or lateral. Take knee extension: at the end of extension, as the movement on the shorter, lateral femoral condyle is finished, the longer, medial femoral condyle keeps rotating which gives rise to the motion of a screw. The knee hinges, its glides, and rotates like a screw, which when tightened is locked in place. Once the knee is locked in place or screwed home, it cannot rotate medially or laterally. However, anything that is locked, eventually needs to be unlocked.

Before looking in detail at the screw-home mechanism (SHM) and how we lock and unlock the knee, we must understand the terminology of open and closed chain movements. If the foot is on the ground and we flex our knee, this is a closed chain movement. With a closed chain movement, because the foot is on the ground, the tibia is stable, and the femur is the bone that rotates. If we are sitting in a chair with our lower limb extended, and our foot off the floor, when we flex the knee, this is an open chain movement. With an open chain movement, when we flex the knee, the femur is stable, and the tibia is rotating.

It is easy to see this on your own body. Start in a standing position, with all your weight on your lower right limb. Notice that your left lower limb will be just hanging there, it is straight but relaxed. In addition, your left knee is not in full extension and is not screwed home—it is almost fully extended but not quite. Now shift your weight to your left lower limb and you will feel your left knee go into full extension and screw home. If you have shorts on, it is easier to appreciate what is happening. As your left knee locks into place—moves to full extension—you will see that your left femur is internally (medially) rotating. This internal rotation of the femur is because of the longer length of the medial femoral condyle with its greater range of movement.

With the left knee fully extended, screwed home, and locked in place, now shift your weight back to your right limb. As you do this you will notice that you are starting to flex the left knee ever so slightly and the femur is now externally rotating. Remember the foot is on the ground, so this is a closed chain movement, with a stable tibia, and the femur rotating. The movement is called unlocking the knee. While it might seem logical to attribute the initial flexion of the knee to the hamstrings, it is instead a small muscle deep in the popliteal fossa called the popliteus that is responsible for unlocking the knee and starting flexion. Once the knee is unlocked, the hamstrings take over.

Popliteus

The *popliteus* is a small triangular shaped muscle deep within the superior portion of the posterior leg that unscrews the knee joint. It has a wide attachment to the tibia and runs up laterally to a point on the lateral condyle of the femur, and the lateral meniscus. In extension the tendon lies posterior to the lateral collateral ligament. As the knee flexes, the popliteus tendon comes to lie deep to the lateral collateral ligament. Its function is to unlock the knee joint in the initial stages of flexion. It is also involved in rotation.

If your leg is straight, with your foot off the ground, the popliteus unscrews the joint with medial rotation of the tibia. With the foot on the ground, it laterally rotates the femur. In addition, the popliteus tendon attaches to the lateral meniscus and during flexion it pulls the meniscus slightly posterior.

Q Angle

The abridged version of the *Q angle of the knee* is that it is the angle between the quadriceps tendon above the patella, and the patellar tendon below the patella. The longer version is that one line is drawn straight down the shaft of the femur from the ASIS to the center of the patella, and a second line is drawn down the tibia from the center of patella to the tibial tubercle. In a standing position the normal angle between these two lines is about 14° for males and about 17° for women (Fig. 6.31).

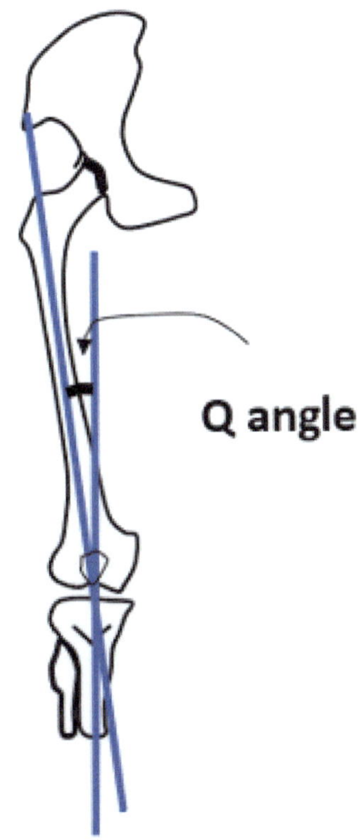

Fig. 6.31 Q Angle. Angle is taken between two lines. The first line is drawn from the ASIS to the patella (quadriceps tendon). The second line is drawn from the patella down through the tibial tuberosity (patellar tendon). A normal angle for men is 12° and for females is 17° [13, 14]

Genu Valgus or Genu Varum

The terms *valgus* or *varum* refer to positions of joints. To determine if the joint is a valgus or varum, start with the joint in question. Any joint is going to be where two bones meet—there will be a proximal bone and a distal bone with the joint between them. If the distal bone of the joint is pointed laterally this is a valgus joint. With valgus think of the "L" in valgus for lateral, and the distal bone pointing *lateral*. Conversely, if the distal part of the joint is pointed medially then it is a varum joint.

Take the knee, varus knee (genu varum) is when the knee is pointed laterally or bow legged—the tibia is deviated medially. The weight of the body is now on the medial part of the knee joint. On the other hand, with a valgus knee (genu valgum) the knee joint is pointed medially or knock kneed—remember the tibia is pointed laterally. With a genu valgum position, the weight of the body is now on the lateral knee joint.

Another way to remember genu valgum is to think of a piece of gum. With the knees deviated medially, almost touching each other, try and imagine a piece of gum holding the together, and the knees are in a val*gum* or valgus position.

The Leg and Foot

There are three compartments of muscles in the leg, the: anterior, posterior, and lateral. The posterior compartment is further subdivided into a superficial and a deep compartment (Fig. 6.32).

Posterior Leg

In the superficial compartment there are three muscles: *gastrocnemius, soleus*, and *plantaris*. All three come together to form the *calcaneal (Achilles) tendon* which is inserted onto the calcaneus. They are all involved with plantar flexion. Deep to these three muscles are *Tom, Dick, and Harry*, standing for **T**ibialis posterior, Flexor **D**igitorum longus, and Flexor **H**allucis longus. Tibialis posterior is a strong inverter, while the names of the other give away their actions. One is a flexor of the big toe, and one is a flexor of the other four toes. All three travel around the medial malleolus deep to the flexor retinaculum in a compartment called the *tarsal tunnel.* Within the tunnel there is also a nerve, artery and vein: the posterior tibial artery, posterior tibial vein, and tibial nerve. Putting the muscles and neurovascular bundle all together gives us the longer mnemonic of **T**om, **D**ick, **A**nd **V**ery **N**ervous **H**arry, with the AVN part standing for the artery, vein, and nerve. Note there are variations on the mnemonic. For instance, some authors just refer to

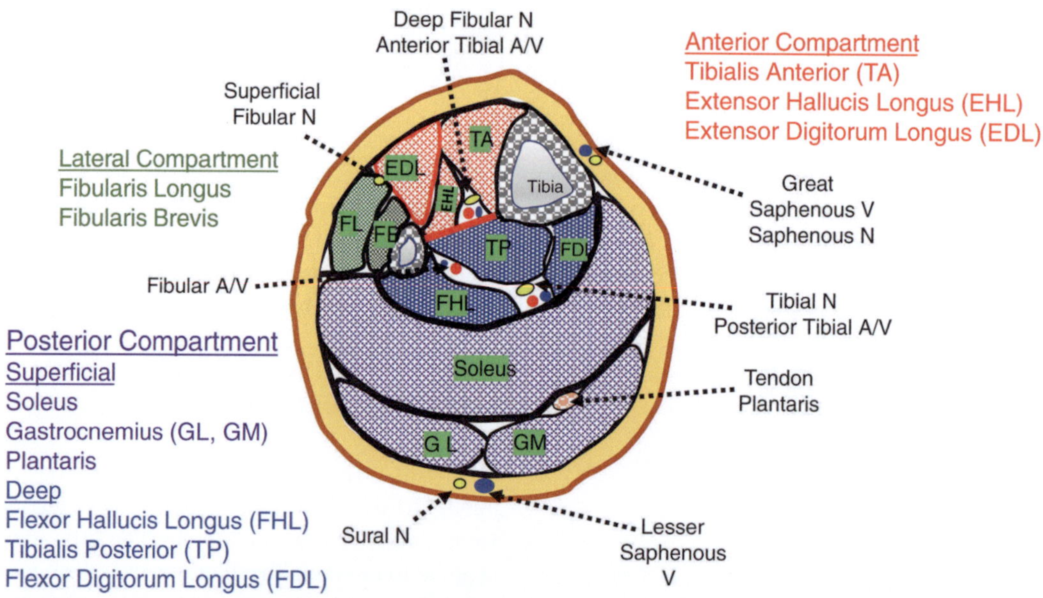

Fig. 6.32 Cross section through the leg. The anterior compartment includes the tibialis anterior, extensor hallicus longus, and extensor digitorum longus. Also in the anterior compartment, and running together, are the deep fibular nerve and anterior tibial artery. The lateral compartment includes fibularis longus and brevis. The superficial posterior compartment includes the soleus and gastrocnemius. The deep posterior compartment includes tibialis posterior, flexor digitorum longus, and flexor hallucis longus. The nerve and artery of the posterior compartment are the tibial nerve and posterior tibial artery [13, 14]

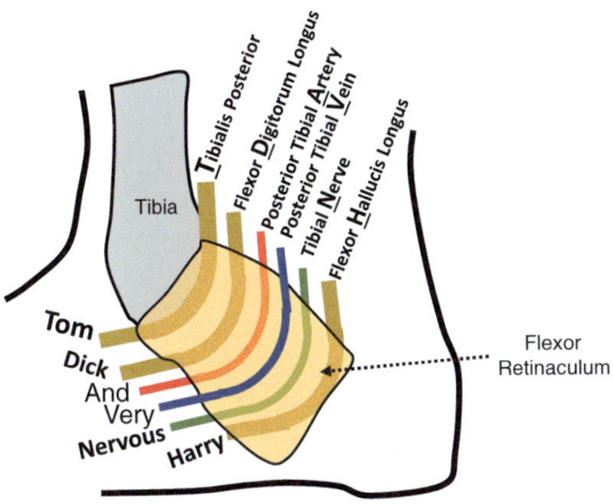

Fig. 6.33 Tom, dick, and harry. At the medial malleolus, the tendons and nerves destined for the sole of the foot pass through the tarsal tunnel. The order of the tendons can be remembered by the saying "Tom, Dick, and Very Nervous Harry." [13, 14]

the order of the tendons and use Tom, Dick, and Harry (Fig. 6.33).

The tendons of *tibialis posterior* and the *flexor digitorum longus* pass posterior to the medial malleolus in a groove on the posterior surface of the distal tibia. They then start to curve anterior and diverge in different directions. The tibialis posterior passes proximal to the sustentaculum tali and inserts onto the navicular. The flexor digitorum longus passes medial to the *sustentaculum tali* which is a shelf projecting medially from the talus. The flexor hallucis longus passes under the sustentaculum tali. Part of the deltoid ligament (Tibiocalcaneal L) attaches to the sustentaculum tali, as does the spring ligament. Just posterior to the flexor digitorum longus is the posterior tibial artery and tibial nerve.

The flexor hallicus longus tendon passes posterior to the tibial nerve and posterior tibial artery. In dancers, this tendon can become overly thick from extended use.

The artery of the posterior leg is the *posterior tibial artery* which is a continuation of the popliteal artery. High up in the posterior compartment, this posterior tibial artery gives of the *anterior tibial artery* which pierces the interosseus membrane to emerge into the anterior compartment. The posterior tibial artery also gives off the *fibular artery* which lies in the lateral side of the posterior leg. At the medial malleolus, the posterior tibial artery runs through the *tarsal tunnel* to enter the foot where it divides into the *lateral and medial planter arteries*. The *posterior tibial vein* and its branches run parallel to the posterior tibial artery. *Tarsal tunnel syndrome* involves entrapment of the neurovascular bundle in the tarsal tunnel.

The tibial nerve is a branch of the sciatic which runs with the posterior tibial artery through the posterior compartment. It supplies all the muscles of the posterior compartment and then travels through the tarsal tunnel to enter the foot and divide into the lateral and medial plantar nerves.

It is important to keep in mind that the mnemonic of Tom, Dick and Harry only works at the medial malleolus. If you are looking at the muscles in the calf, the mnemonic does not work. Also keep in mind that, in the sole of the foot the tendons of flexor digitorum longus and flexor hallicus longus cross each other (Henry's knot), which means the muscle ending on the medial foot comes from the lateral leg, and the muscle ending on the lateral foot comes from the medial leg—whichever side the muscle inserts on means that it originates from the opposite side. Think of the flexor hallicus longus going to the big toe, which is medial, meaning that it arises from the lateral leg—the fibula. And the flexor digitorum longus ends at the four smaller toes which are lateral, meaning that the muscle originates from the medial side—the tibia. The tibialis posterior muscle sits in the middle of the compartment and arises from both the tibia and fibula (Fig. 6.34).

Anterior Leg

The anterior leg compartment contains three muscles, all of which are easy to palpate on your own ankle. At the dorsum of the ankle the tendons of these three muscles are held down by the extensor retinaculum. The most medial muscle is the tibialis anterior muscle which is a strong inverter and dorsiflexor. Shin splints are micro tears of the tibialis anterior muscle. Moving laterally, the next muscle is the extensor hallucis lon-

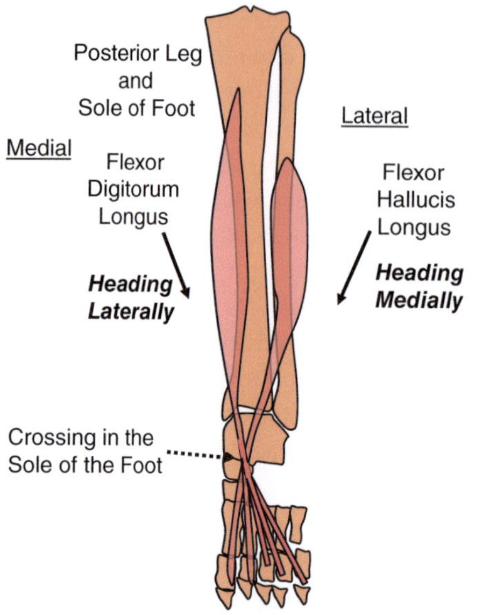

Fig. 6.34 Two tendons crossing. The FDL starts medial and ends lateral. The tendon of FHL starts lateral and ends medially. The tendon of tibialis posterior is not shown but its insertion is between these two muscles [13, 14]

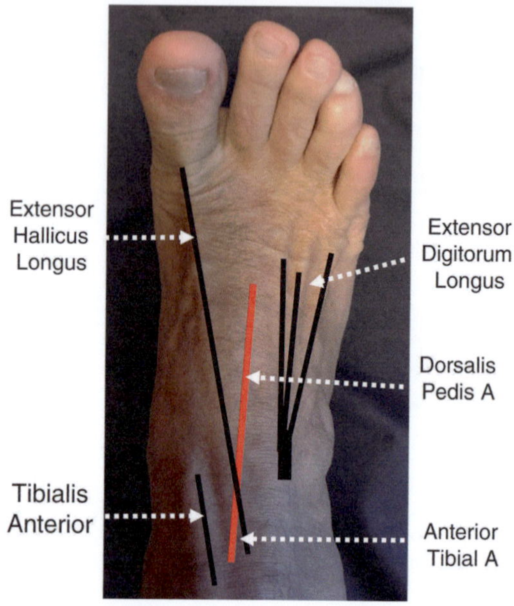

Fig. 6.35 Dorsum of foot. The dorsalis pedis pulse can be felt just distal to the navicular between the tendons of the extensor hallicus longus and the extensor digitorum longus [13, 14]

gus, and then the extensor digitorum longus. The tendons of extensor digitorum proceed to the distal phalanx of each of the four lateral toes. In addition, there is a slip of this muscle that drops down to the fifth metatarsal that is named the *fibularis tertius*.

The artery of the anterior leg is the *anterior tibial artery* which arises from the popliteal artery in the posterior thigh, and then crosses from the posterior compartment to the anterior compartment by passing through the interosseus membrane. It then runs down the anterior leg with the deep fibular nerve between the tibialis anterior and extensor hallucis longus. Proximal to the ankle joint it dives under the extensor hallucis longus and then enters the dorsum of the foot between extensor hallucis longus and extensor digitorum longus and is now called the *dorsalis pedis artery*. The dorsalis pedis then runs down the dorsum of the foot and gives off the *arcuate artery* which is the arterial arch on the dorsum of the foot. The pulse of the dorsalis pedis can be felt lateral to the extensor hallicus longus tendon. If you start at the medial malleolus and move laterally across the dorsum, you have two tendons—the tibialis anterior and the extensor hallicus longus—and then the pulse of dorsalis pedis artery. The dorsalis pedis artery gives off a deep plantar artery which meets up with the plantar arch (Figs. 6.34 and 6.35).

Lateral Leg

There are two muscles in the lateral leg. The *fibularis longus and brevis*. They both arise from the fibula with the longus slightly higher than the brevis. The fibularis longus enters the sole of the foot posterior to the lateral malleolus and crosses deep to the *long plantar ligament* in a tunnel to insert onto the first metatarsal and the medial cuneiform. The fibularis brevis also arises from the fibula and inserts onto the tuberosity of the fifth metatarsal. Both muscles are evertors of the foot (Fig. 6.36).

Sciatic Nerve and Branches in the Leg

In the lower limb, all the muscles below the knee are innervated by the sciatic nerve. Compared to

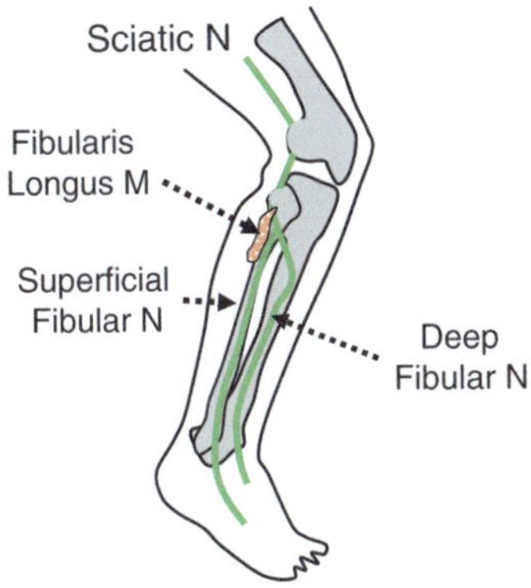

Fig. 6.36 Nerves of the leg. The common fibular nerve enters the lateral leg deep to the peroneus longus muscle and splits into the superficial and deep fibular nerves. The superficial fibular innervates the muscles of the lateral leg. The deep fibular innervates the muscles of the anterior leg [13, 14]

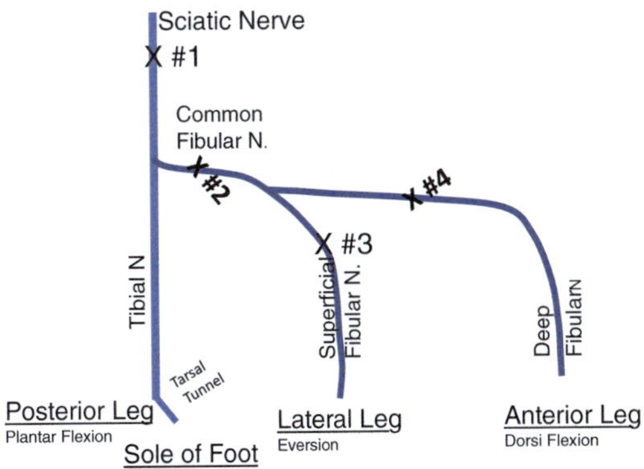

Fig. 6.37 Leg compartments and nerves. An injury to the sciatic nerve will result in a complete loss of motor function below the knee. Injuries to the common fibular will result in loss of the lateral and anterior leg compartments [13, 14]

the upper limb, this is very different. Consider, for instance, if you lesion either the radial, ulnar, or the median nerve in the arm then you will lose some but not all motor function below the elbow. However, if you lesion the sciatic nerve in the thigh, you will lose *all* motor function from the knee down, and almost all the sensory function (Fig. 6.37).

In the posterior thigh, the sciatic nerve splits into the *common fibular* and *tibial nerves.* The common fibular nerve passes around the neck of the fibula between the origins of extensor hallucis longus and fibularis longus. The nerve is very superficial here and easily damaged in injuries to the lateral leg. For instance, in a soccer player who gets kicked on the lateral leg, and fractures the neck of the fibular, the common fibular nerve is at risk. At the fibular head, the common fibular nerve splits into the *superficial fibular* and the *deep fibular nerves*. The superficial fibular nerve innervates the lateral compartment (fibularis longus and brevis), while deep fibular nerve goes to the anterior compartment.

Lesions to the deep fibular nerve will result in loss of dorsiflexion. This loss of dorsiflexion can lead to a "foot drop" meaning that when the patient walks, they have difficulty lifting their toes off the ground. They will now counteract this foot drop by lifting their leg higher than normal to keep their toes off the ground. The deep fibular nerve can be compressed by a poorly fitted cast or a ski boot that is too tight.

To think about nerve injuries and motor function of the leg, one should put on an engineer's hat and think of an electrical schematic. As mentioned above, if you lesion the sciatic then all three compartments of the leg are lost, if the common fibular is damaged then both the anterior and lateral compartments are lost, and if the deep fibular nerve is damaged then the anterior compartment is lost, and with damage to just the superficial fibular nerve then the lateral compartment is lost. Now we also need to go in reverse here and think about patient scenarios. If a patient has difficulties with eversion, then you would equate this to the lateral compartment which is superficial fibular nerve. If both eversion and dorsiflexion are compromised, then you would conclude that the lateral and anterior compartments are affected, which would result from an injury to the common fibular nerve (Fig. 6.37).

Ankle Joints

The *talocrural joint* or "ankle joint" is a mortis joint with the tibia and fibula each making one side of the joint, with the talus in the middle. Like a hinge, this joint allows the talus to pivot so that the ankle can plantar and dorsiflex. On the medial side of the joint is the strong tough deltoid ligament preventing excessive eversion, On the lateral side is a set of ligaments preventing excessive inversion. They are listed here in order of most likely to be involved in an inversion sprain: *anterior talofibular, calcaneofibular*, and *posterior talofibular*. The joint is weakest and most susceptible to injury in plantar flexion (Fig. 6.38).

Moving from the leg and the talocrural joint into the foot, as an overview, the foot can be divided into three sections, the forefoot, midfoot, and hindfoot. The forefoot is involved with the toe-off phase of gait. The midfoot is mainly involved with the rotational stability. The hindfoot is involved with absorbing the shock and loads on the foot during walking (Fig. 6.39).

The *subtalar joint* is below the talocrural joint and is formed from the talus sitting on top of the calcaneus and navicular. Running from the sustentaculum tali of the calcaneus to the navicular is the all-important "spring" ligament or *plantar calcaneonavicular ligament*. The talus is like the top piece of a medieval arch bounded on either side by navicular and calcaneus. The weight of the body pushing down on the *talus* wants to push the navicular and calcaneus out of the way, but they are held together by the *spring ligament*.

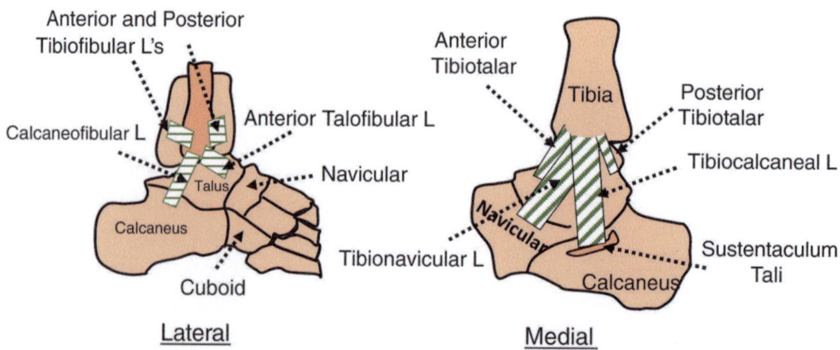

Fig. 6.38 Ankle ligaments. Panel (**a**) is the lateral view showing the anterior talofibular ligament which is the most often injured ligament on an inversion sprain—<u>A</u>lways <u>T</u>orn <u>F</u>irst. The second most common is the calcaneofibular ligament. Panel (**b**) is the medial view with the four ligaments making up the deltoid ligament [13, 14]

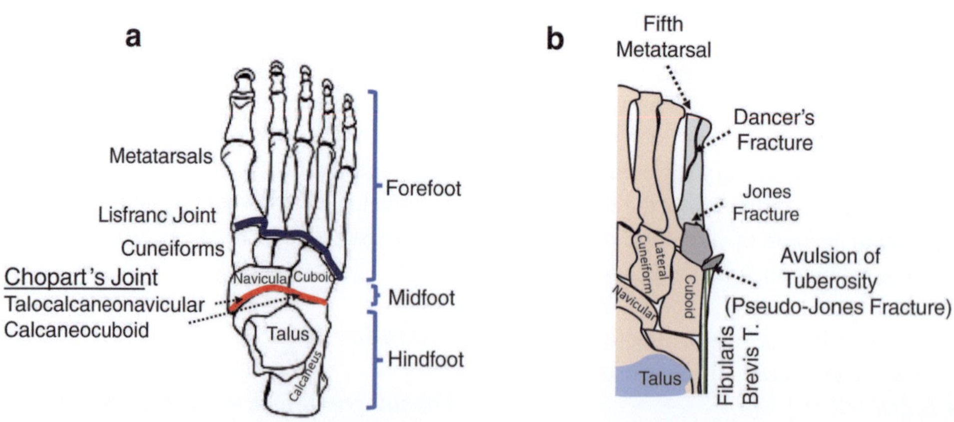

Fig. 6.39 Foot and ankle joints. Panel (**a**) Chopart's Joint is made up of the talocalcaneonavicular and calcaneocuboid joints. The Lisfranc joint is between the tarsal bones and the proximal metatarsals. The subtalar joint is between the talus and calcaneus. Panel (**b**) Fractures of the fifth metatarsal. Strains on the fibularis brevis can lead to an avulsion fracture of the tuberosity (pseudo-Jones fracture). A Jones fracture is to the proximal metatarsal. A Dancer's fracture is a spiral fracture through the metatarsal shaft [13, 14]

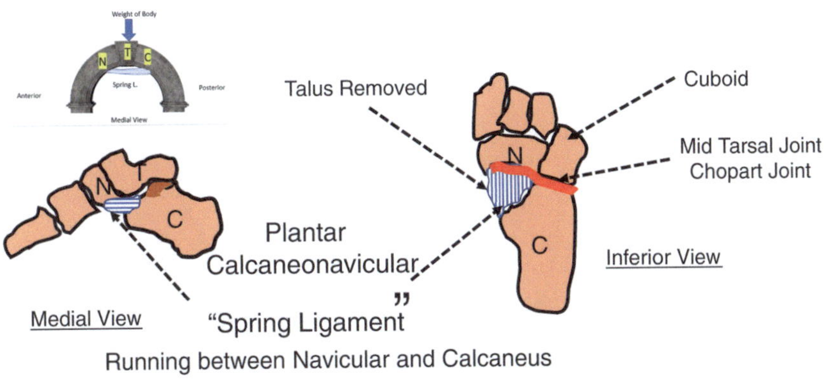

Fig. 6.40 Spring ligament. The spring ligament runs from the calcaneus to the navicular. The talus is sitting on top of it. The weight of the body is coming down through the talus and onto the spring ligament. The mid tarsal or Chopart's joint is the joint between hindfoot and midfoot [13, 14]

The talus is sitting on top of the ligament and is supported by the ligament, but the ligament itself does not attach to the talus (Fig. 6.40).

The *Chopart joint* or *midtarsal* or *transverse tarsal joint* is composed of the talonavicular and the calcaneocuboid joints. The Chopart joint separates the hindfoot from the midfoot and is involved in inversion and eversion (Fig. 6.41).

The *Lisfranc joint* is between the proximal metatarsals and the tarsals—the three cuneiforms and the cuboid. The second metatarsal abuts the middle cuneiform but then is nestled between the medial and lateral cuneiforms. The most important ligament here is the shock absorbing Lisfranc ligament running obliquely from the lateral side of the medial cuneiform laterally to the medial side of the base of the second metatarsal.

Ankle Fractures

There are two common inversion injuries at the ankle that are helpful to compare. As mentioned above, inversion sprains, which most of us have had at one point, tend to damage the *anterior talofibular ligament*—think of the mnemonic, **A**lways **T**orn **F**irst. However, if the force is severe enough, there can be two ankle fractures with an inversion injury. The inversion force can result in a fracture of the distal one-third of the fibula. Plus, the patient can have an avulsion fracture of the tuberosity of the fifth metatarsal (Jones fracture).

Besides inversion injuries, there are eversion injuries at the ankle. A common one involves the deltoid ligament and its attachment. With excessive eversion, three is a strong force exerted on the deltoid ligament, which because of its strength does not tear. Instead, its attachment to the medial malleolus (distal tibia) is avulsed. In addition, there is often a fracture of the distal fibula. This is referred to as a *Pott's fracture* (Fig. 6.41).

A *trimalleolar fracture* involves the distal tibia and fibula where there are fractures to the medial and lateral malleoli, plus another fracture line through the distal tibia. This is also known as a *cotton fracture.*

Excessive inversion of the ankle can also lead to an *avulsion fracture of the tuberosity of the fifth metatarsal.* In many cases the patient will also have a fracture of the distal fibula in the region of the lateral malleolus.

A *Maisonneuve fracture* is a fracture of the proximal fibula that results from an inversion injury. There will be severe disruption of the ankle ligaments. With this injury, because an x-ray typically focuses on the ankle, the higher fracture can go undetected.

There are three potential fractures to the fifth metatarsal (Fig. 6.41):

1. An *avulsion fracture of the tuberosity* of fifth metatarsal results from excessive strain on the tendon of fibularis brevis where it attaches to

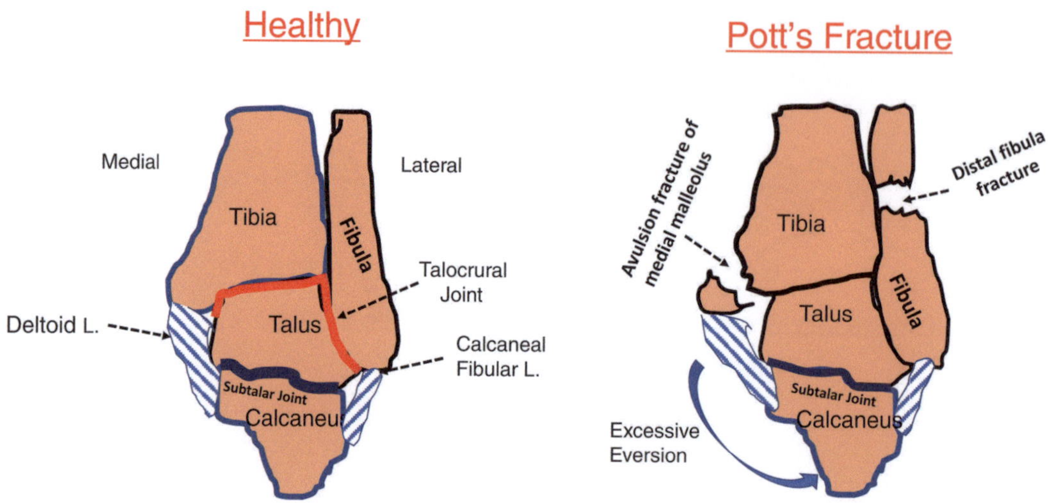

Fig. 6.41 Talocrural joint. The talocrural joint is the mortise joint with the talus sandwiched between the tibia and fibula. The deltoid ligament is located on the medial side, and the calcaneal fibular ligament is on lateral side. The subtalar joint is between the talus and calcaneus. With excessive eversion, an avulsion fracture of the medial malleolus can occur. In addition, there is often a fracture of the distal fibula [13, 14]

the tuberosity. This is considered a pseudo-Jones fracture (Zone I).

2. A *Jones fracture* is slightly more anterior along the fifth metatarsal (Zone II).
3. A *Dancer's fracture* is a spiral fracture along the distal metatarsal (Zone III).

The Foot

The organization of the foot is like the hand. In the hand we have one compartment of muscles acting on the thumb and another compartment on the little finger, likewise in the foot we have muscles organized into one compartment acting on the big toe and another compartment on the little toe. While the hand muscles are involved in fine motor control, the foot muscles are involved both with supporting the weight of the body, and with gait. The big toe does not have complicated movements like the thumb. When dissecting the sole of the foot, the first prominent structure you encounter is the plantar fascia which is a thick tough layer equivalent to the palmar aponeurosis.

The muscles of the foot are conveniently divided into four layers. The number to remember here is "32"—Three, Two; Three, Two. There are three muscles in the first layer, two in the second, three in the third, and two in the fourth. In the layers with three muscles, we have bookends.

The *first layer,* with three muscles, includes bookends, meaning that the muscles on the lateral and medial sides are similar, while the one in the middle is different. On the lateral side is the *abductor digit minimi brevis*, and on the medial side is the *abductor hallucis,* while the muscle in the middle is the *flexor digitorum brevis*. The abductors are the bookends, and the flexor is in the middle (Fig. 6.42).

In the *second layer*, there are two muscles, the *quadratus plantae* and the *lumbricals*. There are also two tendons in this layer, the tendon of *flexor hallucis longus* and *flexor digitorum longus*. These two tendons cross each other (Henry's knot) on their way to their insertions. Between the first and second layer, at the medial margin of the foot, we see the posterior tibial artery and tibial nerve emerging from the tarsal tunnel and entering the sole of the foot. And it is here between the first and second layers that both the artery and nerve divide into *lateral* and *medial plantar nerves and arteries*.

The lateral plantar artery runs from medial to lateral crossing the quadratus plantae, and it then

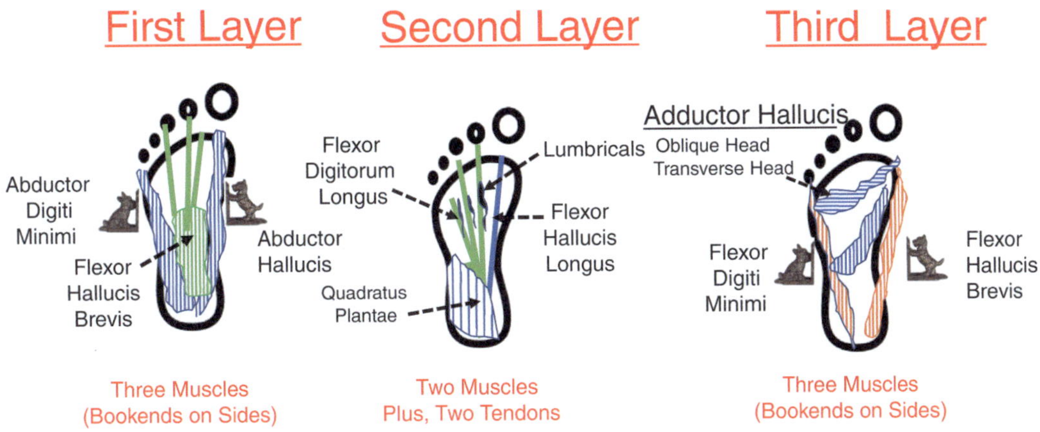

Fig. 6.42 Foot muscles. The muscles of the foot are arranged in four layers (the image shows the first three layers). In the layers with three muscles, there are bookends meaning the muscles on the sides are similar, with the odd man out in the middle. The first layer is bookended on the sides with the abductor digit minimi and the abductor hallicus, while sandwiched between them is the flexor hallucis brevis. In the second layer are two muscles the quadratus plantae and the lumbricals. Both these muscles are attached to the tendon of flexor digitorum longus. In addition, the tendon of flexor hallucis longus is also in this layer. In the third layer are the bookends of flexor hallucis brevis and flexor digit minimi which are sandwiching the adductor hallucis. In the fourth layer (not shown) are the dorsal and plantar interossei [13, 14]

gives rise to the deep plantar arch which in turn passes deep to the adductor hallucis. Rising from the plantar arch are the plantar metatarsal arteries, which give rise to the common planter digital arteries and then the planter digital arteries going out to the distal toes. The tendon of flexor hallucis longus passes under the sustentaculum tali, a medial projection of the calcaneus that supports the talus (sustains the talus).

The *quadratus plantae* is a thin muscle running from the calcaneus to the tendon of flexor digitorum longus, and its role is to keep the angle of these long tendons running as straight as possible down the axis of the toes. The lumbricals arise from the tendon of flexor digitorum longus and run towards the toes.

A *bunion* occurs at the metatarsal phalangeal joint. With aging, the action of the flexor hallicus longus tends to pull the distal phalanx of the first toe laterally which results in the metatarsal phalangeal joint moving medially. This is known as a hallux valgus. Think of the distal toe moving **L**aterally or va**L**gus.

In the ***third layer***, there are three muscles, and we are back to our bookends. On the medial side is the *flexor hallucis brevis*, and on the lateral side is the *flexor digiti minimi brevis*. In the middle is *the adductor hallucis*. The flexor bookends are on either side while the adductor is in the middle. The adductor hallucis has two heads: a transverse head, and an oblique head. Diving deep to the adductor hallucis is the lateral plantar artery turning into the plantar arch.

In the ***fourth layer*** there are two muscles, the dorsal and plantar interossei. In the hand, the axis of rotation for abduction/adduction is the third finger, while in the foot it is the second toe. A major function of most of the muscles in the sole of the foot is to maintain the arch of the foot. They are aided in this function by the ligaments of the foot. In a person who stands all day, the muscles can become tired and strained, which puts more pressure on the ligaments, which leads to the ligaments stretching, the bones moving, and the development of flat feet. As the arch weakens, or falls, the navicular bone will be displaced medially.

A *hammer toe* involves abnormal bending of the middle toe joint and usually happens to the second toe, but others can be affected. The toe becomes bent at the middle and assumes a hammer-like shape. Instead of pointing forward,

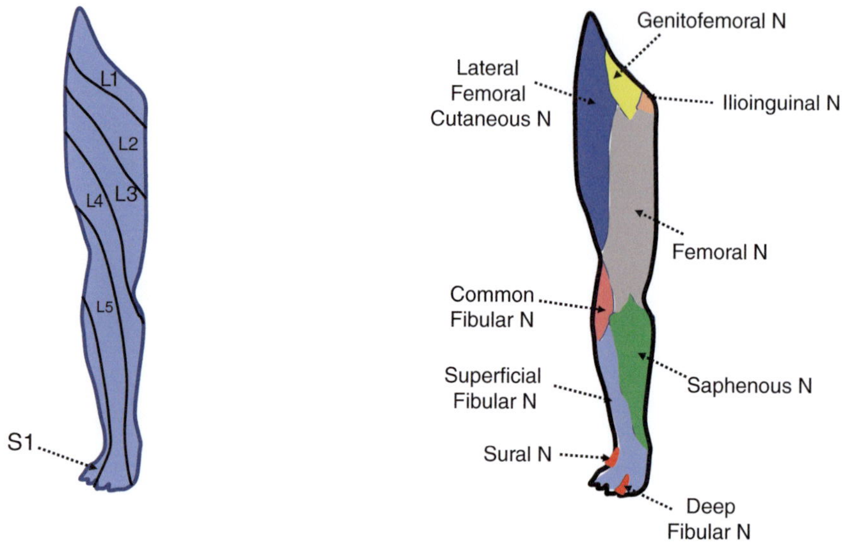

Fig. 6.43 Roots versus peripheral nerves. Panel (**a**) is the dermatome map of the lower limb. Panel (**b**) is the peripheral nerve map of the lower limb [13, 14]

the toe will be pointing downward. It often comes from wearing high heel shoes and will result in a callus forming on the dorsum of the toe. Closely related to hammer toe, is *mallet toe* which affects the distal toe joint (Fig. 6.43).

Nerves and Arteries in the Sole of the Foot

The tibial nerve passes through the tarsal tunnel and enters the sole of the foot on the medial side where it divides into lateral and medial plantar nerves. The lateral plantar nerve is equivalent to the ulnar nerve of the hand, while the medial plantar nerve is equivalent to the median nerve. Whereas the median nerve innervates three and half muscles in the hand and the ulnar nerve innervates all the others; in the foot the medial plantar nerve innervates three and quarter muscles and the lateral plantar innervates all the others.

The *medial plantar nerve* passes between the flexor digitorum brevis and abductor hallicus. It innervates both those muscles plus the flexor hallicus brevis, and the first lumbrical (one of the four lumbricals or 1/4). It gives off *common plantar digital nerves* which divide into proper planter digital nerves which carry sensation from the palmar surface of the big toe, and the second, third, and medial half of the fourth toe.

The *lateral plantar nerve* passes between the flexor digitorum brevis and the quadratus plantae, and then continues towards the lateral side where it curves back medially to pass deep to the adductor hallicus. It innervates the abductor digiti minimi, flexor digiti minimi brevis, quadratus plantae, the lumbricals, the dorsal and plantar interossei and the adductor hallicus. It gives off a *common plantar digital nerve* which then gives off *proper plantar digital nerves* which carry sensation from the fifth toe and the lateral half of the fourth toe.

The medial and lateral plantar nerves on the plantar surface also ascend at their most distal reaches to cross over to the dorsum of the foot to innervate the distal toes on the dorsum of the foot.

The *inferior calcaneal nerve* (Baxter's Nerve) is the first branch of the lateral plantar nerve. It arises in the vicinity of the bifurcation of the tibial nerve. It runs between the quadratus plantae and the flexor digitorum brevis where it can become compressed leading to chronic heel pain. The pain is like the pain felt from plantar fasciitis, however, with Baxter's nerve entrapment the pain is felt more on the inside of the heel and the pain tends to be more persistent, while plantar fasciitis is usually worse in the morning, or after sitting for extended times.

Morton's neuroma occurs from the metatarsals rubbing against each other and pinching the nerves which leads to the nerve becoming swollen and scarred. This most often occurs to the nerves located between the third and fourth toes where branches of the medial and lateral plantar nerves meet.

The *plantar arch* gives off plantar metatarsal arteries. It also forms an anastomosis with the dorsalis pedis artery located on the dorsal surface of the foot. The location of the plantar arch deep in the foot makes it difficult to stop the bleeding from lacerations—for instance steeping on a nail.

Plantar Fasciitis

Just deep to the skin of the sole is the very thick, tough *planter aponeurosis* that runs from the calcaneus to the toes. With age this layer can tighten, leading to pain in the sole of the foot, which is usually worse after extended periods of sitting. For instance, patients will usually say the pain is worse in the early morning, and that as they move around during the day it will lessen. Over time these patients often develop a calcaneal spur from the fascia pulling at its attachment point. Stretching can help to relieve the pain. For office workers, one suggestion is to roll their foot back and forth during the day on top of a tennis ball.

Lumbar Disc Herniations

The most common disc herniations in the lower limb region are either L4, L5, or S1. With a disc injury you want to think of three tests. The first is the reflex test (Fig. 6.45), the second is the muscle test—the myotome (Table 6.1), and the third is the sensory loss related to a dermatome. Not every level has a good reflex test.

Dermatomes and Peripheral Nerve Map of Lower Limb

The dermatome map shows which *spinal cord levels* are responsible for sensation from the lower limb. The peripheral nerve map shows which *peripheral nerves* are responsible for sensation from the lower limb. For a more in-depth discussion of the difference, chapter seven compares root injuries to peripheral nerve injuries. When it comes to the lower limb and dermatomes, the most important roots are: L4 is medial foot; L5 is dorsum of the foot; and S1 is the lateral foot. In addition, L1 is the inguinal region (Fig. 6.43).

For the peripheral nerve map, note that the medial leg and medial foot are saphenous nerve territory. The dorsum of the foot is mostly the superficial fibular nerve, although the first dorsal web space is the deep fibular nerve. On the dorsum of the foot, the deep fibular nerve does not innervate the distal toes. The dorsum of the toes is innervated by the medial and lateral planter nerves. The lateral foot is the sural nerve. The *sural nerve* receives contributions from both the tibial and common fibular nerves and runs down the posterior leg to the lateral foot. It can be injured in Achilles tendon repair (Figs. 6.43, 6.44 and Table 6.2).

Valga Versus Vara

An Anatomy Study Break—The Chicken Bone Case

One of the earliest medical malpractices cases in the United States is referred to as the chicken-bone case, and the lawyer defending the doctor was Abraham Lincoln. On October 17, 1855, in Bloomington, Illinois, there was a large fire that consumed an entire block. Samuel Fleming broke both his femurs when a chimney collapsed on him. He was subsequently treated by four doctors for his subtrochanteric fractures. At first, his recovery was uneventful, but 16 days after the

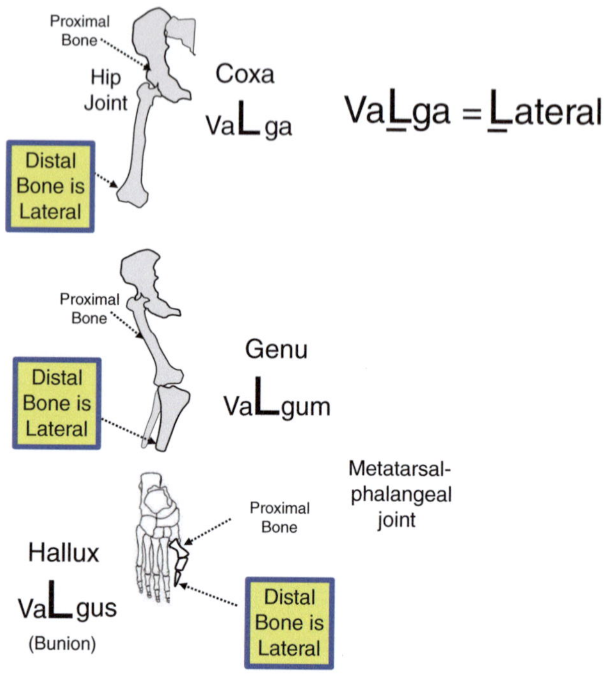

Fig. 6.44 Valgus versus vera. To differentiate between Varus and Valgus look to the distal portion of the distal bone of the joint in question. With Coxa Valga, the distal femur is lateral. With Genu Valgum, the distal tibia is lateral. With Hallux Valgus the distal toe is lateral. For Vara, everything would be reversed [13, 14]

	L4	L5	S1
Reflex Test	Patellar tendon	No Good Reflex	Achilles Reflex
Muscle Test	Dorsiflexing Ankle	Dorsiflexing Toes	Plantarflex Ankle
Sensory Loss	Lateral thigh, medial leg, and medial foot	Lateral leg, dorsum of Foot	Posterior thigh, lateral leg, and lateral foot

Fig. 6.45 Lumbar Disc Herniations

Table 6.1 Lower limb myotomes

Level	Rhyme	Action
C2	Look at your shoe	Neck flexion
C3	A fallen tree	Neck lateral flexion
C4	I'm not sure	Shoulder shrug
C5	Arms out wide	Shoulder abd/elbow flex
C6	Smell your wrist	Wrist ext/elbow flex
C7	No zombies in heaven or brint it on	Wrist flex/elbow ext/ finger ext
C8	You're doing great	Thumb ext/finger flexion/ulnar deviation
T1	One and done	Finger abduction

accident he complained about pain in his right leg. The pain progressed to the point where 24 days later, Dr. Freese attempted to reset the right femur. The patient was administered chloroform and Dr. Freese, along with two assistants, a cabinet maker, and a medical student, broke the bone and reset it. The patient recovered, but the leg was still badly misshapen, and in March of that year the patient filed a $10,000 lawsuit against the doctor.

During the trial both sides presented technical evidence from several doctors. Mr. Lincoln said little during the trial, but throughout the trial he had a small, blue velvet bag in front of him that he occasionally fidgeted with. At the summation, he approached the jury and from the bag he pulled out two chicken bones—one from a young chicken and one from an older chicken. The purpose of the demonstration was to show the jury that young bones were supply and slightly bendable, while the old bones were brittle and easy to break. Lincoln knew that the jury was made up of mostly farmers, and rather than base his defense

Table 6.2 Summary of Lower Limb Nerves

Nerve	Sensory deficit	Motor deficit	Typical causes
Ilioinguinal L1	Groin	Weak ant wall	Hernia surgery
Genitofemoral L1–2	Anteromedial thigh	Cremaster	Surgery
Lateral femoral Cutaneous L2–3	Lateral thigh	None	ASIS trauma
Femoral L2–4	Anterior thigh/knee	Quadriceps	Trauma, pelvic mass
Saphenous L3–4	Medial knee/leg	None	Entrapment medial epicondyle
Obturator L2–4	Medial thigh	Adductors of thigh	Pelvic mass
Superior gluteal L4-S1	Buttock	Gluteus medius and minimus. Trendelenburg gait	Trauma
Inferior gluteal L5–S2	Buttock	Difficulty with standing	Fall
Sciatic	Posterior thigh, leg except for medial side	Hamstrings and all muscles below the knee	Trauma
Common fibular L4–S2	Dorsum and lateral foot	Anterior, lateral leg	Fracture of fibular head, baker's cyst
Superficial fibular L4, 5 and S1	Dorsum of foot	Lateral leg	Trauma
Deep fibular L5, S1 and 2	First dorsal web space	Anterior leg	Ski boot syndrome, cast
Tibial L4-S3	Sole of foot	Posterior compartment	Tarsal tunnel Fractures

on technical jargon, he used an analogy which he knew the jury could relate to. After 18 hours of deliberation, the jurors could not reach a consensus. The plan was to have another trial but based on unforeseen circumstances, the second trial never took place.

Further Reading

1. Dibra FF, Prieto HA, Gray CF, Parvataneni HK. Don't forget the hip! Hip arthritis masquerading as knee pain. Arthoplasty Today. 2017;4(1):118–24.
2. Ekstrand J, Dijk CN. Fifth metatarsal fractures among male professional footballers: a potential career-ending disease. BMJ Sports Med. 2013;47:723–4.
3. Falvey EC, Franklyn-Miller A, McCrory PR. The Greater Trochanter: a pathoanatomic approach to the diagnosis of chronic, proximal, lateral, lower pain in athletes. Br J Sports Med. 2009;43:146–52.
4. Fox KM, Magaziner J, Hebel R, Kenzora JE, Kashner TM. Intertrochanteric versus femoral neck fractures: differential characteristics, treatment, and sequelae. J Gerontol. 1999;54A(12):M635–40.
5. Grimaldi A, Fearon A. Gluteal tendinopathy: integrating pathomechanics and clinical features in its management. J Orthop Sports Phys Ther. 2015;45(11):910–22.
6. Grose AW, Gardner MJ, Sussman PS, Helfet DL, Lorich DG. The surgical anatomy of the blood supply to the femoral head. J Bone Joint Surg. 2008;90-B (10):1298–303.
7. Hallen LG, Lindahl O. The "screw-home" movement in the knee joint. Acta Orthop Scand. 1966;37:97–106.
8. Houston CS, Swischuk MD. Varus and valgus—no wonder they are confused. NEJM. 1980;302:471–2.
9. Hogervorst T, Bouma H, de Vos J. Evolution of the hip and pelvis. Acta Orthop. 2009;80(sup336):1–39.
10. Hoveidaei AH, Sattarpour R, Dadgostar H, Razi S, Razi M. Unhappy triad of the knee: what are the current concepts? World J Orthop. 2023;14(5):268–74.
11. Hubbard C. Lincoln and the chicken bone case: August '98 American history feature. Historynet 1998.; Available at: Lincoln and the Chicken Bone Case: August '98 American History Feature (historynet.com)
12. Kozin SH. Correlation between external rotation of the glenohumeral joint and deformity after brachial plexus birth palsy. J Ped Orthop. 2004;24(2):189–93.
13. Leo J. Medical neuroanatomy for the boards and clinic: finding the lesion. 2nd ed. Cham: Springer; 2024.
14. Leo J. Clinical anatomy and embryology: a guide for the classroom, clinic, and clinic. 2nd ed; 2024.
15. Morgan T, Stevens SD, Palmer T. Popliteus dysfunction and manual therapy. Athletic Therapy Today. 2007;12(6):16–9.

16. Moore K, Daley AF, Agur A. Moore clinically oriented anatomy. 7th ed. New York: Lippincott Williams and Wilkins; 2014.
17. Rosse C, Gaddum-Rosse P. Hollinshead's textbook of anatomy. 5th ed. New York: Lippincott-Raven Publishers; 1997.
18. Standring S. Gray's anatomy: the anatomical basis of clinical practice. London: Elsevier; 2005.
19. Vincent G, Adachi JD, Schemitsch E, Tarride JE, Ho N, Wani RJ, Brown J. Postfracture survival in a population-based study of adults aged ≥ 66yr: a call to action at hospital discharge. J Bone Min Res. 2024;8(5)
20. Welck M, Zinchenko R, Tudor F. A painful foot: Lisfranc fracture-dislocations. The BMJ. 2016; 352. March.

7 The Upper Limb

Introduction

The organization of the upper limb is based on compartments. All the details will follow, but before getting into the specifics it helps to have an overview of these compartments. When you lose a nerve, you typically lose a compartment, or two, and if you know the function of that compartment then the nerve palsies are easier to understand. Both the arm and forearm each have anterior and posterior compartments. The posterior arm and posterior forearm are radial nerve territory, the anterior arm is musculocutaneous nerve territory, and the anterior forearm is innervated by the median nerve except for one and a half muscles—the flexor carpi ulnaris, and half of flexor digitorum profundus. And in the hand, the median nerve innervates three-and-a-half muscles, while the ulnar innervates everything else (Fig. 7.1). The "three" refers to the three thenar muscles, and the "half" refers to two of the four lumbricals.

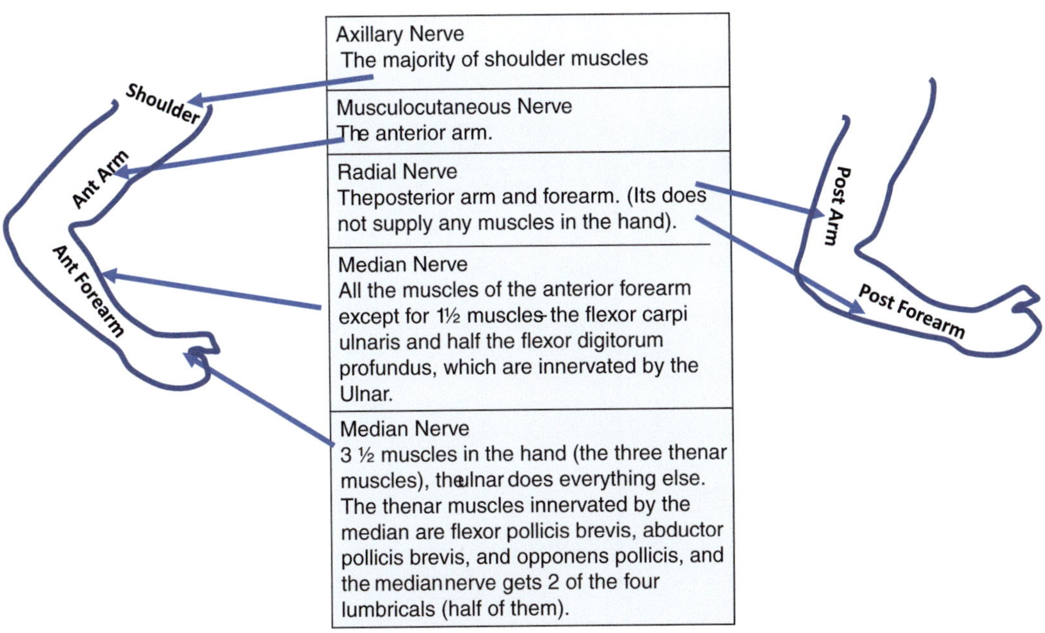

Fig. 7.1 Overview of nerve supply to upper limb [8, 9]

J. Leo, *Gross Anatomy, Neuroanatomy, and Embryology for Medical Students*,
https://doi.org/10.1007/978-3-031-87151-1_7

The Shoulder

There are several muscles that attach the upper limb to the trunk.

1. The *trapezius* is a large flat trapezoid-shaped muscle that originates from a line running down the posterior midline from the skull and along the cervical, and thoracic vertebrae. It inserts along the spine of the scapula. It is divided into upper, middle, and lower divisions. The trapezius can move the scapula in several different directions. If we look at the location of each division and the orientation of their muscle fibers, the muscle actions should make sense. The superior division elevates the scapula, the middle division retracts it, and the inferior division depresses the lateral corner of the scapula (Fig. 7.2).
2. The *rhomboid major* and *rhomboid minor* together form a thin sheet of muscle originating along the midline from the C7 to T5 spinous processes. The fibers continue to the medial border of the scapula and are involved in retraction. They are innervated by the dorsal scapular nerve.
3. The *levator scapulae* is a strap like muscle originating from the transverse processes of C1-C4 and inserting onto the superior portion of the medial border of the scapula. When it fires it will pull this medial angle superiorly, which tilts the glenoid cavity inferiorly. It is innervated by the dorsal scapular nerve.
4. The *pectoralis major* arises from the sternum, ribs, and medial portion of the clavicle. Its muscle fibers head towards the humerus but on the way the fibers rotate such that the inferior fibers end up forming the posterior lamina of the tendon while the superior fibers form the anterior lamina of the tendon. The tendon attaches to the medial lip of the intertubercular groove on the humerus. It is innervated by the medial and lateral pectoral nerves. *Poland Syndrome* is a rare congenital defect that results in a missing or underdeveloped body part. The most common anomaly involves agenesis of the pectoralis major muscle.
5. The *pectoralis minor* arises from ribs 3–5 and inserts onto the coracoid process and is involved in stabilizing the shoulder. It is innervated by the medial pectoral nerve.
6. The *deltoid muscle* has three heads which overlie the shoulder. The three heads are named for their relative locations: the anterior portion is over the clavicle, the intermediate portion over the acromion, and the posterior

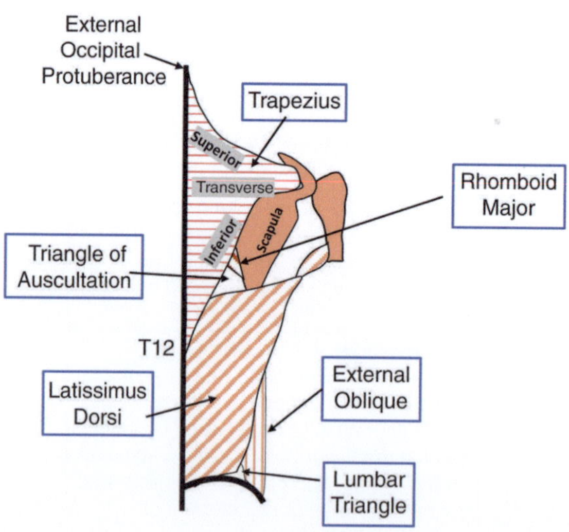

Fig. 7.2 Superficial back. Trapezius has a long origin, running from the external occipital protuberance all the way down to T12 spinous process. It inserts onto spine of scapula. There are three parts to it: Superior, Transverse, and Inferior. The latissimus dorsi runs from the spinous process of T6 to L5 to insert onto the intertubercular sulcus. As it approaches the humerus, the tendon twists so that the superior fibers go inferior, and inferior fibers go superior. The lumbar and auscultation triangles can be seen [8, 9]

portion over the scapula. Each head arises from the structure it covers, and all three heads insert onto the deltoid tuberosity. Its actions are abduction, flexion, and extension. It is innervated by the axillary nerve.

7. The latissimus dorsi runs from the spinous processes of T6 to L5 to the intertubercular sulcus. As it approaches the humerus, the tendon twists so that the superior fibers go inferior, and the inferior fibers go superior. It is sometimes referred to as the "swimming muscle" as at the shoulder, it extends, adducts, and internally rotates. An interesting variation is the presence of an *axillary arch muscle* also known as Langer's muscle which is an extra slip of the latissimus dorsi that runs from the lateral border of the latissimus dorsi across the neurovascular bundle of the axillary artery and brachial plexus to intermingle with fibers of the pectoralis major. Some of the slips attach to the capsule of the shoulder joint.

The Shoulder Joint

The shoulder joint is made up of three joints: the acromioclavicular, the glenohumeral, and sternoclavicular.

The *acromioclavicular ligament* is the attachment between the lateral end of the clavicle and the acromion. Surrounding the joint is a weak capsule which is surrounded by the superior and inferior capsular ligaments. In addition, the joint is strengthened by the *coracoclavicular ligament* which in turn is composed of two parts. The medially located *conoid ligament* is shaped like a fan, and the more lateral *trapezoid ligament* is shaped like a quadrangle. The clavicle is suspended from the scapula by the coracoclavicular ligament (Fig. 7.3).

Dislocation of the acromioclavicular joint often follows blows to the shoulder in traffic accidents or sporting injuries. The severity of a shoulder separation occurs on a spectrum but can involve the acromioclavicular ligament, coracoclavicular ligament, or both.

1. A mild sprain of the acromioclavicular ligament may not show up on an x-ray and will not cause a shoulder deformity.
2. A minor tear of the acromioclavicular ligament can result in a mild misalignment of the collar bone.
3. A complete tear of the acromioclavicular and coracoclavicular ligaments will lead to the shoulder sagging and a large bump over the shoulder.

You can test someone else's shoulder mobility, or your own, by asking them to reach behind their back and touch the opposite shoulder with their hand (Apley Scratch Test). It should be symmetrical for each side.

The Clavicle

The clavicle is a long thin S-shaped bone that, via the sternoclavicular joint, attaches the upper limb to the axial skeleton. The conoid tubercle is a bony

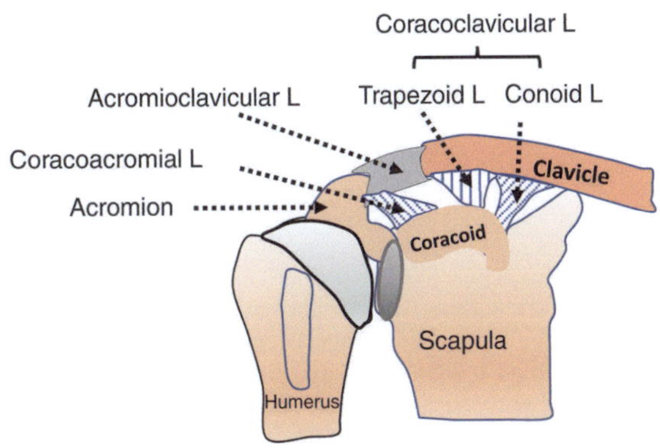

Fig. 7.3 Shoulder ligaments. The coracoclavicular ligament is composed of two parts: trapezoid and conoid. The coracoacromial ligament connects the coracoid process to the acromion [8, 9]

prominence on the lateral one-third of the clavicle that serves as the attachment point for the conoid ligament. The clavicle is the most often fractured bone in the body. Superomedially it is attached to the sternocleidomastoid, and inferolaterally it is attached to the pectoralis major. Fractures to the clavicle often occur following a fall on the outstretched hand. The patient will typically present with the medial portion of the scapula pulled superiorly by the sternocleidomastoid, and the lateral portion pulled inferiorly by the pectoralis major.

The Manubrium

The *manubrium* is a quadrangular shaped structure that articulates with the clavicle, first rib, second rib, and the sternum. The *sternoclavicular joint* between the manubrium and the clavicle has an articular disk between the two bony features. On either side of the joint are the anterior and posterior sternoclavicular ligaments. Running across the manubrium from one clavicle to another is the *interclavicular ligament*. Running from the clavicle to the first rib is the *costoclavicular ligament* (Fig. 7.4).

Between the first rib and the manubrium is a strong immobile synchondrosis that allows the clavicle and manubrium to move together. Starting with rib 2 and moving down the sternum, the remaining joints are synovial joints. Note that anteriorly, rib 2 articulates with both the manubrium and sternum, while ribs 2–7 articulate just with the sternum.

Rotator Cuff

The four rotator cuff muscles surround and hold the humeral head in place against the glenoid fossa. They are often referred to as the SITS muscles. They all insert on the superior aspect of the humerus in the region of the greater and lesser tuberosities (Fig. 7.5).

1. The *supraspinatus* originates from the supraspinous fossa and inserts on the superior aspect of the greater tuberosity. It is innervated by the suprascapular nerve. It is responsible for the first 15° of shoulder abduction. If it is injured, the patient can initiate abduction by swinging their hip and pushing the upper limb laterally, or they can lean towards the damaged side which will result in the upper limb being abducted 10–15° relative to the trunk. They can use other muscles to keep the abduction going.
2. The *infraspinatus* has a wide origin from the infraspinous fossa of the scapula and comes to a point to insert on the posterior aspect of the greater tuberosity. It is innervated by the suprascapular nerve (Fig. 7.6).
3. The *teres minor* is very closely related to the infraspinatus and seems to be part of infraspi-

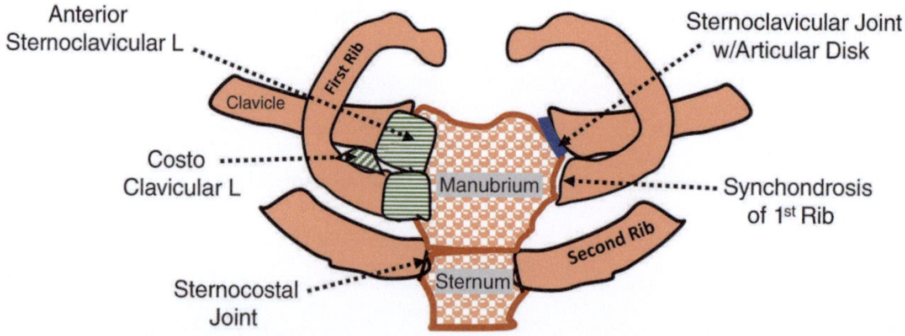

Fig. 7.4 Manubrium. The manubrium joins the first two ribs and the clavicle. The sternoclavicular joint is between the manubrium and the clavicle. There is an articular disk between the two bones. The first rib joins the manubrium just inferior to the clavicle. The second rib joins the manubrium and the sternum.[8, 9]

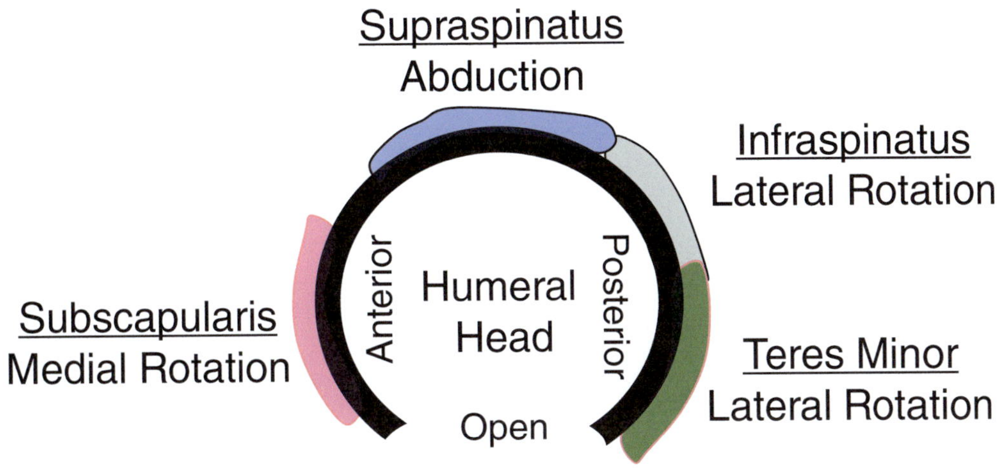

Fig. 7.5 Rotator cuff or SITS muscles. In this view the examiner is looking at the side of the shoulder. Note the supraspinatus elevates or abducts at the shoulder. The infraspinatus and teres minor are lateral rotators. The subscapularis is a medial rotator. The inferior portion of the cuff is open. Dislocations will often move inferior at this weak point [8, 9]

Fig. 7.6 Posterior shoulder. Three of the four rotator cuff muscles (SITS muscles) Supraspinatus, Infraspinatus, and Teres minor are visible. Subscapularis is not visible [8, 9]

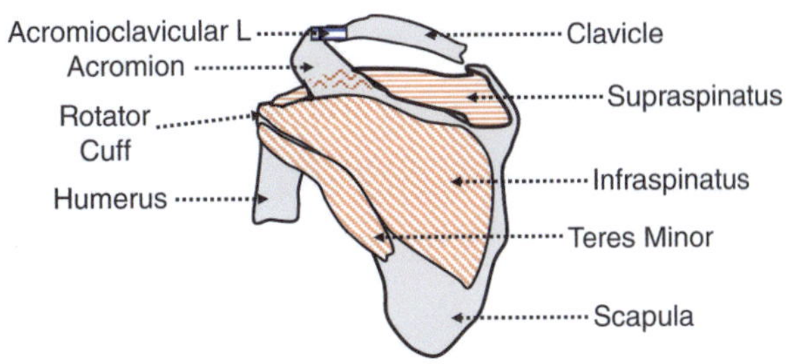

natus. It inserts on the greater tuberosity. It is a lateral rotator at the shoulder.

4. The *subscapularis* muscle is located on the inner surface of the scapula in the subscapular fossa. It inserts on the lesser tuberosity. It is a medial rotator of the shoulder. It is innervated by the upper and lower subscapular nerves (Fig. 7.7).

Note that in the above discussion, three of the SITS muscles, the supraspinatus, infraspinatus, and the teres minor all insert on the greater tuberosity. Fractures of the greater tuberosity can compromise these three muscles. Meanwhile the subscapularis attaches to the lesser tuberosity so fractures here would involve the subscapularis.

Abduction of the Upper Limb

To discuss abduction of the upper limb, start with an individual standing up with their upper limb loosely hanging by their side. When they go from this position to moving their upper limb straight over their head, several muscles are involved. The supraspinatus is responsible for the first 15° of abduction, and then the deltoid takes over and moves the upper limb to the 90° position. At this point, the glenoid cavity is pointing out to the side. To continue moving the upper limb to straight over the head, the serratus anterior and trapezius contribute by rotating the scapula so that the glenoid cavity now pivots to point more superiorly.

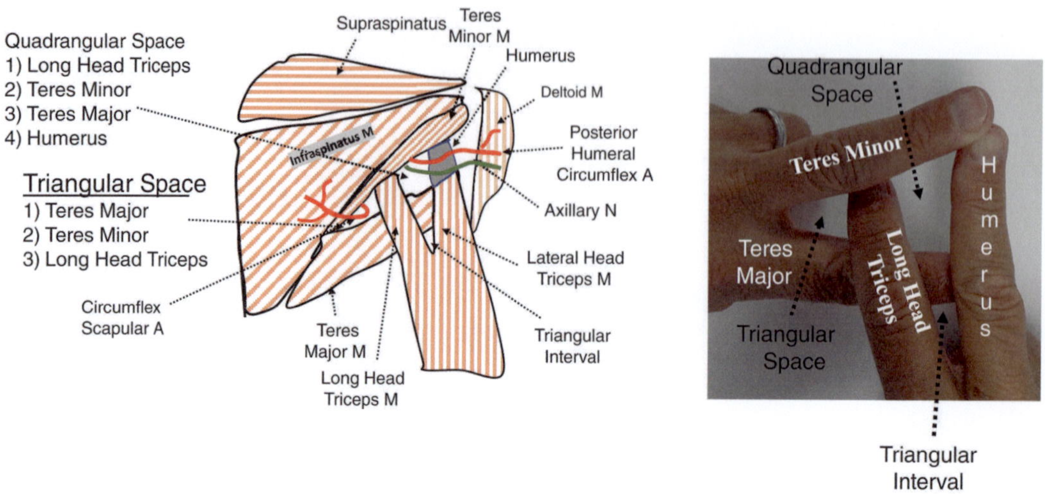

Fig. 7.7 Triangular and quadrangular spaces [8, 9]

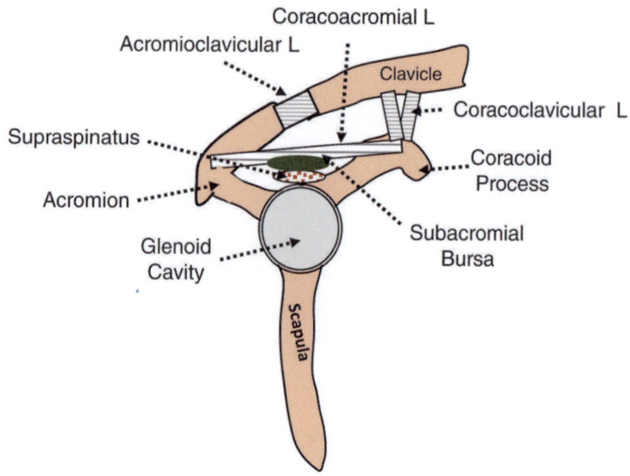

Fig. 7.8 Coracoacromial arch. The arch is made up of the acromion, the coracoacromial ligament, and the coracoid process. Under it, is the subacromial bursa and the tendon of supraspinatus [8, 9]

Painful Arc Syndrome refers to a patient who complains of pain on attempted abduction of the upper limb. The source of the pain can come from several different structures. The supraspinatus tendon lies in a small tight space between the acromion and the humeral head. Also in this small space is the *subacromial bursa* (Fig. 7.8).

Pain in this region can come from the impingement of either of these structures. Besides inflammation, impingement can also result from bone spurs forming on the bones around the space (Fig. 7.9). Damage to the supraspinatus tendon can be tested by the *Empty Can Test*, also known as the *Jobe Test*. The patient is asked to abduct and medially rotate the upper limb with the thumb pointing towards the ground—think of emptying a can where you hold the can as far away from your body (abduction) and then turn the can upside down (medial rotation). If the patient complains of pain with this movement, it indicates damage to the supraspinatus tendon.

Supraspinatus is the most injured of the SITS muscles which can lead to pain in the shoulder. The tendon can become frayed or torn away at its origin. In some cases, there will be crackling sensations on shoulder movement.

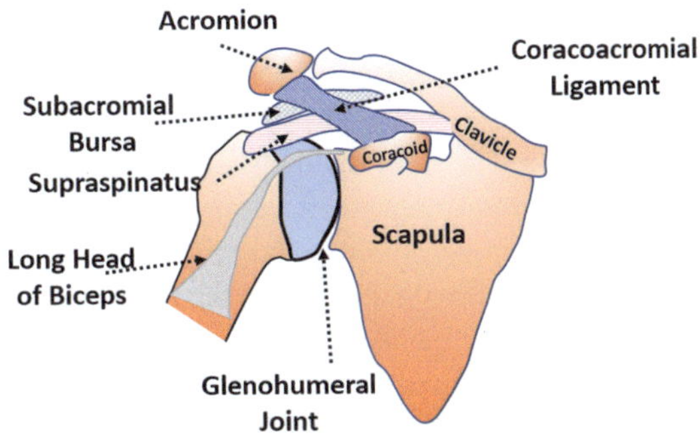

Fig. 7.9 Subacromial space. The subacromial space is bounded superiorly by the coracoacromial ligament. The humeral head is inferior. Within the space is the tendon of supraspinatus and the subacromial bursa [8, 9]

Glenohumeral Joint

The glenohumeral joint is the most mobile joint in the body, and the most common site for dislocations. The humeral head is the ball, and the glenoid fossa is the socket of the ball-and-socket *glenohumeral joint*. The socket is strengthened by the *glenoid labrum*. The joint is strengthened by the *superior, middle, and inferior glenohumeral ligaments*. The humeral head can be dislocated anteriorly, posteriorly, or inferiorly. The most common direction starts inferior with a rupture of the inferior glenohumeral ligament. The humerus then comes to lie anterior. The patient will often present with a lump on the anterior shoulder which represents the head of the humerus coming to lie deep to the pectoralis minor. *Adhesive capsulitis,* also known as frozen shoulder, refers to the joint becoming tight and stiff usually from immobility.

SLAP Tear and the Long Head of the Biceps

The long head of the biceps enters the glenohumeral joint and attaches to the *supraglenoid tubercle*. A slap tear refers to a tear of the *superior labrum* on either side—anterior and posterior of the attachment of the long head of the biceps tendon thus the mnemonic **S**uperior **L**abrum **A**nterior **P**osterior. Slap tears can occur because of trauma such as car accidents or falling on the outstretched hand, or from repetitive overuse injuries such as weightlifting (Fig. 7.10).

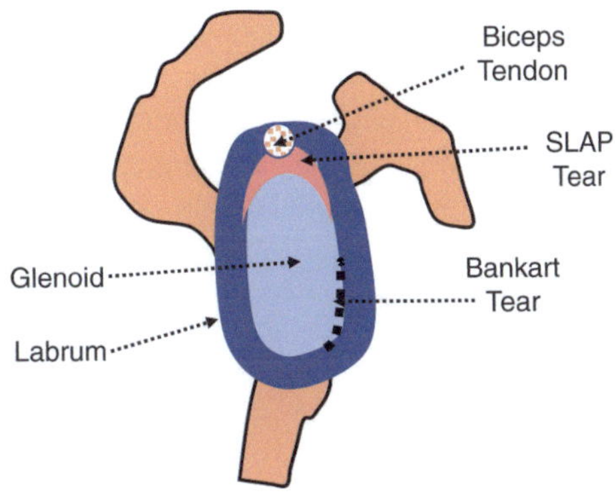

Fig. 7.10 Labrum tears. Bankart tears occur on the anterior inferior margin of the labrum. SLAP tears occur anterior and posterior of the biceps' insertion [8, 9]

Bankart Tears

A Bankart tear occurs at the anterior labrum usually following a shoulder dislocation, especially in those under 30 years of age (Fig. 7.10).

Scapula

In Latin, *scapula* means shovel. It is a flat-shaped bone that resembles a triangle. The top corner and bottom corners are appropriately named the superior and inferior angles. The three borders are also appropriately named as superior, medial, and lateral borders. The coracoid process is a rounded prominence jutting anterior. Surgeons sometimes refer to this as the "lighthouse of the shoulder" because it is best to stay lateral to it as the neurovascular structures are found on the medial side. The anterior surface of the scapula is made up of the scapular fossa. Along the posterior surface is the spine of the scapula that ends in the acromion. The spine divides the posterior surface into a supraspinous and infraspinous fossa. On the lateral corner of the scapula is the glenoid fossa which joins with the head of the humerus to form the glenohumeral joint. Along the lateral portion of the superior border is the scapular notch, which in turn is covered by the superior transverse scapular ligament. Running inferior to the ligament is the suprascapular nerve. Running superior to the ligament is the suprascapular artery—the army goes over the bridge, and the navy goes under the bridge. Running along the medial border of the scapula is the dorsal scapular artery and nerve (Fig. 7.11).

Collateral Circulation Around Shoulder

There is an extensive anastomotic network around the shoulder joint which can provide an alternate pathway for blood to go around a blockage in the axillary artery. In the case of a blockage, you want to think about what arteries are proximal to the blockage and what arteries are distal to the blockage. There are two prominent arteries proximal to the blockage that contribute to the network. The suprascapular artery comes off the thyrocervical trunk and heads to the scapular notch. In addition, the dorsal scapular artery comes off the subclavian artery and heads toward the medial angle of the scapula. Coming off just distal to the blockage is the subscapular artery,

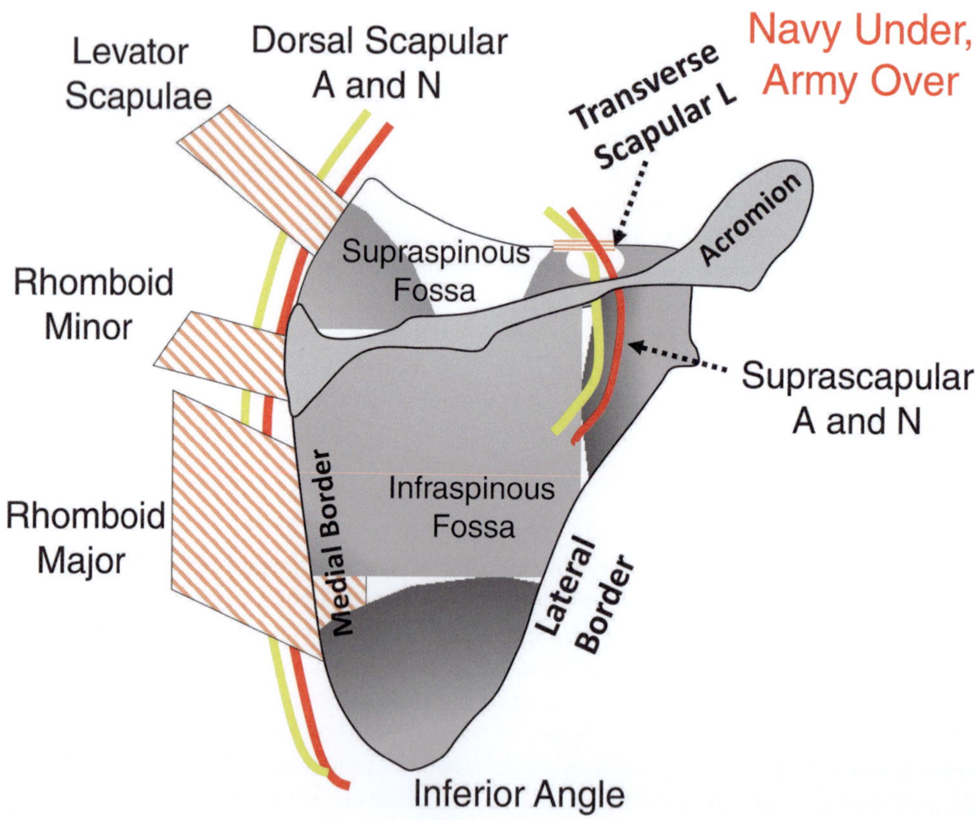

Fig. 7.11 Posterior scapula. Note the dorsal scapular nerve and artery passing deep to the levator scapulae and then running along the medial border of the scapula. The suprascapular nerve and artery enter the supraspinous fossa at the scapular notch, with the nerve going under the transverse scapular ligament and through the notch, and the artery going superior to it—navy under the bridge, army over the bridge [8, 9]

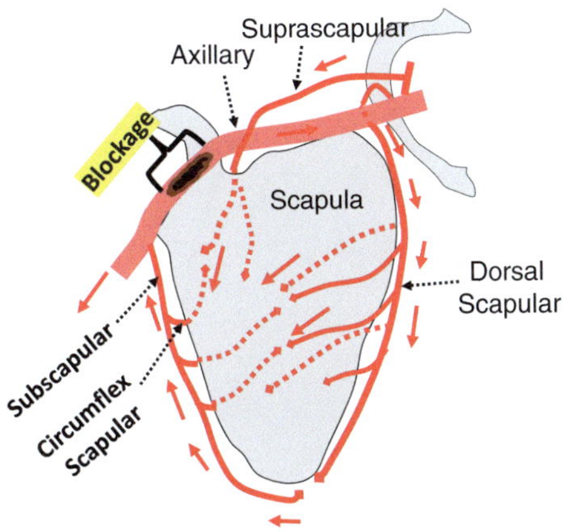

Fig. 7.12 Blockage in axillary artery. The extensive anastomosis between the dorsal scapular, the circumflex scapular, and the suprascapular arteries allows blood to travel down the upper limb. In the figure there is a blockage of the axillary artery. The arrows show the blood bypassing the blockage. Remember the last branch of the axillary artery is the subscapular artery. In the example above, blood is flowing retrogradely along the subscapular to complete the bypass. Note that not all the branches of the axillary artery are shown in this diagram [8, 9]

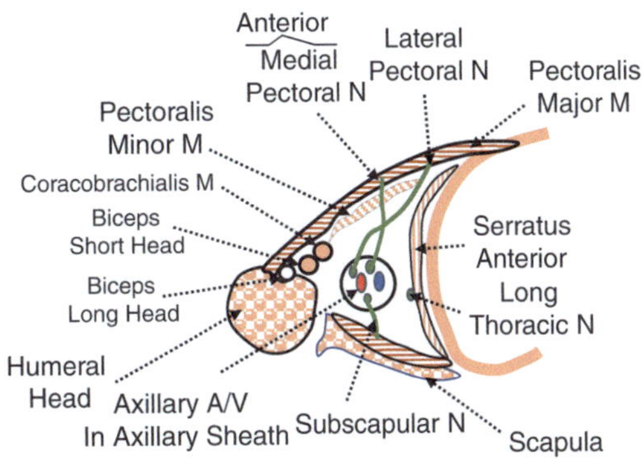

Fig. 7.13 Axilla. The axilla is bounded by the serratus anterior, the pectoralis major and the subscapularis. The axillary sheath is seen surrounding the axillary artery and vein [8, 9]

which splits right away into the thoracodorsal and the circumflex scapular artery. It is the circumflex scapular which contributes to the shoulder joint. With an axillary artery blockage, blood will go down the suprascapular and dorsal scapular arteries, and from there into the circumflex scapular artery, the subscapular artery, and then into the axillary artery just distal to the blockage (Fig. 7.12).

Axilla

The *axilla* is a triangular shaped area bounded by the serratus anterior medially, the pectoralis major anteriorly, and the subscapularis muscle posterior. The axilla contains the axillary artery, axillary vein, cords of the brachial plexus, and the axillary nodes. Some authors refer to the thin layer of fascia encompassing the neurovascular structures as the axillary sheath, but its existence is debated (Fig. 7.13).

Clavipectoral Fascia

The *clavipectoral fascia* is a strong layer that starts from the clavicle and heads inferiorly to wrap around the pectoralis minor, and then continues inferiorly to blend in with the axillary fascia. Between the pectoralis minor and the clavicle, the lateral thoracic artery and the cephalic vein pierce the fascia. Deep to the fascia is the axillary artery along with the medial, lateral, and posterior cords of the brachial plexus. The medial cord gives off the medial pectoral nerve, and the lateral cord gives off the lateral pectoral nerve both of which travel anteriorly. When these two nerves reach the anterior abdominal wall, note that the lateral pectoral nerve is found medial to the medial pectoral nerve. Keep in mind that nerves are named for where they come from. Although the medial pectoral nerve is found laterally, it gets its name because it comes from the medial cord, and likewise the lateral pectoral nerve comes from the lateral cord (Fig. 7.14).

Axillary Artery

The *axillary artery* runs from the first rib to the inferior border of teres minor. There are three

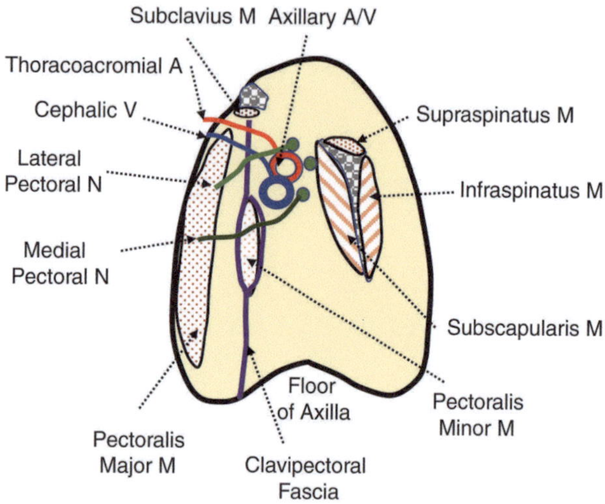

Fig. 7.14 Clavipectoral fascia. Extension of the investing deep cervical fascia. It is pierced by the thoracoacromial artery, and the cephalic vein. Within the axilla is the axillary artery, axillary vein, and the cords of the brachial plexus [8, 9]

parts to the axillary artery based on its relationship to the pectoralis minor muscle. The pectoralis minor muscle runs from the ribs medially to the coracoid process of the scapula and overlies the axillary artery. The first part of the artery is proximal to pectoralis minor, the second part of the artery is posterior to pectoralis minor, and the third part is distal to pectoralis minor. There are six branches of the axillary artery, and it is organized very conveniently. There is one branch off the first part, two branches off the second part, and three branches off the third part (Fig. 7.15).

First Part of Axillary Artery

1. The *supreme thoracic artery* goes to the superior thoracic wall.

Second Part of Axillary Artery

2. The *thoracoacromial artery* comes off right at the superior border of pectoralis minor and pierces the clavipectoral fascia. It has several branches: pectoral, acromial, clavicular, and humeral.
3. The *lateral thoracic artery* runs to the lateral thoracic wall and supplies the lateral breast. It runs with the long thoracic nerve which innervates the serratus anterior muscle. During breast surgery, the lateral thoracic artery may need to be ligated. If the surgeon damages the long thoracic nerve the patient will have a winged scapula.

Third Part of Axillary Artery

4. The *subscapular artery* comes off the medial side of the axillary artery and splits into the circumflex scapular artery, which travels through the triangular space, and the thoracodorsal artery, which continues to the medial inferior scapula. The thoracodorsal artery runs with the thoracodorsal nerve which innervates the latissimus dorsi muscle.
5. The *anterior humeral circumflex artery* comes off the lateral side of the axillary artery and heads to the anterior surface of the neck of the humerus.
6. The *posterior humeral circumflex artery* comes off right next to the anterior humeral circumflex artery and these two arteries form an anastomosis. Of the two, the posterior humeral circumflex is usually larger, and it runs through the quadrangular space with the axillary nerve.

Brachial Plexus

The brachial plexus arises from the ventral roots of C5, C6, C7, C8, and T1. In some individuals, C4 or T2 may contribute (Fig. 7.16).

1. The *long thoracic nerve* comes from branches of the C5, C6, and 7 roots and supplies the serratus anterior.

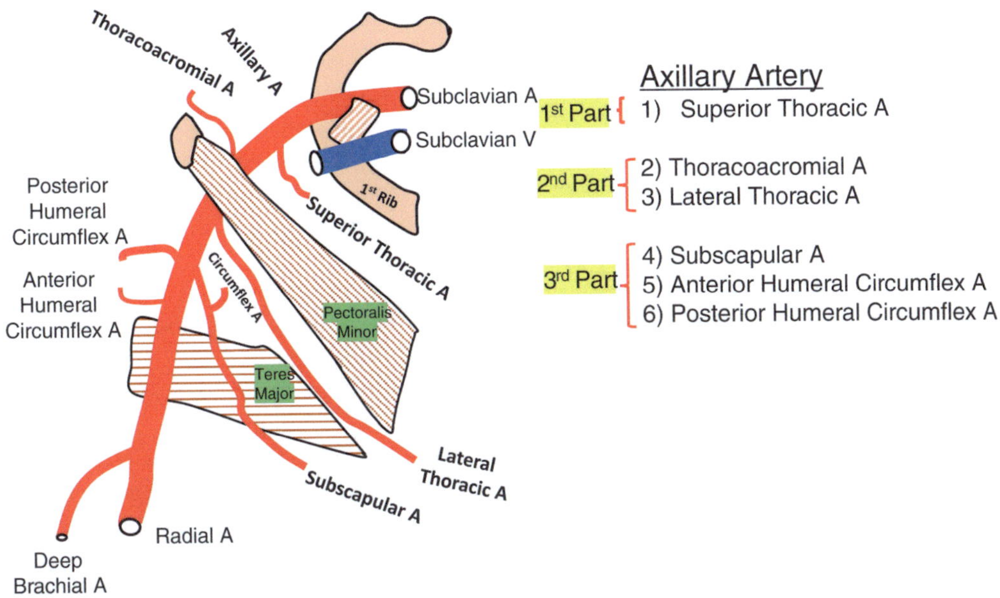

Fig. 7.15 Axillary artery. There are three parts to the axillary artery based on its relationship to the pectoralis minor muscle. It has six branches. Off the first part is one branch, off the second part are two branches, and off the third part are three branches [8, 9]

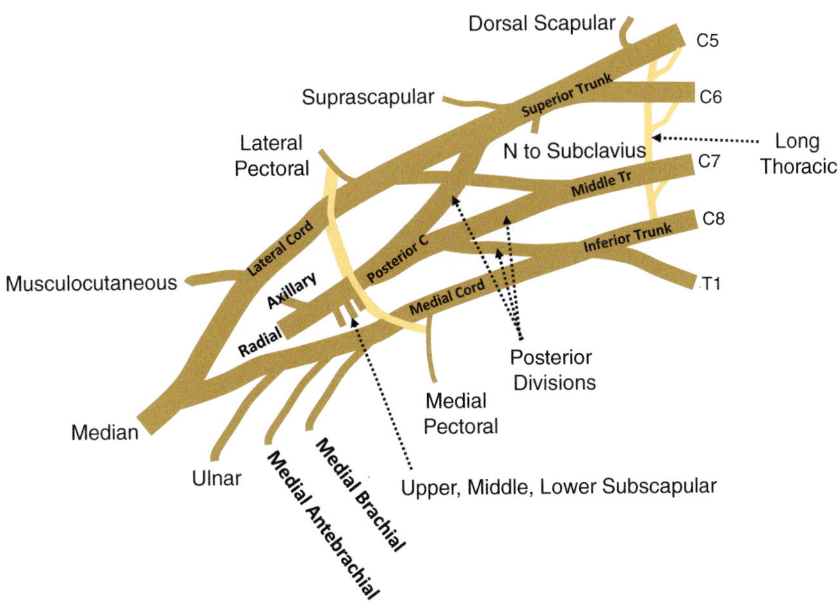

Fig. 7.16 Brachial plexus. The brachial plexus arises from the roots of C5-T1, which in turn gives rise to the trunks, divisions, cords and branches [8, 9]

2. The *dorsal scapular nerve* come directly from the C5 root and supplies the rhomboid major and minor muscles plus the levator scapulae muscle.
3. The *nerve to subclavius* comes from the roots of C5 and C6 and innervates the subclavius muscle.

The roots then form the trunks. The superior trunk (upper trunk) comes from C5 and C6, the middle trunk from C7, and the inferior trunk (lower trunk) from C8 and T1. The trunks lie in the scalene triangle with the subclavian artery. They are susceptible here to impingement and fractures of the first rib.

1. The *suprascapular nerve* arises from the superior trunk and innervates the supraspinatus and infraspinatus muscles.
2. The *nerve to subclavius* also arises from the upper trunk.

Each trunk split into two divisions, an anterior and a posterior division.

The lateral cord is formed by the combination of the anterior divisions of the superior and middle trunks, the posterior cord is formed from all three posterior divisions, and the medial cord comes from the anterior division of the inferior trunk. The cords are named for their relationship to the axillary artery. The cords go on to form the branches to the upper limb muscles. There are five main branches and several smaller branches.

The posterior cord gives rise to two of the five main branches, the axillary and radial nerves. It also gives rise to three smaller branches lined up in a row: the upper, middle, and lower subscapular nerves.

1. The *axillary nerve* innervates several muscles of the shoulder, the deltoid, and the teres minor muscles. In addition, it is responsible for sensation on the lateral aspect of the upper arm—an area sometimes referred to as the "sergeant's stripes" or "regimental badge."
2. The *radial nerve* innervates the muscles of the posterior arm and posterior forearm.
3. Both the *upper and lower subscapular nerves* innervate the subscapularis muscle. The lower subscapular nerve also innervates the teres major muscle.
4. The *middle subscapular nerve,* also known as the thoracodorsal nerve, innervates the latissimus dorsi muscle.

The lateral cord sends a contribution to the median nerve, and it also forms:

1. the *musculocutaneous nerve* which supplies the anterior forearm muscles. The musculocutaneous nerve then continues past the elbow as the lateral cutaneous nerve of the forearm.
2. The *lateral pectoral nerve* which goes to the pectoralis major.

The medial cord gives off the medial cutaneous nerve of the forearm and the medial cutaneous nerve of the arm and sends a contribution to the median nerve. It also forms:

1. the *ulnar nerve* which supplies one and a half muscles in the anterior forearm and many of the hand muscles.
2. The *medial pectoral nerve* which goes to the pectoralis minor and major.

The *intercostobrachial nerve* carries sensory information from the medial arm. It comes from the T2 level, and it intermingles with the medial cutaneous nerve of the arm. Patients who have a heart attack often complain of pain in the left arm. This is because the visceral afferents from the heart travel back to T2 leading to the pain being referred to the arm.

The Compartments of the Upper Limb

Anterior Arm Compartment

The anterior compartment of the arm contains three muscles all innervated by the musculocutaneous nerve. The muscles have several functions

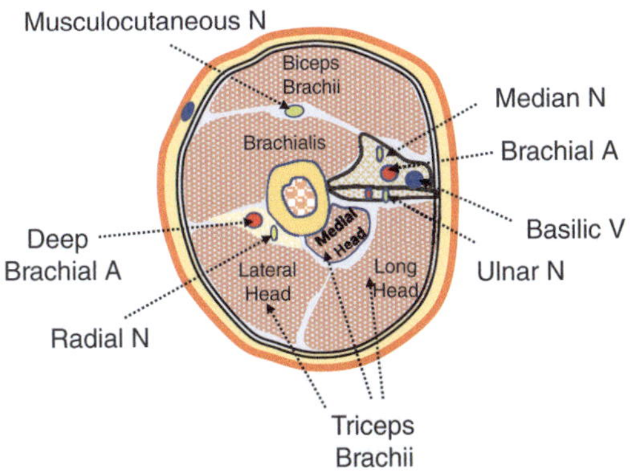

Fig. 7.17 Cross section of the arm. On the posterior side are the three heads of the triceps. On the anterior side are the biceps and brachialis. On the medial side note the median nerve, brachial artery, and basilic vein. The musculocutaneous nerve is located between the biceps brachii and the brachialis. The radial nerve and the deep brachial artery wrap around the humerus in the radial groove [8, 9]

at the shoulder and are the main flexors at the elbow (Fig. 7.17).

1. The *biceps brachii muscle* has two heads. The long head arises from the supraglenoid tubercle and runs through the glenohumeral joint cavity to go over the superior surface of the humerus. It then travels through the intertubercular groove covered by the *transverse humeral ligament*. The short head arises from the coracoid process and joins the long head in the upper third of the arm. The biceps continues to the radial tuberosity. The bicipital aponeurosis runs from lateral to medial to insert on the ulnar fascia. The best way to think about the action of the biceps is opening a wine bottle with a corkscrew. The biceps is a flexor at the elbow and a supinator. When you are removing the cork from a wine bottle, you are flexing and supinating. The muscle also acts at the shoulder as an abductor. In some patients, the long head of the biceps can avulse the supraglenoid tubercle of the scapula. The muscle belly will then pull the tendon inferiorly which leads to a large bump in the anterior arm known as a *Popeye deformity*.
2. The *coracobrachialis muscle* arises at the coracoid process with the short head of the biceps. It inserts on the medial side of the humerus. It is a flexor and adductor at the shoulder.
3. The *brachialis muscle* runs from the humerus to the ulna and is a flexor at the elbow. It is sometimes referred to as the "workhorse" of the elbow since it is the only pure flexor at the joint. Its motor innervation is from the musculocutaneous nerve. In some cases, the radial nerve can be seen entering the muscle, but these radial nerve fibers are thought to carry information about proprioception and not somatomotor fibers to the muscle. Academically this is interesting, but the radial nerve innervation to the brachialis has little relevance to clinical scenarios. When thinking about clinical scenarios, the brachialis is innervated by musculocutaneous nerve.

Posterior Arm Compartment

The posterior compartment of the arm is involved with extension at the shoulder and the elbow. All the muscles of the posterior compartment are innervated by the radial nerve.

1. The *triceps muscle* has three heads. The long head arises from the infraglenoid tubercle, the medial head from the humerus, and the lateral head from the humerus. The three heads meet, and the triceps attaches to the olecranon process of the ulna. Just under the skin, over the olecranon process, at the insertion of the triceps is the olecranon bursa. Resting on one's elbow while sitting at a desk for prolonged periods can lead to olecranon bursitis—student's elbow. The triceps contributes to extension at the shoulder (via the long head) and is the main extensor at the elbow.

Arteries of the Upper Limb

The brachial artery gives off the profunda brachii artery (deep brachial artery) which wraps around the humerus between the medial and lateral heads of the triceps in the triangular interval. It runs with the radial nerve. Behind the humerus the

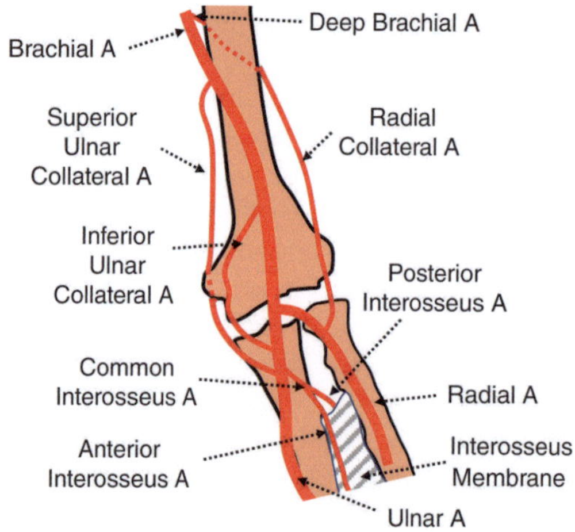

Fig. 7.18 Forearm arteries. The common interosseus artery splits into anterior and posterior interosseus arteries. The radial collateral artery arises from the profunda brachii artery and passes anterior to the lateral epicondyle. The superior and inferior ulnar collateral arteries head towards the medial side of the elbow joint [8, 9]

artery splits into the middle collateral artery and the radial collateral artery, which follows the radial nerve (Fig. 7.18).

Unless you are a vascular surgeon the collateral circulation around the elbow is probably not high on the "items to know for anatomy." But, just in case, the brachial artery also gives off the *superior ulnar collateral artery* which travels posterior to the medial epicondyle with the ulnar nerve. The superior ulnar collateral anastomoses with the *posterior ulnar recurrent* artery which is a branch of the ulnar artery. In a similar fashion the *inferior ulnar collateral artery* arises from the brachial artery and travels anterior to the elbow joint to meet up with the *anterior ulnar recurrent artery* which is a branch of the ulnar artery.

On the radial side, the *radial collateral artery* comes off the deep brachial artery, runs anterior to the elbow, forms an anastomosis with *radial recurrent artery*, and then joins the radial artery. A *middle collateral artery* also comes off the radial collateral artery and runs behind the elbow to become the *recurrent interosseus artery*.

Nerves of the Posterior Compartment

The *musculocutaneous nerve* is the continuation of the lateral cord. It enters the superior aspect of the coracobrachialis and continues down the arm between the biceps brachii and the brachialis muscles. It supplies these three muscles,

The radial nerve is a branch of the posterior cord. It travels with the profunda brachii artery in the radial groove deep to the lateral head of the triceps. The median nerve travels with the brachial artery on the medial side. Likewise. the ulnar nerve is located medially. Neither the ulnar nor the median nerve innervate any muscles in the arm (Table 7.1).

The Elbow Joint

At the elbow, the *capitulum* of the humerus meets with *radial head*, while the *trochlea* of the humerus rests in the *trochlea notch* of the ulna. The anterior prominence of the trochlea is the coronoid fossa of the anterior distal humerus. The posterior process of the superior ulna is the *olecranon*, which on extension moves into the olecranon fossa on the posterior distal humerus.

With the elbow flexed to 90°, the olecranon process forms an isosceles triangle with the medial and lateral epicondyles. On extension these three points line up in a row. With elbow injuries these relationships are disrupted.

On the lateral side, the *radial collateral ligament* maintains stability. On the medial side, the ulnar collateral ligament is composed of the anterior, lateral, and posterior bands (bundles). *Tommy John Surgery* refers to restoration of the ulnar collateral ligament by using a ligament harvested from somewhere else in the body. Often the palmaris longus tendon is used for grafting. The surgery was first performed on the baseball player Tommy John in 1974. The ulnar nerve enters the elbow around the medial epicondyle and crosses the ulnar collateral ligament. (Note, do not confuse the ulnar collateral ligament and

Table 7.1 Pathways and landmarks for the three major nerves of the upper limb as they pass through the arm, elbow, forearm, and wrist [8, 9]

	Ulnar nerve	Median nerve	Radial nerve
Arm	Passes medial to brachial artery, enters the posterior compartment and then joins the superior ulnar collateral artery.	Found lateral to brachial artery in cubital fossa.	Runs with profunda brachial artery in radial groove.
Elbow region	Passes posterior to the medial epicondyle and then passes through the cubital tunnel	Passes between the two heads of pronator Teres	Located anterior to the lateral epicondyle.
Forearm	Deep to flexor carpi ulnaris. Runs with ulnar artery	Between the flexor digitorum superficialis and flexor digitorum profundus. Gives off anterior interosseus nerve which runs with anterior interosseus artery.	Splits into superficial and deep branches. Deep branch pierces supinator to reach posterior compartment. The superficial branch runs under brachioradialis.
Wrist	Lateral to pisiform. Travels through Guyon's canal and splits into superficial and deep branches	Passes through the carpal tunnel. Gives off recurrent branch to the thenar muscles.	Superficial branch enters superficial to the extensor retinaculum and send branches to the thumb and index finger

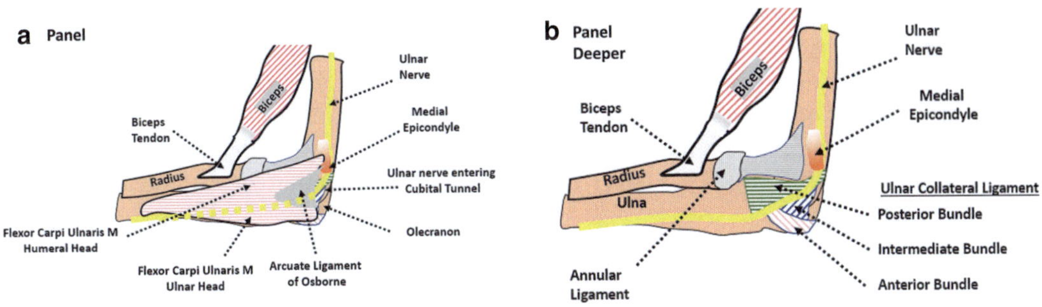

Fig. 7.19 Medial elbow. Panel (**a**) shows the ulnar nerve entering the cubital tunnel which is deep to the arcuate ligament of Osborne. In Panel (**b**) the flexor carpi ulnaris has been removed to show the ulnar nerve wrapping around the medial epicondyle. The ulnar collateral ligament has three divisions [8, 9]

its three sections with the lateral ulnar collateral ligament—they names are similar, but they are different).

Wrapping around the radial head is the *annular ligament* which allows the radial head to spin within the ligament for supination and pronation. The ligament is attached to the notch of the ulna making up the *proximal radioulnar joint* which is encased by the articular capsule. In adults this ligament is strong, however in infants it is weaker and a strong pull on the arm can subluxate (dislocate) the radial head. Over the years this has unfortunately taken on the pejorative term of *nursemaid's elbow*.

The *terrible triad of the elbow* refers to an injury of the elbow joint that involves: (1) a radial head fracture, (2) a fracture of the ulnar coracoid process, and (3) a posterior dislocation of the elbow joint. It typically results from trauma where large forces push on the extended and supinated elbow joint; for instance, a car accident where the hand strikes the dashboard. In addition to the three structures mentioned above, the collateral ligaments of the elbow can also be injured.

As the ulnar nerve approaches the medial elbow, it enters the cubital tunnel with the ulnar collateral ligament making up the floor, and the cubital tunnel retinaculum making up the ceiling. Nerve impingement in this area is common (Fig. 7.19).

As the nerve emerges from the tunnel, it dives deep to the arcuate ligament (of Osborne) that lies between the two heads of the flexor carpi ulnaris.

In summary, as the three major nerves to the forearm and hand cross the elbow, they all pierce a muscle which can be a source of aggravation: the ulnar nerve travels between the two heads of flexor carpi ulnaris; the median nerve travels between the two heads of the pronator teres; and the deep radial nerve pierces the supinator muscle.

Cubital Fossa

The *cubital fossa* is found on the anterior surface of the elbow. It is a triangular shaped space transmitting several structures from the arm to the forearm. It is bounded by the medial border of brachioradialis, the lateral border of pronator teres, and a horizontal line across the elbow. The order of the structures from lateral to medial is the biceps tendon, the brachial artery, and the median nerve. This gives us the mnemonic TAN for tendon, artery, and nerve. However, realize that the radial nerve is also found in the far lateral side of the compartment where it divides into superficial and deep branches (Fig. 7.20).

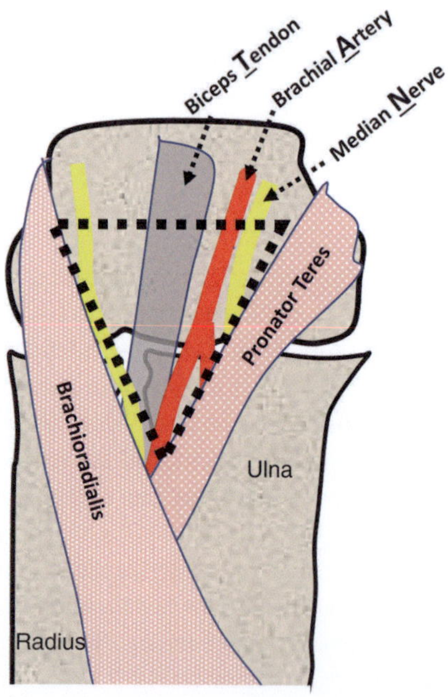

Fig. 7.20 Cubital fossa. The fossa is bound by the medial border of the pronator teres, the lateral border of the brachioradialis and a line above the elbow. Within the fossa, from lateral to medial is the biceps Tendon, the brachial Artery, and the median Nerve. Remember TAN for the order of the structures [8, 9]

Forearm

Many of the muscles responsible for hand movements arise in the forearm. The common flexor origin is located on the medial epicondyle and many of the extensors are located on the lateral epicondyle. Keep in mind that in most cases when you talk about muscles to the thumb and little finger there are redundant muscles—a longus and a brevis. And in some cases, losing one muscle, say the longus, does not mean the associated movement is lost, because the associated brevis takes over, or vice versa (Fig. 7.21).

Flexion of the fingers involves moving your fingertips towards your palm, while extension involves moving the fingertips away. Abduction of the fingers involves spreading your fingers apart, while adduction involves moving them closer together.

Because of the thumb's rotation, its movements are in a plane that is 90° to the fingers. Flexion of the thumb involves moving it in towards the little finger and crossing over the palm, while extension involves spreading it out laterally (Fig. 7.22).

Abduction of the thumb involves moving the thumb away from the hand at a right angle to the palm, while adduction brings it back into the palm (Fig. 7.23).

Anterior Forearm

There are five muscles that arise together from the common flexor origin along the medial epicondyle and travel in the anterior forearm towards the hand. Starting with the most lateral muscle:

1. The *pronator teres muscle* has two heads. One head arises from the humerus, and one from the ulna tuberosity. They merge to insert onto the radius. It is a flexor and a pronator of the elbow. Median nerve.
2. The *flexor carpi radialis muscle* arises from the common flexor tendon and inserts onto the radial tuberosity and the bases of the second and third metacarpals. It is a flexor at the elbow and an abductor at the wrist. Median nerve.

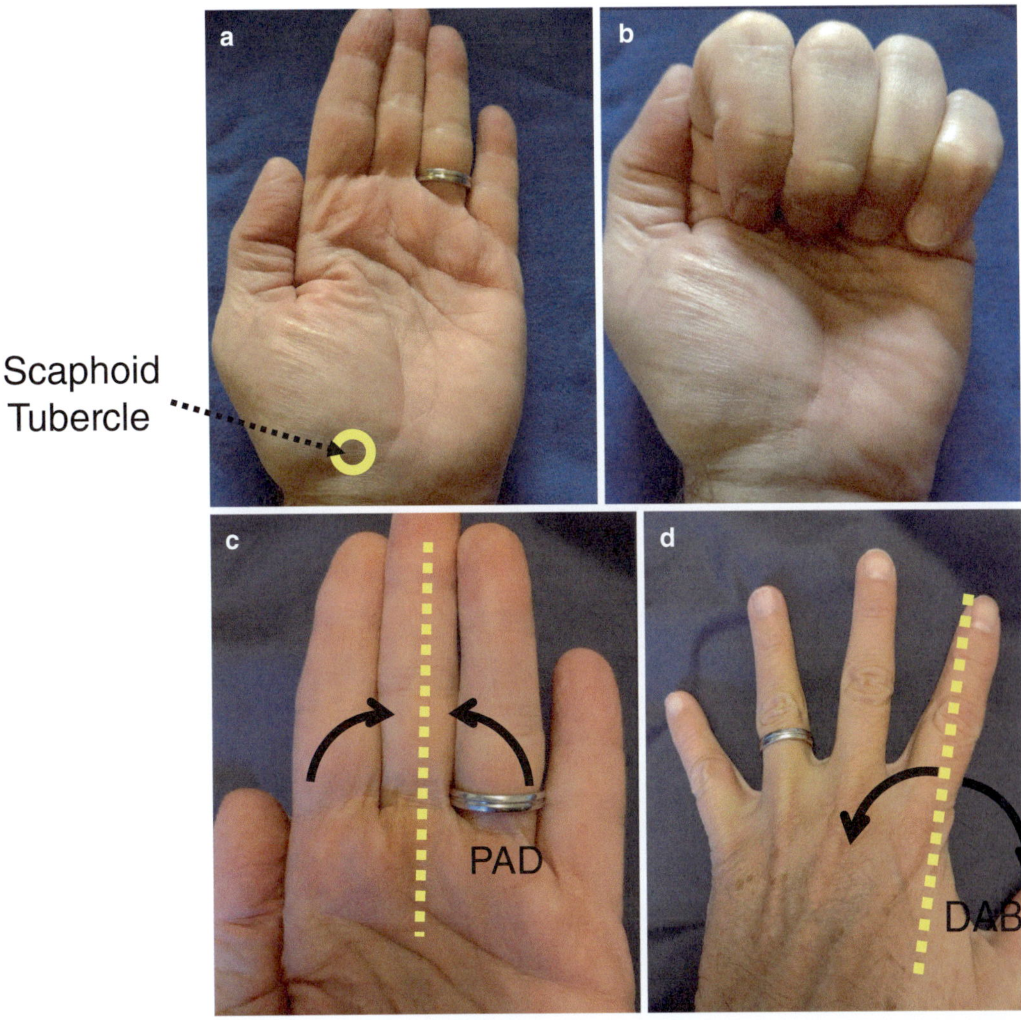

Fig. 7.21 Finger movements. Panel (**a**) Extension of the fingers. Panel (**b**) Flexion of the fingers., Panel (**c**) Adduction (Palmar Interossei), Panel (**d**) Abduction (Dorsal interossei) [8, 9]

3. The *palmaris longus muscle also* arises from the common flexor origin and inserts into the palmar aponeurosis. Median nerve.
4. The *flexor carpi ulnaris muscle* also arises from the common flexor origin and inserts onto the fifth metacarpal, the hook of the hamate and the pisiform. It is a flexor at the elbow and an adductor at the wrist. Ulnar nerve
5. The *flexor digitorum superficialis muscle* has two heads. A humeroulnar head which arises in part from the common flexor tendon but in part from the coronoid process of the ulna. It also has a radial head arising from the radius. The tendons travel down the arm to insert on the middle phalanges of digits 2–5. Its action is flexion of the metacarpal phalangeal and proximal interphalangeal joints. It is innervated by the median nerve. Note that when it comes to organizing these muscles some authors place this muscle in an intermediate compartment. It is just a matter of how you would like to organize it. When it comes to learning the nerves, it seems easier to put it in the superficial compartment for the simple fact that if you place your palm on medial epicondyle and flair out your fingers you have the five superficial flexors—four does not work

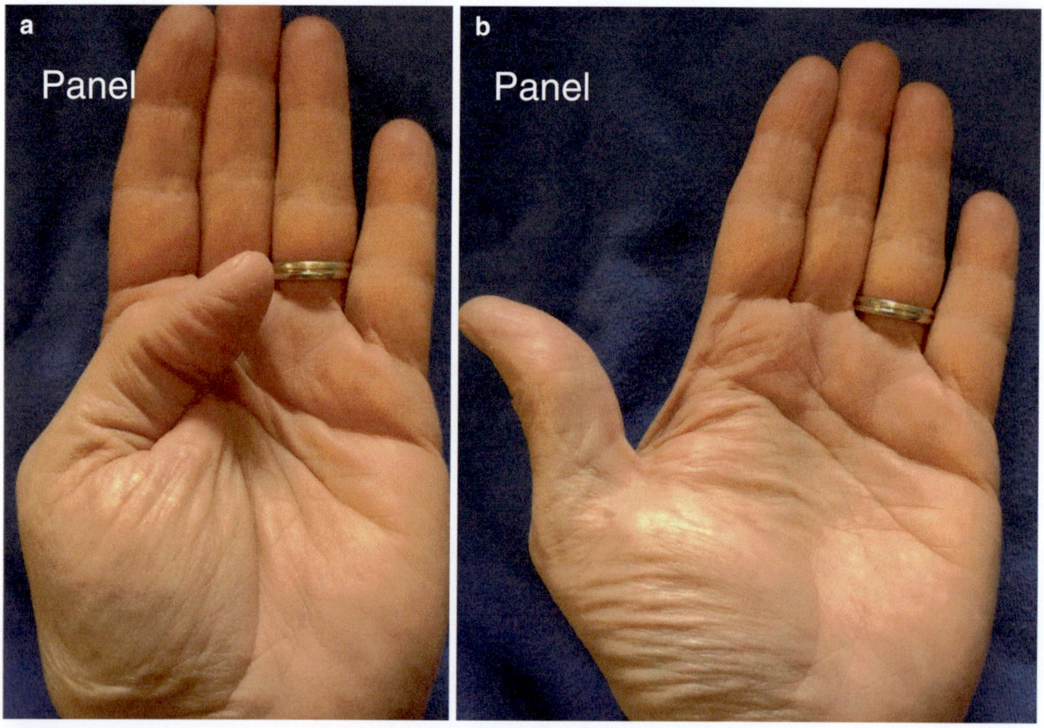

Fig. 7.22 Panel (**a**) flexion of the thumb. Panel (**b**) extension of the thumb [8, 9]

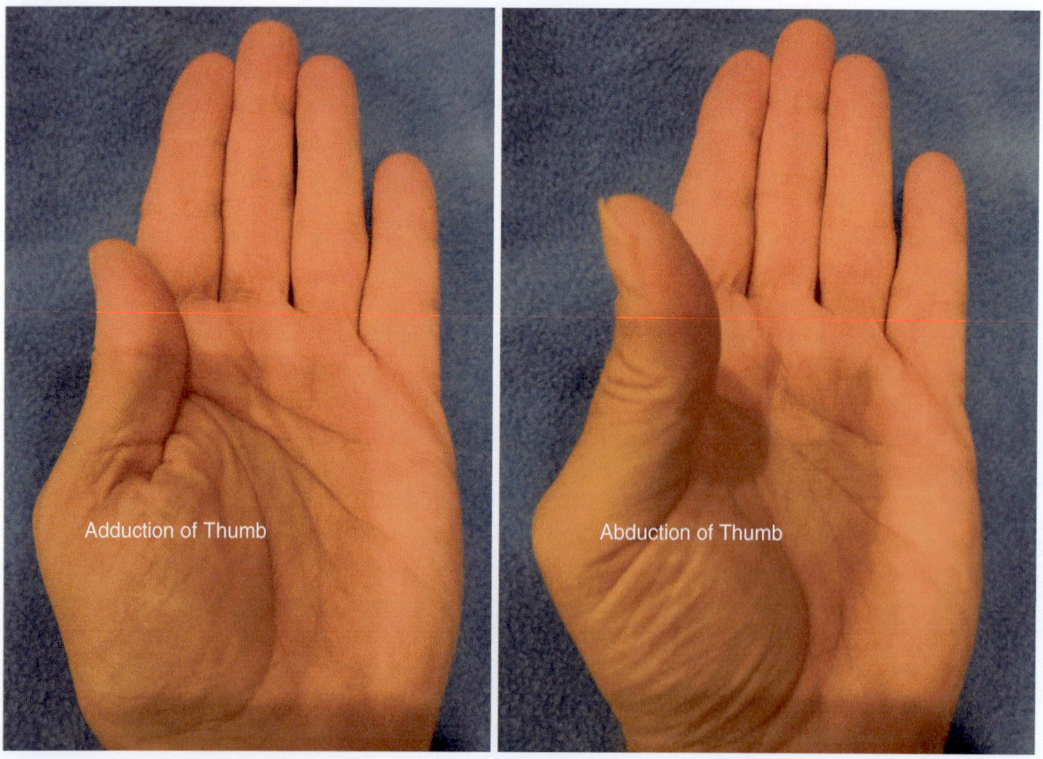

Fig. 7.23 Thumb adduction and abduction [8, 9]

quite as well with this scheme. Repetitive injuries to the medial epicondyle, or *medial epicondylitis* come from continuous flexion of the forearm. These are sometimes referred to as *Golfer's Elbow* (Figs. 7.24 and 7.25).

Deep Forearm Compartment

In the deep forearm there are three muscles, which are innervated by the anterior interosseus nerve, except for half of the flexor digitorum profundus:

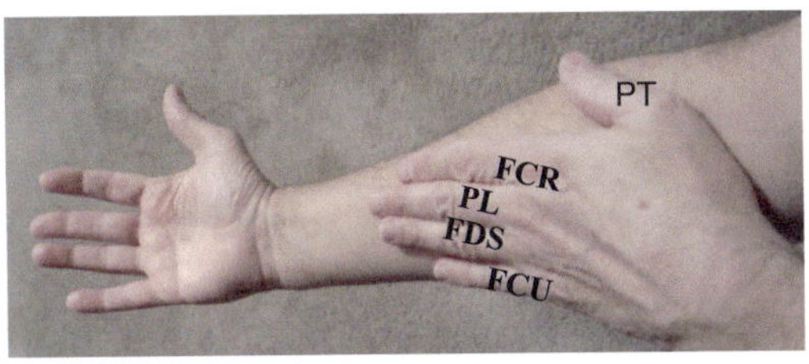

Fig. 7.24 Common flexor origin. There are five superficial flexors originating from the the medial epicondyle. If you lay you hand on the medial elbow, your five fingers represent the five muscles. *PT* pronator teres, *FCR* flexor carpi radialis, *PL* palmaris longus, *FDS* flexor digitorum superficialis, *FCU* flexor carpi ulnaris [8, 9]

1. The *flexor digitorum profundus* arises from the ulna and the interosseus membrane and inserts into the distal phalanges of the fingers. It flexes all the joints it crosses: the wrist, metacarpophalangeal, proximal interphalangeal, and distal interphalangeal.
2. The *flexor pollicis longus* arises from the radius and interosseus membrane and inserts into the distal phalanx of the thumb.
3. The *pronator quadratus* runs from ulna to radius and is a pronator (Fig. 7.25).

Flexor Digitorum Superficialis and Flexor Digitorum Profundus Insertions

As the four tendons of *flexor digitorum superficialis* approach the proximal phalanges each tendon splits into two bands that attach to the sides of the middle phalanges. This split allows the tendon of *flexor digitorum profundus* of each finger to travel through the split and continue to the distal phalanges. The tendons of both muscles are held down close to the fingers by fibrous flexor sheaths. The sheaths are composed of a

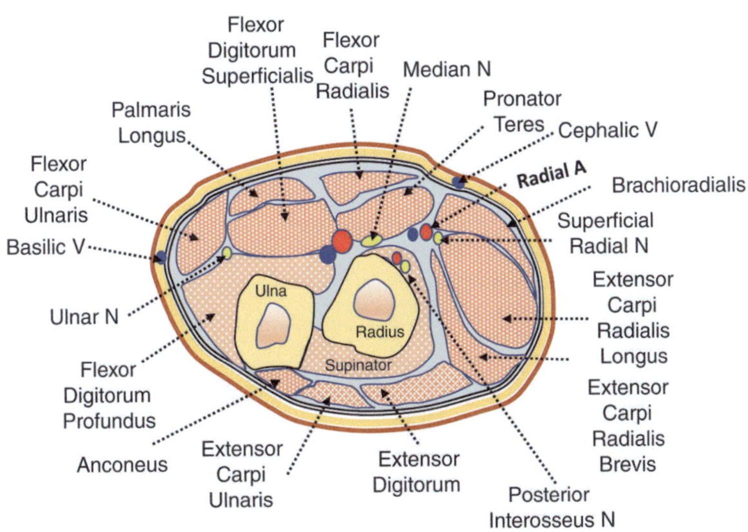

Fig. 7.25 Cross section through the superior forearm. In the anterior forearm, arising from the medial epicondyle is the flexor carpi ulnaris, palmaris longus, flexor digitorum superficialis, pronator teres, and flexor carpi radialis. Deep to these superficial muscles note the flexor digitorum profundus arising from the ulna. Arising from the lateral epicondyle is the extensor carpi ulnaris, extensor digitorum, and extensor carpi radialis longus and brevis. The supinator runs from the ulna to the radius on the posterior side [8, 9]

combination of ligaments, some that encircle the bone and others that form a crisscross pattern enclosing the tendons. A *trigger finger* refers to a sharp sound that comes from the finger when it is flexed and extended. The sound comes from a growth on the tendon which makes a snapping noise as it moves through the ligaments around the finger.

Dupuytren's Contracture

Just under the skin of the palm is a strong tough fibrous membrane, the palmar fascia. In some cases, this fascia becomes thick and tight, which leads to flexion of the fingers. This closely resembles claw hand in appearance, but it is not a nerve injury. The symptoms are more severe in the fourth and fifth digits.

Neurovascular Compartment in Forearm

The brachial artery enters the forearm and divides into the radial and ulnar arteries. The ulnar artery continues medially and lies beneath the flexor carpi ulnaris. It runs with the ulnar nerve. The ulnar artery gives off the common interosseus artery which quickly divides into anterior and posterior interosseus arteries. The *posterior interosseus artery* gains access to the posterior forearm by traveling over the interosseus membrane, moving from the anterior to posterior compartment, and then traveling down the posterior surface of the interosseus membrane where it runs with the *posterior interosseus nerve* which is a branch of the radial nerve.

The *anterior interosseus artery* runs in front of the interosseus membrane with the anterior interosseus nerve which is a branch of the median nerve.

The *radial artery* travels from the cubital fossa down to the wrist between the brachioradialis and the flexor carpi radialis tendons, where its pulse can be felt. Just below the elbow, the radial artery gives off the radial recurrent artery which meets up with the radial collateral artery.

The *radial nerve* enters the forearm in the lateral region of the cubital fossa. It splits into superficial and deep branches. The deep branch becomes the *posterior interosseus nerve,* while the superficial branch travels down towards the anatomical snuff box. (Some authors say that the radial nerve splits into the deep branch and the superficial branch, and that the deep branch quickly turns into the posterior interosseous nerve).

The *median nerve* enters the cubital fossa medial to the brachial artery and then travels between the two heads of the pronator teres. In the forearm it gives off two branches, the anterior interosseus nerve and the palmar cutaneous branch (Fig. 7.26).

The median nerve continues down the forearm between the flexor digitorum superficialis and the flexor digitorum profundus. The anterior interosseus nerve travels down the forearm between the flexor digitorum profundus and the flexor pollicis longus to reach the pronator quadratus. A test for the anterior interosseus nerve is to ask the patient to make an "Ok" sign. The successful move is based on the flexor digitorum profundus tendon to the second digit, and the flexor pollicis longus tendon going to the thumb, both of which are innervated by the anterior interosseus nerve. Damage to the nerve will result in more of a pinch than an "Ok" sign (Figs. 7.27 and 7.28).

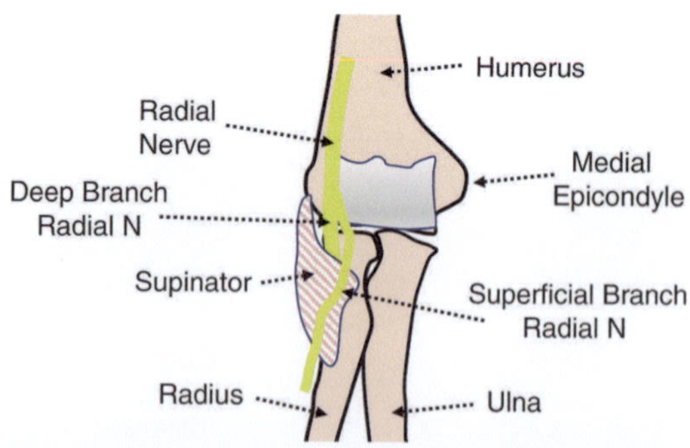

Fig. 7.26 Radial nerve. The radial nerve enters the elbow region and divides into a superficial and deep branch. The deep branch pierces the supinator muscle and enters the posterior forearm as the posterior interosseus nerve. The superficial branch continues to the hand and crosses the snuff box [8, 9]

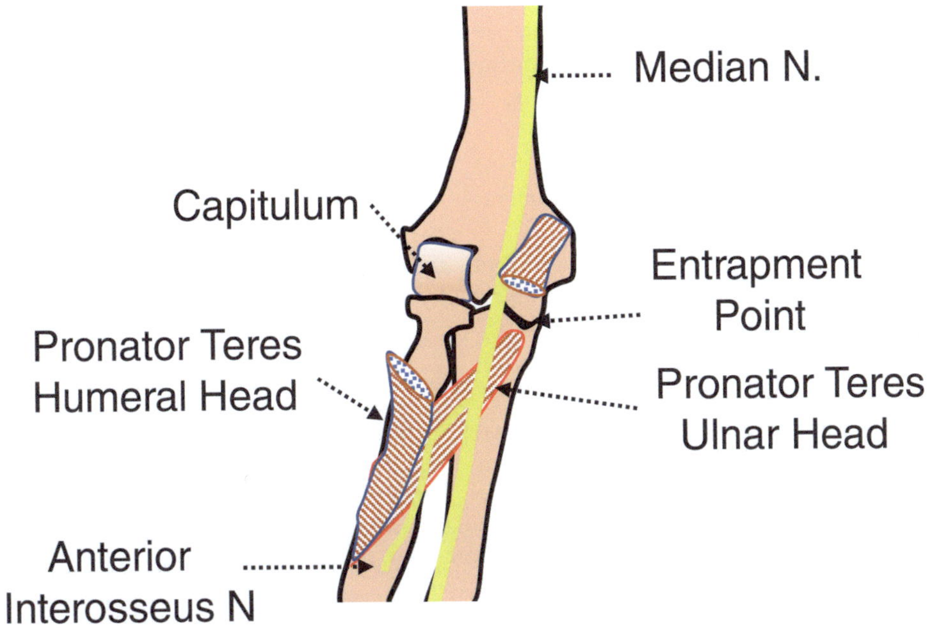

Fig. 7.27 The median nerve. The median nerve enters the elbow region between the two heads of the pronator teres. At this point, the nerve can be become entrapped. The anterior interosseus nerve comes off the median nerve between the two heads of pronator teres [8, 9]

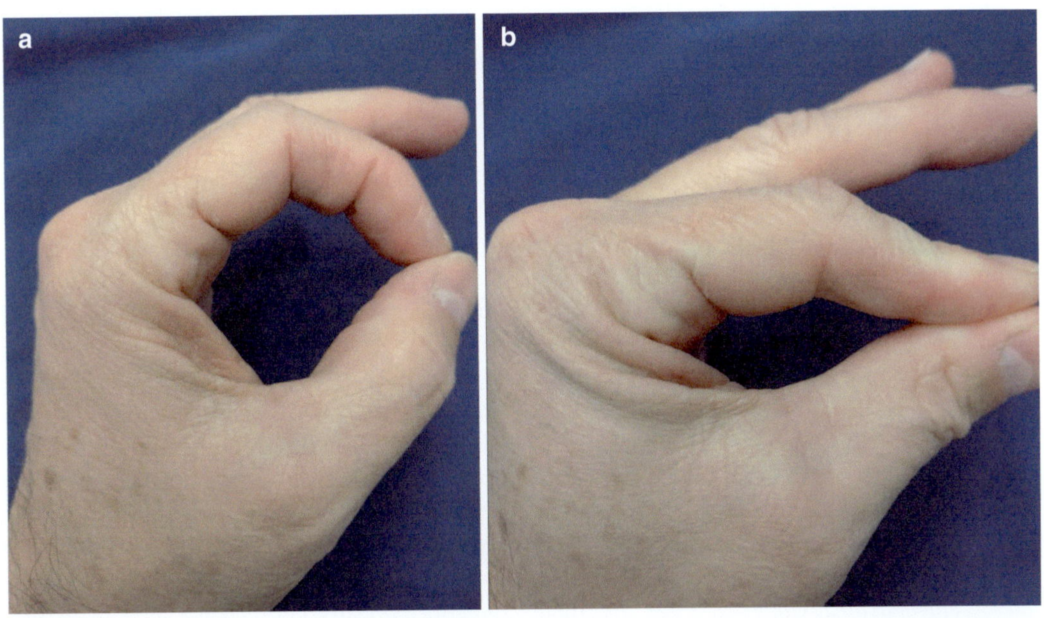

Fig. 7.28 Anterior interosseus nerve. Panel (**a**) shows normal anterior interosseus nerve function. Panel (**b**) shows the fingers of a patient with anterior interosseus nerve palsy [8, 9]

Posterior Forearm

The muscles of the posterior forearm are all innervated by the radial nerve. Many of them are involved in extension of the wrist and fingers.

1. The *extensor carpi radialis longus* runs from the lateral supracondylar ridge of the humerus to the second metacarpal.
2. The *extensor carpi radialis brevis* runs from the lateral supracondylar ridge to the third metacarpal. The muscle lies deep to the extensor carpi radialis longus. The two of them together extend and abduct at the wrist.
3. The *extensor digitorum* arises from the lateral supracondylar ridge and inserts into the extensor expansion. It is an extensor of the wrist and digits.
4. The *extensor digiti minimi* is an extension of the extensor digitorum that sends a tendon to the fifth digit. It extends the wrist and the fifth digit.
5. The *extensor carpi* ulnaris runs from the lateral epicondyle to the fifth metacarpal.
6. The *anconeus* is a small triangular shaped muscle in the superior portion of the posterior forearm that blends in with the triceps.
7. Finally is the *brachioradialis***.** The brachioradialis is somewhat of an outlier. It arises from the lateral side of the humerus near the other extensors; however it is a flexor. It runs down the forearm and attaches to the radial tuberosity. When the arm is in the neutral position, the brachioradialis is a flexor at the elbow. Imagine you have just picked up a can of soda from a table. At this point your hand is in the neutral position. When you move your hand towards your mouth it is the brachioradialis that is responsible for this movement. Think of it as your soda drinking muscle.

These muscles that arise from the lateral elbow can become aggravated in overuse scenarios what involve continuous extension of your elbow such as playing tennis, thus the term "tennis elbow" or *lateral epicondylitis. Ganglion cysts* are fluid filled sacs that can appear on tendons anywhere in the body, however they are usually found on the hand, and most of these occur on the extensor tendons on the posterior wrist.

Posterior Forearm Muscles to Thumb

There are three muscles that originate in the forearm and travel through the forearm on their way to the thumb. As they cross the wrist, they form the anatomical snuff box. They are all innervated by the radial nerve.

1. The *extensor pollicis longus* arises from the ulna and inserts on the distal phalanx of the thumb. As it crosses the distal radius it makes a turn around the *dorsal tubercle* (Lister's tubercle). The tubercle acts like a pulley to increase the leverage for the muscle. A hyperextension injury can fracture the tubercle leaving a sharp edge which can tear the tendon. A *mallet finger* refers to an injury that tears the distal end of the extensor pollicis longus tendon with a transverse tear just before its insertion onto the distal phalange. A common injury is a baseball player sliding into the base with their upper limb extended such that the distal phalanges strike the base with a hard impact that tears the extensor tendon. With the tendon torn, the fingertip will be stuck in a flexed position.
2. The *extensor pollicis brevis* arises from the radius and inserts onto the distal phalanx of the thumb.
3. The *abductor pollicis longus* arises from the ulna and the radius and inserts onto the first metacarpal bone.

The *snuff box* is bound by the extensor pollicis longus and the extensor pollicis brevis. The floor of the snuff box is the *scaphoid and trapezium.* Crossing deep to the tendons in the snuff box is the radial artery where the pulse can be felt. Crossing superficially, above the tendons, is the superficial branch of the radial nerve and the cephalic vein. *Wartenberg's Syndrome* refers to constriction of the superficial radial nerve in the forearm, typically between the tendons of brachioradialis and extensor carpi radialis longus (Fig. 7.29).

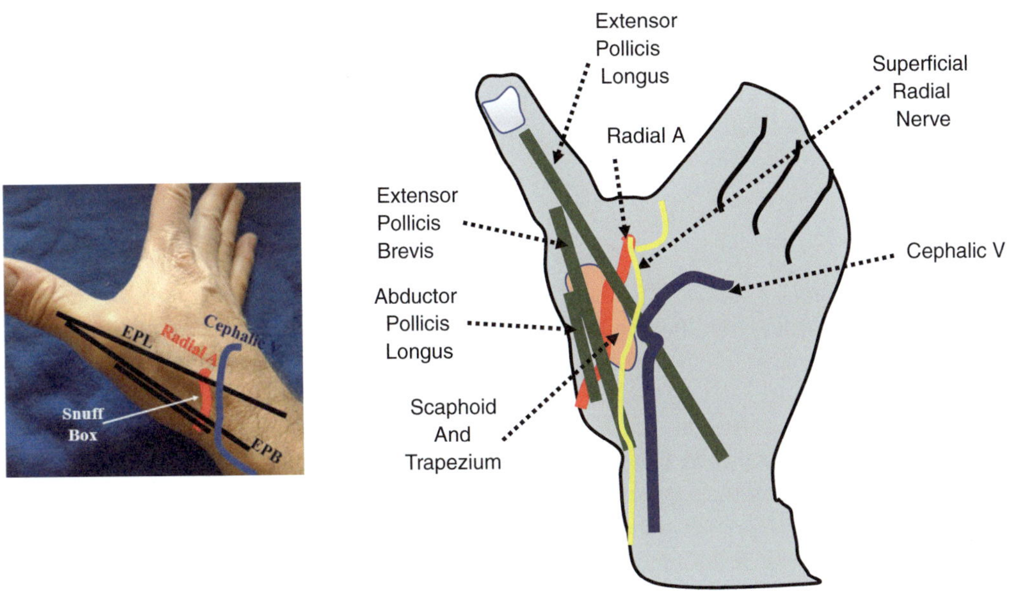

Fig. 7.29 Snuff box. The anatomical snuff box bounded by the extensor pollicis longus and brevis. The floor is made up of the trapezium and scaphoid. The radial artery crosses deep to the tendons, while the superficial radial nerve and cephalic vein cross superficially [8, 9]

The tendons of the abductor pollicis longus and the extensor pollicis brevis pass in a fibrous tunnel along the radius and deep to the extensor retinaculum. Repetitive motion injuries can occur here leading to *De Quervain's syndrome,* which is thickening of either the tendons, the sheaths, or in some cases both. This leads to pain on flexion of the thumb and wrist (Finkelstein's test.)

Distal Radioulnar Joint

The *distal radioulnar joint* is between the sigmoid notch of the radius and the head of the ulna. The joint allows pronation and supination of the forearm. An articular disk holds the two bones together and separates the distal radioulnar joint from the radiocarpal joint. The *articular disk* along with several smaller ligaments from the *triangular fibrocartilage complex* known as the TFCC for short. The TFCC connects the lunate, triquetrum, and ulna. The TFCC is the structure between the ulna and the carpal bones and can be injured from trauma (type I) or overuse (type II). In addition to pain and swelling of the medial wrist, patients will often report a clicking or popping feeling with wrist movement.

The *fovea* of the wrist is a point on the medial wrist between the styloid process and the tendon of flexor carpi ulnaris tendon. Remember the tendon of flexor carpi ulnaris passes over the pisiform. If the examiner can elicit pain by pressing on this region, it suggests damage to the TFCC and the distal radioulnar joint.

The Hand

The palm of the hand is organized around three compartments: the thenar compartment containing the small muscles of the thumb, the hypothenar compartment containing the small muscles of the fifth digit, and the middle compartment situated between the thenar and hypothenar compartments. The abridged version of the motor nerve supply to the hand is that the median nerve innervates three and half muscles and the ulnar innervates the rest. The median nerve innervates the 3 thenar muscles and two of the four lumbricals (1/2 of the lumbricals). The ulnar nerve innervates everything else. Note that the "everything else" includes the muscles in the hypothenar compartment, the interossei, two of the four lumbricals, and the adductor pollicis.

Carpal Bones

There are eight carpal bones arranged in two rows of four each. The first row, moving lateral to medial is the *scaphoid, lunate, triquetrum, and pisiform* (Fig. 7.30).

The radius articulates with the scaphoid and lunate. Falls on the outstretched hand typically result in a fracture of either the scaphoid, the distal radius, or the clavicle. The individual bone that is fractured is typically a result of the patient's age. In a teenager the clavicle is the most often fractured bone. In an elderly person the most common fracture occurs at the distal radius (Colle's fracture). In a middle-aged person, the most common fracture is to the scaphoid.

The danger of a scaphoid fracture comes from the fact that the blood supply to the scaphoid enters the bone at its distal segment. So with a fracture, the proximal segment now devoid of its blood supply will undergo avascular necrosis. Scaphoid fractures will lead to pain in the snuff box and can take up to 2 weeks to appear on an x-ray. The scaphoid tubercle can be found just distal (1 cm) to the wrist folds. The tendon of flexor carpi radialis passes over it (Fig. 7.15).

In addition to the scaphoid fracture, another common injury following a fall on the outstretched hand is an anterior dislocation of the lunate which on a radiograph appears as a triangular shaped piece of bone pushed anterior. Anterior dislocations of the lunate often compress the median nerve leading to similar symptoms as carpal tunnel syndrome.

The second row of carpal bones contains the *trapezium, trapezoid, capitate, and hamate.* The hook of the hamate and the pisiform protect the ulnar nerve. The hamate and pisiform also serve as an attachment for several muscles and ligaments. The carpal bones all have interesting names (Table 7.2).

Metacarpals

The metacarpals connect the carpal bones to the phalanges forming the scaffold for the intermedi-

Table 7.2 Origin of names of carpal bones

Carpal bone	Meaning
Scaphoid	Canoe
Lunate	Moon
Triquetrum	Three sided
Pisiform	Pea
Trapezium	Quadrilateral
Trapezoid	Quadrilateral
Capitate	Compact head
Hamate	Hook

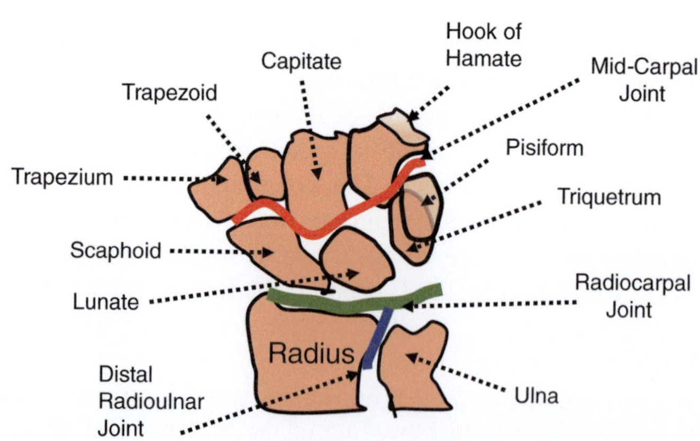

Fig. 7.30 Carpal bones [8, 9]

ate compartment. The interossei muscles also attach to these bones. The axis for abduction and adduction is through the third finger. The palmar interossei are responsible for adduction, and the dorsal interossei for abduction. A *boxer's fracture* is to the distal metacarpals, usually of the fifth metacarpal. A *Bennett fracture* is to the base of the first metacarpal (the thumb), it can go along with a fracture of the trapezium.

Thenar Compartment

The thenar compartment contains three muscles, all of which are innervated by the recurrent branch of the median nerve which passes between the two heads of the flexor pollicis brevis.

1. The *flexor pollicis brevis* has a superficial (Median N) and a deep head (Ulnar N). It arises from the flexor retinaculum and the trapezium, and it inserts onto the proximal phalanx of the thumb. It is a flexor of the thumb at the metacarpophalangeal joint.
2. The *abductor pollicis brevis* arises from the scaphoid and trapezium, and it inserts onto the proximal phalanx of the thumb.
3. The *opponens pollicis* arises from the trapezium and inserts onto the proximal phalanx of the thumb.

The recurrent branch of the median nerve is sometimes referred to as "the million-dollar nerve"– a reference to how much a physician could be held liable if it is cut during a surgical procedure. Shortly after the median nerve passes though the carpal tunnel it gives off the recurrent branch which travels between the two heads of the flexor pollicis brevis. At this point, the nerve is just under the skin and can be easily injured in lacerations of the thenar compartment. In this scenario, the patient would lose the function of the three thenar muscles. If this patient is in your office and you want to test whether the nerve is damaged, you test opposition. This is because, although the patient would lose the flexor pollicis brevis, they would still be able to flex their thumb because the flexor pollicis longus is intact. Likewise, although the patient would lose the abductor pollicis brevis, they would still have function of their abductor pollicis longus. In other words, keep in mind that for flexion and abduction of the thumb there is both a longus and a brevis, but for opposition there is no longus or brevis, just a single opponens pollicis—for the opponens there is no redundancy.

The Hypothenar Compartment

There are three muscles in the hypothenar compartment. They all act on the fifth digit and are innervated by the deep branch of the ulnar nerve.

1. The *flexor digiti minimi* arises from the hamate and inserts into the proximal phalanx of the fifth digit.
2. The *abductor digiti minimi brevis* arises from the pisiform and inserts into the base of proximal phalanx of fifth digit.
3. The *opponens digiti minimi* arises from the hamate and inserts into the metacarpal of the fifth digit.

Intermediate Compartment

Between the hypothenar and thenar compartments is the adductor pollicis. It has an *oblique head* arising from the second and third metacarpals, and a *transverse head* arising from the third metacarpal. The two heads merge to insert onto the proximal phalanx of the thumb. Note that it is a thenar muscle, meaning that it acts on the thumb, but it is not *located* in the thenar compartment. It is in the intermediate compartment. It brings the abducted thumb back towards the second digit. It is innervated by the deep branch of the ulnar nerve which can be seen coming off the ulnar nerve medially and going laterally to go between the two heads of the muscle.

Palmar and Dorsal Interossei

There are four *palmar and four dorsal interossei*. To test the interossei you can ask the patient to abduct and adduct the fingers. The palmar interossei are responsible for adduction (PAD). The dorsal interossei are responsible for abduction (DAB). The axis for these movements is through the third digit, meaning that when the other fingers are brought towards the third finger this is adduction, while movement away from the third digit is abduction. Because the third digit is the axis, whichever way it moves is away from the axis and considered abduction. All the interossei are innervated by the T1 spinal level traveling via the ulnar nerve.

Lumbricals

The lumbricals are unique in that they do not attach to bone, but instead run from one tendon to another tendon. On the palmar side they are attached to the tendon of the flexor digitorum profundus, and on the dorsal side they are attached to the extensor digitorum. When they contract, they flex the metacarpophalangeal joint and extend the interphalangeal joints. The two lumbricals on the medial or ulnar side are innervated by the ulnar nerve, and the two lumbricals on the lateral or radial side are innervated by the median nerve.

Ulnar Nerve at the Wrist

At the wrist, the ulnar nerve enters *Guyon's canal,* which is bounded posteriorly by the transverse carpal ligament (the floor), anteriorly by the palmar carpal ligament (the roof) and medially by the pisiform bone and flexor carpi ulnaris tendon. The nerve travels with the ulnar artery at this point. Impingement here can occur in bike riders who rest their hand on their bike handles, or office workers, who rest their hands on their desks. As the ulnar nerve continues into the hand it splits into a superficial branch, which is sensory, and a deep branch which supplies the muscles. The motor branch travels into a second opening referred to as the pisohamate hiatus which is distal to Guyon's canal. The floor of the pisohamate hiatus is the pisohamate ligament, and the roof is made up by the fibrous arch. Along with the deep branch of the ulnar nerve, the deep branch of the ulnar artery runs through the *pisohamate hiatus.* The superficial branch of the ulnar nerve can be found just medial to the hamate. (Fig. 7.31).

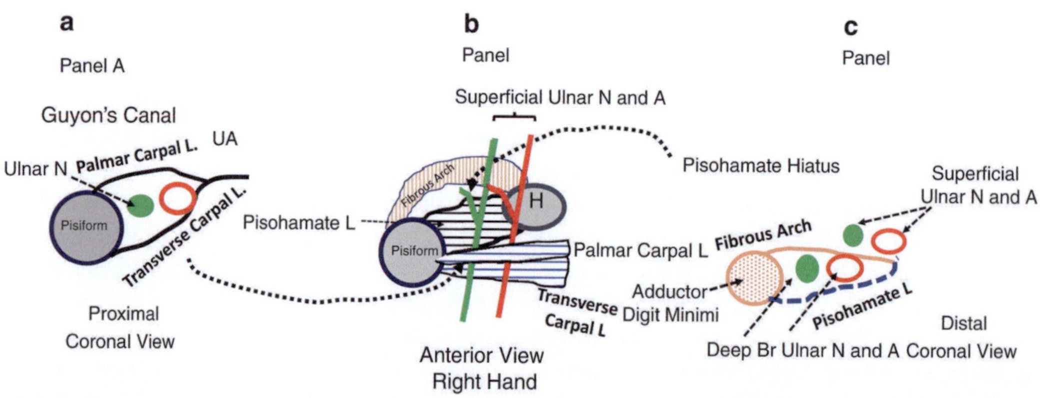

Fig. 7.31 Pathway of ulnar nerve. Panel (**a**) an axial view of ulnar nerve in wrist, shows the boundaries of triangular shaped Guyon's canal: Roof is palmar carpal L, floor is the transverse carpal L., and medial border is pisiform. Panel (**b**) shows the palmar view with the ulnar nerve and artery passing deep to the palmar carpal ligament (anterior boundary) in Guyon's canal, emerging from the canal and passing over the pisohamate L., and then splitting into superficial deep and deep branches to pass on either side of the fibrous arch from hypothenar muscles. Panel (**c**) is a distal axial view, showing the deep branches passing under the fibrous arch to enter the pisohamate hiatus, while the superficial branches pass superficial to the arch [8, 9]

Froment's Sign

In a healthy individual when you place a piece of paper between their thumb and second digit, they can hold the piece of paper firmly in place with their entire thumb fully adducted against the finger by using their adductor pollicis and first dorsal interossei muscle. In a patient with an ulnar nerve palsy, they can hold the paper in place, but the thumb is held in a slightly different position. Because they have lost the adductor pollicis, they use their flexor pollicis longus muscle which is innervated by the median nerve to flex the distal phalangeal joint of the thumb. Instead of using the surface of the entire medial thumb they are only using the tip of the thumb to hold the paper (Fig. 7.32).

Claw Hand

In a healthy individual the lumbricals and interossei muscles are involved with flexion of the metacarpal phalangeal joints and extension of the interphalangeal joints. With an injury to the ulnar nerve, all the interossei and the medial two lumbricals are lost. The metacarpal phalangeal joints are now extended, and the interphalangeal joints are flexed. The fingers assume a claw like position, and the clawing will be more severe in the medial two fingers because the lumbricals are lost in those fingers, but they are intact in the lateral two fingers.

Claw hand can result from an injury to the ulnar nerve at either the elbow or the wrist. Interestingly, the claw hand will be more severe if

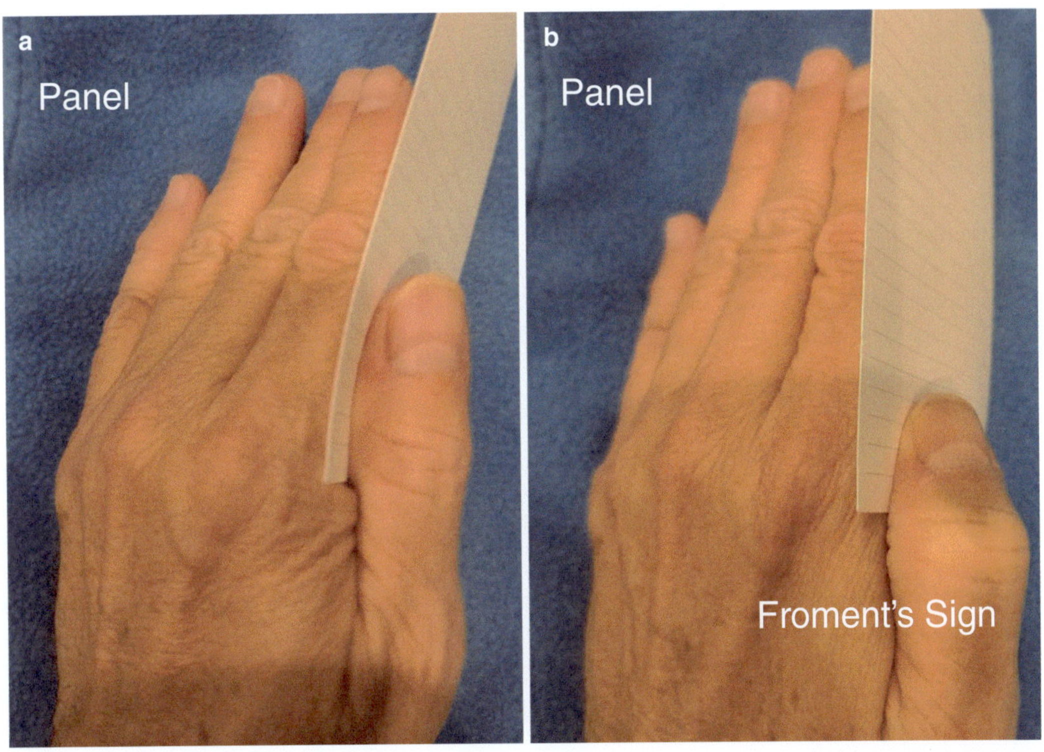

Fig. 7.32 Froment's sign. Panel (**a**) shows normal ulnar function when holding the piece of paper. The person is adducting the thumb with adductor pollicis. In Panel (**b**), the patient has an ulnar nerve palsy and instead of using their adductor pollicis, they hold the paper by flexing the metacarpal phalangeal joint of the thumb with their flexor pollicis longus which is innervated by the median nerve. The bump at the metacarpal phalangeal joint is Froment's sign [8, 9]

the ulnar nerve is compromised at the wrist as compared to an injury at the elbow—this is referred to as the *ulnar paradox*. This seems counterintuitive since usually, the closer the injury is to the midline the more severe the symptoms are. However, when the ulnar nerve is cut at the wrist this leaves the flexor digitorum profundus intact. Since this muscle is involved in flexion, the activity in this muscle will contribute to the claw hand appearance. If the nerve is cut at the elbow, then the patient loses the flexor digitorum profundus and digits 4 and 5 will open a bit.

One point to emphasize about claw hand: If the ulnar nerve is damaged the patient will exhibit the claw hand at rest. In other words, they may walk into your office with an obvious claw hand. If you are walking down the street behind them, you can observe the claw hand. You do not need to conduct a motor test to observe the claw hand. If they have a claw hand and you suspect ulnar nerve pathology, the motor task you would check is abduction/adduction of the fingers. The patient with ulnar palsy would lose this ability since they have lost the interossei.

Another minor issue with ulnar nerve palsy is that the fifth finger—the little finger- will be abducted because the third palmar interossei is compromised. This muscle wants to adduct the fifth finger, without it the finger is abducted. This is referred to as *Wartenberg's sign*—not to be confused with Wartenberg's syndrome which involves compression of superficial branch of the radial nerve.

The Median Nerve at the Hand and Wrist

The median nerve enters the wrist between the palmaris longus and flexor carpi radialis, deep to the transverse carpal ligament (flexor retinaculum) in the carpal tunnel. The floor of the carpal tunnel are the carpal bones. There are ten structures in the carpal tunnel—nine tendons and a nerve. There are the four tendons of the profundus (FDP), the four tendons of superficialis (FDS), one tendon of flexor pollicis longus, and the one median nerve.

Note that back in the forearm, the median nerve gives off the *palmar cutaneous branch of the median nerve* which carries sensation from the proximal palm. This cutaneous branch passes superficial to the carpal tunnel. With compression of the median nerve in the carpal tunnel the patient will have reduced function of the thenar muscles along with pins and tingling sensation along digits 1–3 and the lateral half of digit 4. Sensation from the proximal palm will be intact because the palmar cutaneous nerve is spared because of its location over the carpal tunnel.

Just past the carpal tunnel, the median nerve gives off two motor branches: the recurrent branch, and the palmar digital branch which innervates the two lateral lumbricals. It also gives off a palmar digital cutaneous branch which carries sensation from digits 1–3 and the lateral half of digit 4. In addition to the motor and sensory deficits, in a carpal tunnel patient there are two tests to aid in the diagnosis (Fig. 7.33):

1. *Tinel's sign* is elicited by tapping on the anterior forearm in the vicinity of the median nerve. In a carpal tunnel patient, pins and needle sensations will be felt in the hand.
2. In *Phalen's test*, both hands are flexed at the wrist with the dorsal surfaces placed again each other. This puts pressure on the carpal tunnel. Pain felt in the hand is considered a positive test for carpal tunnel compression. Phalen's test is sometimes referred to as the reverse prayer test.

Of note is that carpal tunnel symptoms are like the symptoms seen in thoracic outlet syndrome—both patients will complain of problems with their hand. However, thoracic outlet compression will affect both median and ulnar nerves, while carpal tunnel compression only affects median nerve territory.

Nerves and Arteries on Palmar Wrist

The ulnar nerve and artery enter the wrist just lateral to the flexor carpi ulnaris muscle. They are both superficial to the flexor retinaculum. The

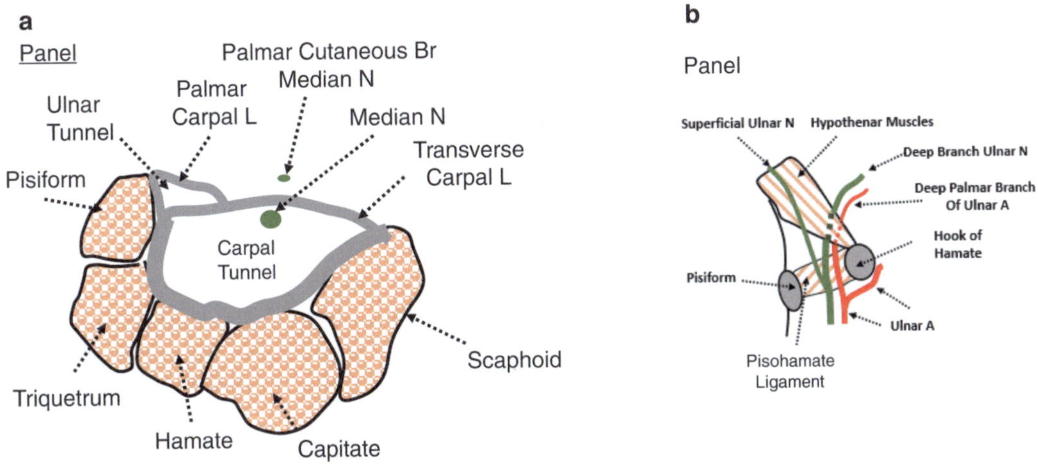

Fig. 7.33 Carpal bones. The proximal carpal bones showing the carpal tunnel with the transverse carpal ligament (roof). Panel (**a**) The ulnar tunnel is also seen on the medial side with the palmar carpal ligament forming the roof. Panel (**b**) is distal to Guyon's canal and shows the ulnar nerve superficial to the pisohamate ligament where it splits into two branches. The ulnar artery runs lateral to the hamate [8, 9]

radial artery enters the wrist just lateral to the flexor carpi radialis. The radial artery pulse can be felt between flexor carpi radialis and brachioradialis. The median nerve enters the wrist deep to the flexor retinaculum.

There are two arterial arches in the hand—a superficial and a deep arch. The main source of the *superficial palmar arch* is the ulnar artery, the main source of the *deep palmar arch* is the radial artery, however, both the radial and ulnar arteries contribute to both arches. *Allen's test* involves compressing the two arteries and then releasing the pressure on either one. If there is sufficient patency of the arteries, then blood traveling on either artery should be sufficient to fill the entire hand (Fig. 7.34).

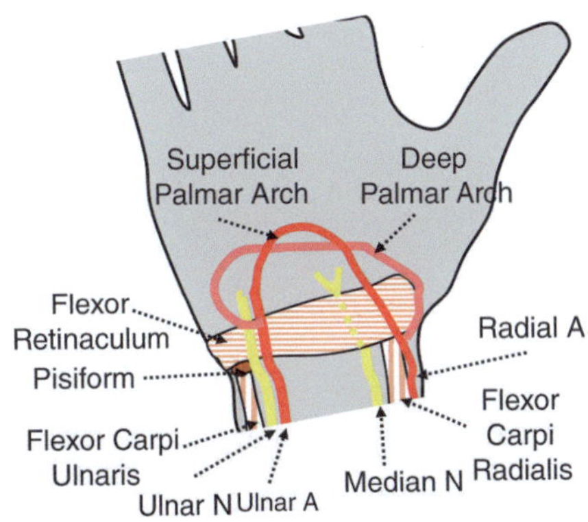

Fig. 7.34 Wrist relationships. Note the ulnar nerve and artery are lateral to the flexor carpi ulnaris. The radial artery is lateral to the flexor carpi radialis. The median nerve goes deep to the flexor retinaculum, while the ulnar nerve goes superficial [8, 9]

Median Nerve Palsy

There are high injuries and low injuries to the median nerve. Let us start with a high injury. As an example, take an injury just above the elbow. In this case the patient would lose most of the flexors located in the anterior forearm. These patients will often be said to have "the pope's blessing sign", or the "sign of benediction." This is easily confused with claw hand which is seen with an ulnar palsy. If you look at a picture of the two, they look similar, but there is a major difference.

As mentioned before, a patient with claw hand walks around with claw hand. When they walk into your office you can see the claw hand. You do not have to ask them to do something with the hand to elicit the claw hand. However, the patient with the sign of benediction does not walk around with this appearance. The sign of benediction refers to a motor test and the patient does not exhibit this sign until you test them. To explain this, we need to focus on the eight long tendons going to the four fingers. Each finger has two tendons running down the palmar side—one tendon of FDP and one tendon of FDS. If you ask a healthy person to flex digits 2–5, they are using all eight tendons. In a patient with a median nerve palsy, only two tendons are functioning—the two tendons of FDP going to digits 4 and 5. So, when you ask this person to flex their fingers, they can only flex digits 4 and 5, resulting in the hand resembling a religious figure blessing the crowd (Fig. 7.29).

A patient with median nerve palsy is sometimes said to have an "ape hand" because they lose opposition of the thumb and over time the thenar muscles will atrophy.

A patient with a low injury will have a similar set of signs and symptoms but they will not have the sign of benediction—because the flexor digitorum longus is still functioning.

Ulnar Collateral Ligament and Gamekeeper's Thumb

The metacarpophalangeal joint of the thumb is supported by the *ulnar collateral ligament.* The ligament is prone to hyperextension injuries, such as a skier falling and landing on their outstretched thumb. A high incidence was also seen in Scottish gamekeepers who killed their prey, such as rabbits, by pushing down on their necks with an outstretched thumb, thus the name gamekeeper's thumb (Fig. 7.35).

Nerves to Fingers

In the hand, on the palmar side, both the median and ulnar nerves give rise to *common palmar digital nerves*. As these nerves approach the metacarpal phalangeal joints, they split into

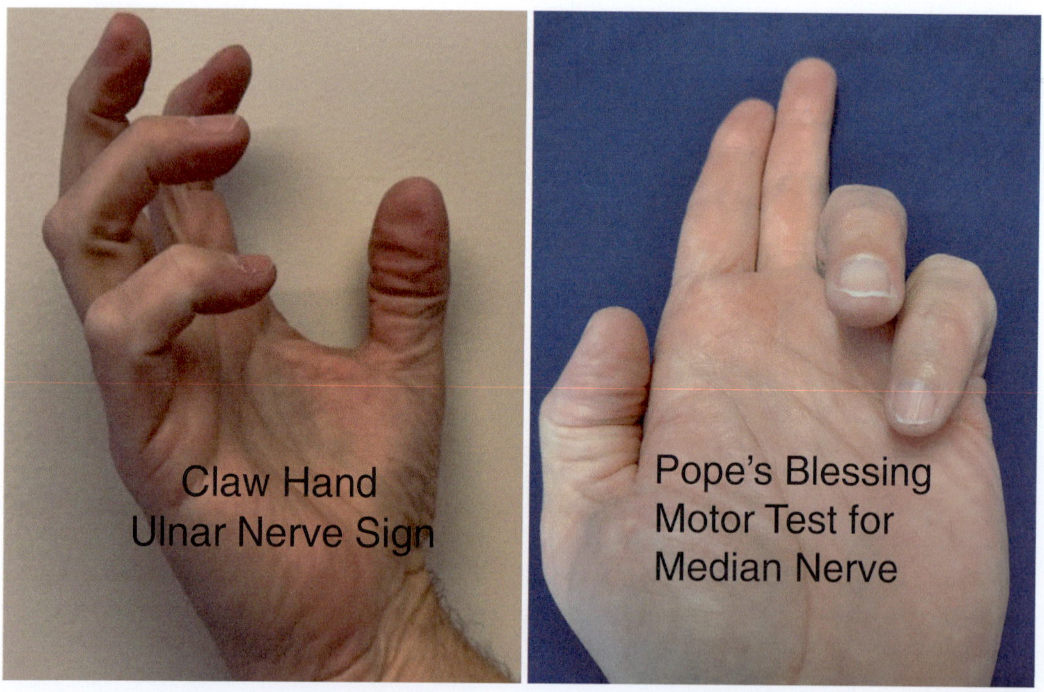

Fig. 7.35 Claw hand and Pope's blessing. Claw hand is a sign for ulnar nerve palsy. Pope's blessing is what happens in a patient with a median nerve palsy on attempted finger flexion. The only two tendons working are the two tendons of flexor digitorum profundus on the ulnar side [8, 9]

proper palmar digital nerves which travel down and innervate the palmar side of the digits. However, the proper palmar digital nerves also give rise to the dorsal branches of the palmar digital nerves which cross the fingers from anterior to posterior to innervate the distal fingertips (nailbeds) on the dorsal side of the hand. Keep in mind that on the dorsal side of the hand, the skin of the proximal and middle phalanges is innervated by the median and ulnar nerves that come from the palmar side of the hand (Fig. 7.36).

Everything Is Not Always So Straightforward

In the upper limb, as the median and ulnar nerves are traveling towards the hand, occasionally there are some small nerve fibers that run from one nerve to the other. This can happen in both the forearm (Martin-Gruber anastomosis) and in the wrist (Cannieu-Riche's anastomosis). For instance, the deep belly of the flexor pollicis brevis may receive branches from both median and ulnar nerves. For a first year student the crucial point here is that you should concern yourself with the typical scenarios for nerve damage. However, just be aware that variations can complicate the real world scenarios.

Upper and Lower Tunk Injuries

Two other injuries that can result in nerve deficits are upper and lower trunk injuries. These injuries occur following strain on the shoulder which can damage the roots emerging from the spinal cord. To think about these injuries, you can mimic this yourself. If you are standing with your left upper limb hanging down by your side, take your right hand and push down on your left shoulder. You should feel it get tighter in your neck area. Injuries that push down on your shoulder will damage the superior part of the plexus which is C5-C6, while the lower part of the plexus is relaxed. *These are superior trunk injuries.*

To mimic *lower trunk injuries*, if you fully abduct your left upper limb, with your hand and fingers trying to touch the ceiling, you should feel tightness in your armpit (the upper thoracic region in the mid axillary line), while the upper part of your shoulder relaxes. It is the lower part of the brachial plexus, C8-T1, that is injured.

1. *Lower trunk injuries* that damage C8-T1 will lead to weakness in the hand in both median and ulnar nerve territories. In addition, the patient may present with Horner's syndrome resulting from damage to the preganglionic sympathetic fibers that emerge at the T1 level

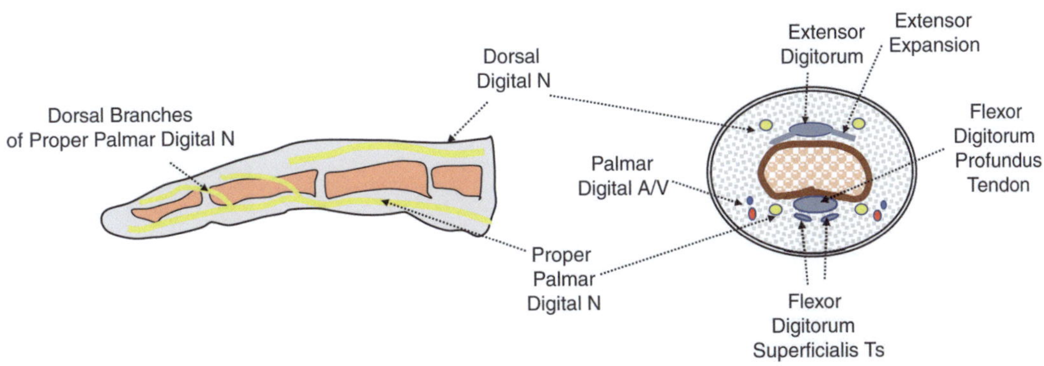

Fig. 7.36 Nerves to fingers. The proper digital nerves are on the palmar side with the palmar digital artery and vein. The proper palmar digital nerves send dorsal branches from the palmar side to the dorsal side to innervate the nail beds. The dorsal digital branches are only on the proximal dorsal side of the fingers [8, 9]

to jump on the ascending sympathetic trunk on their way to the head. Lower trunk injuries can occur during a delivery when the upper limb is pulled, or when a child is playing on a jungle gym and swings by their hands on the bars, etc.

2. *Upper trunk injuries* that damage C5–6 roots will lead to damage in the shoulder and arm regions. In addition, in about 50% of these injuries C7 is damaged. If we look at what nerves are affected, what these nerves normally do, and what happens when they are damaged, we can think through the symptoms. C5 and C6 fibers get into the axillary and suprascapular nerves which will normally abduct (deltoid) and laterally rotate (infraspinatus and teres minor) the shoulder. Without the deltoid and the lateral rotators, the upper limb will be adducted and medially rotated. C5 roots also make their way into the musculocutaneous nerve, which is involved in supination and flexion. Without this nerve, the upper limb will be extended at the elbow and pronated. The upper limb will hang by the side and will be pronated. This is sometimes referred to as "waiter's tip" sign which refers to the waiter walking by the table with their hand out subtly asking for a tip.

   Note that in an adult with an upper trunk injury, the medial rotation at the shoulder might not be obvious—the pronated wrist and flexed hand is more prominent. You can test this on yourself: With your upper limb hanging straight down, and your forearm in the waiter's tip position, now medially rotate at your shoulder and you will notice that it is a subtle sign—barely noticeable, especially if you have a shirt on.

   On the other hand, in an infant with an upper trunk injury, because their bones are still growing, the absence of the lateral rotators will eventually lead to a permanently malformed glenohumeral joint with obvious excessive medial rotation of the shoulder. To prevent this, it is important to treat early in infants, typically with a nerve graft. C7 is often used in these cases since none of the major upper limb actions rely strictly on C7, so moving the C7 nerve does not leave a group of muscles devoid of a nerve supply. This is all assuming C7 is intact.

Distal Fractures of the Radius

Falling on an outstretched extended hand can lead to a fracture of the distal radius (transverse fracture) known as *Colle's fracture*—or a "Dinner Fork Deformity." Looking at the injured radius from the side it resembles a dinner fork with a bump on it. The bump is made by the proximal segment pushed anteriorly, and the distal segment pushed posteriorly.

A *Smith's fracture* most likely occurs from a fall on the flexed hand. In contrast to Colle's fracture, the distal segment of the radius will be displaced towards the palmar side.

Fractures of the Humerus

There are four common fractures that can damage associated arteries and nerves (Fig. 7.37):

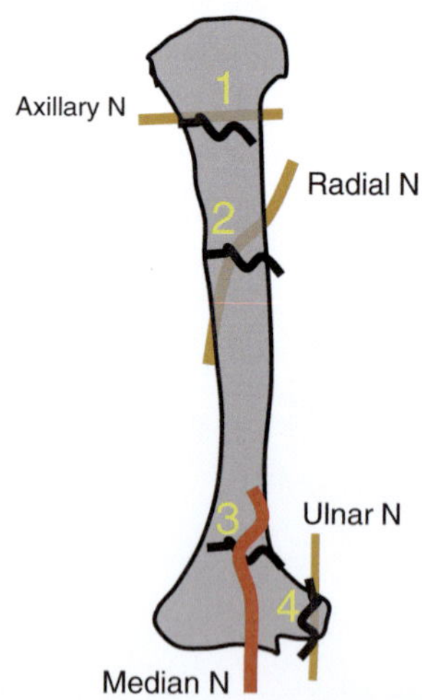

Fig. 7.37 Humerus fractures. There are four common fractures to the humerus, all of which can damage a different nerve. (1) Surgical Neck: Axillary nerve, (2) Midshaft: Radial nerve, (3) Supracondylar: Median nerve, (4) Medial Epicondyle: Ulnar nerve [8, 9]

1. A fracture of the *surgical neck* can damage the axillary nerve and the posterior humeral circumflex artery.
2. *A mid-shaft* humeral fracture can damage the radial nerve and the profunda brachii artery. Keep in mind that the muscles in a compartment are usually innervated at the superior portion of the compartment. So when it comes to a radial nerve fracture at the mid-shaft of the humerus this means that the triceps is intact. This patient would still be able to extend at the elbow, but they would have a deficit of wrist and finger extension. The patient would have "wrist drop" meaning that without extension of the wrist, the wrist would be stuck in flexion. Besides a fracture at this point, Saturday night palsy refers to compression of the radial nerve along the humerus which leads to loss of extension of the wrist and fingers. The term *Saturday night palsy* is named for the person who comes home from the bar on Saturday night and falls asleep in a chair with their arm resting all night on the top of the chair. This leads to a temporary compression of the radial nerve and subsequent radial nerve palsy signs. Poorly fitting crutches can also aggravate the radial nerve here.
3. A *supracondylar fracture* is to the distal humerus, and it can damage several different nerves, but the median nerve is the nerve to be affected. In addition, the brachial artery can be compressed which leads to a loss of blood flow to the forearm. This can lead to shortening of the forearm muscles which results in the hand, wrist, and fingers being flexed into a claw-like position. This is referred to as *Volkmann's contracture.*
4. A fracture of the *medial epicondyle* can damage the ulnar nerve and the superior ulnar collateral artery.

Peripheral Nerve Map of the Upper Limb

In addition to the motor deficits in the hand following injuries, patients will often have detrimental sensory deficits. Sensation from our fingers is important for day-to-day activities. On the palmar side, the median nerve supplies the thumb and digits 1–3, and the lateral half of 4. The ulnar nerve carries sensation from the hypothenar region and the medial half of digit 4 and all the palmar surface of digit 5 (Fig. 7.32).

On the dorsum of the hand, the radial nerve is responsible for a patch of skin centered around the first dorsal webspace. In addition, the proximal dorsal side of the digits are innervated by the radial and ulnar nerves (Fig. 7.38).

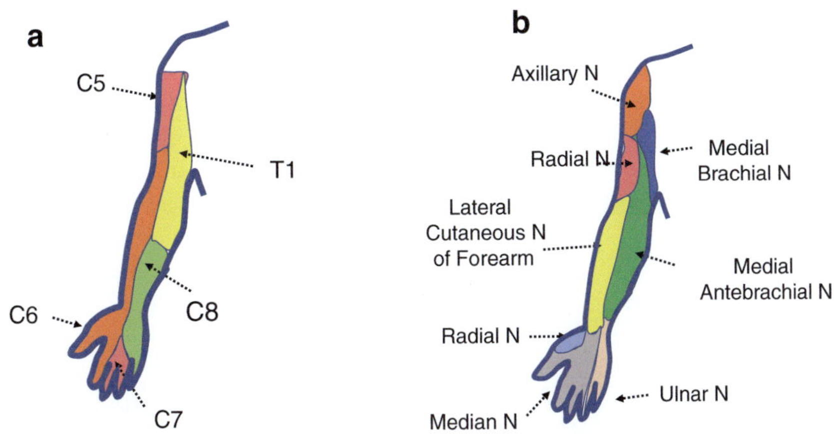

Fig. 7.38 Roots vs peripheral nerves. Panel (**a**) shows the dermatomes of the upper limb. The thumb is C6, middle fingers are C7, and pinky is C8. Panel (**b**) shows the peripheral nerve map of the upper limb [8, 9]

Dermatomes of Upper Limb

Note that the thumb is C6, middle fingers are C7, pinky is C8, and the armpit is T1. With radiculopathies you want to think about the *dermatome map*, with peripheral nerve injuries you want to think about the *peripheral nerve map*. For a more in-depth discussion see the chapter on the back. If you think of making a "6" by pinching your thumb and second digit it can be a reminder that the thumb dermatome is C6 (Fig. 7.32).

As an example of how knowing the difference between dermatomes and peripheral nerve is important, compare a lesion of the lateral cutaneous nerve to a lesion of C6. In both cases the lateral forearm will be affected but with a C6 root lesion that thumb will also be affected but with a lesion to the lateral cutaneous nerve of the forearm, the thumb will be spared.

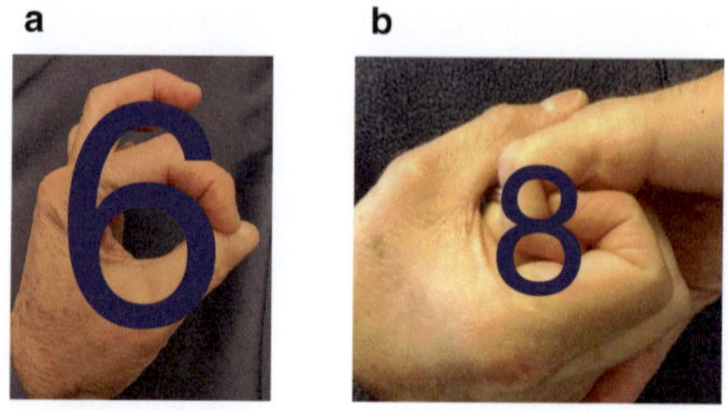

Fig. 7.39 Tricks to remember root levels. Panel (**a**) If you make a pinching motion with your thumb and second digit, you are making what looks like a "6." The thumb is the C6 dermatome. Panel (**b**) If you put your fingers together and make a "fig. 8" it should help you remember that flexion of the fingers, the myotome, is C8 [8, 9]

Table 7.3 Upper limb myotomes (motor function)

Level	Rhyme	Action
C2	Look at your shoe	Neck flexion
C3	A fallen tree	Neck lateral flexion
C4	I'm not sure	Shoulder shrug
C5	Arms out wide	Shoulder abd/elbow flex
C6	Smell your wrist	Wrist ext/elbow flex
C7	No zombies in heaven or Brint it on	Wrist flex/elbow ext/ finger ext
C8	You're doing great	Thumb ext/finger flexion/ulnar deviation
T1	One and done	Finger abduction

Myotomes of the Upper Limb

When it comes to the nerve root levels of the upper limb, the shoulder is C 4, 5. The elbow is C 5, 6, 7, and 8. The wrist is C 6, 7, 8, and T1. Flexion of the fingers is C 8. A straightforward way to remember this is to interlock your flexed fingers from both hands together and see that you are making an "8" (Fig. 7.39). Abduction and adduction of your fingers is a test for T1 (Table 7.3). Table 7.3 highlights the myotomes involved with various movements at each upper limb joint. Note that the shoulder abduction is C5, elbow flexion is C5 and C6 while elbow extension is C6 and C7. At the wrist, note that C6 and C7 are both involved with flexion and extension. At the fingers, C8 does flexion, while T1 does abduction and adduction of the fingers.

Upper Limb Root Injuries

When the roots to the upper limb are injured as they leave the spinal cord there will be a characteristic pattern of deficits. The patient will have a weakness in muscles innervated by that group (myotome), a specific sensory loss (dermatome), and in most cases, but not all, a deficit (hyporeflexia) in a specific reflex. For C8 and T1 there is no good reflex test. The *Spurling test* can be used to assess cervical radiculopathy. The patient's neck is side-bent and rotated towards the damaged side, and then the examiner places downward pressure to the top of the head. Pain down the upper limb indicates a possible radiculopathy. In the chapters on the back and the lower limb there is a more extensive discussion about root injuries in general, at this point the focus is just on the upper limb (Fig. 7.40 and Table 7.4).

Hand and Finger Grips

There are several positions of the hand and fingers that humans use daily (Fig. 7.41).

Fig. 7.40 Upper Limb Radiculopathies

Root	Muscle Weakness	Sensory Deficit	Decreased Reflex
C5	Deltoid, Biceps	Lateral Arm	Biceps
C6	Wrist Extension	Lateral Forearm, Thumb	Brachioradialis
C7	Finger Extension	Index Finger	Triceps
C8	Finger Flexion	Medial Hand, Medial Forearm	None
T1	Abduction/Adduction of the Fingers (Interossei)	Medial Arm	None

Table 7.4 Spinal Cord Levels of Upper Limb Nerves

Nerve	Level
Suprascapular	C5 6
Dorsal scapular	C5
Long thoracic	C5–7
Thoracodorsal	C6–8
Axillary	C 5–6
Radial	C5–8
Median	C 5–8
Ulnar	C8–T1
Musculocutaneous	C5–7

Pincer Grip: The best example of this is threading a needle. You will hold the thread between your thumb and index finger.

Tripod Grip: The best example of this is holding a pen. Unlike the pincer grip which uses two fingers, the tripod grip uses three fingers.

The Key Grip: This grip also involves two fingers but compared to the pincer grip it is used for power. Besides holding a key, it is also used when holding and using a screwdriver.

Power Grip: When you want to hold something in your wrist, such as a baseball bat, you use all your fingers plus your thumb. Importantly the wrist is in a neutral position, meaning that it is straight up and down and not flexed or extended. In a patient with radial nerve palsy and the subsequent wrist drop, the power grip will be weakened (Figs. 7.42, 7.43, 7.44, 7.45 and 7.46).

Summary of Major Nerves to the Upper Limb and Their Lesions

Historical Snippet: The First African American Anatomy Professor in the US

In 1868, Alexander Thomas August was named as an anatomy professor at Howard University becoming the first African American professor at a medical college in the US. He was born in Virginia on March 8, 1825, to free people of color. Although he was free, he was denied entrance to medical school in the United States. He subsequently went to Trinity medical school in Toronto Canada. In 1863, after Lincoln signed the Emancipation Proclamation, Alexander wrote President Lincoln offering his services but was again denied. To make his case, he traveled to Washington DC to make his request in person. This time he was given a chance, and in 1863, after passing the medical license exam, he became a surgeon for the 7th US Colored Infantry. In the history books he is known for many "Firsts," including: the first US Army's African American doctor, the first African American head of a hospital, and the first African American professor of medicine, After the war, he went back to private practice and became an anatomy professor at Howard University. To his list of accolades, should also be: The first African American Anatomy Professor in the US. He died on December 21, 1890, and is buried at Arlington National Cemetery (Fig. 7.47).

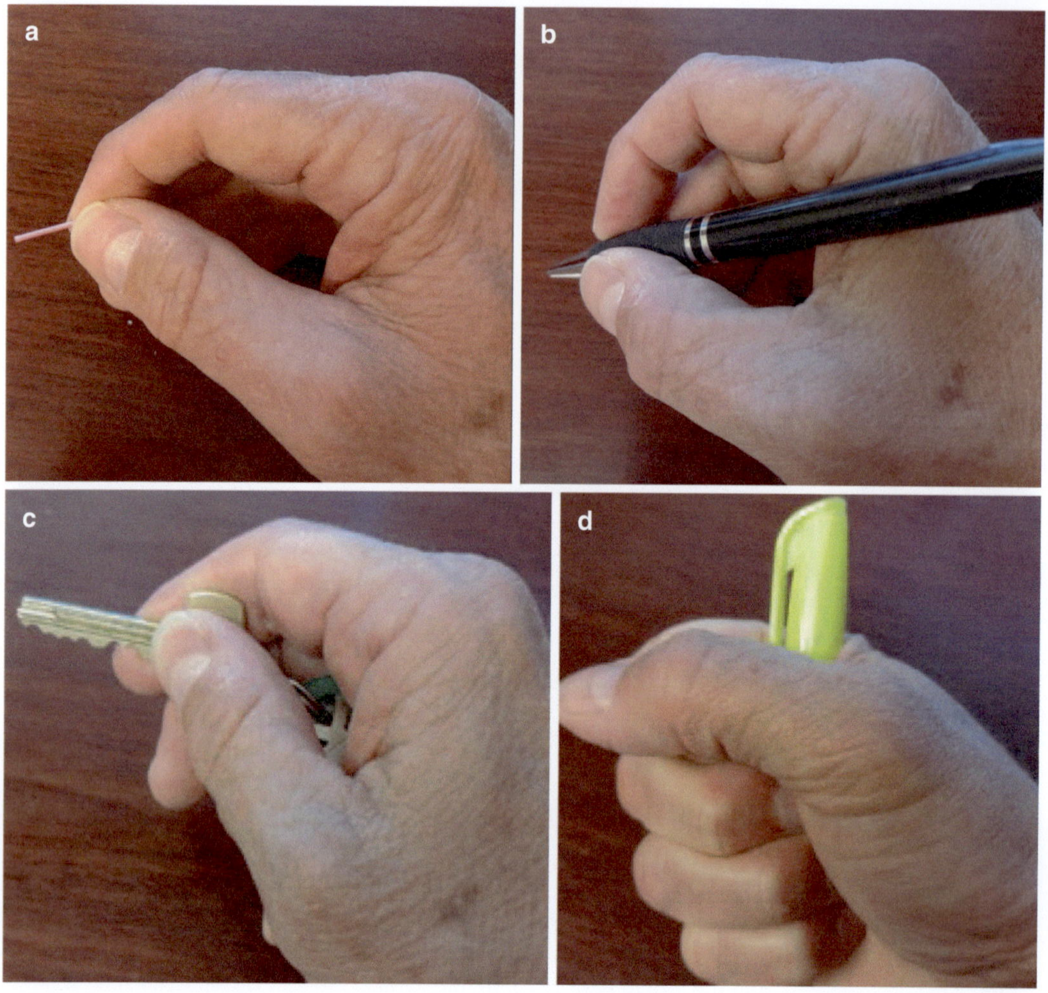

Fig. 7.41 Hand grips. Panel (**a**) Pincer grip. Panel (**b**) Tripod grip. Panel (**c**) Key grip. Panel (**d**) Power grip [8, 9]

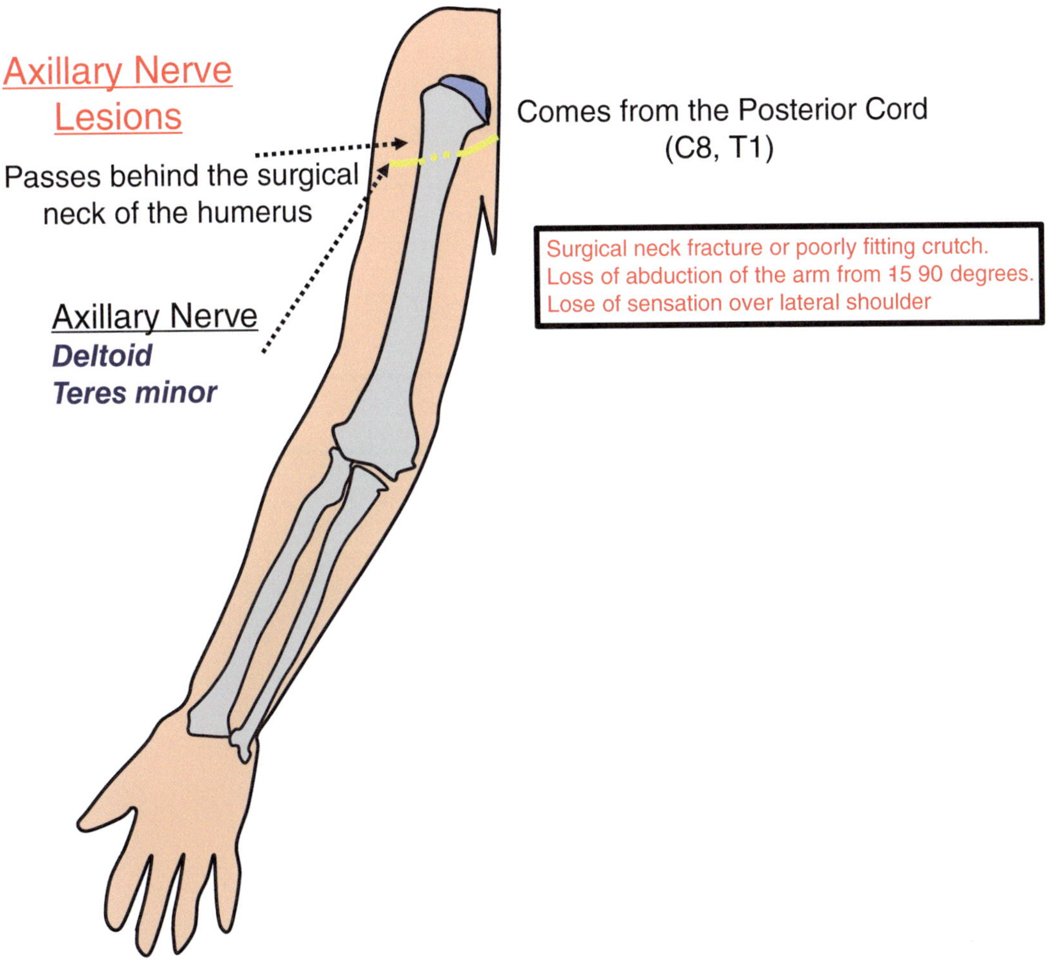

Fig. 7.42 Axillary nerve lesion summary

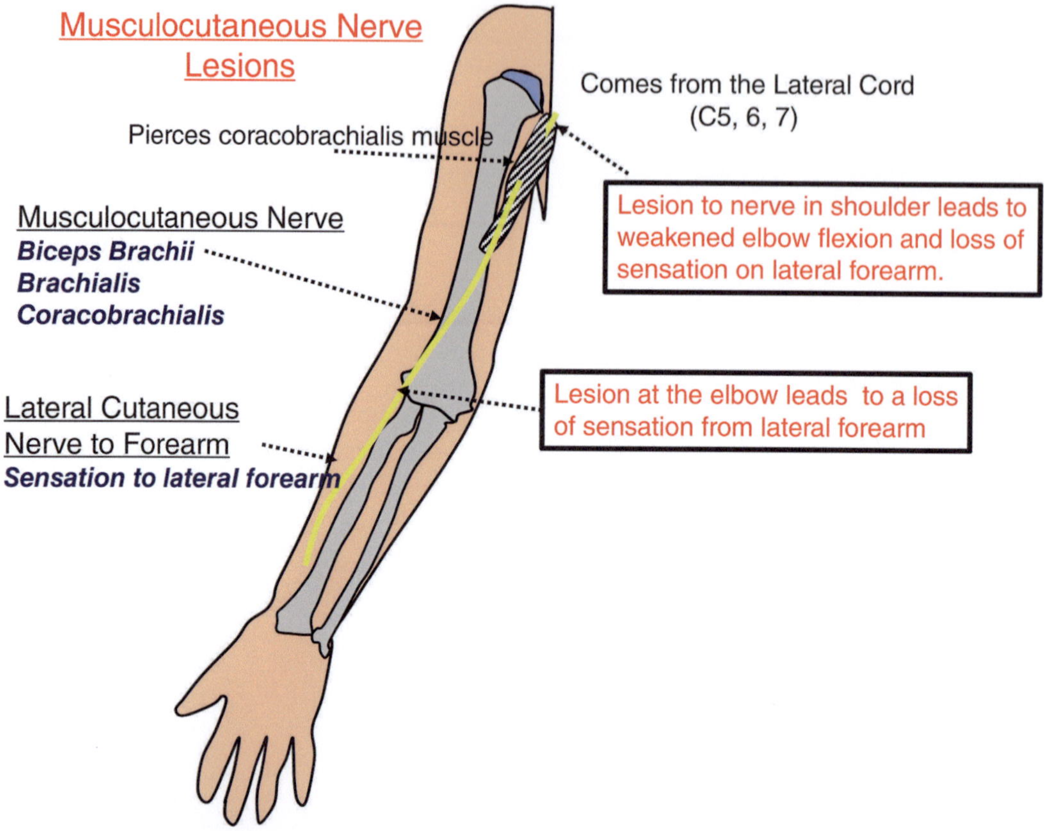

Fig. 7.43 Musculocutaneous nerve lesion summary

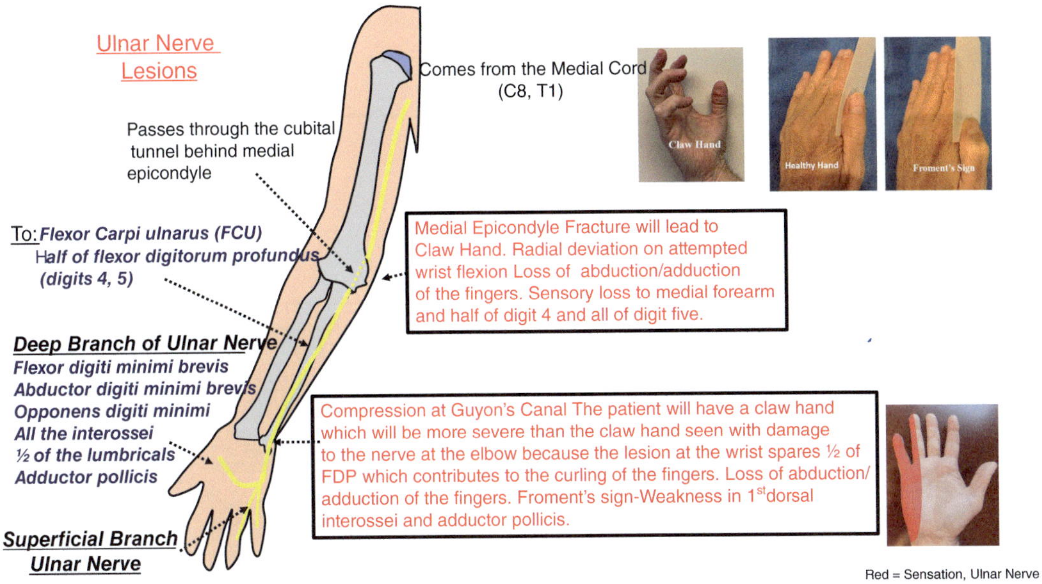

Fig. 7.44 Ulnar nerve lesion summary

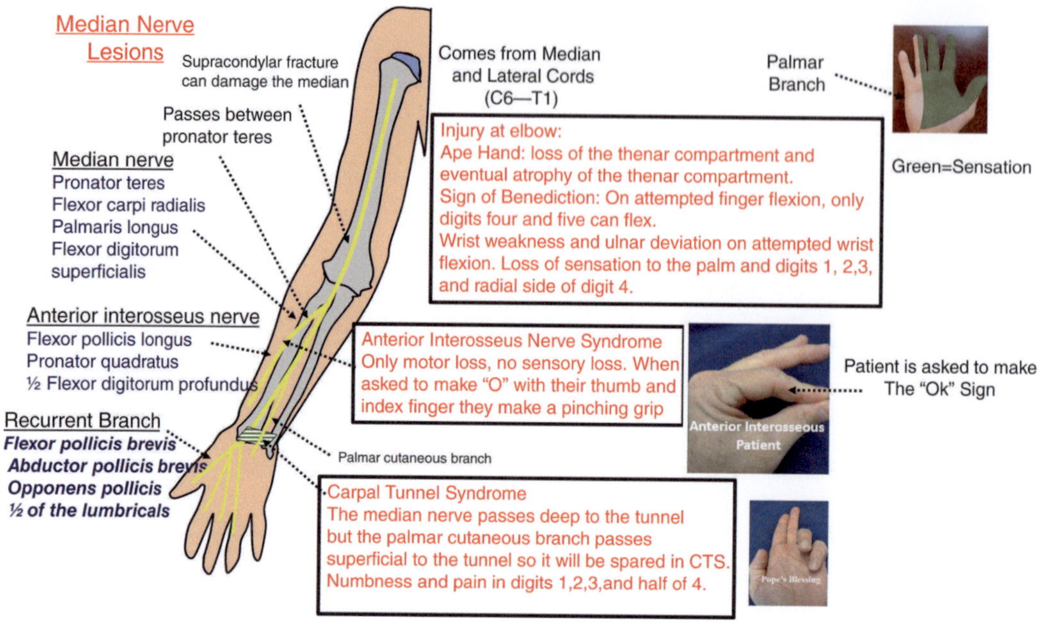

Fig. 7.45 Median nerve lesion summary

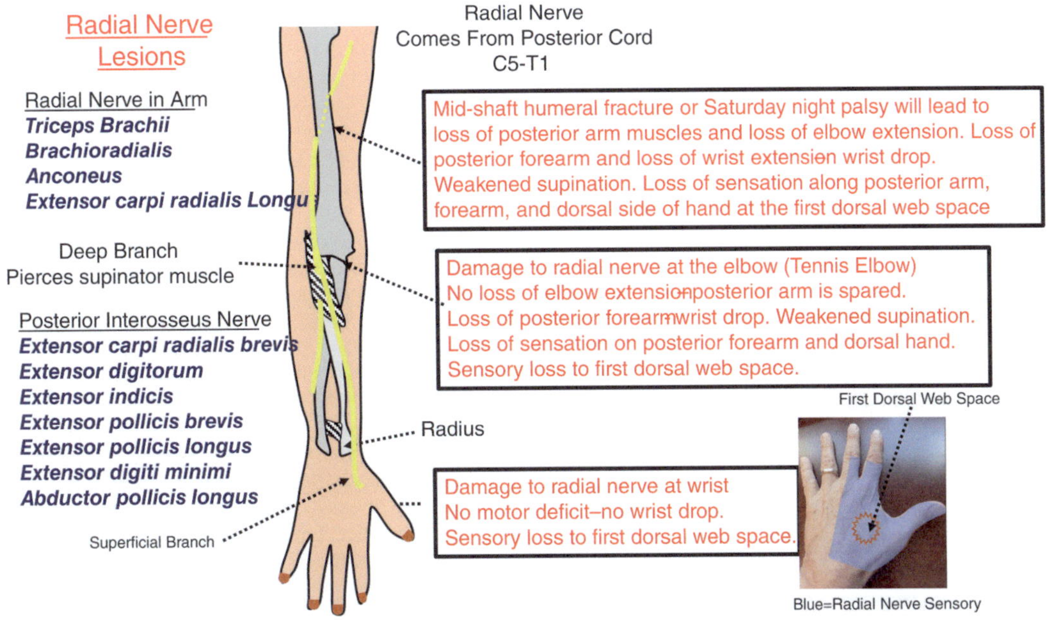

Fig. 7.46 Radial nerve lesion summary

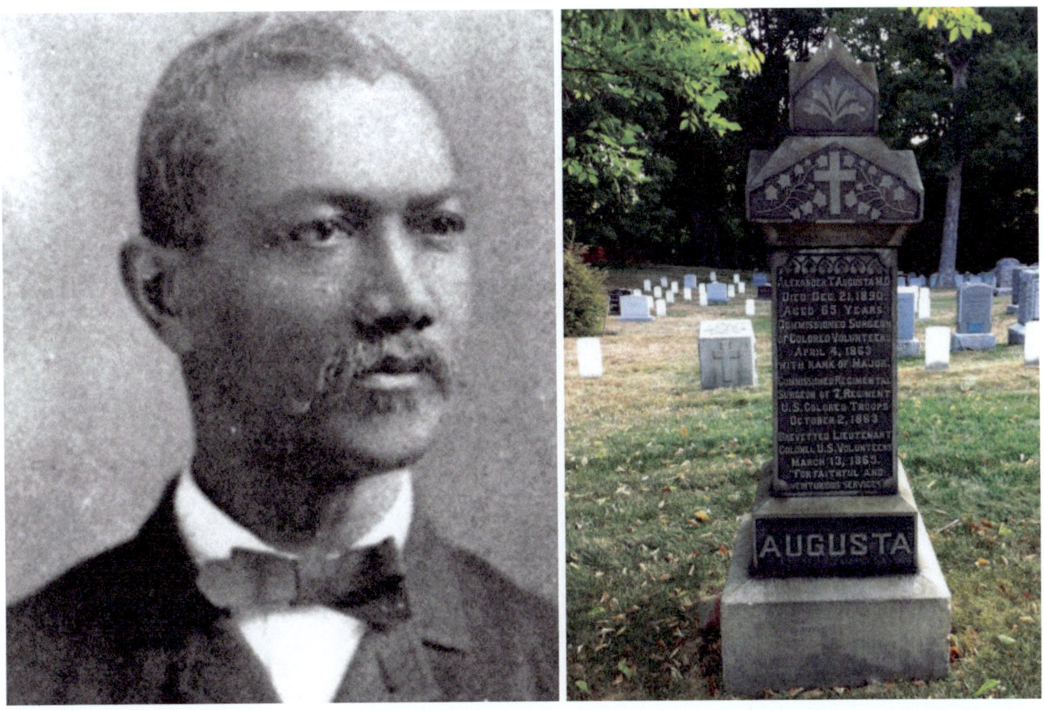

Fig. 7.47 Alexander thomas augusta. First African American Doctor in the United States Army plus, the first African American Anatomy Professor in the US

Further Reading

1. Bharambe V, Arole V. The axillary arch muscle (Langer's muscle): clinical importance. Med J DY Patil Univ. 2013;6(3):327–30.
2. Caetano EB, Nakamichi Y, de Andrade RA, et al. Flexor pollicis brevis muscle. Anatomical and study and clinical implications. Open Ortho. 2017;11:1321–9.
3. Chater M, Camfield C. Erb's palsy—who is to blame and what will happen? Ped Child Health. 2004;9(8):556–60.
4. D'Arcy CA, McGee S. Does this patient have carpal tunnel syndrome? JAMA. 2000;283(23):3110–7.
5. Chidgey LK. The distal radioulnar joint: problems and solutions. J Am Acad Orthop Surg. 1995;3(2):95–109.
6. Gaur NL, Soni JS, Gaur S. The innervation of brachialis muscle by radial nerve in Gujarat region—a human cadaveric study. Int J Anat Res. 2020;8(12):7328–32.
7. Han BR, Yong JC, Yang JS, Kang SH, Choi HJ. Clinical features of wrist drop caused by compressive radial neuropathy and its anatomical considerations. J Korean Neurosurg Soc. 2014;55(3):148–51.
8. Henig GS. The indomitable Dr. Augusta: the first black physician in the US Army. Army Hist. 2013;87(Spring):23–31.
9. Leo J. Medical neuroanatomy for the boards and clinic: finding the lesion. 2nd ed. Cham: Springer; 2024.
10. Leo J. Clinical anatomy and embryology: a guide for the classroom, clinic, and clinic. 2nd ed. Springer; 2024.
11. Maroukis BL, Ogawa T, Rehim SA, Chung KC. Guyon canal: the evolution of clinical anatomy. J Hand Surg Am. 2016;40(3):560–5.
12. Moore K, Dalley AF, Agur A. Clinically oriented anatomy. 7th ed. Baltimore: Lippincott Williams and Wilkins; 2014.
13. Nzeako O, Tahmassebi R, John-Lewis J, Baggott J. The truth about the hand of benediction. Open Access Library J. 11:e11425.
14. Pearl M. Shoulder problems in children with brachial plexus birth palsy: evaluation and management. J Am Acad Orthop Surg. 2009;7:242–54.
15. Razak L. Pathophysiology of pelvic organ prolapse, pelvic floor disorders. Raheela M. Rizvi, IntechOpen; 2018. https://doi.org/10.5772/intechopen.76629. Available from: https://www.intechopen.com/chapters/60935
16. Robertson WC, Eichman PL, Clancy WG. Upper trunk brachial plexopathy in football players. JAMA. 1973;231(14):1480–3.
17. Rosse C, Gaddum-Rosse P. Hollinshead's textbook of anatomy. 5th ed. New York: Lippincott-Raven; 1997.
18. Standring S. Gray's anatomy: the anatomical basis of clinical practice. London: Elsevier; 2005.
19. Stoker GE, Kim HJ, Riew K. Differentiating C8-T1 radiculopathy from ulnar neuropathy: a survey of 24 spine surgeons. Global Spine J. 2014;4:1–6.
20. Tay SC, Tomita K, Berger RA. The "ulnar fovea sign" for defining ulnar wrist pain: an analysis of sensitivity and specificity. J Hand Surg. 2007;32(4):438–44.
21. Umar M, Qadir I, Azam M. Subacromial impingement syndrome. Orthop Rev. 2012;4(2):e18.
22. Xiao K, Zhang J, Li T, Dong YL, Weng XS. Anatomy, definition, and treatment of the "terrible triad of the elbow" and contemplation of the rationality of this designation. Orthop Surg. 2015;7:13–8.

8 The Back

Occipital Bone

Along the posterior surface of the occipital bone, there are several important landmarks. The bump that you can feel on the back of your skull is the *external occipital protuberance*. The point of the external occipital protuberance is the *inion*. Running laterally from the external occipital protuberance is the *superior nuchal line*. And then inferior and parallel to it is the *inferior nuchal line*.

Atlas (C1)

The *atlas* or C1 sits right below the skull. It does not have a vertebral body or a intervertebral disk. Laterally are the two *lateral masses* with their *superior articular facets* and *inferior articular facets*. The superior articular facets articulate with the occipital condyles to form the *alanto-occipital joint*. The main movements at this joint are flexion and extension—think of a person nodding "yes." The atlas also has an anterior and posterior arch to complete its ring structure. On the superior surface of the posterior arch, on each side, there is a groove for the vertebral artery as it passes from lateral to medial on its way to the foramen magnum. The atlas does not have a spinous process but instead has a posterior tubercle. On its anterior arch there is an articular surface on the posterior side for the articulation with the dens.

Axis (C2)

The most prominent feature of the *axis* (C2) is the superiorly projecting dens (or odontoid process) that lies against the posterior surface of anterior arch of the atlas. The superior articular facets of the axis meet the inferior facets of the atlas (C1) to form the *lateral atlantoaxial joints*. Movement at the atlantoaxial joints mainly involves side-to-side movement—think of person nodding "no." The articulation of the dens with the axis in the midline forms the single *medial atlantoaxial joint* (Fig. 8.1).

J. Leo, *Gross Anatomy, Neuroanatomy, and Embryology for Medical Students*,
https://doi.org/10.1007/978-3-031-87151-1_8

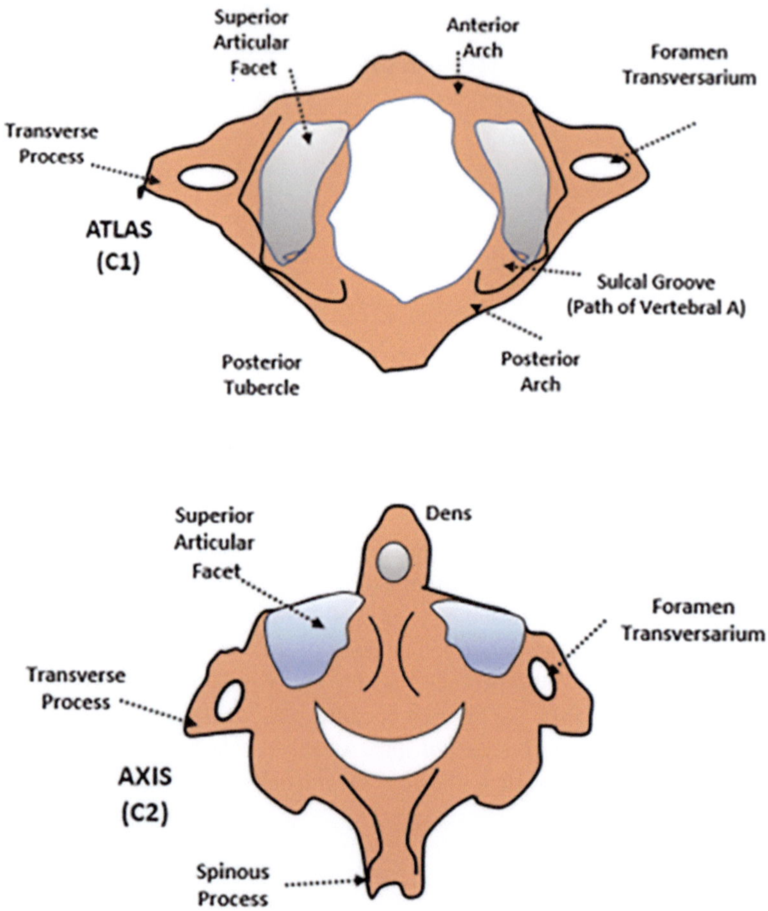

Fig. 8.1 The atlas and axis [5, 6]

Cruciate and Alar Ligaments

The dens is held in place by several ligaments. The most prominent is the cruciate ligament with its four bands resembling a cross. Running horizontally across the dens and holding it in place is the transverse ligment. The superior and inferior bands run vertically to aid in support. Besides the cruciate ligment there is the odontoid ligament made up of apical and alar ligaments. The apical ligament runs from the top of the dens to the occiptal bone, and the alar ligament projects superiorly and diagonally from the dens to the occipital condyles. The tectorial membrane is the extension of the posterior longitudinal ligament from C2 to the skull. The anterior longitudinal ligament continues to the skull as the anterior atlantooccipital membrane. The ligamenta flava continues as the posterior atlantooccipital membrane (Fig. 8.2).

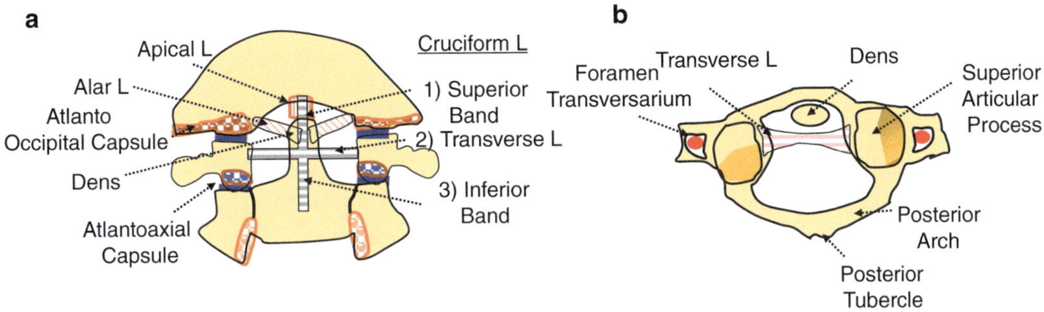

Fig. 8.2 Atlas and axis. Panel (**a**) is a posterior view of the cruciform ligament—shaped like a cross. It has a (*1*) superior band (*2*) transverse ligament, and (*3*) inferior band. The alar ligament attaches to the dens. Panel (**b**) is a superior view of the atlas showing the dens held in place against the atlas by the transverse ligament [5, 6]

Cervical Fractures

The atlas is a ring, and when rings are fractured, just like the pelvis, there are typically multiple fracture lines. A *Jefferson fracture* is a burst fracture to the atlas (C1) following severe trauma—such as diving into the shallow end of the pool or a lake. It usually results in four fracture lines forming a square with a fracture at each corner of the square: two to the anterior arch, and two to the posterior arch. If the patient survives the trauma they will typically recover and have no long term deficits.

A hangman's fracture is a burst fracture that involves the axis (C2). It often occurs when there is significant whiplash with the head being rocked back and forth resulting in a bilateral fractures of the pedicles or pars interarticularis.

Another common fracture of the axis is to the dens and it can from either hyperflexion or hyperextension of the neck—automobile accidents for instance. With a dens fracture the bone typically looses its blood supply resulting in avacular necrosis. There is typically enough space within the canal to accommodate the displaced dens so that the spinal cord is not necessarily compromised. On the other hand, rupture of the transverse ligmament can be life threatening because the dens can now compress the spinal cord with catastrophic results. Compression fractures can damage the C3–C7 vertebrae. The most common cervical fracture is to C5.

Injuries to cervical fractures are life-altering events. The phrenic nerve comes from C3 to C5 which means that patients with complete transections of the cord at C3 or higher will need permanent ventilation to live. If the lesion is below C8 the patient will be able to use crutches. Remember C8 is important for the hands. If the lesion is just below C6 they will not be able to use crutches but they will be able to use a wheelchair. They will need assistance getting into and out of the chair but once they are in the chair they will have some mobility.

Suboccipital Triangle

The suboccipital triangle sits between the base of the skull and the top of the vertebral column. A series of strap-like muscles form a scaffold that needs to balance two opposing jobs. On one hand the muscles must be strong enough to protect the head, brain and spinal cord, but they also need to allow a certain amount of flexibility for the head to move. To understand the suboccipital triangle you need to discuss the bones, ligaments, nerves, and arteries just inferior to the base of the skull.

The borders of the suboccipital triangle are composed of three muscles: (1) the rectus capitus posterior major, (2) the obliquus capitus inferior, and the (3) obliquus capitus superior. In the floor of the triangle, running from lateral to medial, is the vertebral artery. Emerging from the triangle is

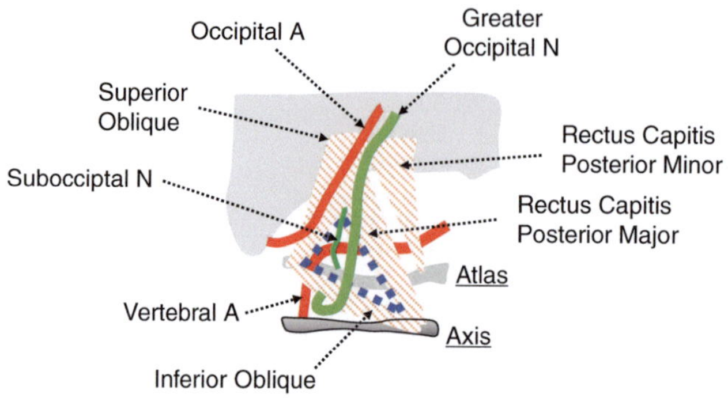

Fig. 8.3 Suboccipital triangle. The suboccipital triangle is bounded by the dotted blue line. In the floor of the triangle is vertebral artery. Below the inferior oblique muscle is the greater occipital nerve (dorsal ramus C2). The suboccipital nerve (dorsal ramus C1) is found within the suboccipital triangle [5, 6]

the suboccipital nerve which is the dorsal ramus of C1. Emerging below the triangle is the greater occipital nerve (Fig. 8.3).

The rectus capitis posterior minor runs from the posterior tubercle of the atlas to the inferior nuchal line of the skull. The rectus capitis posterior major lies lateral and runs from the spinous process of the axis to the skull. The obliquus capitis inferior (inferior oblique) runs from the spinous process of the axis (C2) to the transverse process of the atlas (C1). The obliquus capitus superior (superior oblique) runs from the transverse process of the atlas to the skull.

Back Ligaments

The ligaments of the back surround the vertebral bodies and the vertebral canal. Knowledge of these ligaments can be tested by asking about lumbar punctures and which structures a needle will move through—and which structures it will not move through in various scenarios.

Anterior and Posterior Longitudinal Ligaments

The *anterior* and *posterior longitudinal ligaments* lie on either side of the vertebral bodies. The anterior ligament is in front (anterior) of the vertebral bodies and resists hyperextension of the neck, and the posterior ligaments are behind (posterior) the vertebral bodies and resist hyperflexion. The posterior longitudinal ligament forms the anterior boundary of the vertebral canal.

The *ligmentum flavum* forms the posterior surface of the vertebral canal and runs from C2 to S1. It is a thick, tough ligament connecting the anterior lamina of the vertebra. It blends in with and contributes to the articular capsule of the facet joints. In elderly individuals the ligament can become ossified, which can in turn lead to spinal stenosis. Running between the spinous process of each vertebra is the *interspinous ligament*, and then running like a ribbon or a strap from one spinous process to another is the *supraspinous ligament*.

Note that the spinal canal is bound anteriorly by the posterior longitudinal ligament, and posteriorly by the *ligamentum flava.* During a *laminectomy* to relieve the pressure on the spinal cord, with a posterior approach, the surgeon removes the spinous process and then the lamina in the appropriate region. At this point, the surgeon is looking at the ligamentum flava—remember the ligamentum flava is the posterior border of the spinal canal (Figs. 8.4 and 8.5).

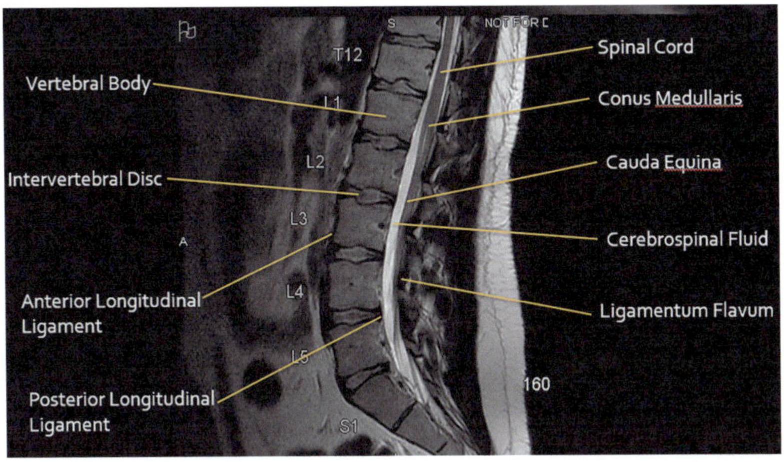

Fig. 8.4 MRI spine. The vertebral bodies are surrounded by the anterior and posterior longitudinal ligaments. The spinal canal which houses the spinal cord is surrounded by the posterior longitudinal ligament and the ligamentum flavum. The conus medullaris, the end of the spinal cord, can be seen at the L1 level. Coming out of the conus medullaris is the cauda equina [5, 6]

Fig. 8.5 Lumbar vertebra. The vertebral bodies are bounded by the anterior and posterior longitudinal ligaments. The red arrow is running down the vertebral canal, which is bounded by the posterior longitudinal ligament and the ligamentum flavum [5, 6]

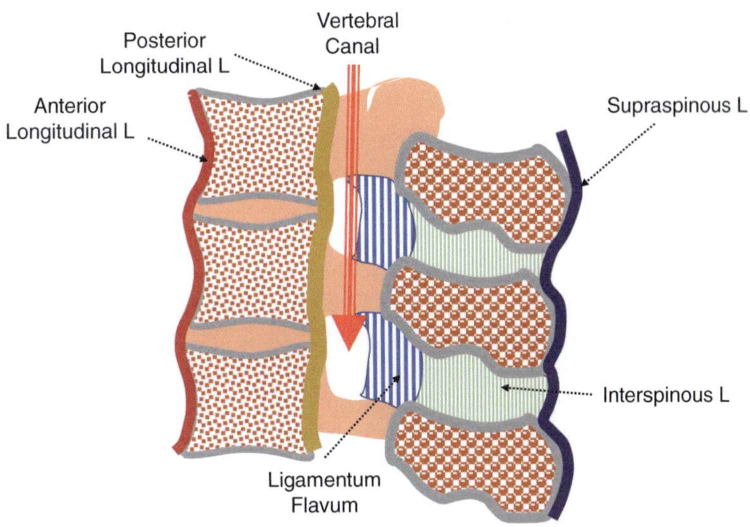

Spinal Meninges

In the cranium the dura is tightly adherent to the skull. The *thecal sac* is the space enclosed by the dura. Outside of the thecal sac is the *epidural space*. From the earlier discussion of the skull, remember that there is no epidural space in the cranium, however in some conditions, such as trauma to the pterion, fluid can drain between the skull and dura and create a space—an epidural hematoma. In the cranium there is a potential space. However in the spinal column there is a true space between the vertebra and the dura. The spinal nerves and venous plexuses travel through this space. This allows anesthesia to be placed into the epidural space to regionally block pain sensation. The anesthesia can be administered at the L2 vertebra either directly in the midline or slightly off the midline. Another location is in the midline just below the S4 spinous process of the

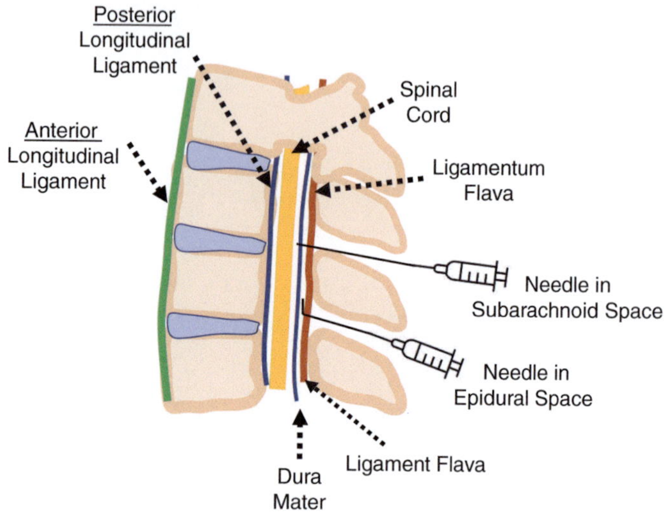

Fig. 8.6 Vertebral body ligaments. The spinal cord is bounded by the dura. The needle in the subarachnoid space had to travel through the ligament flavum and the dura. The needle in the epidural space is between the ligamentum flavum and the dura mater [5, 6]

sacrum. If you place your finger just below the S4 spinous process it will be bound on either side by the right and left sacral cornua. This marks the *sacral hiatus* through which you can gain access to the epidural space.

In the epidural space around the spinal cord there is a valveless *internal vertebral plexus* which carries blood back to the heart from regions such as the pelvis. It can also serve as a conduit for malignant cells which can lead to cancer of the pelvic organs spreading to the lungs, and eventually to the brain. Deep to the dura is the arachnoid, and then the subarachnoid space.

A needle destined for the epidural space will not go as deep as one destined for the subarachnoid space. It will go through the skin, supraspinous ligament, interspinous ligament, and then the ligamentum flava (Fig. 8.6).

Lumbar punctures are usually performed between L3 and L4, or L4 and L5 vertebrae. The L4 vertebra is horizontally across from the highest point of the iliac crest. A needle inserted in the midline to gain access to the subarachnoid space will go through the: supraspinous ligament, interspinous ligament, ligamentum flava, the dura mater, and finally the arachnoid, As the needle moves into the space it will encounter resistance at both the ligamentum flavum, and the dura mater. Note that the needle should not go through the posterior longitudinal ligament, and clearly not through the anterior longitudinal ligament (Fig. 8.7).

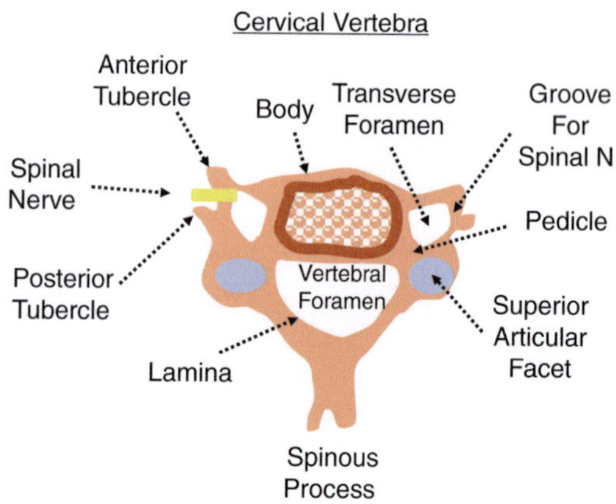

Fig. 8.7 Cervical vertebra. The transverse processes have anterior and posterior tubercles. The spinal nerve travels between the anterior and posterior tubercles. Note the bifid spinous process [5, 6]

Cervical Vertebrae

The cervical vertebrae going from C3 to C7 all have openings in the transverse processes. These *foramen transversarium* transmit the vertebral artery. The spinous processes of C3–C6 are notched or bifed. The C7 vertebra has an elarged spinous process referred to as the *vertebral prominens,* but it is flat instead of notched. The *nuchal ligament* runs from the skull to the C7 spinous process. The superior facet faces backward, upward, and slightly medially. The inferior facet faces forward, downward, and laterally (Fig. 8.6).

The *carotid tubercle* is the anterior tubercle of C6 which is a bony prominence that can be palpated. It separates the carotid artery from the vertebral artery. The common carotid artery runs anterior to the tubercle and its pulse can be felt here. Posterior to the tubercle is the vertebral artery crossing to enter the foramen transversarium of C6.

Thoracic Vertebrae

There are 12 thoracic vertebrae. The T1 vertebra resembles the cervical vertebrae but as you proceed down the column they become larger, with T12 being the largest. T1–T9 all have a demifacet so that each rib articulates with two vertebral bodies. T10–12 all have full facets. The facet joints of the thoracic vertebrae are oriented in superior to inferior direction. The superior articular facet faces anteriorly and meets up with an inferior articular facet facing posteriorly. The vertebral artery runs anterior to the thoracic vertebral bodies. Aneurysms of the thoracic aorta can erode the anterior left lateral edges of the vertebral bodies from T5 to T8. *Jumped Facets* refers to the facet joints becoming locked together following trauma. It most often occurs in the lower cervical in the region of C4 and C6 (Figs. 8.8 and 8.9).

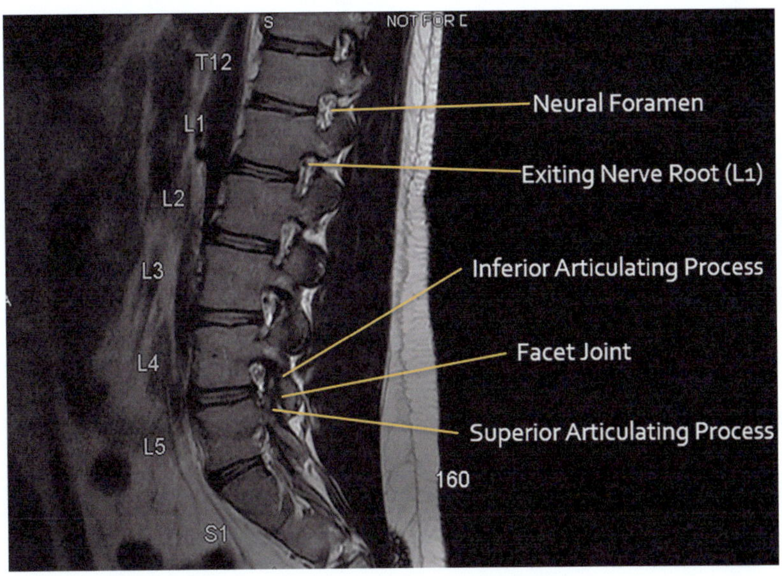

Fig. 8.8 The neural foramina are found between the superior and inferior articular processes. If you look closely at the L1 nerve root you can see that it is emerging just superior to the intervertebral disk between L1 and L2. If there is herniated disc between L1 and L2 it will not hit the L1 root, but it would hit the L2 root [5, 6]

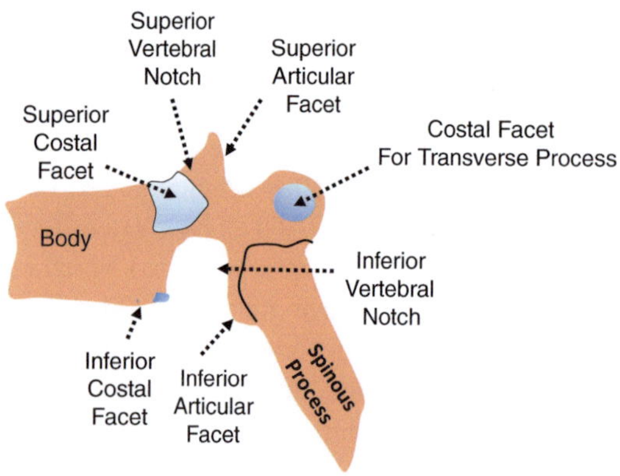

Fig. 8.9 Thoracic vertebra. The superior articular facet will meet the inferior articular facet from the vertebral body above. The inferior articular facet will meet the superior facet from the vertebra below. There is a costal facet on the transverse process for meeting the tubercle of a rib. The superior and inferior costal facets on the body join with the head of the rib [5, 6]

Lumbar Vertebrae

The five lumbar vertebrae are the largest vertebral bodies with L5 being the largest. On the lumbar vertebra the superior articular facets face posteromedial. The inferior facet faces anterolateral. The joints are in a sagittal plane to resist axial rotation. The spinous processes are flat.

Ribs

There is also a tubercle on each rib that articulates with the transverse process of the same numbered rib forming the *costotransverse joint* which is covered by the ligament of the head of the tubercle.

Costovertebral Joints

The ribs join the vertebral bodies posteriorly to make up the costovertebral joints. There is slight variation in the nature of the joints between various ribs and the vertebral bodies. The vertebral bodies of T1 and T10 have costal facets where the rib meets the middle of the vertebral body. However, ribs 2–9 have demifacets (half a facet joint) located on the edges of the vertebral body where the rib meets two vertebral bodies. So, ribs 2–9 each meet with two vertebral bodies—the rib at that level and the one below. For instance, rib 5 articulates with T5 and T6. And vertebral bodies T11 and T12 have full costal facets but these are located on the pedicles of the vertebral bodies. The radiate ligament sits between the head of the rib and the vertebral body (Figs. 8.10 and 8.11).

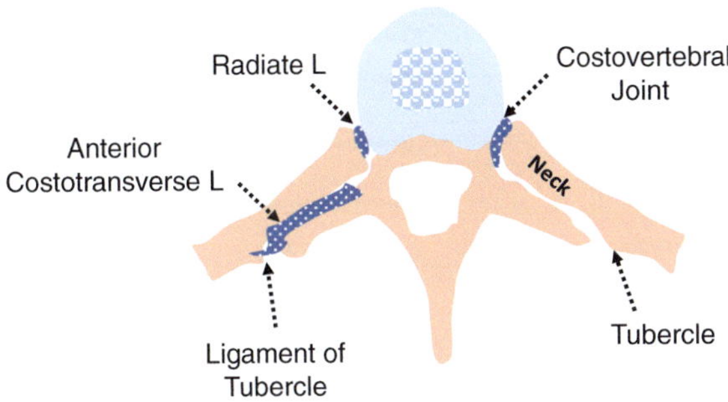

Fig. 8.10 The T6 vertebral body and its connection with the rib 6. Note the costovertebral joint where the head of the rib meets the vertebra. The tubercle of the rib meets the transverse process which is covered by the ligament of the tubercle which continues anterior as the anterior costotransverse ligament. The radiate ligament attaches the head of the rib to the vertebra [5, 6]

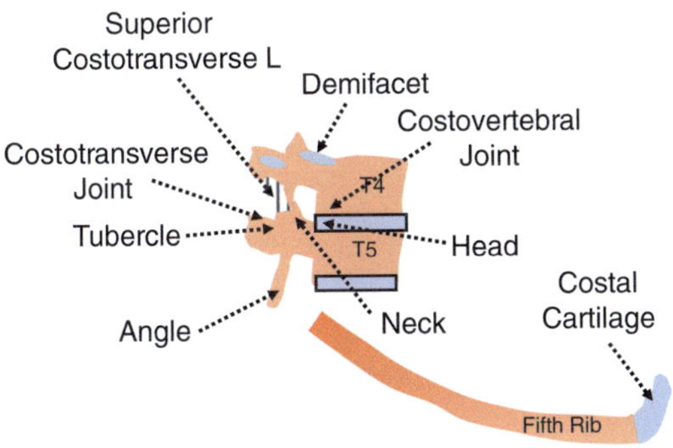

Fig. 8.11 Rib and vertebra. The head of the rib five articulates with the inferior costal facet of T4 and the superior costal facet of T5 to form the costovertebral joint. The transverse costal facets articulate with the tubercle to form the costotransverse joint [5, 6]

Table 8.1 Rule of three's

Vertebral body level	Spinous process = transverse process	Example
T1–T3	SP at level of TP	T2 SP is at level of T2 TP
T4–T6	SP ½ level below TP	T5 SP is halfway between T5 and T6
T7–9	SP one level below TP	T8 SP is at level of T9 TP
T10	Same as T7-T9 SP one level below TP	T10 SP is at level of T11 TP
T11	Same as T4-T6 SP ½ level below TP	T11 SP is between T11 and T12
T12	Same as T1-T3 SP at level of TP	T12 SP is at level of T12

From T1 to T3, the spinous process of a vertebral body lies at the same level as its transverse process. From T4 to T6 the spinous process slopes downward to lie halfway between its level and the one below. From T7 to T9, the spinous process slopes down to the next level. The example shows the spinous process of T8 sloping downward one level to lie adjacent to the T9 vertebral body and the T9 transverse process [5, 6].

Palpating the Spinous Processes and the Rule of Three's

When you run your hand down the middle of the back you can feel the spinous processes. Keep in mind that the spinous process are sloping downward. As you move down the thoracic vertebrae the angle of the slope increases. If you are at the T1–T3 level, you can run your finger from a spinous process out to the side and palpate the same numbered transverse process—there is little slope in this area. If you are at the T2 SP and move to the side then you are palpating the T2 TP. However, if you jump down to the T4-T6 spinous process you will see that the SP lies ½ level below its TP. And if you are at T 7–9 then the SP is one level below the TP—for instance, T8 SP is at the level of T9 TP (Table 8.1 and Figs. 8.12 and 8.13).

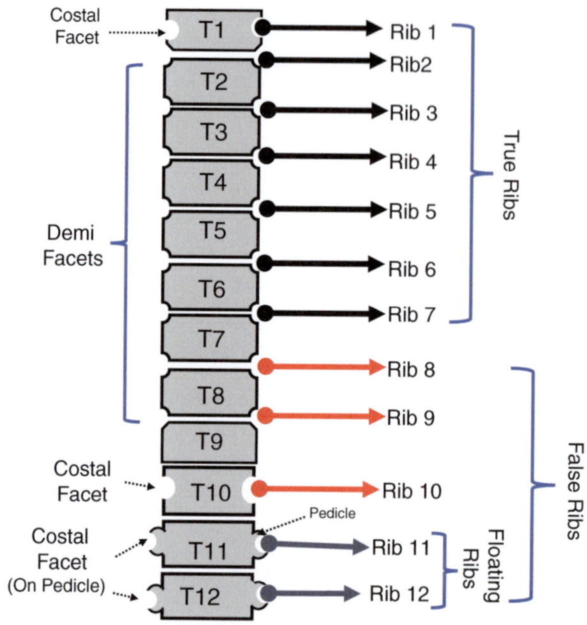

Fig. 8.12 Costovertebral joints. The posterior articulation of the ribs is highlighted in this figure. Vertebral bodies of T1, T10, T11, and T12 have costal facets. The vertebral bodies of T1–T9 have demi facets. Note that T1 has both costal and demi facets, while T10–T12 only have costal facets. For T10 the costal facet is on the body. For T11 and T12 the costal facet is on the pedicle. Where there is a demi facet there is an articulation between one rib and two vertebral bodies. Where there is a costal facet there is an articulation between one rib and one vertebral body [5, 6]

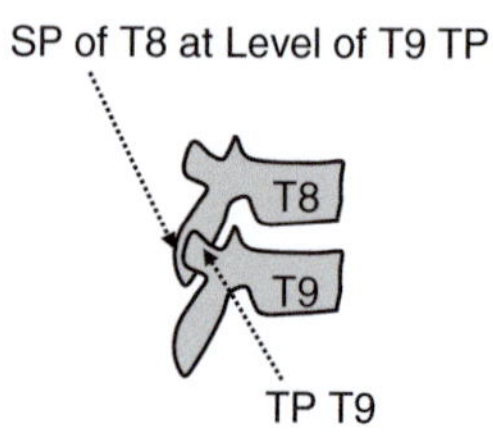

Fig. 8.13 Rule of three's. From T7 to T9, the spinous process slopes down to the next level. The example shows the spinous process of T8 sloping downward one level to lie adjacent to the T9 vertebral body and the T9 transverse process [5, 6]

Geelhoed's Rule

Some authors have questioned the feasibility of using the *Rule of Three's* when it comes to accurately identifying the spinous and transverse processes during palpation. In response to this, one group has proposed the simpler idea that the thoracic transverse processes are at the level of the spinous process of the adjacent superior vertebra. This is referred to as *Geelhoed's Rule.*

Disk Herniations

The spinal cord ends at the L1 (or L2) vertebral body. In the anatomy lab, when you do a laminectomy of L1 and expose the spinal cord you are looking at the end of the cord (conus medullaris), which is the S 2, 3, 4 spinal cord level. You will also see the cauda equina at this point which is the collection of nerve roots from the lumbar and sacral regions traveling down in the vertebral canal alongside the spinal cord to eventually exit via their respective intervertebral foramen, In the cervical region, the spinal nerves exit above the equivalent vertebral body. So, the C1 nerve exits above the C1 level (the atlas) and the C2 nerve exits above C2 (the axis). This pattern continues down to the level of the C7 vertebra where the C7 nerve exits above the C7 vertebral body, and the

C8 nerve between C8 and the T1 vertebrae. And then starting with the thoracic vertebra the nerve exists below the equivalent vertebral body, with the T1 nerve exiting below T1 vertebral body.

The disks located between the vertebral bodies are composed of a tough circumferential outer layer—the *annulus fibrosus*—and a jelly like soft inside—the *nucleus pulposus* (a remanent of the notochord). The disks are kept between the vertebral bodies by the *anterior* and *posterior longitudinal ligaments*. However, as we age, the ligaments can become weak. This usually happens at the lateral portion of the posterior longitudinal ligament, so that herniated disks most often herniate posterolateral. The disk then hits the spinal nerve which is passing right beside it (Figs. 8.14 and 8.15).

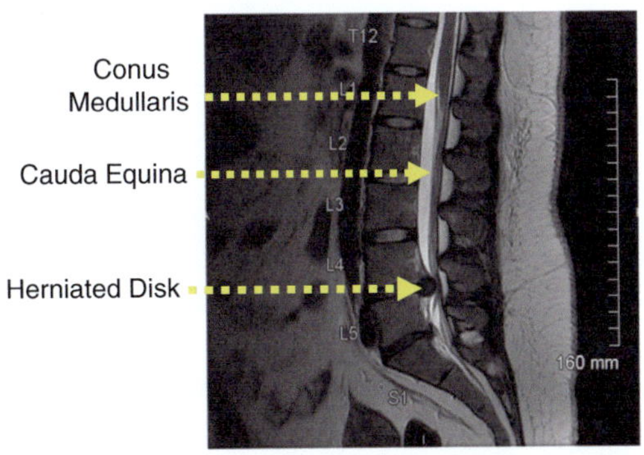

Fig. 8.14 Herniated disk and cauda equina

In the cervical region the nerves travel at right angles to exit the spinal cord. If there is a disk herniation between C3 and C4 it will hit the C4 nerve. However, in the lumbar region because the nerves must travel down to exit at their appropriate level, a disk herniation say between L4 and L5 will hit the L5 nerve. In most cases, especially on exams, the disk herniation in this example will spare S1. But keep in mind that in the real world if the disk herniation is large enough it could hit the S1 nerve (Figs. 8.15 and 8.16).

Looking at two vertebrae from a posterior view, imagine we have cut the pedicles of each vertebra with a bone saw. We can see the pedicles jut out from the top edge of each vertebra. The intervertebral foramen is between the pedicles of two adjacent vertebrae. If we focus on the L4 and L5 vertebrae, we see a disk between the two, and exiting at the top of the foramen is the L4 nerve. If this disk herniates then it will *not impinge* the L4 root, which is exiting above the disk, but *will impinge* the L5 root as it passes by the disk to exit one level down. In other words, a disk herniation between L4 and L5 will hit the nerve exiting one level down, which is L5. In some cases, a lumbar

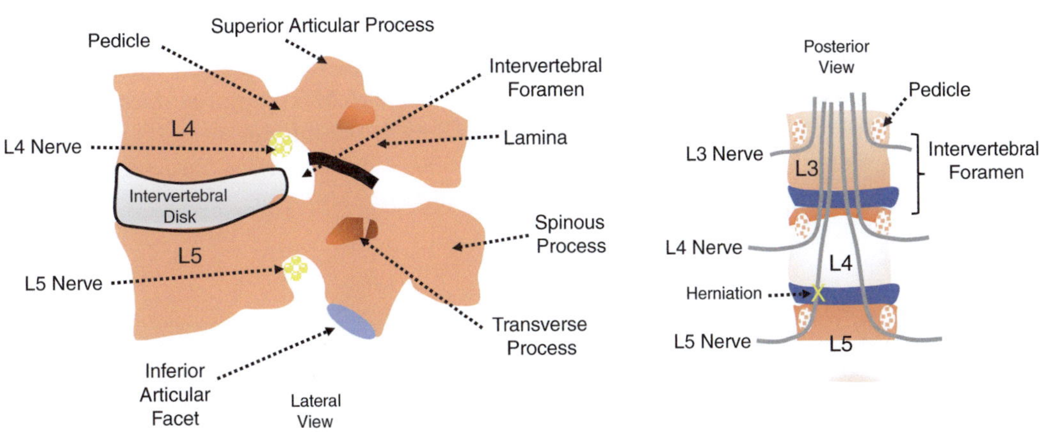

Fig. 8.15 Two views of the nerves and vertebral body relationships. Note the L4 spinal nerve exits at the superior margin of the intervertebral foramen. If the disk between L4 and L5 herniates it will hit the L5 nerve [5, 6]

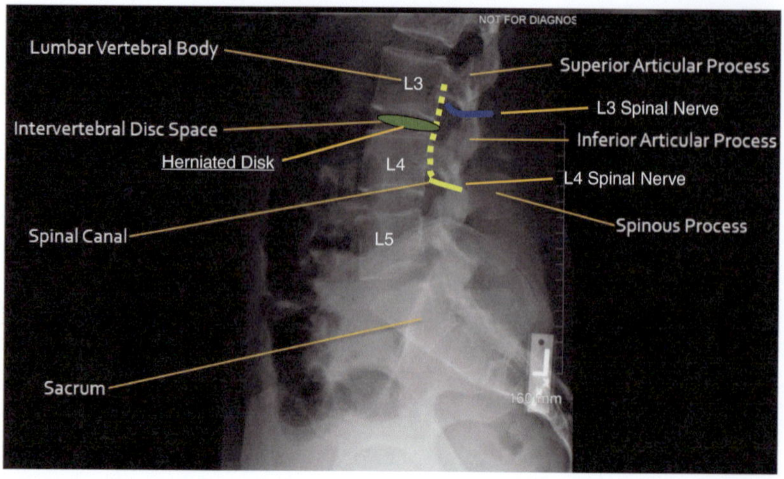

Fig. 8.16 Herniated disk. The L3 spinal nerve is exiting the neural foramen between L3 and L4 but note that it exits above the herniated disk. If the disc herniates posteriorly, it will hit the L4 nerve as it descends on its way to exit one level below, but not the L3 nerve [5, 6]

disk will herniate at the far lateral edge of disk, in which case the nerve will compress the nerve exiting at that level. For instance, a disk herniation at the far lateral edge of L4/5 will hit the L4 nerve.

Spondylolisthesis Versus Spondylolysis

The *pars interarticularis* is the small piece of bone between the superior and inferior articular facets. *Spondylolysis is* a stress fracture along the lytic line in the pars interarticularis—at the collar in the Scottie dog picture. The most common site is L5. *Spondylolisthesis* is when one vertebra slides forward over the vertebra below it (listhesis = to slip). *Ankylosing spondylitis* refers to fused vertebra. The patient will have a hunched forward position (Fig. 8.17).

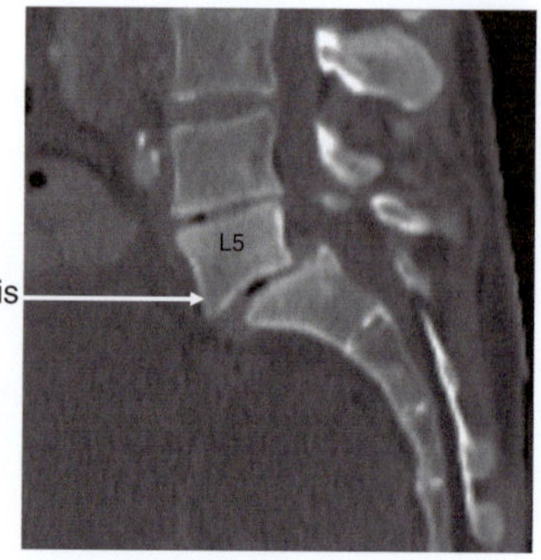

Fig. 8.17 Spondylolisthesis. In this image one can see how the L5 vertebral body in this patient has slipped forward from its typical position just atop the sacrum [5, 6]

On a radiograph a straightforward way to picture a spondylolysis is to think of a picture of a Scottie dog. The fracture of the pars interarticularis occurs at the dog's collar. The eye is the pedicle. Making up the facet joint, the front foot is the inferior articular process and ears are the superior articular process (Fig. 8.18).

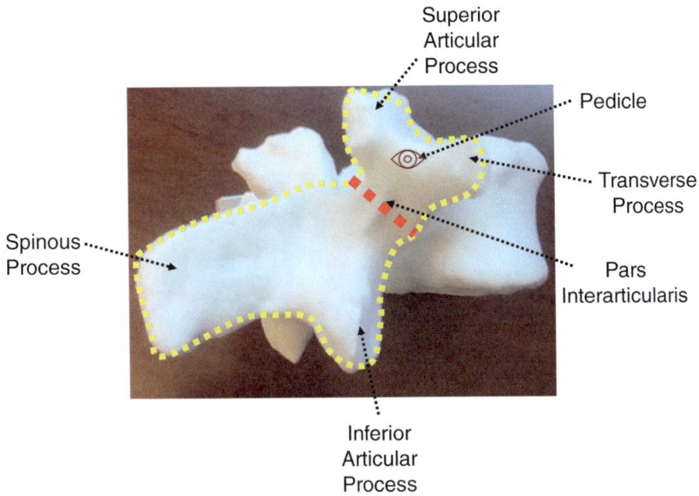

Fig. 8.18 Scottie dog and spondylolysis. The dog's collar is the pars interarticularis which is the site of spondylolysis. The facet joint is between the superior articular facet (the dog's head) and the inferior articular process (the dog's front foot) of vertebra above it [5, 6]

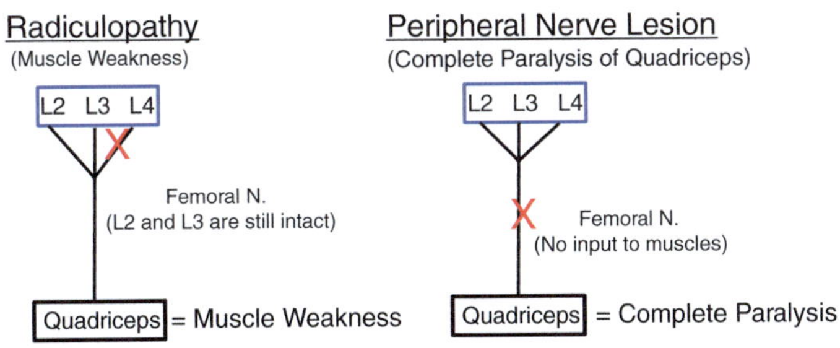

Fig. 8.19 Radiculopathy versus Peripheral Nerve Lesion. Panel (**a**) The femoral nerve receives contributions from L 2, 3, and 4. If the L4 root is damaged then the quadriceps will be weak because L2 and 3 are still intact. Panel (**b**) If the femoral nerve is severed then the quadriceps will be completely (100%) paralyzed [5, 6]

Disk Herniations Versus Peripheral Nerve Trauma

It is important to understand the difference between cutting a peripheral nerve versus cutting a root (radiculopathy). To understand the difference in clinical presentation between the two, we need to keep in mind two points: (1) that any individual root goes to several distinct levels, and (2) every nerve receives contributions from multiple levels. As an example, take the femoral nerve; it receives contributions from L2, L3, and L4 roots (Fig. 8.19).

If the femoral nerve is cut, then the muscles supplied by the femoral nerve—the quadriceps—will be completely paralyzed. Conversely, if the L4 root is damaged, because the femoral nerve still gets a contribution from L2 and L3, the quadriceps will not be paralyzed but will be weak. In addition, with femoral nerve damage you want to think about the *peripheral nerve map*, but with a compromised root you want to think about the *dermatome map* (Figs. 8.12 and 8.13).

On the other hand, if you cut a peripheral nerve then the muscles innervated by that nerve will exhibit complete flaccid paralysis. Note that in the case of a muscle that is innervated by two nerves (not common), that the second nerve can send a signal to the muscle (Fig. 8.20).

Take cutting L4 as an example, (Fig. 8.20), there will be weakness of several different muscle groups but not complete paralysis. This is

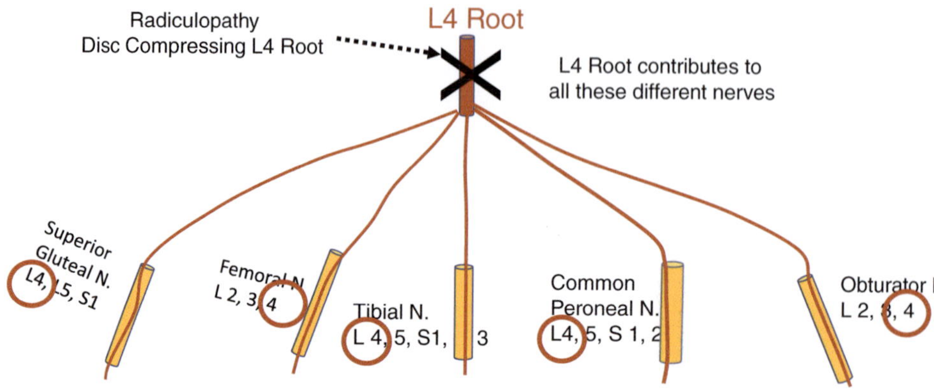

Fig. 8.20 Root damage. The L4 root travels into several different nerves, but any given nerve receives contributions from several different levels. Thus, each nerve that gets a branch from L4 will be weakened, but because of these other contributions, their muscle groups will not be completely paralyzed. One question for the clinician then, is what nerve gets most of its supply from L4. For the femoral nerve, the most important root is L4 which is why with a radiculopathy of L4, the quadriceps will be noticeably weak [5, 6]

because L4 fibers make their way into several different nerves.

In the chapters on the upper and lower limbs, there is a detailed explanation of radiculopathies at each level.

Keep in mind that with a herniated disc that compresses a peripheral nerve, when it comes to motor function, the patient will have lower motor neuron deficits. For instance, their reflexes at the level of the nerve compression will be reduced or absent. In contrast, a lesion that compresses the actual spinal cord, which is referred to as *cervical myelopathy* will typically lead to upper motor neuron deficits from the lesion on down. For instance, compression of the cervical spinal cord could lead to Babinski's sign on one side or possibly both sides.

Abormal Curves of Spine

Kyphosis is an exageration of the thoracic curvature, usually resulting from osteoporosis. Lordosis is an exageration of the lumbar curvature usually resulting from a spondylolisthesis or pregnancy. Scoliosis is a lateral curvature (Table 8.2).

Table 8.2 Summary of the relationship of structures to vertebral body levels

Vertebra level	Structures
C4	Bifurcation of common carotid
C6	Start of esophagus and trachea
C7	Vertebral prominens
T2	Superior border of scapula
T2/3	Suprasternal notch, top of aortic arch and the origin of three main branches of the aorta. Left brachiocephalic vein crossing from left to right in front of these three branches
T4	Aortic arch ends
T4	Sternal angle, bifurcation of trachea
T7	Inferior angle of scapula
T8	Caval opening, IVC, and right phrenic nerve
T10	Esophageal hiatus, R/L vagus nerves
T12	Aortic hiatus, azygous vein, thoracic duct, celiac trunk
L1	Superior mesenteric artery, renal veins, end of spinal cord
L3	Inferior mesenteric artery
L4	Abdominal aorta bifurcation
L5	Start of IVC
S2	End of dural sac

100 key anatomy words

1	Infratemporal fossa nerve	V3
2	Pterygopalatine fossa nerve	V2
3	Bell's palsy, where is lesion?	Facial canal
4	Claw hand	Ulnar nerve
5	Pope's blessing	Median nerve
6	Mallet finger	Tear of extensor digitorum longus
7	Callot's triangle, what artery?	Cystic artery
8	Most posterior structure in hepatoduodenal ligament	Portal vein
9	Trauma, lower limb laterally rotated	Femoral neck fracture
10	Dashboard injury, lower limb medially rotated	Posterior hip dislocation
11	Anterior layer rectus sheath Above pectinate line	External abdominal oblique, internal abdominal oblique, transversus abdominus muscles
12	Lesser omentum subdivisions	Hepatoduodenal, hepatogastric ligaments
13	Ulcer of the first part of duodenum	Gastroduodenal artery and hepatic duct.
14	Between SMA and aorta	Left renal vein, uncinate process, duodenum
15	Jugular foramen syndrome	CN IX, X, and XI
16	Otic ganglia	Parasympathetics to parotid
17	Running with superficial temporal artery	Auriculotemporal nerve
18	Landmark for inguinal hernias	Inferior epigastric artery
19	SLAP tear, tendon?	Glenoid labrum near where long head of the biceps inserts
20	First 10–15% of shoulder abduction	Supraspinatus
21	Cavernous sinus nerves?	CNs III, IV, and VI and V1 and V2, not V3
22	Medial strabismus, nerve damaged?	CN VI
23	Jefferson fracture	C1—Atlas
24	Dislocated lunate, symptoms?	Mimics carpal tunnel
25	Handlebar palsy	Ulnar nerve
26	DeQuervain syndrome	Extensor pollicis brevis and abductor pollicis longus
27	Pope's blessing	Motor test for median nerve
28	Claw hand	Ulnar nerve sign
29	Right to left shunts	Transposition of great vessels, persistent truncus arteriosus, tetralogy of Fallot
30	Tetralogy of Fallot	Interventricular septal defect, hypertrophied right ventricle, overriding aorta, pulmonary hypertension
31	Base of heart	Left atrium
32	Dermatome of thumb	C6
33	Unhappy triad	Medial collateral, medial meniscus, ACL
34	Tarsal tunnel nerve	Tibial nerve
35	Pott's fracture	Medial malleolus and distal fibula
36	Fracture of femoral neck	Lower limb laterally rotated
37	Posterior hip dislocation	Lower limb medially rotated
38	Pes Anserinus	Sartorius, gracilis, semitendinosus
39	Subclavian steal syndrome	Blockage of subclavian artery proximal to vertebral A
40	Carotid tubercle	Anterior tubercle of C6. Common carotid A is anterior, vertebral A is posterior
41	Posterior humeral circumflex A	Runs with axillary nerve
42	Posterior superior iliac spine	End of dura, S2 vertebra, middle of sacroiliac joint, dimples of Venus
43	Pudendal nerve block	Ischial spine, sacrospinous ligament
44	Pulse in snuff box	Radial artery
45	Gamekeeper's thumb	Ulnar collateral ligament
46	Froment's sign	Ulnar nerve
47	Pronator Teres syndrome	Median nerve
48	Midshaft humeral fracture	Radial nerve, wrist drop
49	Supracondylar fracture	Median nerve
50	Emergency airway opening	Cricothyrotomy
51	Piriform recess	Internal laryngeal nerve
52	Posterior Cricoarytenoid	Only muscle that opens the glottis
53	Aortic aneurysm, horse voice	Left recurrent laryngeal nerve
54	Esophageal hiatus	T10, esophagus and right and left vagus nerves
55	Duodenal ulcer	Gastroduodenal artery
56	Arteries to terminal esophagus	Left gastric artery

(continued)

57	Lesser sac	Between stomach/lesser omentum and pancreas
58	Nutcracker syndrome	SMA and aorta sandwiching the left renal vein
59	Lienorenal ligament: dorsal or ventral mesentery?	Dorsal mesentery
60	Scalene triangle boundaries	Anterior and middle scalene muscles and first rib
62	Beginning of portal vein behind what organ?	Pancreas
63	Femoral hernia and pubic tubercle	Femoral hernia lateral to PT
64	Adductor hiatus	Femoral A becomes popliteal A. Opening in adductor magnus
65	Most important ligament for medial arch in foot	Plantar calcaneonavicular (spring) L
66	Subtalar joint	Talus and calcaneus
67	Chopart joint	Talonavicular and calcaneocuboid ligaments
68	Bunion	Hallux valgus
69	Nerves traveling through tendinous ring in orbit	CNs III, VI and nasociliary
70	Gag reflex	CN IX afferent, CN X efferent
71	Pott's fracture	Tibia (med malleolus) and fibula
72	Dorsalis Pedis pulse, where?	Lateral to extensor hallucis longus.
73	Posterior rectus sheath, superior to arcuate line	Internal abdominal oblique and Transversus Abdominus
74	Trachea ends	T4/T5
75	Rib notching	Coarctation of aorta
76	Gastrosplenic ligament: Dorsal or ventral mesentery?	Dorsal
77	Machine-like murmur	PDA
78	Cremaster muscle: What layer?	Internal abdominal oblique muscle
79	Lowest point peritoneal cavity in females	Rectouterine pouch
80	Supracondylar fracture	Median nerve
81	Whiplash injury	Anterior longitudinal ligament
82	Waiter's tip	Upper trunk injury
83	Spondylosis	Pars interarticularis
84	Deep fibular nerve sign	Foot drop
85	Foramen Spinosum	Middle meningeal artery
86	Amnion, what layer	Ectoderm
87	Deep inguinal ring	Fascia transversalis
88	Pelvic diaphragm muscles?	Levator ani and coccygeus
89	Membranous urethra, what space?	Deep perineal space
90	CN IV palsy, head tilt?	Head tilt away from the side of lesion
91	Prostate: endo, ecto, or meso?	Endo
92	Superior part of vagina: endo, ecto, or meso	Endo
93	Stab wound to the right of sternum at rib 4	Right atrium
94	Stab wound to left of sternum, rib 4	Right ventricle
95	Loop of Henle: In medulla or cortex of kidney?	Medulla
96	Left to right shunts	ASD, VSD, PDA
97	Radial head dislocation	Annular ligament
98	Sensation to first dorsal web space	Radial nerve
99	Abduction/ adduction of fingers	Ulnar nerve
100	Sensation between first and second toes	Deep fibular nerve

Further Reading

1. Boone JM, Abrahams PH, Meiring JH, Welch T. Lumbar puncture for the generalist. S Afr Fam Pract. 2004;46(2):38–42.
2. Drake RL, Vogl W, Mitchell AW. Gray's anatomy for medical students. New York: Elsevier; 2005.
3. Geelhoed M, McGaugh J, Brewer PA, Murphy D. A new model to facilitate palpation of the level of the transverse processes of the thoracic spine. J Orthop Sports Phys Ther. 2006;36(11):876–81.
4. Hoppenfeld JD, Hoppenfeld S. Orthopaedic neurology: a diagnostic guide to neurologic levels. Philadelphia: Wolters Kluwer; 2018.
5. Leo J. Medical neuroanatomy for the boards and clinic: finding the lesion. 2nd ed. Cham: Springer; 2024.
6. Leo J. Clinical anatomy and embryology: a guide for the classroom, clinic, and clinic. 2nd ed. Cham: Springer; 2024.
7. Moore K, Dalley AF, Agur A. Clinically oriented anatomy. 7th ed. Baltimore: Lippincott Williams and Wilkin; 2014.

8. Razak L. Pathophysiology of pelvic organ prolapse. In: Rizvi RM, editor. Pelvic floor disorders. IntechOpen; 2018. https://doi.org/10.5772/intechopen.76629. Available from: https://www.intechopen.com/chapters/60935.
9. Riascos R, Bonfante A, Cotes A, Guirguis M, Hakimelahi R, West C. Imaging of atlanto-occipital and atlantoaxial traumatic injuries: what the radiologist needs to know. RSNA. 2015;35(7):2121–34. Available at: Imaging of atlanto-occipital and atlantoaxial traumatic injuries: what the radiologist needs to know | RadioGraphics. rsna.org
10. Rosse C, Gaddum-Rosse P. Hollinshead's textbook of anatomy. 5th ed. New York: Lippincott-Raven; 1997.
11. Standring S. Gray's anatomy: the anatomical basis of clinical practice. London: Elsevier; 2005.
12. Westbrook JL. Anatomy of the epidural space. Anaesth Intensive Care Med. 2012;13(11):551–4.

Part II

Neuroanatomy

9 The Three Long Tracts in the Spinal Cord

Introduction

When you see a patient, or an exam scenario, one of the first questions you will ask yourself is: Is the lesion in the CNS or the PNS? If the signs and symptoms point to one or more of the three long tracts being compromised, then you will be thinking about the CNS. The three long tracts are the: (1) corticospinal, (2) dorsal columns, and (3) spinothalamic. The corticospinal tract is a descending motor pathway, while both the dorsal columns and spinothalamic tracts are ascending sensory pathways. As these tracts travel to or from the cerebral cortex, all three decussate at some point in the CNS. What makes life complicated for students is that all three tracts cross at different locations in the CNS.

Before getting into the specifics, consider the big picture by first focusing on the difference between a lesion in the cortex, spinal cord, or brainstem.

1. By the time we get to the cortex, all three tracts have crossed so a lesion in the cortex will lead to contralateral signs for all three tracts. The patient would have contralateral motor deficits, contralateral dorsal column signs, and contralateral spinothalamic tract signs. But on the way to the cortex, because the tracts decussate at distinct locations, patients can present with mixed signs and symptoms.
2. Consider a patient with motor deficits on one side of the body, and pain and temperature deficits on the other side of the body. Most likely, this patient has a spinal cord lesion, with motor deficits on the ipsilateral side, and the pain and temperature loss on the contralateral side. In addition, the dorsal column deficits will be found on the ipsilateral side.
3. Next, consider a patient with an alternating pattern of motor deficits, meaning that they have some motor deficits on one side of the body and some motor deficits on the other side of the body. This is sometimes referred to as an *alternating hemiplegia*. Most likely, this patient has a lesion in the brainstem.

For this first chapter, we will focus on the three long tracts in the spinal cord. We will then devote a significant amount of time to the brainstem and then finish with the cortex. For thinking about how we function as human beings, obviously the cerebral cortex is the most complicated part of the CNS, however, the cortex lesions are straightforward. For our purposes, when it comes to lesions, the brain stem is the most complicated piece of the CNS, and the most important for making a correct diagnosis.

J. Leo, *Gross Anatomy, Neuroanatomy, and Embryology for Medical Students*,
https://doi.org/10.1007/978-3-031-87151-1_9

Corticospinal Pathway

The major motor pathway is a two-neuron pathway consisting of upper motor neurons (UMNs) and lower motor neurons (LMNs) (Fig. 9.1). The UMN tract, also called the corticospinal tract, begins with cell bodies in the precentral gyrus and projects down through the corona radiata, internal capsule, cerebral peduncle, and then to the caudal medulla, where about 90% of the fibers decussate at the pyramidal decussation. Once the fibers decussate, they enter the lateral funiculus of the spinal cord and continue down as the lateral corticospinal tract. The 10% of fibers that do not decussate travel down the cord as the anterior corticospinal tract. For the purposes of understanding the clinical scenarios, we are going to focus on the lateral corticospinal tract.

There are approximately one million fibers in the corticospinal tract as it moves down from the cortex, through the brainstem, the caudal medulla, and then the spinal cord. These fibers are known as upper motor neurons (UMNs) and are like a major highway transporting information to various locations. Along the path of this highway, a small group of fibers, like exit ramps, will peel off at each level and project to the anterior horn cells which are the beginning of the lower motor neurons (LMNs). The lower motor neurons project out as the ventral roots, to eventually form the motor component of the peripheral nerves.

Keep in mind that the pyramidal decussation is not a demarcation for the UMN and LMN neuron designation. Sometimes students make the mistake of thinking that the term "UMN" refers to the corticospinal tract above the pyramidal decussation, and the term "LMN" refers to tract below the pyramidal decussation and that all the fibers in the cord are LMNs. But this is not the case. Even below the decussation, you will find upper motor neurons. In fact, at every level of the spinal cord, you will find both UMNs and LMNs. Or another way to think of it is that if you have a patient who has UMN signs on the right, that does not necessarily mean that there is a lesion in the left cortex. The lesion could be in the left cortex, but it could also be in the right spinal cord.

Damage to UMNs will lead to a distinct set of symptoms compared to damage to the LMNs. If the patient has UMN signs, then the lesion is in the CNS. If the patient has LMNs then the lesion is most likely, but not necessarily, in the PNS. Lower motor neurons begin in the ventral horn, which is in the CNS, and leave on the ventral root to join a spinal nerve. The majority of a LMN is in the PNS but a small part of it is in the CNS. A lesion to the ventral horn can result in

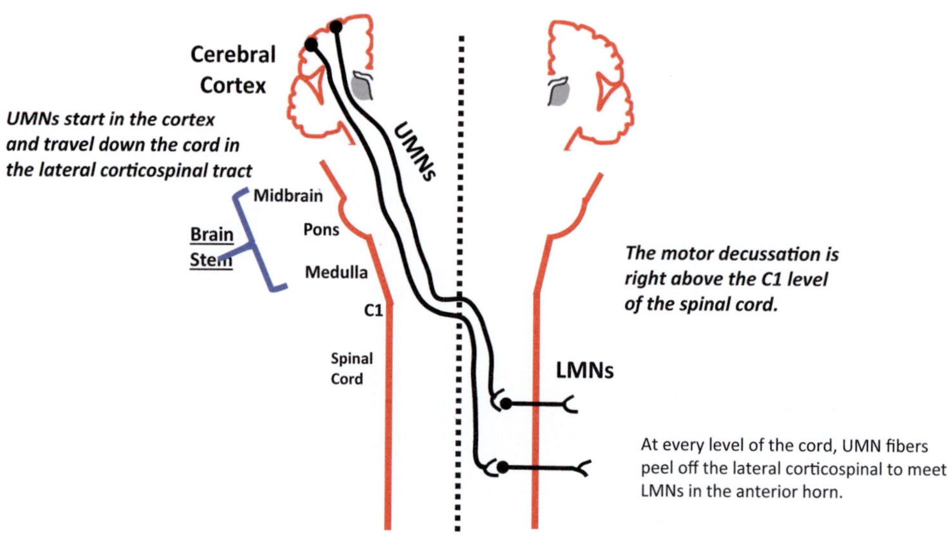

Fig. 9.1 Motor pathway. Upper motor neurons meeting lower motor neurons in the spinal cord [14, 15]

LMN signs even though the lesion is in the CNS. Polio leads to lesions in the CNS, but it targets anterior horn cells resulting in LMN symptoms, such as hyporeflexia and decreased tone.

The hallmark sign of an UMN lesion is Babinski's sign. In a normal healthy individual, if the bottom of their foot is scratched, they will plantar flex their toes. In a patient with a lesion to the UMN pathway (or in a newborn) the toes will dorsiflex. In addition, UMN lesions will lead to spastic paralysis, hyperreflexia, increased muscle tone, and priapism. Patients with UMN lesions will be hemiplegic, meaning that they are not completely paralyzed. On the affected side their arm will be adducted, and their forearm held close to their chest. The farther out on a limb you go, the more important the corticospinal is for fine movement. An example would be someone with a lesion to UMNs in the internal capsule, reaching up to grab an item from a shelf. With their shoulder muscles they can start their upper limbs moving towards the shelf, but because their hands are more severely affected, they will have problems picking up the item. The same is true for their lower limbs. The UMN patient will be able to walk by swinging their lower limbs at the hip, but movement at their knees and ankles will be weaker. When they walk, they will swing their lower limbs at the hip with their limb swinging laterally.

Babinski's sign is the most often used reflex to denote an UMN neuron injury, but there are other areas of the lower limb that can be stroked that will lead to upgoing toes. The Chaddock sign involves stroking the lateral foot, Oppenheim sign involves stroking the anterior medial tibia, and Gordon sign involves squeezing the gastrocnemius. Any of these tests that lead to an upgoing toe are indicative of an UMN injury.

Hoffmann's sign is also an UMN sign but it occurs in the upper limb. With an UMN patient, if you squeeze the tip of their third finger it will often lead to flexion of the second finger and thumb.

Note that in the clinical world, while you might hear clinicians refer to Babinski's sign as either positive or negative, there is no need to word it like this. Babinski's is either present or not, a patient either has Babinski's or does not, you do not need to qualify it be either positive or negative.

Cross Section of Spinal Cord

When you look at a cross section through the spinal cord you see the dorsal side with the dorsal horns and the ventral side with the ventral horns (Fig. 9.2). If you stick your finger on the hot stove, the sensation travels on the spinal nerve towards the spinal cord. The sensation then travels on the dorsal root, with its associated dorsal root ganglion, and then enters the spinal cord to synapse in the dorsal horn. The ventral horn on the other hand is the location of the cell bodies for the LMNs or efferent fibers. These fibers travel on the ventral root to join the spinal nerve and then project to the muscle. If the ventral roots are cut, there will be a motor deficit; if the dorsal roots are cut there will be a sensory deficit; and if the spinal nerve is cut there will be both a motor and sensory deficit.

Patients with LMN lesions will have complete flaccid paralysis of the muscles affected. They will also exhibit absent or reduced reflexes and decreased muscle tone. They will also have fasciculations and fibrillations, which are small twitches of the muscle. Fasciculations are visible and have been described as looking like worms under the skin. Fibrillations occur in individual muscle fibers and are not visible (Table 9.1).

As an example of how to think about the loss of reflex with a LMN lesion, take the quadriceps. With a LMN injury, say to the femoral nerve innervating the quadriceps, because the wire is cut there is no electrical signal to the muscles. So, when you tap on the patellar tendon there is no way that the quadriceps muscles can move. With no electrical signal, there will be reduced tone to the muscles, and over time the muscles will atrophy. However, if you cut the UMN anywhere between the premotor cortex and the anterior horn, the LMN is still intact, and when you tap on the tendon, the afferent signal comes into the cord, synapses with the LMN or efferent fiber, and the leg extends. In fact, when the reflex fires it will be hyperactive. This

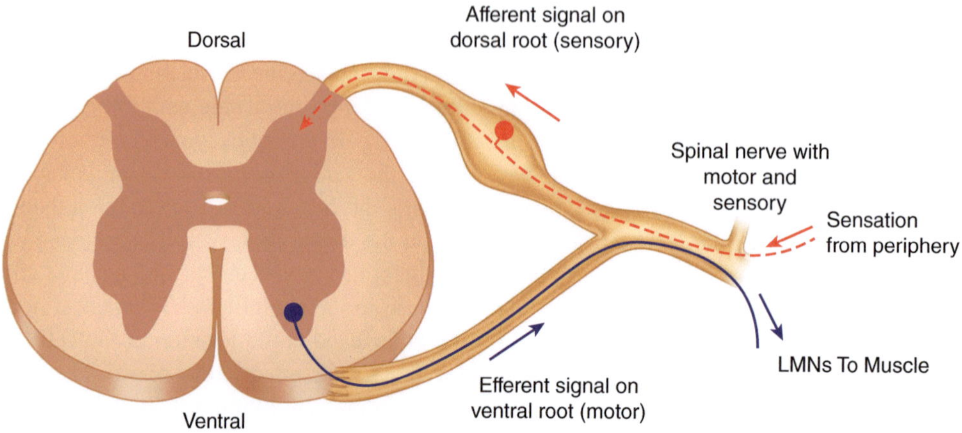

Fig. 9.2 Spinal cord cross section. On the dorsal side, primary afferents travel on dorsal roots to the dorsal horn. Their cell bodies are in the dorsal root ganglion. On the ventral side, the efferent fibers, which are LMNs, travel on ventral roots to the spinal and then to muscles [14, 15]

Table 9.1 Upper and lower motor neuron deficits

Upper motor neuron deficit	Lower motor neuron deficit
Spastic paralysis	Flaccid paralysis
Hyperreflexia	Areflexia
Babinski's sign, clonus	No Babinski
Increased muscle tone	Decreased muscle tone
Muscle weakness	Fasciculations (worm-like)
Disuse atrophy of muscles	Atrophy
Decreased speed of voluntary movements	Fibrillations (not visible)
Hoffmann's sign	
Priapism	

sounds counterintuitive but in a healthy individual when the tendon is tapped, one of the jobs of the cortex is to inhibit, or check, the reflex. With an UMN deficit, this cortical inhibition is lost, and the reflex is hyperactive.

Here is another way to think of it. As an example, take a patient with a hemisection of the right cord at C5. The spinal cord below C5 is not completely atrophied. It still has a blood supply, is getting oxygen, and is still functioning tissue. But the patient has lost the ability of the cortex to send information down to L4 where the femoral nerve begins. If you give this patient a command to move their leg, they understand you, and they try to send the information from primary motor cortex down to L4, but they cannot get the information past the cord lesion. Yet, if you tap on their patellar tendon, the afferents carry the information into the cord and form a synapse with the LMN cell body. Thus, because the reflex loop is still intact, the leg moves. The reflex loop does not need cortical influence.

Both UMN and LMN deficits can lead to muscle atrophy, however with an UMN neuron injury

Table 9.2 Grading muscle strength

Grade	Description
0/5	No muscle movement
1/5	Barely detectable movement
2/5	Movement with gravity eliminated
3/5	Movement against gravity
4/5	Movement against gravity and light resistance
5/5	Normal strength

you will hear the term "disuse" atrophy. The difference is that with a LMN injury because there is no input to the muscle and it is devoid of any input, it will atrophy. With the UMN injury, the muscle still has an electrical signal coming into it, it has just lost the cortical input to make coordinated movements, which will lead to the patient not using the muscle. With these UMN patients the goal of physical and occupational therapy is to develop exercises to so that the patient uses these muscles to minimize the potential "disuse atrophy."

It is important to understand the different symptoms between UMN and LMN lesions, such as hyperreflexia and hyporeflexia, however you also need to be familiar with how these terms are reported. Muscle strength is reported on a scale from zero to five, with five being "normal" and zero being no muscle contraction—or paralysis. A score of three is active movement against gravity without any resistance (Table 9.2).

Deep Tendon Reflexes

Deep tendon reflexes are tested by short, sharp, "taps," on tendons. The main reflexes are the biceps (C5–6), brachioradialis (C6), triceps (C7 and 8, mostly C7), patellar (L4), and Achilles (S1). The reflexes are graded on a scale of 1+ to 4+, with a 2+ being "normal." Hyperreflexia would be either a 3+, meaning a brisk response, or a 4+ being clonus. On the other end, a 0 is an absent response, and 1+ is a reduced reflex. The + sign simply denotes that it is the reflex test grade, not to be confused with the score on the strength grade. Hyperactive reflexes indicate a UMN lesion. Absent reflexes indicate a LMN injury (Table 9.3).

Table 9.3 Grading reflexes

Grade	Description
4+	Very brisk response, hyperactive, with clonus
3+	Brisker than average
2+	Average, normal
1+	Diminished response
0	No response

Table 9.4 Reflexes

Reflex	CNS level
Biceps	C **5** & 6
Brachioradialis	C5 & 6
Triceps	C **7** & 8
Patellar	L 2, 3, & **4**
Achilles	S1
Cremasteric	T12, **L1**
Plantar	**S1** & 2
Gluteal	L4, 5, S1, S2

Rather than use the terms hyperreflexia or hyperreflexia, the clinician or the question writer might use the numerical grading and state that the patient's biceps reflex was 4+ or the quadriceps reflex was 1+.

The major reflexes which are part of the neurological exam are included in Table 9.4.

Cerebral Peduncle, Basis Pontis, and Pyramid

It is important to pay attention to the location of these fibers within each level of the brainstem. In the midbrain the fibers are in the middle one third of the cerebral peduncle, in the pons there are in the basis pontis, and in the medulla they are in the pyramid (Fig. 9.3).

C5 Hemisection

Delving further into the example of a hemisection at C5, note that when the cord is cut at C5 then both UMNs and LMNs are damaged—you have cut both the corticospinal highway and the exit ramps. In this example there is an accident on the highway right at the point where the exit ramp leaves the road. The UMN pathway is the

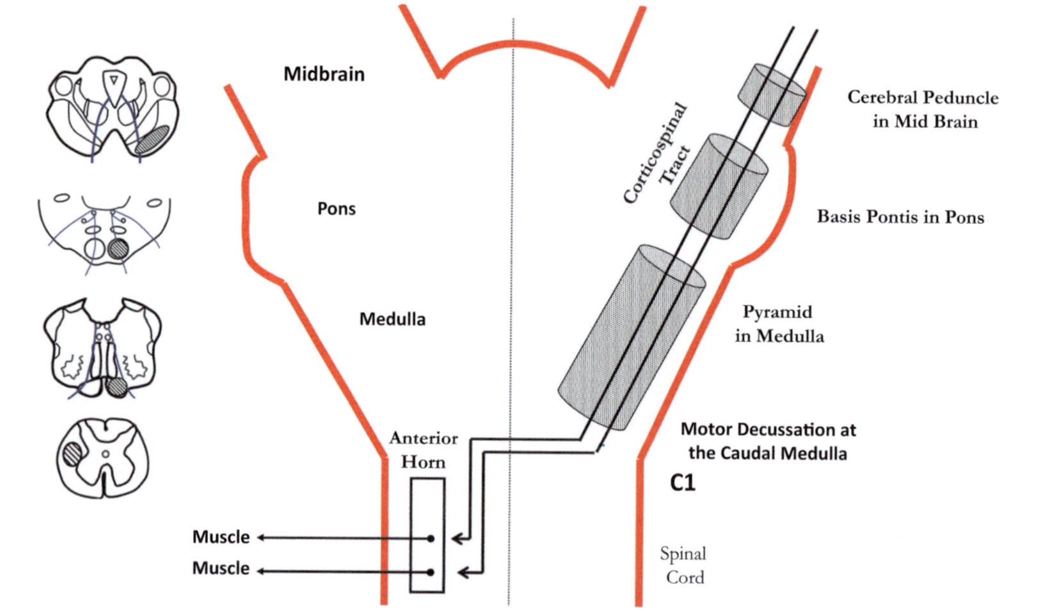

Fig. 9.3 Location of corticospinal tract. Upper motor neurons descending from cerebral cortex to spinal cord [14, 15]

highway with its one million neurons coming down the cord. Remember, at each level of the cord, some fibers will peel off at the exit ramps to innervate LMNs. With the lesion at C5, from the biceps point of view you have cut a LMN, but from the quadriceps point of view you have cut an UMN. Granted from the biceps point of view you have really cut both a LMN and an UMN but cutting the LMN will override any more subtle UMN issues. Think of your car and compare a dead battery to a blown engine. If your engine is destroyed, then whether the battery works or not is immaterial. If the LMNs are cut, it does not matter about the UMNs, there is simply no signal getting to the muscle.

With the lesion at C5, the biceps reflex will be absent or decreased (1+) while the quadriceps reflex will be increased (4+). In addition, the patient would have Babinski's sign. And all the motor signs would be on the ipsilateral side (Fig. 9.4).

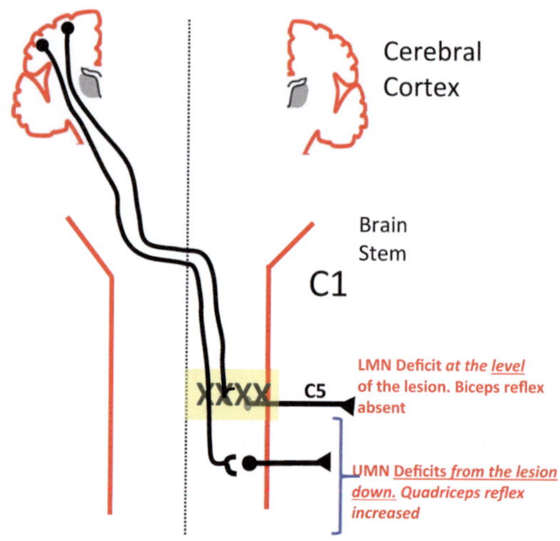

Fig. 9.4 Hemisection. Lesion at C5 level of the spinal cord. From the biceps point of view the LMN is cut. From the quadriceps point of view the UMN is cut [14, 15]

Spinothalamic

The spinothalamic tract carries pain, temperature, and vague touch information from the periphery to the cerebral cortex (Fig. 9.5). We do not use the term UMN and LMN when referring to sensory tracts, instead we use the term primary, secondary, and tertiary neurons. The primary afferent begins somewhere in the periphery with a receptor. Take stepping on a tack with your big toe as an example. The pain sensation from

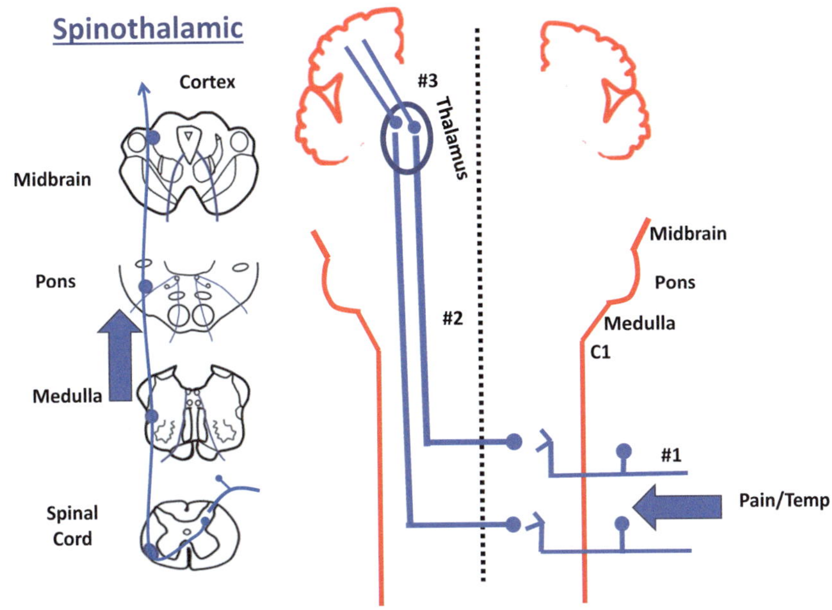

Fig. 9.5 Spinothalamic pathway [14, 15]

the tack fires the primary afferents whose fibers project along the medial plantar nerve, into the sciatic nerve, and then onto the lumbosacral plexus. As the fiber approaches the cord it has a cell body (pseudounipolar neuron) in the dorsal root ganglion (DRG) at the L4 level. The fiber, still the primary afferent, enters the spinal cord and ascends for one or two segments before terminating in the dorsal horn, where it meets the secondary neuron.

The secondary neuron then sends a fiber which decussates in a structure called the anterior white commissure and ascends the cord in the spinothalamic tract, which continues through the medulla, pons, and midbrain to eventually end in the thalamus, specifically the Ventral Posterior Lateral (VPL) nucleus of the thalamus. (See the thalamus chapter for more details.)

From the VPL, the tertiary neuron, also referred to as the thalamocortical pathway, projects to the primary somatosensory cortex, also known as the postcentral gyrus. Note that the secondary fibers pass through the lateral side of the medulla, pons, and midbrain. Lesions to the spinothalamic tract will lead to hemianesthesia on the contralateral side of the body.

Dorsal Columns

The dorsal columns carry information about vibration, conscious proprioception, fine touch, and two-point discrimination (Fig. 9.6). Like the spinothalamic it is also a three-neuron pathway. An important landmark here is T6 of the cord. Fibers that carry information from the lower limb enter the cord below T6 and ascend in the *fasciculus gracilis*. Fibers from the upper limb enter the cord above T6 and ascend in the *fasciculus cuneatus*. These two pathways, fasciculus gracilis and fasciculus cuneatus, are together known as the dorsal columns. In the caudal medulla the fibers from the fasciculus gracilis terminate in the nucleus gracilis, and fibers in the fasciculus cuneatus terminate in the nucleus cuneatus. Consider that a fiber carrying vibration information from the big toe would start in the big toe, ascend to the cord, enter the cord, ascend in fasciculus gracilis, and then terminate in nucleus gracilis in the caudal medulla near the base of the skull. In other words, this is a long neuron, running almost the entire length of the body.

After the primary afferents synapse in the nucleus gracilis or cuneatus, the secondary affer-

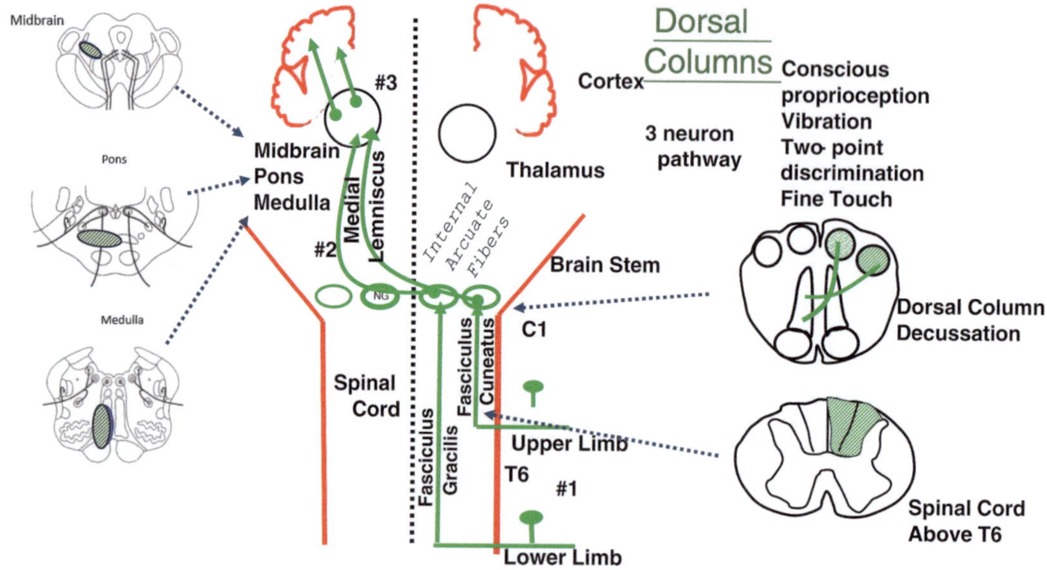

Fig. 9.6 Dorsal column pathway. The decussation is at the caudal medulla [14, 15]

ents emerge from the two nuclei (gracile and cuneate) as *internal arcuate fibers*, decussate to the opposite side, and form the *medial lemniscus* which sits on top of the pyramids (CST) in the medulla. The medial lemniscus fibers then ascend through the pons and medulla and eventually enter the VPL of the thalamus. In the caudal medulla the medial lemniscus is just posterior to the pyramid.

One detail for these two important sensory tracts is that the spinothalamic tract carries "vague touch" information, while the dorsal columns carry "fine touch" information. An example to illustrate the difference comes from having three coins in your pocket. If you have a quarter, a dime, and a nickel in your pocket, and you put your hand in your pocket, using your spinothalamic tract (vague touch) you can feel that there are three coins, but you are unable to differentiate one coin from the others. However, with your dorsal column pathway (fine touch), you can tell the difference between the quarter, the dime, and the nickel.

Damage to the information traveling in the dorsal column/medial lemniscus pathway can occur in the peripheral nerves, the spinal cord, the brainstem, the thalamus, or the cortex. With damage to the dorsal column pathway, either in the nerves, spinal cord or thalamus, the patient is said to have *astereognosis*. With damage to the parietal cortex, the patient is said to have *agnosia*.

Romberg Sign

Damage to the dorsal column system can result in Romberg sign. In a healthy person, both the visual system and the dorsal columns are used to maintain an upright posture. To test the dorsal columns, you will ask the individual to stand up and maintain posture. At this point they are using the visual system and the dorsal columns to maintain posture—even the patient with damage to the dorsal columns can maintain posture. You now ask the person to close their eyes. With damage to the dorsal columns, the patient will sway. In addition, when they walk, because proprioception is impaired, they have a hard time knowing where their legs are, they will be hesitant with the placement of their feet—like walking on a trampoline. The take home point: Romberg sign = dorsal column pathology.

Summary of the Three Long Tracts

At this point, you should be able to take a blank piece of paper and draw out the schematic of these three tracts without thinking about it—it should be a reflex activity (Fig. 9.7). Many patient scenarios will include these tracts. Do not expect a neuroanatomy test question to just ask a specific isolated factoid about one of these tracts. Instead, expect to see these tracts woven together throughout numerous questions. As mentioned earlier, one of the first questions you will ask yourself is: Is the lesion in the CNS or the PNS? In addition to the presence of long tract signs, if a patient has UMN signs, or sensory deficits over a large part of the body, then you suspect that the lesion is in the CNS.

The Long Tracts in the Brain Sem

Medulla

To work through the topography of the brainstem, the first step is to look at the location of these three tracts in the medulla, pons, and midbrain. In the traditional cross-sectional view of the medulla, the medial lemniscus stands vertically on the pyramids like a headless stick person holding their head. The feet rest on the pyramid and the shoulders are on top. The stick figure represents the orientation of the cervical, thoracic, lumbar, and sacral fibers that emerged from the nucleus gracilis and cuneatus as internal arcuate fibers and entered the medial lemniscus.

This stick figure medial lemniscus is holding its head, which represents the sensory fibers in the *ventral trigeminothalamic tract* (VTT). The VTT is carrying information from the trigeminal system– or face. The shoulders of the stick figure, or the top of the medial lemniscus in the orientation on the picture, lie half-way between the pyramids and the floor of the fourth ventricle (Fig. 9.8).

Immediately above the medial lemniscus, going from ventral to dorsal, is the tectospinal tract, the medial longitudinal fasciculus, and hypoglossal (XII) nucleus. Lateral to the medial lemniscus is the inferior olivary nucleus. The inferior olives are prominent structures and useful landmarks. As we move into the pons the stick figure is about to slip on the olives and fall (think of olives as being slippery).

The medulla is also the site of the motor decussation and the sensory decussation. When we say the sensory decussation, we are only referring to the dorsal column decussation—remember the spinothalamic tract crossed in the spinal cord. The motor decussation occurs just a tad higher than the sensory decussation.

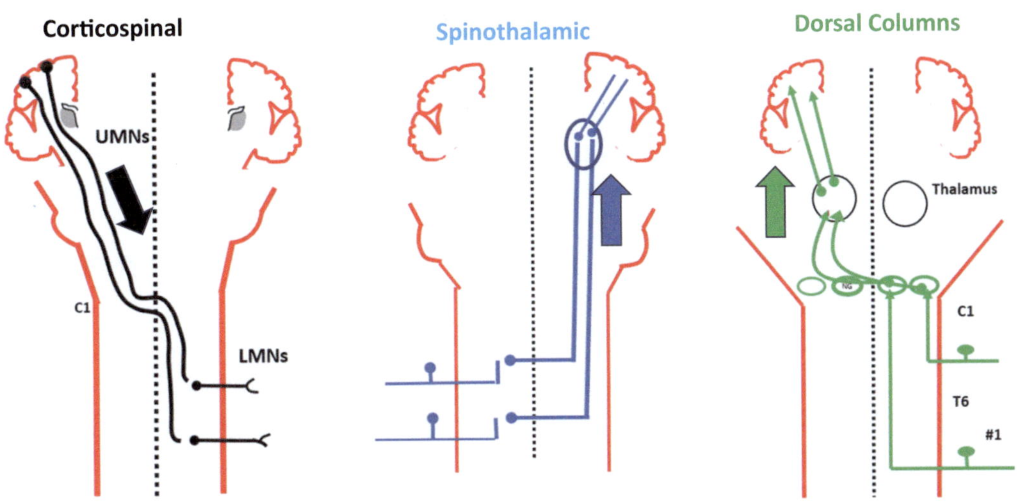

Fig. 9.7 The three long tracts [14, 15]

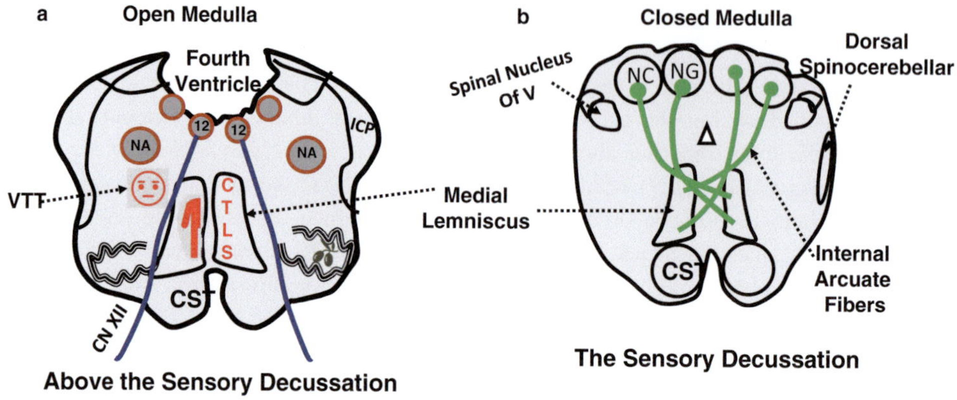

Fig. 9.8 Panel (**a**) Open medulla. The headless man represents the topography of the medial lemniscus with cervical fibers at the top, followed by thoracic, lumbar, and sacral in descending order. This headless man is standing on the pyramid (corticospinal tract). The slippery olives are off to the left. The face fibers are not in the medial lemniscus but are off to the side in the ventral trigeminothalamic tract (VTT). Panel (**b**) Closed medulla. In this section you can see the internal arcuate fibers coming out of nucleus gracilis (NG) and cuneatus (NC) and decussating to end up in the contralateral medial lemniscus [14, 15]

Sensory Decussation

The fibers ascending in the dorsal columns terminate on the dorsal column nucleus—nucleus cuneatus and fasciculus. Coming out of these nuclei are the internal arcuate fibers which cross to the other side and ascend in the medial lemniscus. A lesion to a medial lemniscus at the level of the sensory decussation would affect both sides of the body because of the crossing fibers. As soon as you are above the sensory decussation, a lesion to the medial lemniscus would affect the contralateral side of the body. A lesion to either nucleus gracilis or cuneatus at the level of the sensory decussation would affect the ipsilateral side of the body. Note that at the level of the sensory decussation, one can see the pyramids, and the pyramids are above the motor decussation—in other words, at the level of the sensory decussation we are above the motor decussation.

Decussation of Corticospinal Tract

In the medulla, the corticospinal tract with the UMNs is in the pyramid, which is superior to the decussation. Keep in mind that as the fibers travel down the pyramid, lesions to the pyramid will result in contralateral UMN signs. At the bottom of the pyramid, the inferior portion, the fibers leave the pyramid and cross over to the contralateral side to continue down the spinal cord (Fig. 9.9).

Moving from Medulla into Pons

The pons is characterized by its ventrally located bulbous shape. The corticospinal tract is descending through the basis pontis. The "headless person" (medial lemniscus) has slipped off the "slippery olive" and lies on its back with its foot lateral and shoulder medial. As we move up into the pons, the feet will rise towards the posterior surface. Within the pons are several cranial nerve nuclei as well as the scattered pontine nuclei. These pontine nuclei receive a projection from the cerebral cortex and then project to the cerebellum as the pontocerebellar fibers. On the dorsal side is the fourth ventricle.

In the middle of the pons, we start to see three sensory pathways lined up together in a structure that looks like a boomerang. The most medial pathway is the medial lemniscus, then moving lateral is the spinal lemniscus (spinothalamic), and then the lateral lemniscus (auditory).

Midbrain

The midbrain is characterized by the two peduncles. It looks something like an upside-down

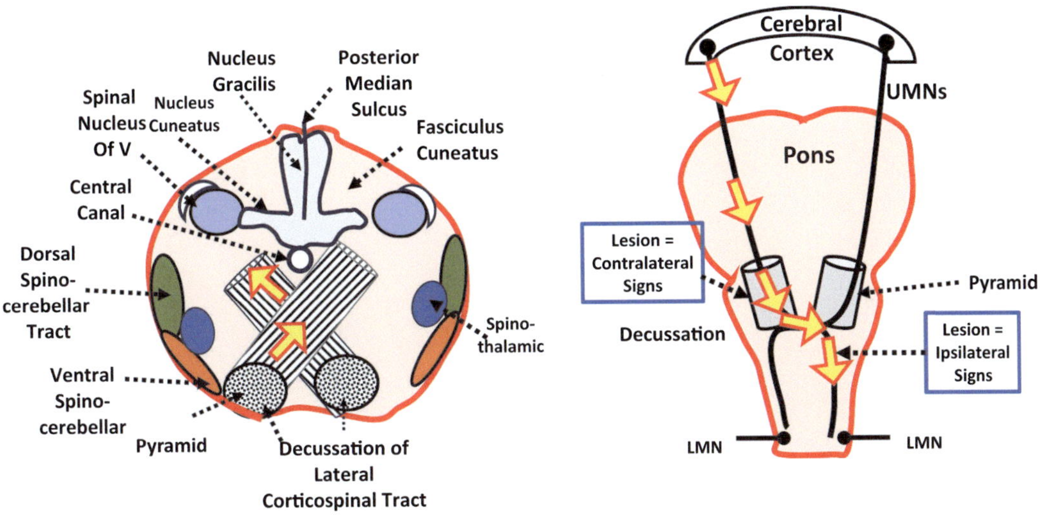

Fig. 9.9 Decussation of the corticospinal tract. The UMNs descend from the precentral gyrus down through the midbrain, pons, and medulla. In the medulla they are in the pyramid. The fibers emerge from the pyramid and cross over at the decussation to the contralateral side of the body. A lesion to the pyramids leads to contralateral signs. A lesion to the tract in the spinal cord leads to ipsilateral signs [14, 15]

mickey mouse, with the peduncles being Mickey's ears, and the red nucleus his eyes. The two peduncles project ventrally and between them is the interpeduncular fossa with CN III coming through it. There are numerous lesions that can occur in this area.

The posterior portion of the midbrain is the tectum, with the superior and inferior colliculus. At the level of the inferior colliculus the medial lemniscus has migrated nearer to the lateral edge of the midbrain. Lateral to the medial lemniscus is the spinal lemniscus, and then the lateral lemniscus. The lateral lemniscus eventually terminates in the inferior colliculus. One way to differentiate the inferior from superior colliculus is that the inferior colliculus resembles a wine glass, with the goblet being the nucleus and the stem being the lateral lemniscus.

At the level of the superior colliculus, we have lost the lateral lemniscus since it terminated in the inferior colliculus. The most prominent structure here is the red nucleus. Here is a straightforward way to remember structures here. Think of the red nucleus as a smiling face, and on the top of the face is a long stocking hat. The bulk of the hat represents the medial lemniscus and the pom-pom on top of the hat is the spinothalamic tract (Fig. 9.10).

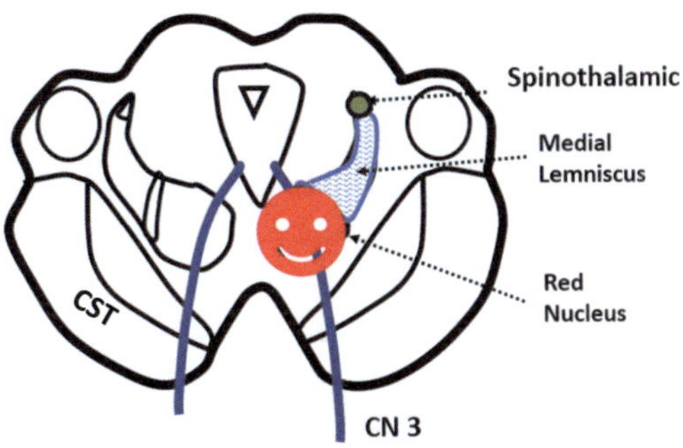

Fig. 9.10 Mid brain. The smiling face represents the red nucleus. The main part of the hat represents the medial lemniscus and the small bob on top of the hat is the spinothalamic tract. The corticospinal tract (CST) is in the middle one-third of the cerebral peduncle [14, 15]

A Test on the Long Tracts

Before continuing, make sure you can do the following exercise (Fig. 9.11). The purpose of this is to be able to relate a cross section view with the longitudinal view. The numbers in the various spinal cord and brain stem sections represent

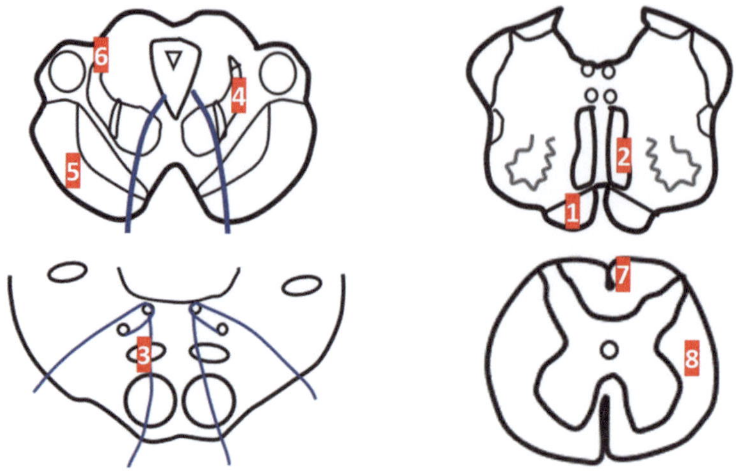

Fig. 9.11 Lesion test. Each number represents a lesion. What are the symptoms, are they contralateral or ipsilateral? And where the cell bodies of origin (CBO) for each tract are located

lesions. For each lesion jot down whether the symptoms are ipsilateral or contralateral, what modality is affected, and where the cell body of origin is located for the fibers in that structure. The point of this exercise is to see the importance of having a visual image in your mind of the tracts. As we discuss the various lesions, these three tracts should be second nature (Table 9.5).

Table 9.5 Key to brainstem and spinal cord lesions

1. Contralateral UMN signs, CBO—precentral gyrus
2. Contralateral dorsal column signs, CBO—nucleus cuneatus and gracilis
3. Contralateral dorsal column signs, CBO—nucleus cuneatus and gracilis
4. Contralateral dorsal column signs, CBO—nucleus cuneatus and gracilis
5. Contralateral UMN signs, CBO—precentral gyrus
6. Contralateral loss of pain and temperature, CBO—dorsal horn
7. Ipsilateral dorsal column signs, CBO—DRG
8. Ipsilateral UMN signs, CBO—precentral gyrus

All the questions above require putting several pieces of knowledge together. For instance, on the most superficial level you need to know what tract you are looking at. Remember you cannot really see the tracts; you just need to know where they are located. Is it the medial lemniscus, corticospinal tract, or another structure? And you also need to know what modality is running in each tract such as motor, pain, or proprioception. But the harder part is looking at the section and the tract and knowing where you are in relation to the decussation. The question you need to ask yourself: Am I above or below the decussation?

If we take a section through the caudal medulla we can walk through each tract. Looking at the pyramid (lesion A) we need to know that since we are in the pyramid then we must be above the decussation. Remember that when the fibers in the corticospinal tract reach the lowest level of the pyramid, they cross over to the descend in the opposite cord. In addition, we should know that the cell bodies are in the precentral gyrus in the frontal lobe (Fig. 9.12).

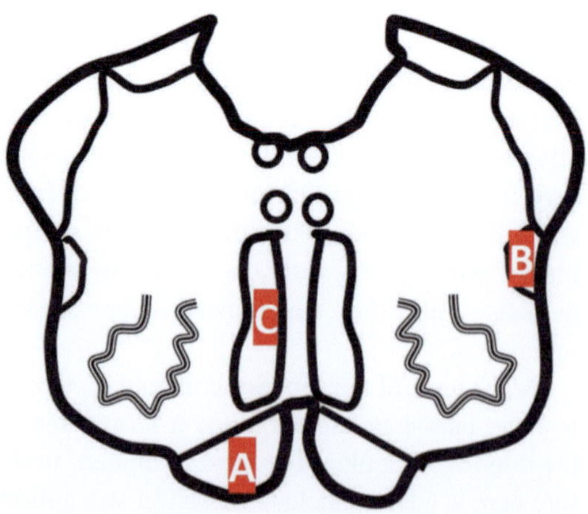

Fig. 9.12 Medulla. At each lesion, note the tract involved, what the symptoms are, and whether the symptoms are on the ipsilateral or contralateral side [14, 15]

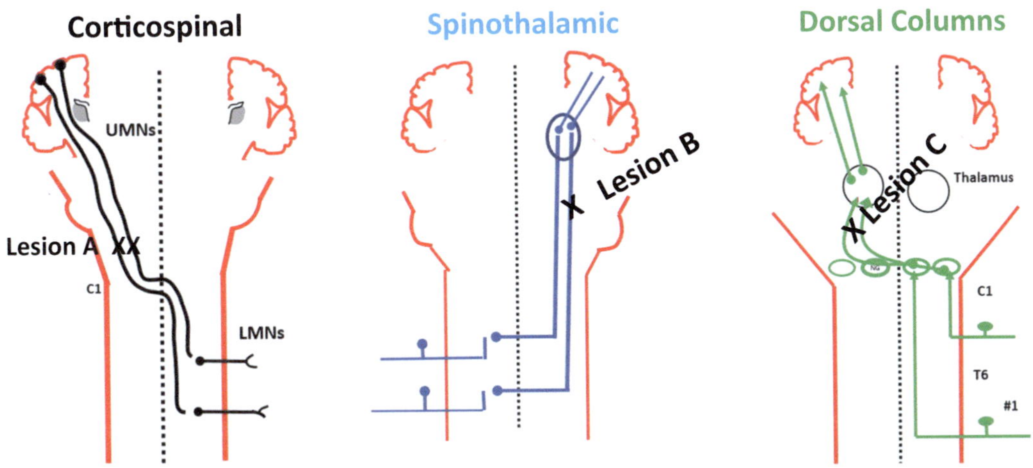

Fig. 9.13 The three long tracts and three lesions [14, 15]

If we look at the lesion in the spinothalamic tract (lesion B), then the symptoms—loss of pain and temperature—will be on the contralateral side. Realize that the lesion is to the second order neurons that originated in the dorsal horn.

If we look at the medial lemniscus (lesion C) we need to know that it carries second order neurons that have their cell bodies in the nucleus gracilis and cuneatus. If we have a small lesion here, then the patient will lose conscious proprioception, two-point discrimination, and vibratory sense from the contralateral limbs (Figs. 9.12 and 9.13).

Jendrassik Maneuver

When testing a lower limb reflex, such as the Achilles tendon, one way to heighten the individual's response is to have them clasp their hands and squeeze (Jendrassik Maneuver). This will often lead to heightened reflex activity in the lower limb. It is not clear why this happens, but one idea is that this maneuver leads to heightened UMN input to the upper cord, which in turn diminishes the UMN input to the lower cord thus removing some of the inhibitory input from the cortex to the lower limb.

Brown Séquard Syndrome

Big Picture The classic way to test your knowledge of the three long pathways is to present a patient scenario of Brown Séquard Syndrome—also referred to as a hemisection of the spinal cord. We have already talked about motor deficits. In the patient scenario below, the patient has a lesion at C5 on the left. This will lead to left side spastic paralysis (ipsilateral side), right side loss of pain and temperature sensation (contralateral), and left side loss of the dorsal column modalities such as proprioception, vibratory sense, and conscious proprioception (contralateral). All these deficits will be evident from the C5 level on down (Fig. 9.14).

The Details The main findings of motor deficits on one side of the body and pain and temperature deficits on the opposite side place the lesion in the spinal cord, but if we look closer to the details, we can be more specific about where exactly in the cord the lesion is located. Consider the motor findings first. If the lesion is at C5, because the anterior horn is damaged you will have LMN signs at that level, so the biceps reflex would be decreased, or absent. But since you have cut the corticospinal tract at that level, from the quadri-

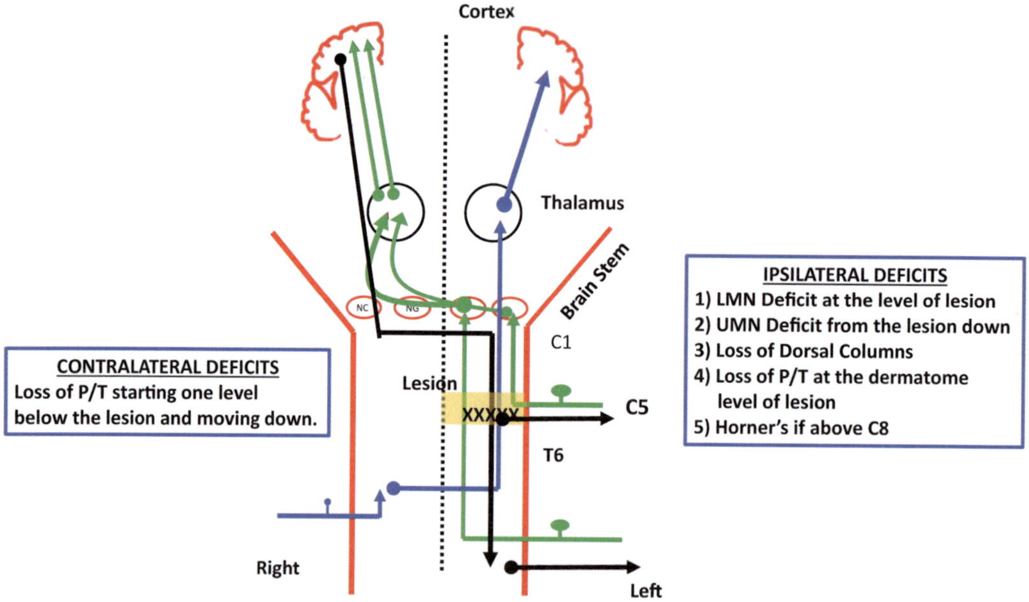

Fig. 9.14 Hemisection of spinal cord at C5 level. UMN signs are ipsilateral. Pain and temperature loss is contralateral. Dorsal column symptoms are ipsilateral [14, 15]

ceps point of view you have cut an UMN, and its reflex will be increased. In fact, any reflex below C5 in this patient should be increased. At the level of the lesion, you will have LMN signs, but from the lesion down you will have UMN signs. In the real world, or on a test question, this is where you appreciate the value of the reflex hammer tests.

In addition, while the patient's major loss of pain and temperature sensation is on the contralateral side of the body, to be more specific the loss of pain starts one level below the lesion due to the primary afferents entering the cords and then ascending one level before synapsing in the dorsal horn. In addition, because the ipsilateral dorsal horn is involved there will be an ipsilateral loss of pain and temperature sensation at the level of the lesion.

And, finally, if the lesion is above T1 there will be an ipsilateral Horner's syndrome because of the loss of the descending fibers from the hypothalamus to the T1 lateral horn (The Ciliospinal Center of Budge).

Syringomyelia

Syringomyelia is another lesion where it is important to understand the neuroanatomy to explain the symptoms. Syringomyelia may be congenital or acquired, with the congenital form often occurring with a Chiari Type I malformation. The acquired form may arise following trauma or for unknown (idiopathic) reasons. Regardless of the cause, to understand the symptoms you need to understand how the spinothalamic tract decussates. In contrast to either the dorsal column pathway or the corticospinal tract that each decussates at one discreet location, the spinothalamic tract decussates at every level of the cord. Whether you are at C5, T5, or L5, you will find crossing fibers of the spinothalamic tract, referred to as the *anterior white commissure.*

The typical patient scenario will be a middle-aged woman who explains that she has lost pain sensation in both hands. There is no sensory deficit in the lower limbs. The lesion in this case is due to an expansion of the central canal which is

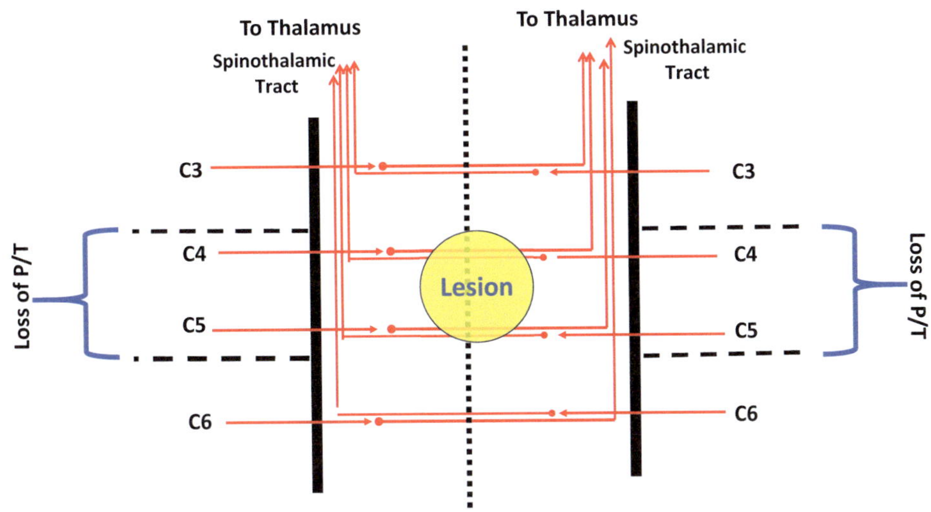

Fig. 9.15 Lesion at anterior white commissure. This is a close-up view of the spinal cord from C3 to C6. Bilateral loss of pain, temperature, and vague touch at the level of the lesion [14, 15]

in the center of the cord, and it usually happens in the cervical cord. The expansion will typically compress the anterior white commissure at several levels—say C5, C6 and C7 (Fig. 9.15).

Because the lesion is compressing the anterior spinothalamic fibers, the dorsal column system remains intact and functioning. Thus, the patient in this scenario will retain the sensations of vague touch. She might report that she can feel the "texture" of objects for instance.

It does not damage the actual spinothalamic tracts which are located out on the lateral side of the cord. If the lesion is in the cervical area, you might here the term a "cape-like loss" of pain and temperature which refers to the C5–C6 and maybe C7 dermatomes. These dermatomes start on your shoulders and come down to your hands. If the lesion is in the thoracic cord, then you might here the term a "belt-like loss" of pain and temperature referring to the fact that the dermatomes such as T3 or T4 resemble a belt.

One caveat is that as the syrinx expands it can impinge on the anterior horn cells which can lead to LMN signs in the muscles of the forearm and hands. It is unlikely that it would hit the corticospinal tract thus the lower limbs would be spared.

Tabes Dorsalis

Tabes Dorsalis is a slow degeneration of the dorsal columns resulting from untreated syphilis. Symptoms include unsteady gait, bladder control problems, progressive degeneration of the joints (Charcot joints), diminished deep tendon reflexes, loss of coordination, and episodes of intense pain. Think of the "Three Ps": Pain, Polyuria, and Paresthesia. Patients will present with: (1) a Romberg sign, meaning that they sway with their eyes closed; (2) an Argyll Robertson Pupil, meaning that the pupils respond to accommodation but not light; and (3) a tabetic gait or foot slap. Because the patient has lost proprioception, they lift their feet higher than normal when they walk, and the foot strikes the floor harder than normal which leads to a slapping noise.

Anterior Spinal Artery

The single anterior spinal artery (ASA) arises from two small branches that come off the vertebral artery. These two small branches immediately unite to form the ASA, which travels down the anterior median fissure of the spinal cord to supply the anterior two-thirds of the cord. As the artery travels down the cord, it receives contributions from the radicular arteries and the *Artery of Adamkiewicz*. Lesions to this artery lead to the bilateral loss of the spinothalamic and corticospinal pathways. The dorsal columns, located posteriorly, will be spared. The ASA can become occluded during surgical procedures to and around the abdominal aorta. Aortic aneurysms, aortic dissections, and atherosclerosis disease of the aorta can all lead to reduced blood flow to the ASA.

The most common site of an ASA lesion is the T4–T8 region. Thus, in the typical scenario the lower limb but not the upper limb will be affected. Bladder and bowel function will usually be disrupted.

If the main anterior spinal artery is occluded the patient will have bilateral signs. However, coming of the anterior spinal artery there are sulcal branches—on both the right and the left sides—which enter the cord. If a sulcal branch is occluded, then only one side of the cord will be affected. In this case, the patient would have ipsilateral motor deficits because the UMNs are damaged, and they would have a contralateral loss of pain and temperature because the spinothalamic tract is damaged. The dorsal columns would not be affected because they are not perfused by the anterior spinal artery. The symptoms would be like a hemisection of the cord, although the dorsal columns would be spared.

Subacute Combined Degeneration

Subacute combined degeneration results from a deficiency of vitamin B12 which leads to degeneration of the corticospinal tracts, dorsal columns, and dorsal spinocerebellar tracts. Patients will present with gait abnormalities, a Romberg sign, muscle weakness, hyperreflexia, spasticity, and impairment of tactile sensation, proprioception, and vibration sense. Because of the loss of the dorsal columns *Lhermitte's sign* may be present. Lhermitte's sign occurs when the patient flexes the neck—chin touching the chest—and they feel an electrical signal shooting up and down their spine.

Central Cord Syndrome

As the corticospinal tract travels down the spinal cord, the fibers destined for the upper limb are medial and they peel off at various levels to travel to the anterior horn cells. Central cord syndrome is a lesion in the central part of the cord that damages these more medial fibers, thus the patient has deficits in the upper limb, while the lower limb is spared. This is sometimes referred to as *sacral sparing*. Because it is typically the corticospinal tract that is affected, sensory information will often be spared, or at least will not be as severely affected as motor function. A likely cause of central cord syndrome is a motor vehicle accident that involves hyperextension of the neck.

Conus Medullaris Syndrome

Time for a thought experiment. Imagine you are in the anatomy lab, and you remove the spinous process and the lamina of the L1 vertebra. What level of the cord are you looking at? You are looking at the sacral cord- or the conus medullaris. Remember the spinal cord ends at the L1 vertebra. Conus medullaris syndrome usually comes from displaced L1 or L2 vertebra. Because the compression will be on both the peripheral nerves (cauda equina) emerging from the cord, and the cord itself, the patient will have a combination of UMN and LMN deficits in the lower limb. They will often have saddle anesthesia and deficits with the bladder and bowel. Conus lesions can be subdivided into a low cone injury or a high cone injury (Fig. 9.16).

Cervical Myelopathy

Cervical myelopathy results from compression of the cervical spinal cord. There are several probable causes, such as: (1) thickening of the posterior longitudinal ligament, (2) a tumor, (3) radiation, or (4) vascular issues. It can lead to a combination of UMN deficits because it compresses the cord, and LMN deficits because it compresses one or more of the cervical nerves.

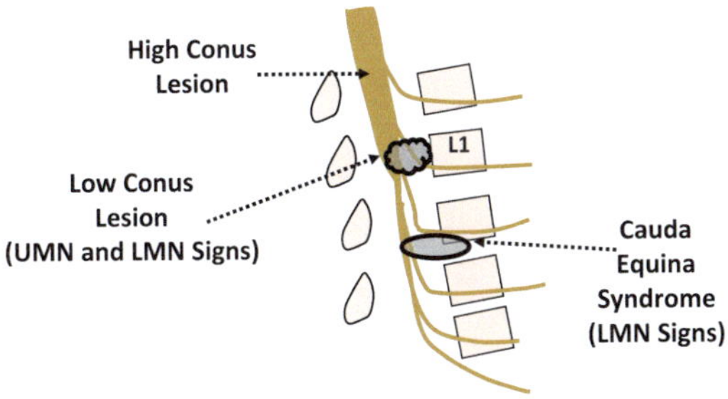

Fig. 9.16 Conus medullaris and cauda equina syndromes. Conus Medullaris Syndrome is the result of lesion to either the high or low part of the cone. Lesions be categorized as high or low conus lesions. Cauda Equina Syndrome is a lesion to the fibers traveling from the cord to where they are exiting the spinal column [14, 15]

Axonal Polyneuropathy

Axonal Polyneuropathy results from damage to peripheral nerves. In patients such as diabetics, whose nerve fibers are compromised, it is the longer axons that first show pathology. This is why diabetics first see this pathology in their feet. As time progresses, the pathology moves up their lower limb. By the time the knee is affected, symptoms are typically starting to appear in the hands.

Guillain-Barré Syndrome

Guillain-Barré is an autoimmune disorder in which the immune system attacks the peripheral nerves, usually following an acute bacterial or viral infection. The patient first reports symptoms in the lower limbs such as weakness and tingling. At first, the symptoms can be mild and may even disappear, however they can also become severe and quickly spread to affect the entire body.

Amyotrophic Lateral Sclerosis

ALS (Lou Gehrig's Disease) starts as small punctate lesions that appear in the anterior horn cells and the corticospinal tracts. It is difficult to diagnose in the initial stages because the symptoms are mild. The patient might have LMN signs on one limb, and UMN signs on another limb, or even another side of the body. An early sign is the presence of fasciculations. The patient may complain of twitches. There are no sensory deficits or higher cortical function deficits. As time goes on, and more lesions appear, the patient will first become wheelchair bound, and eventually become bedridden. Typical symptoms include constipation, drooling, weight loss, and labored breathing.

Friedreich Ataxia

Friedreich ataxia (FA) is the result of an autosomal recessive genetic mutation that affects the nervous system and the heart. The mutation leads to a deficit in frataxin, which is a mitochondrial matrix protein. Symptoms typically start around the age of puberty with the first symptom being a gait deficit due to degeneration of the posterior columns and the associated dorsal root ganglion cells. This is followed by degeneration of the cerebellar Purkinje cells and the dentate nucleus. The corticospinal tract can also be affected. Many FA patients will be short of breath and have heart palpitations. The vertebral column can also be affected resulting in scoliosis. Over time they may also develop *pes cavus*—a high plantar longitudinal arch. The cerebral cortex and higher cortical functions are typically not affected in FA patients. The most common cause of death in FA patients is cardiomyopathy.

Spinal Shock

Immediately after traumatic damage to the spinal cord, the patient will exhibit complete loss of motor and sensory function below the level of the lesion. They will exhibit flaccid paralysis, a loss of tone to the muscles, and no reflex activity, even though the reflex arcs below the lesion are anatomically intact. However, while the specifics vary from patient to patient, the presence of spinal shock is often temporary, and the patient will eventually regain reflex activity and some motor control. The average time to move out of spinal shock to the more permanent presentation is 4–12 weeks.

To illustrate spinal shock, take the example of a 28-year-old male in a motorcycle accident who suffered a hemisection to the right side of the spinal cord at C5. We are going to focus on the motor deficits. You are examining this patient 8 weeks after the injury, and you note an absent biceps reflex and increased patellar tendon reflex—classic motor deficits for this type of patient (LMN signs at the level of the lesion, and UMN signs from the lesion on down). Yet, when this patient was first brought into the Emergency Department, he did not have these signs. Instead, he was in spinal shock and had complete LMN signs from the lesion down. At some point, maybe 4 weeks after the accident, he moved from spinal shock with no reflex activity to the more long-term presentation of LMN signs at the level of the lesion, and UMN signs from the lesion down. When he was brought into the emergency department he had flaccid paralysis, 8 weeks later when you are examining him, he has spastic paralysis.

In the Emergency Department, when the patient is moving out of spinal shock, the first reflexes to return are the bulbocavernosus reflex and the anal wink. Both of which are functional tests for S 2, 3, and 4. In the real world, right after the accident, you might scratch the patient's foot every time you walk into the room to see if Babinski's is returning. In a patient scenario you would be given the results of two physical exams separated by several weeks: one right after the accident with all LMN signs, and one several months later, with LMN signs at the level of the lesion and UMN signs from the lesion down.

Dissociated Sensory Loss

With lesions to the spinal cord or brainstem it is possible to damage only the spinothalamic tract while sparing the dorsal column system. In these cases, the patients will lose pain and temperature but not vibration, proprioception, and two-point discrimination. These patients exhibit dissociated sensory loss. Lateral medullary syndrome is an example of a patient with dissociated sensory loss.

Dermatome, Peripheral Nerve, and Myotome Maps

Myotomes refer to the spinal level or levels that are most important in movements at each limb. A word of warning is in order about the tables below, especially the myotome table (Table 9.6). If you look at these tables in three different books, you might see subtle differences amongst the books. These differences are due to normal human variation that leads to the slight differences in the various studies. However, do not panic because the information on a specific movement in a patient is only one finding amongst many others, and it will not be the sole piece of information that you need to determine where the lesion is located.

When it comes to sensory loss you want to keep two maps in your mind—the dermatome map, and the peripheral nerve map. Most anatomy textbooks will show the two maps side-by-side. With a spinal cord patient, you want to think about the dermatome map. With a lesion to a peripheral nerve such as either the radial or femoral nerve, you need to think about the peripheral nerve map. With the typical neurology patient, you want to focus on the dermatome map. I will leave the PNS lesions and the peripheral nerve map to the gross anatomists, with one exception: the radiculopathies. With a radiculopathy, which is in the PNS, right next to the cord, and before the nerve fibers joins the brachial or lumbar plexuses, you want to think about dermatomes (Table 9.7).

Table 9.6 Myotomes

Spinal level	Movement
C5	Shoulder abduction
C6	Elbow flexion/Wrist extension
C7	Elbow extension/Wrist flexion/Finger extension
C8	Wrist flexion/Thumb extension
T1	Finger abduction/adduction
L2	Hip flexion
L5	Dorsiflexion
S1	Plantar flexion

Table 9.7 Dermatome map

Spinal level	Region
C6	Thumb
C7	Middle fingers
C8	Fifth digit
T1	Armpit
T4	Nipple
T10	Umbilicus
L1	Inguinal
L2, 3	Anteromedial thigh
L4	Medial leg, foot
L5	Anterior leg, dorsum of foot
S1	Lateral foot
S2, 3, 4	Gluteal region

Radiculopathies

Radiculopathies (damage to spinal roots) are often the result of herniated discs. The discs themselves have an outer thick, strong *annulus fibrous*, and an inner core of the softer *nucleus pulposus,* which is the remanent of the embryological notochord. Anteriorly, the disc is held in place by the *anterior longitudinal ligament*, and posteriorly, by *the posterior longitudinal ligament*. The weak link in this region is the lateral portion of the posterior longitudinal ligament. If this ligament is weakened, the nucleus pulposus will herniate in a posterior lateral direction and compress the nerve exiting one level below. The majority of disc herniations are at this posterolateral position, however in approximately 5% of cases, the disc can herniate at the far lateral margin, in which case the herniation will hit the nerve exiting at that level. For instance, a disk herniation at the far lateral margin of the L4/5 disk could hit the L4 nerve, but again this is rare compared to the more typical posterolateral location.

To understand the symptoms of a radiculopathy, before getting into the specifics, make sure you understand the big picture difference between cutting a nerve or a root. When you cut a peripheral nerve, the muscle innervated by that nerve will be completely (100%) paralyzed. For instance, if you cut the femoral nerve then the four quadriceps muscles will be completely paralyzed. However, if you cut the root, the muscle group will be weak. This is because peripheral nerves receive contributions from several different spinal levels, and the femoral nerve gets contributions from L2, L3, and L4. Thus, if just one of these roots is damaged, say L2, the muscles innervated by the femoral nerve will just be weak, because L3 and L4 are still intact.

In the lumbar area, the spinal cord ends at the L1 vertebra. The nerves coming out at the lower cord then travel down as the cauda equina to exit through their appropriate intervertebral foramen. Looking at the vertebrae from the posterior view, imagine we have cut the pedicle of a vertebra with a bone saw. We can see the pedicles at the top of each vertebra. The intervertebral canal is between the pedicles of two vertebrae. If we focus on the L4 and L5 vertebrae, we see a disc between the two, and exiting at the top of the foramen is the L4 nerve. In the most common scenario, if this disc herniates then it will not hit L4, which is exiting above the disc, but will hit the L5 nerve as it passes by the disc to exit one level down. In other words, a disc herniation between L4 and L5 will hit the nerve exiting one level down, which is L5 (Fig. 9.17).

If we move to the cervical area, everything changes (Fig. 9.16). The first thing to note is that the numbering scheme for the nerves is different. The C1 nerve comes out above the C1 vertebra (the atlas), and C2 nerve exits above C2 (the axis), and so forth for the other cervical nerves. These nerves do not have to travel down the vertebral canal before exiting, but instead exit straight out of their respective foramen. If the disc between C3 and C4 is displaced then the nerve that is exiting at this level will be compressed, which is the C4 nerve. In addition, because there are seven cervical vertebrae and eight cervical nerves, when the disc between C7 and T1 herniates it will hit the C8 nerve. With a herniation between T1 and T2, the T1 nerve will be compromised.

The most common disc herniations are in the lower limb region to either L4, L5, or S1. With a disc injury you want to think of three physical findings. The first is the reflex test, the second is the muscle test (the myotome), and the third is the sensory loss related to dermatome. Not every level has a good reflex test (Table 9.8).

Spondylolysis is a stress fracture in the pars interarticularis, at the collar in the Scottie dog

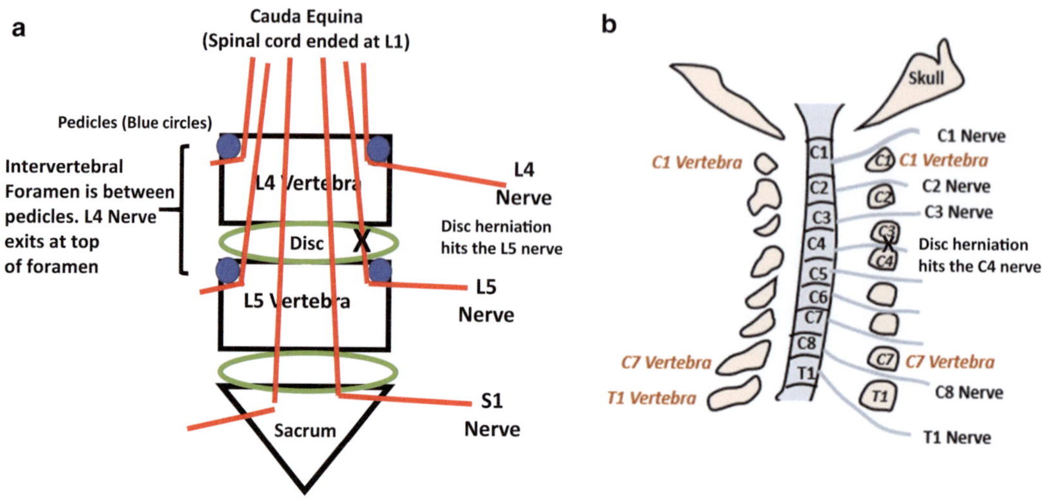

Fig. 9.17 Disc herniation. Panel (**a**) is a herniation between L4 and L5 which hits the L5 nerve. The L5 nerve exits one level inferior. Panel (**b**) shows the cervical nerves exiting above their various vertebral bodies. A disc herniation between C3 and C4 hits the nerve exiting at that level—in this case C4 [14, 15]

Table 9.8 Radiculopathies and major symptoms

	L4	L5	S1
Reflex test	Patellar tendon	No good reflex	Achilles' reflex
Muscle test	Quadriceps	Dorsiflexing toes	Plantarflex ankle
Sensory loss	Lateral thigh, medial leg, and medial foot	Lateral leg, dorsum of foot	Posterior thigh, lateral leg, and lateral foot

picture. The most common site is L5. *Spondylolisthesis* is when one vertebra slides forward over the vertebra below it (*listhesis = to slip). Ankylosing spondylitis* refers to fused vertebrae. The patient will have a hunched forward position. A hangman's fracture is a bilateral fracture at the pars interarticularis of C2.

On a radiograph a straightforward way to picture a spondylolysis is to think of a picture of a scotty dog. The fracture of the pars interarticularis occurs at the dog's collar (Fig. 9.18).

Tarlov Cysts

Tarlov cysts are fluid filled cysts that surround the roots of the spinal cord near the sacral cord. It is more common for them to surround the posterior roots. Patients with Tarlov cysts have a similar presentation to those with other spinal cord problems such as spondylolisthesis or herniated disks.

Some Terminology

The term *analgesia* refers to a loss of pain sensation, while *anesthesia* refers to a loss of all sensation. *Hypoalgesia* refers to a deceased ability to feel pain, while *hypoesthesia,* commonly called numbness, refers to decreased ability to feel all forms of sensation in a part of the body. Examples of hypoesthesia would be carpel tunnel syndrome or meralgia paresthetica. *Paresthesia* refers to an abnormal or spontaneous sensation (tingling or crawling).

Hemiplegia refers to complete paralysis, while *hemiparesis* refers to partial weakness. Hemiparesis is less severe than hemiplegia.

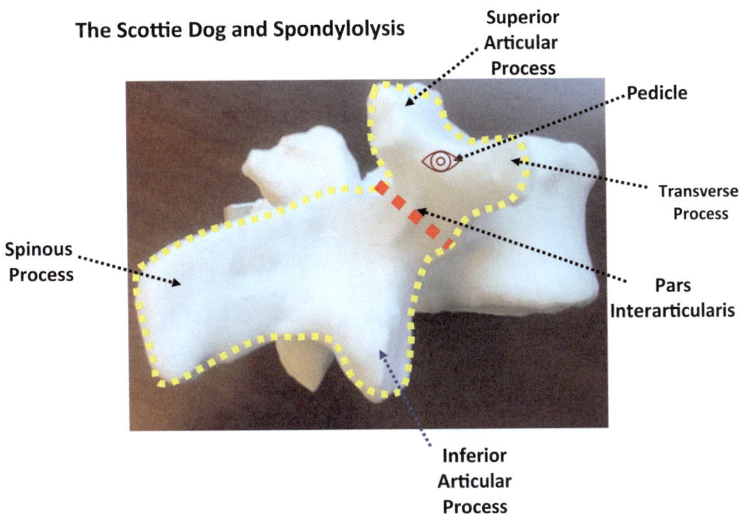

Fig. 9.18 Scottie dog and spondylolysis. The dog's collar is the pars interarticularis which is the site of spondylolysis. The facet joint is between the superior articular facet (the dog's ear) and the inferior articular process of the vertebra above it [14, 15]

Complete vs. Incomplete Spinal Cord Injuries: In some cases, the spinal cord is completely damaged in others it is only partially (incomplete) damaged. The five most common types of *incomplete* spinal cord injuries (or syndromes) are: Brown-Sequard, central cord, anterior cord, conus medullaris, and cauda-equina. The mobility of a patient to walk after a spinal cord injury varies from one patient to another.

Case #1 A 55-year-old female with a history of Hodgkin's disease in remission came to the clinic complaining of trouble using her right hand. She also dragged her right foot when walking. Her symptoms began 4 weeks previously and had gradually worsened. She found it difficult to write and work with her right hand. The left leg and left-hand were numb. She also reported some aching pain over the posterior aspect of the neck.

On examination she was alert, oriented, and cooperative. Proprioception and vibratory sensation were decreased in the right toes, ankle, and fingers. Pinprick and temperature sensation was decreased on the left arm, trunk, and leg, but not on the neck or face. Mild weakness without wasting or fasciculation was present in the right arm and leg. In the lower right extremity, hip flexion and ankle dorsiflexion were weak. Tendon reflexes were increased on the right side, and Babinski's sign was present on that side.

You also note that she has right ptosis and miosis.

Where Is the Lesion?

The findings of right-side UMN symptoms, right-side dorsal column loss, and left-side loss of pain and temperature sensations all suggest that the lesion is in the cervical region of the cord. In addition, because the lesion is above T1 there is an ipsilateral Horner's Syndrome which leads to miosis and ptosis. Horner's syndrome results from damage to the descending hypothalamic fibers projecting from the hypothalamus to the lateral horn at C8.

Same Case But More Information

If we know a little more detail from the neurological exam, we can deduct a more precise localization of the lesion. During reflex testing, you find the following (+2 is normal) (Table 9.9):

During your test for pain and temperature with a pin you find the following:

On the left side she has lost pain and temperature sensation starting on the lateral forearm region, and continuing to the hand, coming up on the medial forearm and then continuing down the thorax, abdomen, and entire left lower limb. On

Table 9.9 Spinal Cord Case and Reflexes

Reflex	Right	Left
Biceps	0	+2
Triceps	+3	+2
Patella	+3	+2
Achille's	+4	+2

the right side she has only lost pain and temperature sensation on a patch of skin of the right shoulder.

From this more detailed information we can localize the lesion to C5. For the reflexes, there is a reduced response for the biceps reflex which is C5 because we have a LMN deficit at this level. But there are increased reflexes from the C6 level on down due to damage of the corticospinal tract. The level of the LMN deficit tells you the level of the lesion.

The patient has lost sensation on the left starting at the lateral forearm. This is the region of the C6 dermatome. The lesion is most likely one level above C6, which would be C5. The lesion at C5 also leads to a small area of pain and temperature loss at the C5 dermatome on the right. On the left, the pain and temperature deficit is starting one level below the lesion. With the lesion at C5, the C5 dermatome is intact, but then the patient has lost pain and temperature from C6 down on the left. However, on the right side, pain and temperature is only lost to the C5 dermatome because there is damage to the primary afferent entering and synapsing at the dorsal horn.

With this amount of detail, we can localize the lesion to the C5 level.

Case #2 You have a 50-year old male with elevated cholesterol levels who presents with the following bilateral signs and symptoms below T2: babinski's sign, spastic paralysis, loss of pain and temperature. He has no problems with proprioception in the lower limbs. His upper limbs are functioning. What artery is affected?

He has most likely had a stroke of the anterior spinal artery.

Case #3 A 45-year-old female was lifting a box and complained of sudden severe pain that went down the back of her right leg up to her foot. The examining physician suspected a prolapsed intervertebral disc between the fourth and fifth lumbar disks. What are the clinical signs that helped her to localize this lesion?

The L5 spinal nerve is compromised. The L5 dermatome is the dorsum of the foot. The motor test for L5 is dorsiflexion of the toes. There is no good reflex test for L5.

Further Reading

1. Afifi AK, Bergman RA. Functional neuroanatomy: text and atlas. New York: McGraw-Hill; 1998.
2. Brazis PW, Masdeu JC, Biller J. Localization in clinical neurology. Philadelphia: Lippincott Williams & Wilkins; 2016.
3. Blumenfeld H. Neuroanatomy through clinical cases. 2nd ed. Hoboken: Wiley-Blackwell; 2010.
4. Brodal P. The central nervous system. 5th ed. New York: Oxford University Press; 2016.
5. Campbell W, Barohn RJ. Dejong's the neurological examination. Philadelphia: Lippincott Williams & Wilkins; 2019.
6. Carpenter M. Core text of neuroanatomy. New York: Williams and Wilkins; 1991.
7. Ertuglu LA, Karacan I, Yilmaz G, Türker KS. Standardization of the Jendrassik maneuver in Achilles tendon tap reflex. Clin Neurophys Prac. 2018;3:1–5.
8. Fuller G. Neurological examination made easy. 6th ed. Edinburgh: Elsevier; 2019.
9. Goldberg S. Clinical anatomy made ridiculously simple. Miami: MedMaster; 1991.
10. Goldberg S. Clinical neuroanatomy made ridiculously simple. Miami: MedMaster; 2002.
11. Hallett M. NINDS myotatic reflex scale. Neurology. 1993;43:2723.
12. Hoppenfeld S. Orthopaedic neurology: a diagnostic guide to neurologic levels. Philadelphia: Lippincott Williams & Wilkins; 1977.
13. Hyun-Yoon K. Revisit spinal shock: pattern of reflex evolution during spinal shock. Korean J Neurotrauma. 2018;14(2):47–54.
14. Leo J. Medical neuroanatomy for the boards and clinic: finding the lesion. 2nd ed. Cham: Springer; 2024.
15. Leo J. Clinical anatomy and embryology: a guide for the classroom, clinic, and clinic. 2nd ed. Cham: Springer; 2024.

16. Masri OA. An essay on the human corticospinal tract: history, development, anatomy, and connections. Neuroanatomy. 2011;10:1–4.
17. Ooi LW, Leong LSX, Tee VWS, CHee YC, Halim SA, Ghani ARI, Idris Z. et al. Deep tendon reflex: The tools and technigues. What surgical neurology residents should know. Malays J Med Sci. 2021;28(2):48–62.
18. Pandolfo M. Friedreich ataxia. JAMA Neurol. 2008;65(10):1296–303.
19. Roper M, Samuels M, Klein J, Prasad S. Adams and Victor's principles of neurology. 12th ed. New York: McGraw Hill; 2023.
20. Splittgerber R. Snell's clinical neuroanatomy. 8th ed. Philadelphia: Lippincott, Williams, & Wilkins; 2018.
21. Swanson PD. Signs and symptoms in neurology. Philadelphia: Lippincott Williams & Wilkins; 1984.
22. Wirz M, Zörner B, Rupp R, Dietz V. Outcome after incomplete spinal cord injury: central cord versus Brown-Sequard syndrome. Spinal Cord. 2010;48:407–14.
23. Woodburne RT, Burkel WE. Essentials of human anatomy. 9th ed. Oxford: Oxford University Press; 1994.
24. Young PA, Young PH, Tolbert D. Basic clinical neuroscience. Philadelphia: Lippincott Williams & Wilkins; 2015.

10 Corticobulbar Tract and Cranial Nerve Nuclei

Corticobulbar

Just like the spinal cord, the cranial nerves have both upper and lower motor neurons. Instead of calling the UMNs the corticospinal tract, we refer to the UMNs of cranial nerves as the *corticobulbar tract.* And the cranial nerve nuclei are analogous to the anterior horn cells of the spinal cord.

In the spinal cord the ventral horn is one long continuous column of cells. It might not seem like this at first because you are used to seeing cross sections of the cord, and when you see a section at say C6, or T2, or L1 the ventral horn looks like a small punctate nucleus, but it is not. Rather, it is one continuous column of cells running from C1 to S4. As you move into the brainstem, this column of cells breaks up into small discrete motor nuclei. Think of the brain stem like a ladder. At the bottom of the ladder is the medulla with the motor nuclei for the lower cranial nerves IX, X, and XII (CN XI is in the cord). In the middle of the ladder is the pons with CNs V, VI, and VII. At the top of the ladder is the midbrain with cranial nerves III and IV. With a patient scenario, you are wondering where on the ladder is the lesion. Is it at the top, middle, or bottom of the brainstem (Fig. 10.1)?

The cranial nerve nuclei and their nerves coming out are analogous to the LMNs emerging from the cord. These cranial nerve nuclei are given directions by the corticobulbar tract—equivalent to corticospinal. There are two differences compared to corticospinal though:

1. While the corticospinal tract decussates at the pyramidal decussation, the corticobulbar does not decussate at one spot, but instead decussates at the level of whichever nucleus the fibers are destined for. For example, the fibers going to the trigeminal motor nucleus will decussate at the level of the trigeminal nucleus in the pons, while the fibers destined for the hypoglossal nucleus will decussate at the level of the hypoglossal nucleus in the medulla, and the fibers destined for the abducens nucleus will decussate at the level of the abducens nucleus (Fig. 10.1).
2. The ventral horn cells in the spinal cord receive a contralateral input from the corticospinal tract, and likewise some of the cranial nerve nuclei receive a contralateral input. However, every rule has exceptions and some of the cranial nerve nuclei receive a bilateral input (Fig. 10.3).

In an earlier section, we looked at the location of the three tracts in the brainstem. We now want to look at the location of the corticospinal and corticobulbar tracts and their relationship to the cranial nerve nuclei. In the medulla the nucleus of the hypoglossal nerve is on the dorsal surface right near the fourth ventricle but LMN fibers

J. Leo, *Gross Anatomy, Neuroanatomy, and Embryology for Medical Students*,
https://doi.org/10.1007/978-3-031-87151-1_10

Fig. 10.1 Corticobulbar tract. Projections to cranial nerve motor nuclei [11, 12]

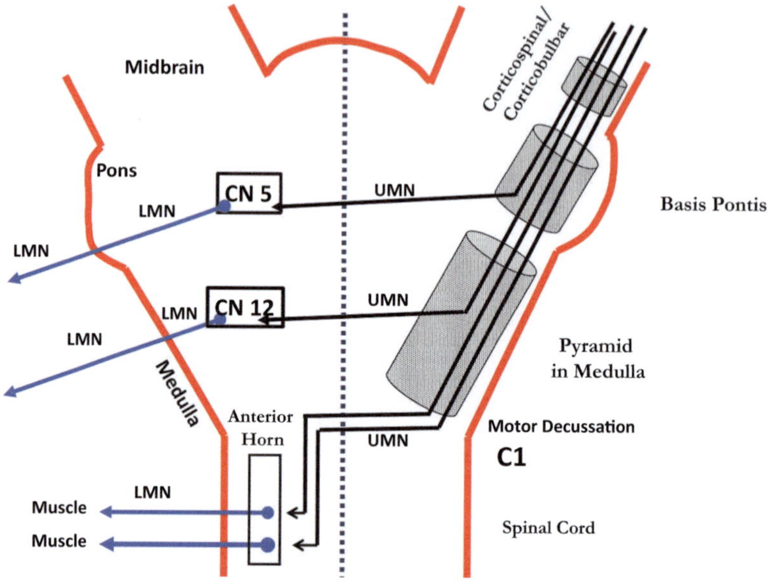

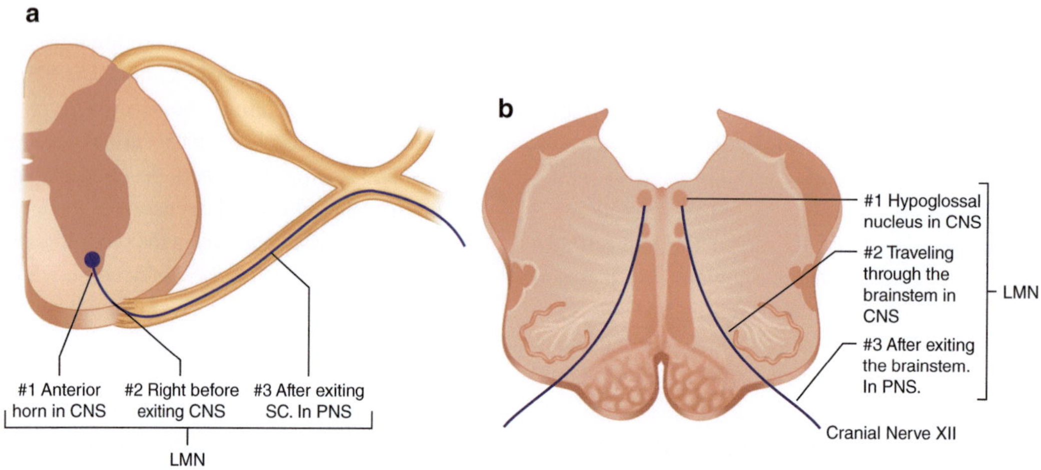

Fig. 10.2 Comparison of Spinal LMNs and Cranial Nerve LMNs. Panel (**a**) Three parts of the LMN going to a limb muscle. The anterior horn (part #1) sends fibers towards spinal nerve (part #2) which in turn exit the CNS to enter the PNS (part#3) Panel (**b**) Three Parts to LMNs of CN XII. Note that the nucleus of CN XII (part #1) sends fibers out through the medulla (part #2), and the fibers then exit the medulla to travel onto (part #3) the tongue muscles—styloglossus, hyoglossus, and genioglossus. A lesion at any one of these parts would have an ipsilateral effect, with the tongue deviating towards the ipsilateral side [11, 12]

coming out of the hypoglossal nucleus project ventrally and travel alongside the medial lemniscus and the corticospinal tract before exiting between the pyramid and inferior olive.

A closer look at the hypoglossal nucleus and the fibers coming out of it illustrates the idea of LMNs of the cranial nerves (Fig. 10.2). There are really three sections of the LMN of CN XII: (1) there is the nucleus with the cell body, which is the start of the LMN, (2) there are the fibers coming out of the nucleus that run through the medulla horizontally on their way to their exit point from the CNS, and (3) the fibers that have left the CNS and are now in the PNS and are traveling to the tongue muscles. All three of these sections are part of the LMN. Every motor cranial nerve has the same basic organization. This organization is equivalent to the LMNs in the spinal cord which also have three parts: (1) the anterior horn, with the cell body or the start of the LMN, (2) the fibers coming out of the anterior horn cell travelling to the exit point from the cord, and (3) the fibers that have left the cord and are now in the PNS and on their way to the muscle. A lesion to any of these three parts of either the spinal nerve or the hypoglossal nerve will lead to LMN symptoms (Fig. 10.2).

Nucleus Ambiguus

Nucleus ambiguus lives about halfway between the inferior olive and the inferior cerebellar peduncle (Fig. 10.3). You cannot see it—which is why it is called "ambiguus." Even though it is invisible, you need to know where it is located. It is the motor nucleus for CNs IX and X. Coming out of it are fibers which go to both CN IX and CN X to supply the pharynx, larynx, and palate. This is an example of how one cranial nerve nuclei can be involved with more than one nerve. A lesion to the nucleus ambiguus will lead to *dysphagia* (swallowing deficits) and *dysarthria* (speech deficits).

The nucleus ambiguus receives a bilateral corticobulbar input, thus the muscles of larynx and pharynx will typically be unaffected when there is a lesion in the cortex. For instance, if the right cortex is injured, the corticobulbar projection to the left nucleus ambiguus could be destroyed, however there is also a projection from the right side of the cerebral cortex to the nucleus, so it will still be functioning. A structure with a bilateral input has a back-up, thus if one input is damaged, the back-up coming from the other side can cover for it.

As we move into the pons, the corticospinal tract lives in the basis pontis. In the middle of the pons is the medial lemniscus and spinothalamic tract (sometimes referred to as the spinal lemniscus). We can also see the motor nuclei of CNs V,

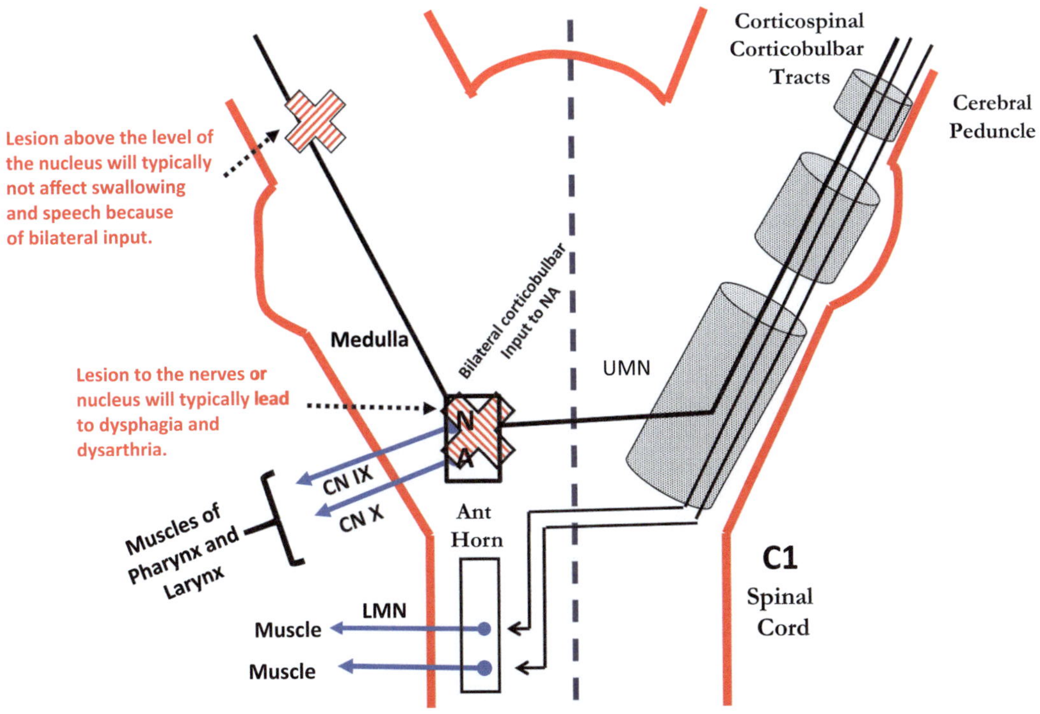

Fig. 10.3 Nucleus ambiguus (NA). Bilateral corticobulbar projections to NA. From NA, fibers of CN IX and CN X project to pharynx and larynx [11, 12]

VI, and VII and their LMN fibers running from nuclei to their exit points.

Facial Colliculus

An interesting relationship, with clinical implications, is the proximity of CN VI and CN VII in the pons (Fig. 10.4). If you are standing in the fourth ventricle and look down at the floor you will see a bump, known as the facial colliculus. This protuberance is made up of the LMN fibers of CN VII and the nucleus of CN VI. You can see in the cross section how the fibers of CN VII come out of its nucleus and run dorsally to wrap around the nucleus of CN VI, and then turn ventrally to exit the pons. A lesion to the nucleus of VI would also affect the fibers of CN VII.

As you move into the midbrain, there are two nerves, CNs III and IV (Fig. 10.5) which are involved with the eye muscles. The motor nucleus of CN III projects ventrally and passes through the red nucleus and then passes close to the corticospinal tract located in the cerebral peduncle. Cranial nerve III exits between the two cerebral peduncles in a space appropriately named the *interpeduncular fossa*. The corticobulbar input to cranial nerve nuclei is addressed in the next chapter.

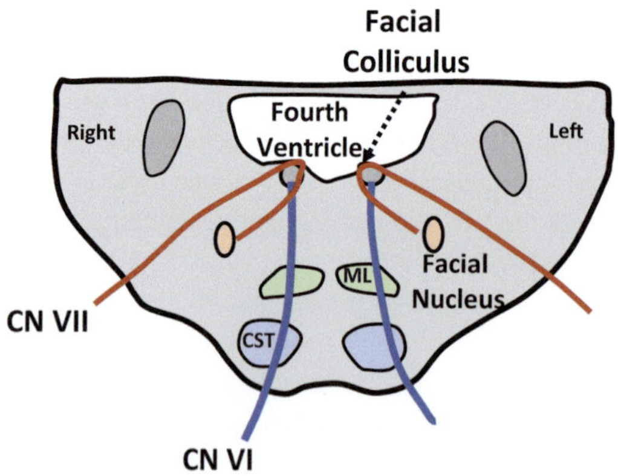

Fig. 10.4 Cross section through pons. The facial colliculus is made up of the fibers of CN VII (the genu of the facial nerve) passing around the nucleus of CN VI [11, 12]

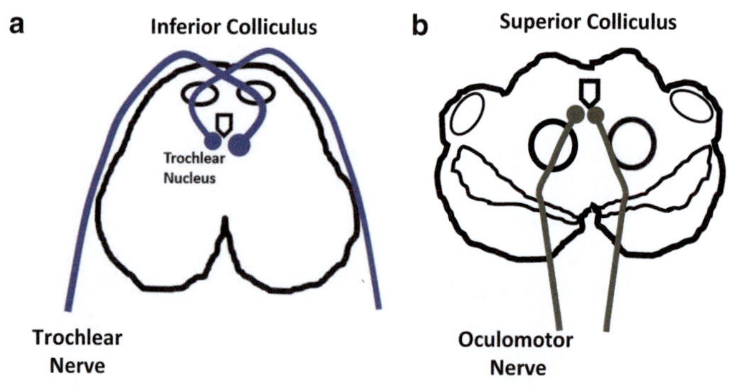

Fig. 10.5 Cross sections through the midbrain. Panel (**a**) is at the level of the inferior colliculus and CN IV. Note the LMN fibers coming out of the trochlear nuclei decussate before leaving the midbrain. Panel (**b**) is at the level of the superior colliculus and CN III. Note CN III passes through the red nucleus [11, 12]

Cranial Nerve V

The trigeminal ganglion sits in a depression on the floor of the middle cranial fossa referred to as Meckel's cave. Think of the ganglion as a three fingered glove representing V1 (Ophthalmic), V2 (Maxillary), and V3 (Mandibular). All three divisions have sensory fibers with cell bodies in the trigeminal ganglion, while V3 has a motor component to the muscles of mastication. A useful mnemonic to follow the three branches out of the skull is **SRO** or **S**tanding **R**oom **O**nly which refers to the fact that: V1 goes through the **S**uperior orbital fissure, V2 through foramen **R**otundum, and V3 through foramen **O**vale.

The trigeminal nerve has four separate nuclei in the brainstem (Fig. 10.6). The pain and temperature fibers enter along V1, V2, and V3 and have their primary cell bodies in the trigeminal ganglion, which then enter the medulla and descend for a short distance in a tract called the spinal tract of V (equivalent to the tract of Lissauer in the cord). These fibers terminate in the spinal nucleus of V (equivalent to the dorsal horn in the cord). The secondary afferents then project out of the nucleus, decussate, and enter the ventral trigeminothalamic tract (VTT) (equivalent to the spinothalamic tract) to ascend to the ventral posterior medial nucleus of the thalamus. Fibers carrying information about touch also have their cell bodies in the trigeminal ganglion but when these fibers enter the cord, they terminate in the main sensory nucleus of V. From there the secondary afferents decussate and enter the VTT on their way to the thalamus, and then go from the thalamus to the postcentral gyrus.

Proprioceptive fibers of CN V are unique, as their primary afferent cell bodies are not in the PNS but in the CNS. The primary afferents travel through the trigeminal ganglia but do not have a cell body in the ganglia. Their first cell body is in the mesencephalic nucleus (inside the CNS) which then sends a collateral to the motor nucleus to form a reflex circuit. This circuit is the jaw-jerk reflex. The motor nucleus of the trigeminal nerve is just medial to the main sensory nucleus and sends fibers out through the trigeminal ganglion onto V3 (not onto V1 or V2). The jaw jerk reflex involves tapping on the chin with the mouth open. If the jaw suddenly and forcefully shuts this suggests a deficit with CN V.

For clinical scenarios, of particular interest is the close relationship of the spinal nucleus of V to the spinothalamic tract. In lateral brain stem injuries both these structures can be lesioned. This will lead to an ipsilateral loss of pain and temperature sensation to the face, and contralateral loss of pain and temperature sensation to the body—from the neck down (Fig. 10.7).

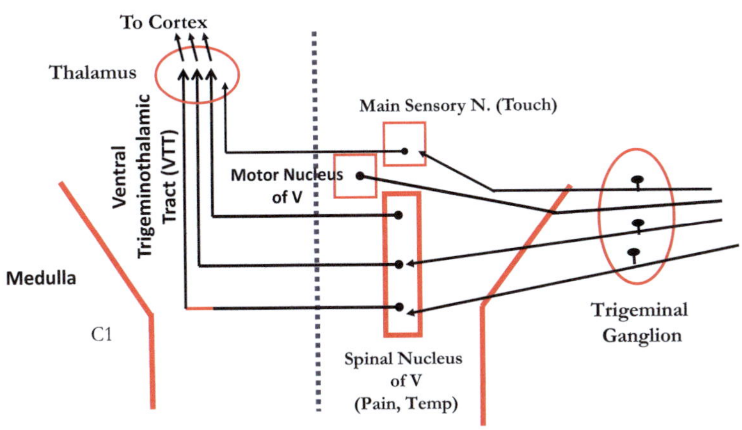

Fig. 10.6 Trigeminal nuclei. Primary afferents for pain and temperature have their cell bodies in the trigeminal ganglion and project to the spinal nucleus of CN V. Fibers carrying touch project to the main sensory nucleus. From these two nuclei, the fibers decussate and travel up the VTT to the thalamus. Motor nucleus sends efferents to muscles of mastication. Mesencephalic nucleus is not shown [11, 12]

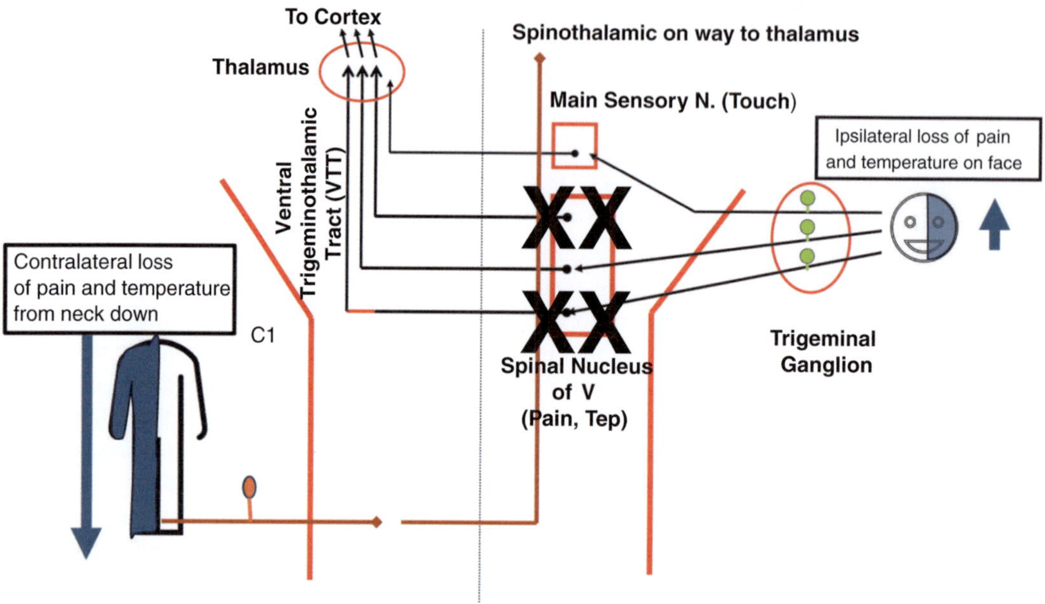

Fig. 10.7 Lateral medullary syndrome ipsilateral loss of pain and temperature from face, and contralateral loss of pain and temperature from the limbs [11, 12]

Trigeminal Neuralgia, or tic douloureux, refers to chronic excruciating pain emanating from the face due to disruption of CN V. Patients often first go to the dentist thinking they have an infected molar. Most cases are caused by compression of the superior cerebellar artery, which lies adjacent to the nerve as it exits the brainstem. It can also result from a latent herpes simplex virus residing in the trigeminal ganglion that during an outbreak leads to pain typically along V2 and V3 divisions. MS patients with a deterioration of the myelin sheath can also present with trigeminal neuralgia.

Spinothalamic Tract vs. Ventral Trigeminothalamic Tract

It can help with understanding pain and temperature transmission by comparing pain and temperature coming into the CNS from the limbs versus the face. The primary afferent for pain and temperature from the limbs is in the dorsal root ganglion, while for the face it is in the trigeminal ganglion. After these primary afferents enters the CNS they can travel for a short segment—either in Lissauer's tract for the limbs or the spinal tract of V for the face. The primary afferent then synapses in either the substantia gelatinosa or the spinal nucleus of V. The second order neuron then travels in either the spinothalamic tract or the ventral trigeminothalamic tract (VTT). The spinothalamic tract synapses in the ventral posterolateral nucleus (VPL) of the thalamus, and the VTT in the ventral posteromedial nucleus (VPM) of the thalamus. From the thalamus, the thalamocortical tracts then project to the appropriate area of the primary sensory cortex found in the postcentral gyrus (Fig. 10.8).

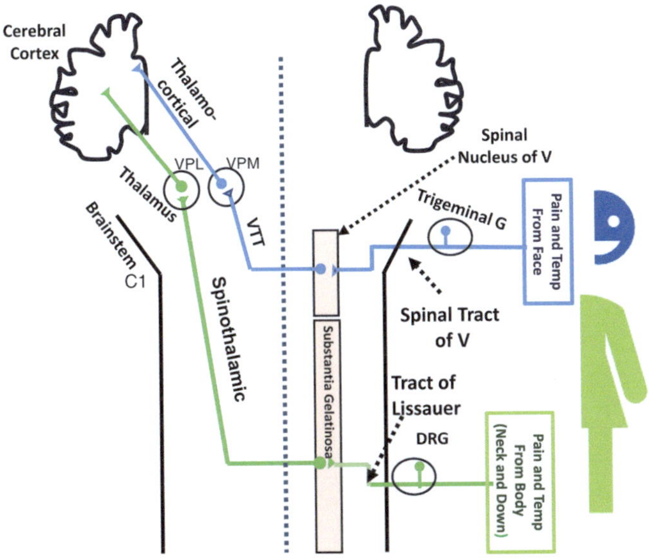

Structure	Pain and Temp from Body	Pain and Temp from Face
Primary Afferent	Dorsal Root Ganglion	Trigeminal Ganglion
First Pathway	Lissauer's Tract	Spinal Tract of V
First Synapse	Substantia Gelatinosa	Spinal Nucleus of V
Second Order Neuron	Spinothalamic	Ventral Trigemino Thalamic
Thalamic Nuclei	VPL	VPM
Third Order Neuron	Thalamo-Cortical	Thalamo-Cortical

Fig. 10.8 Pain and temperature sensation from the body (green) compared to the face (blue). The two pathways have the same functional organization—we just give them different names [11, 12]

Corticobulbar Projections to Cranial Nerve VII

The facial motor nucleus is in the pons, and it can be divided in half. The upper part of the nucleus supplies the upper part of the face, and the lower part of the nucleus supplies the lower part of the face. The cortical control of the nucleus arises in the face area of the precentral gyrus which projects down as the corticobulbar pathway. Of clinical importance is the fact that the upper part of the nucleus receives a bilateral cortical input, while the lower part of the nucleus only receives a contralateral input (Fig. 10.9).

Thus, a lesion to the cortex will result in the loss of the contralateral lower facial muscles. However, since the upper part of the facial nucleus receives information from both sides, it will still function. Granted the muscles might be weaker but the patient will still be able to close their eye and smile on that side. If the lesion is to the nucleus in the brainstem, then the patient will lose both the upper and lower facial muscles on the ipsilateral side (Fig. 10.9).

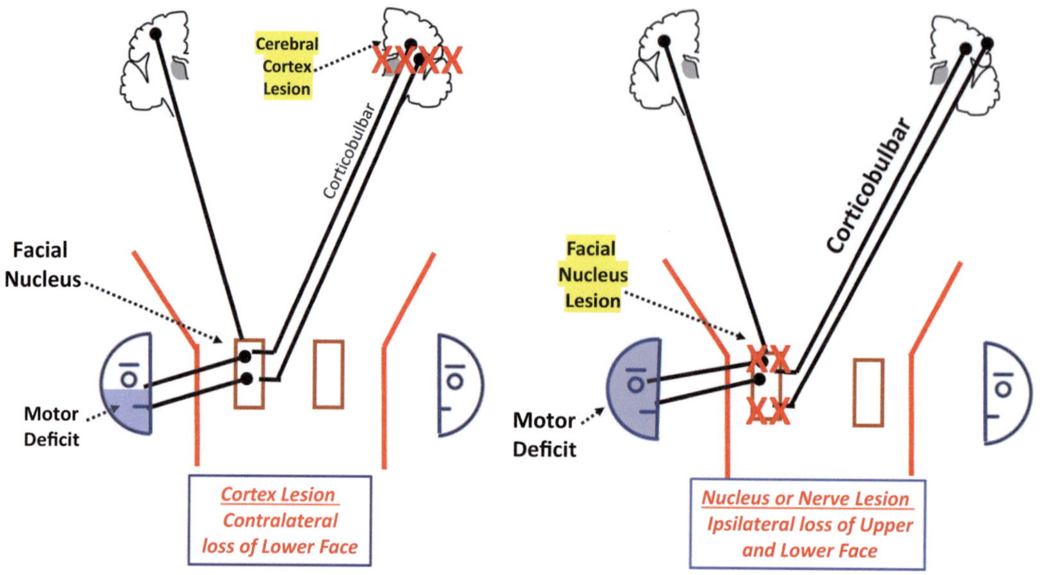

Fig. 10.9 Corticobulbar input to facial motor nucleus. The upper part of the nucleus receives a bilateral input. The lower part of nucleus receives a contralateral input. In panel (**a**) the patient has a cortex lesion which leads to a loss of the contralateral lower facial muscles. In panel (**b**) the patient has a brainstem injury which leads to an ipsilateral loss of upper and lower facial muscles [11, 12]

Cranial Nerve XI

The spinal accessory nucleus is in the cervical spinal cord. Realize that this is nothing more than the anterior horn from C1 through C5 and is the origin of lower motor neurons of CN XI that leave the nucleus and then ascend parallel to the cord and enter the skull through the foramen magnum. They then exit the skull through the jugular foramen and project to the sternocleidomastoid (SCM) and the trapezius muscles.

Based on clinical findings, the corticobulbar fibers are unique to the accessory nerve. Some have suggested that the portion of the accessory nucleus sending fibers to the trapezius muscle receives a *contralateral* corticobulbar input, but the portion of the nucleus going to the sternocleidomastoid (mainly the sternomastoid portion) receives a *bilateral* corticobulbar input. Therefore, lesions in the cortex may lead to a loss of the trapezius but not sternocleidomastoid.

Besides its distribution to the sternocleidomastoid and trapezius, CN XI has a *cranial portion.* These fibers originate from nucleus ambiguus and come out of the brainstem with CN X, but they quickly peel off from CN X and jump on CN XI for just a moment. In other words, some of these fibers from CN X jump from X to XI but then quickly come back to X. All this is happening within the skull. This piece that goes from X to XI and back to X is the recurrent laryngeal nerve branch of CN X. Remember from embryology that CN X comes from pharyngeal arch 6, except for its recurrent branch which comes from pharyngeal arch 4 (Fig. 10.10).

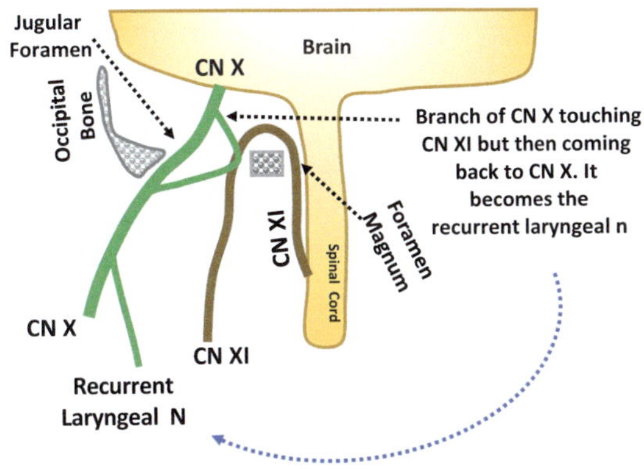

Fig. 10.10 Cranial Portion of CN XI. The accessory nerve arises from rootlets of the C1–C5 spinal cord and ascends into the foramen magnum to enter the skull with the spinal cord. In the skull, There is a branch of CN X that touches CN XI but then immediately goes back to CN X. This branch then continues as the recurrent laryngeal nerve [11, 12]

Cranial Nerve XII

The hypoglossal nucleus lies in the caudal medulla near the fourth ventricle. Fibers from the nucleus pass through the medulla between the pyramid and the inferior olive. Once they emerge from the skull through the hypoglossal canal, the nerve passes in the anterior triangle of the neck to innervate the hyoglossus, genioglossus, and the styloglossus. The only tongue muscle which is not innervated by CN XII is the palatoglossus which is innervated by CN X. Lesions to CN XII will lead to the tongue protruding towards the side of the lesion.

Jugular foramen syndrome results from a mass or trauma that compromises CNs IX, X, and XI. The patient will be dysarthric, dysphagic (CN IX and X) and have a weakened gag reflex (CN IX and X). And on attempted elevation of the chin, it will deviate to the ipsilateral side (weak side). The lesion will also compromise the ipsilateral otic ganglion (CN IX) leading to reduced parotid gland secretion. If the mass is large enough it may also compromise the superior cervical ganglion leading to ipsilateral Horner's syndrome.

Further Reading

1. Afifi AK, Bergman RA. Functional neuroanatomy: text and atlas. New York: McGraw-Hill; 1998.
2. Brazis PW, Masdeu JC, Biller J. Localization in clinical neurology. Philadelphia: Lippincott Williams & Wilkins; 2016.
3. Brodal P. The central nervous system. 5th ed. New York: Oxford University Press; 2016.
4. Blumenfeld H. Neuroanatomy through clinical cases. 2nd ed. Hoboken: Wiley-Blackwell; 2010.
5. Carpenter M. Core text of neuroanatomy. New York: Williams and Wilkins; 1991.
6. Campbell W, Barohn RJ. Dejong's the neurological examination. Philadelphia: Lippincott Williams & Wilkins; 2019.
7. DeToledo JC, David NJ. Innervation of the sternocleidomastoid and trapezius muscles by the accessory nerve. Neuroophthalmol. 2001;21(3):214–6.
8. Fuller G. Neurological examination made easy. 6th ed. Edinburgh: Elsevier; 2019.
9. Goldberg S. Clinical anatomy made ridiculously simple. Miami: MedMaster; 1991.
10. Goldberg S. Clinical neuroanatomy made ridiculously simple. Miami: MedMaster; 2002.
11. Leo J. Medical neuroanatomy for the boards and clinic: finding the lesion. 2nd ed. Cham: Springer; 2024.
12. Leo J. Clinical anatomy and embryology: a guide for the classroom, clinic, and clinic. 2nd ed. Cham: Springer; 2024.
13. Ropper M, Samuels M, Klein J, Prasad S. Adams and Victor's principles of neurology. 12th ed. New York: McGraw Hill; 2023.
14. Splittgerber R. Snell's clinical neuroanatomy. 8th ed. Philadelphia: Lippincott, Williams, & Wilkins; 2018.
15. Swanson PD. Signs and symptoms in neurology. Philadelphia: Lippincott Williams & Wilkins; 1984.
16. Woodburne RT, Burkel WE. Essentials of human anatomy. 9th ed. Oxford University Press, Oxford; 1994.
17. Young PA, Young PH, Tolbert D. Basic clinical neuroscience. Philadelphia: Lippincott Williams & Wilkins; 2015.

Abducens Nerve Lesions 11

Cranial Nerve VI

Of all the cranial nerves, the abducens nerve has the longest course within the skull, and it is subject to injury at numerous locations within the cranial vault. A common cause of injury to it comes from increased intracranial pressure which stretches the nerve.

The abducens nucleus is in the caudal pons right in front of the fourth ventricle. Its fibers run horizontally through the brainstem and then exit the brainstem and then make a sharp turn to travel superiorly between the pons and the clivus, deep to the dura mater, in Dorello's canal. They then enter the cavernous sinus, travel through the superior orbital fissure, and reach the lateral rectus muscle. There are numerous locations where CN VI can be lesioned (Fig. 11.1).

Of considerable clinical importance is that when there is a lesion to the abducens nucleus there is a deficit with both eyes. This is an exception to the typical scenario where if you lesion a cranial nerve nucleus you would simply affect the muscles on one side of the body. The details of this are explained below.

When you approach a patient with a deficit of the eye muscles you should break down your exam into two parts. The first part of the exam is when the patient is sitting in your office and you notice, or suspect, that something is amiss with the eyes. For instance, at rest maybe one of the eyes has a medial or lateral deviation and you become curious. The second part of the exam is when you formally test the muscles by asking the patient to follow your finger as you move them through the test. We will first look at the actions of the eye muscles and their respective nerves. We will then look at how you would test the muscle and nerves. To do this we are going to look at two pictures to discuss the eye muscles.

J. Leo, *Gross Anatomy, Neuroanatomy, and Embryology for Medical Students*,
https://doi.org/10.1007/978-3-031-87151-1_11

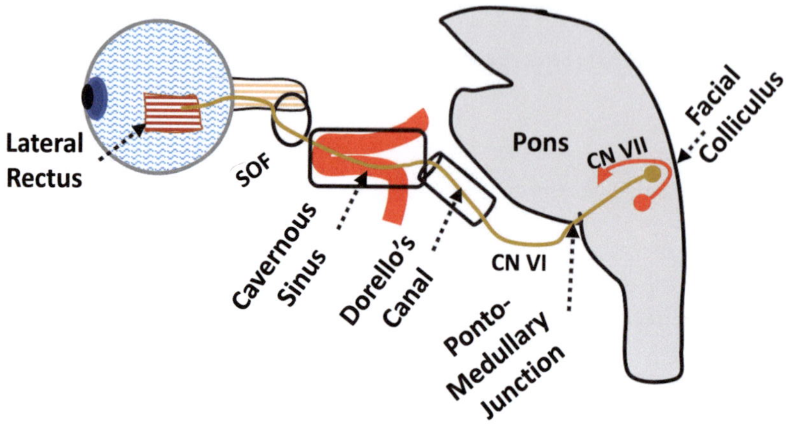

Fig. 11.1 Pathway of CN VI. The abducens nucleus sends fibers that emerge from the pontomedullary junction and run superiorly on the clivus. The fibers pierce the dura to enter Dorello's canal and then run to the cavernous sinus where they are lateral to the internal carotid artery. They then run through the superior orbital fissure (SOF) to enter the orbit [12, 13]

Actions

The first picture shows *the actions* of the muscles (Fig. 11.2). This is the picture that you would see in a typical anatomy textbook. After all, anatomists like to talk about actions or functions. Note that medial rectus and lateral rectus each have only one action. The lateral rectus pulls the eye laterally (abduction), and medial rectus pulls the eyes medially (adduction). However, the other four muscles each have three actions. Superior oblique pulls the eye down and out, while inferior oblique pulls the eye up and out. And the superior rectus pulls the eye up and in, while inferior rectus pulls the eye down and in. Yet, we also need to pay attention to the often ignored intorsion and extortion movements. Intorsion is when the 12 o'clock position of your eye rotates towards your nose, and extortion is when it rotates away from the nose.

Do not confuse intorsion and extortion with medial and lateral movements. Intorsion and extorsion involve the eyes rotating within the eye socket. While you are reading this, tilt your head to the left. If you did not have intorsion and extorsion your world (the page) would tilt, but you know that the world stays level This is because when you tilt your head to the left, your left eye intorts and your right eye extorts. As you walk down the street, your head is in constant motion in various planes. This ability to intort and extort allows your eyes to compensate for these head movements so that the world does not bob around and make you dizzy. When you look at the picture showing the actions of the muscles you can see that there are two intorters (superior oblique and superior rectus), and two extorters (inferior oblique and inferior rectus).

The action picture for the eye muscles is important to understand because it explains what happens with the eyes at rest when there is a nerve lesion.

Cranial Nerve VI Lesion

The eye is a democracy. To look straight ahead you need to have equal tension on medial and lateral rectus. If you have a deficit with the lateral rectus, then the medial rectus will take over and move the eye medially. The patient will have a medial strabismus. If they have a deficit with medial rectus, then lateral rectus takes over and they will have a lateral strabismus.

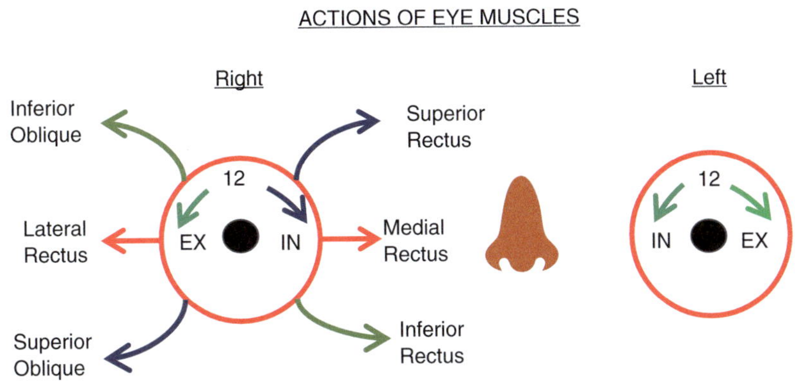

Fig. 11.2 Actions of eye muscles. For instance, the superior oblique moves the eye down, out, and intorts. The inferior rectus moves the eye in, down, and is an extorter. Superior oblique and superior rectus are intorters, while inferior oblique and inferior rectus are extorters [12, 13]

Cranial Nerve III Lesion

If you have a lesion to CN III, then you would lose all the eye muscles except lateral rectus and superior oblique which will lead to the eye projecting down and out—a lateral strabismus. Because CN III has parasympathetic fibers the patient will also have ptosis (droopy eyelid) and mydriasis (dilated pupil).

Cranial Nerve IV Lesion

With a lesion to the right trochlear nerve (CN IV) the patient loses the superior oblique, one of the two intorters. With weakened intorsion, the right eye will now be extorted. With the right eye extorted the patient now has two visual fields. To bring the world back to one visual field, the patient will lean away from the lesion side—in this case towards the left. This movement brings the right eye up to level, and since the muscles on the left are working the left eye will intort. Keep in mind that you cannot look at a patient's eyeball and see intorsion and extortion. *Brown's syndrome* involves pathological shortening of the tendon of the superior oblique muscle which leads to an inability of the muscle to function normally. These patients will have a hard time with intorsion and elevation—looking in and up.

Amblyopia

During development if one eye does not develop as fast as the other the patient can have a lazy eye or amblyopia. In these cases the healthy eye takes over and the other eye can drift. One way to correct this is to put a patch on the healthy eye so that the patient uses the other eye.

Testing

The next figure depicts the H test which shows how to test the eyes (Fig. 11.3). This is the picture that you would see in a typical clinical exam textbook. To test the MR and LR you ask the person to look medially or laterally. However, if you want to test the right SO, first you ask the patient to look left, and then once the eye is pulled in, you ask the person to look down. The only way the adducted eye can look inferiorly is with SO. The first part of the test, when the patient looked medially, isolated the SO. From this medial position, the only way the patient can look inferiorly is with SO, and the only way they look superiorly is with IO. Ideally when you test the eye movements you keep on the H lines, and do not take the diagonal shortcuts.

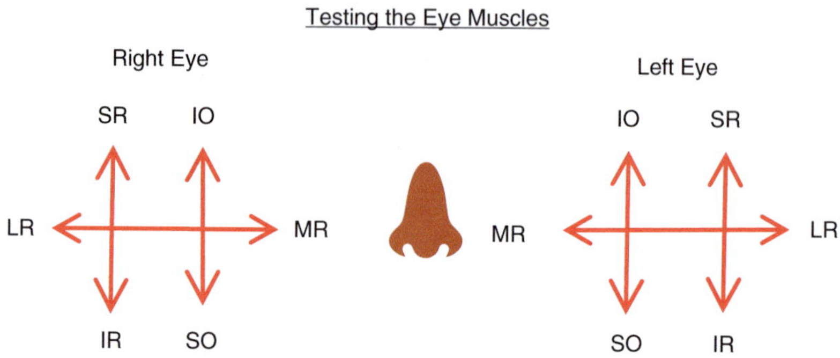

Fig. 11.3 Testing of eye muscles. Diagram of the H-test. To test superior oblique the patient first looks in and then down [12, 13]

Cortex Control from Frontal Eye Field

Understanding the lateral gaze pathway is essential for understanding lesion scenarios. Before getting into the details, we will start with the big picture. Start off looking at something in your room, like a wall clock. If you move your head horizontally to the left, but want to stay focused on the clock, your eyes will slowly move to the right (slow phase). If you keep moving your head to the left, eventually your eyes will quickly follow your head rotation (the fast phase). We can refer to these two movements of the eyes as the slow phase and the fast phase. The slow phase is under control by your vestibular system, and you use this all the time when you are walking around. Without it you would be dizzy. With a head turn, the slow phase of the eye movement, which occurs first, is opposite the head turn.

Eventually, your eyes follow your head. This is the fast phase and it is under control by your cortex. In contrast to the slow phase, you will notice that during the fast phase, your eyes do not take in everything in the visual world as they move. At one point your eyes are looking straight ahead, and the next moment you are looking off to the side, and during this movement your eyes did not see everything in between. We are first going to examine the fast phase in detail. In the vestibular chapter we will look at the slow phase in detail.

Disruptions along this pathway can lead to rhythmic oscillation of the eyes which is known as nystagmus. To the untrained observer, the patient with nystagmus will have "fluttering" or the eyes moving "to and from." However, the trained clinician will see more details in this pathological movement, and they will notice that the eyes are not just fluttering, but that they are moving slowly in one direction, and quickly in the other direction. And the direction of the slow and fast phase is an important clue to where the lesion is located.

Fast Phase of Nystagmus

The frontal eye fields are two bilateral structures that sit in the frontal lobe just anterior to the precentral gyrus. When one FEF fires, it drives the eyes towards the contralateral side. For instance, when the right frontal eye field fires, the eye will move to the left. Tonic activity from both frontal eye fields keeps the eyes looking straight ahead. Therefore, if there is a lesion to the right frontal eye field the eyes will drift right—they cannot look to the left, so the eyes drift to the right.

Let us look at the details of moving the eyes to the right. The signal starts in the left FEF and projects to the right paramedian pontine reticular formation (PPRF). The PPRF is small and sits right next to the abducens nucleus. Some textbook authors will show the PPRF in their schematic, while others will leave it out. For the purposes of clinical neuroanatomy, it does not really matter one way or the other. Both the PPRF and abducens nucleus are small structures and practically sit on top of each other. For our purposes, to understand the lesions, think of them as the same structure.

We are going to look at numerous lesions to this pathway, and we will look at how the eyes will appear at rest, and what the eyes will do when you test them. The key point is that lesions to the abducens nucleus effects both eyes.

The abducens nucleus projects to the ipsilateral lateral rectus nucleus, but it also projects via the medial longitudinal fasciculus (MLF) to the contralateral oculomotor nucleus and then to the medial rectus (Fig. 11.4). This system ensures that both eyes will move together to one side—a lateral gaze. We need to discuss four different lesions to this system, and we need to compare the position of the eyes will be at rest versus their position on attempted lateral gaze.

Lesion 1: Left Frontal Eye Field *Lateral Gaze Paralysis*. In a patient with a lesion to the left frontal eye field, at rest you will note that their eyes have a slow drift to the left (Fig. 11.5). When

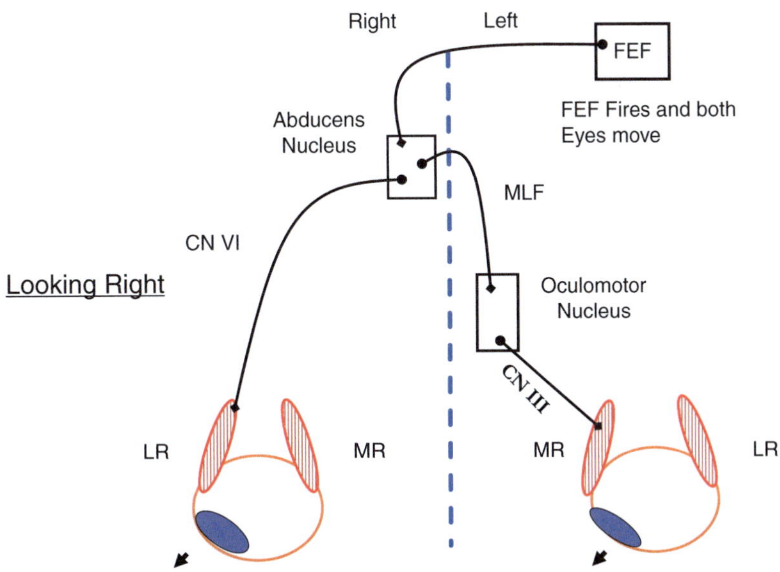

Fig. 11.4 Horizontal gaze pathway in healthy individual [12, 13]

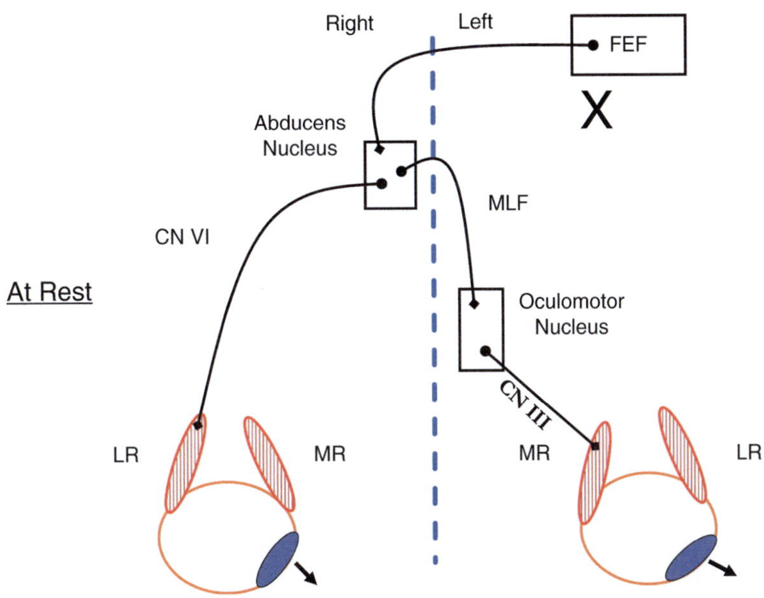

Fig. 11.5 Lesion #1 to frontal eye field. Eyes at rest deviate towards the lesioned side [12, 13]

you ask them to look to the right, they can move their eyes to the midline but no further (Fig. 11.6).

Lesion 2: Right Abducens Nerve *Ipsilateral Paralysis of Ocular Abduction*. In a patient with a lesion to the fibers of CN VI the patient will only have a deficit with one eye. At rest, this eye will be medially deviated (Fig. 11.7).

and when asked to laterally the best they can do is bring the eyes to the midline (Fig. 11.8). This is paralysis of ipsilateral ocular abduction. Their left eye will function normally.

Lesion 3: Right Abducens Nucleus *Lateral Gaze Paralysis*. In a patient with a lesion to the

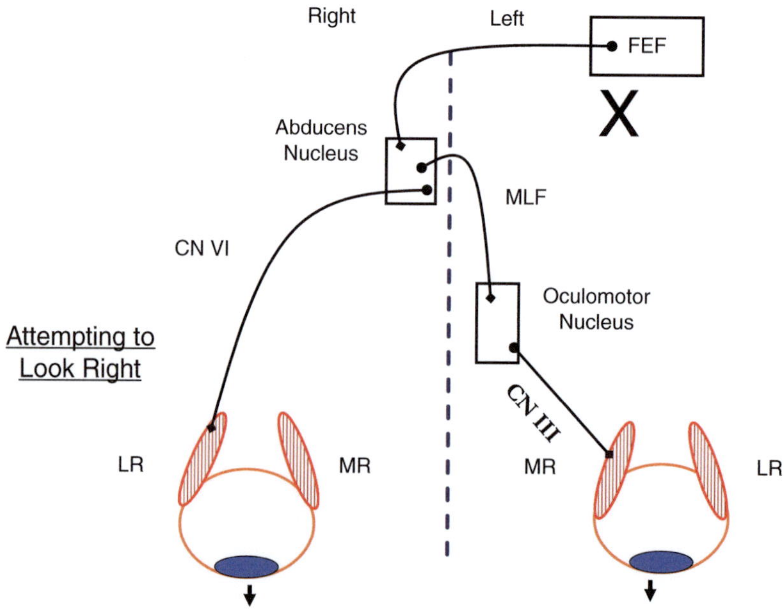

Fig. 11.6 Lesion #1 frontal eye field lesion. Patient attempts to look right. Best the eyes can do is midline [12, 13]

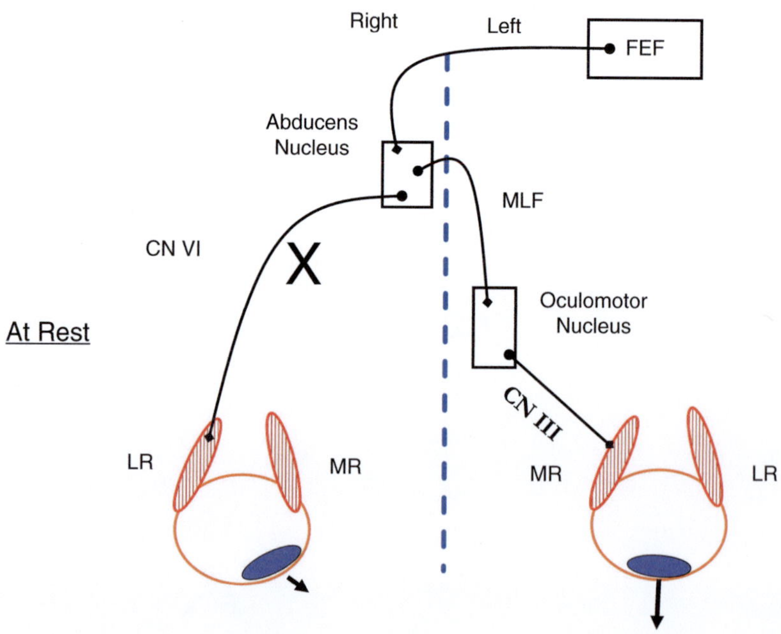

Fig. 11.7 Lesion #2 abducens nerve lesion. At rest, medial strabismus of ipsilateral eye [12, 13]

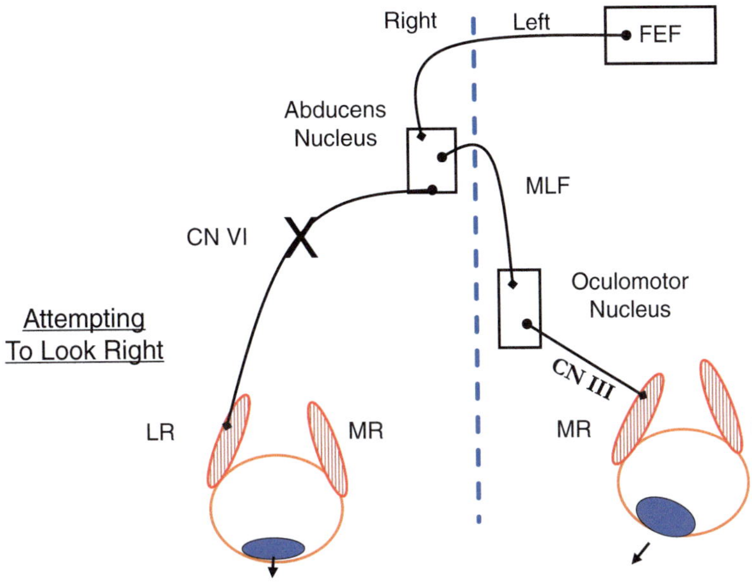

Fig. 11.8 Lesion #2 abducens nerve lesion. On attempted lateral gaze, best the right eye can do is midline [12, 13]

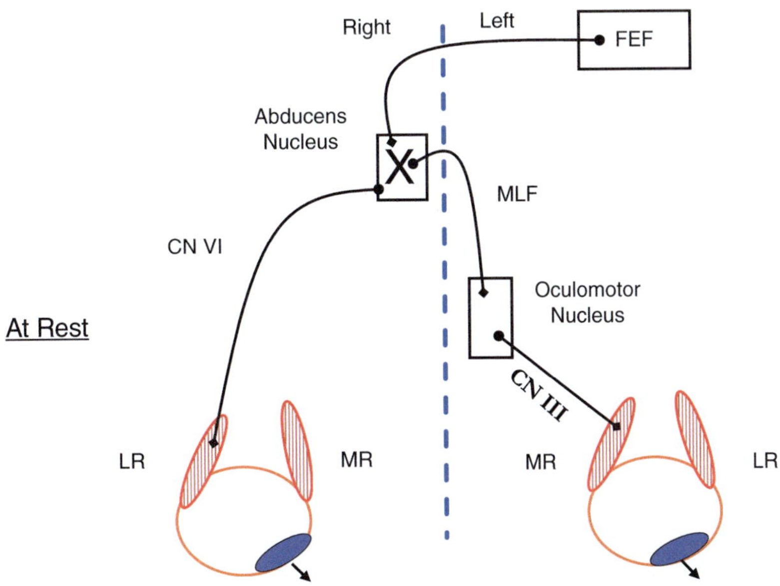

Fig. 11.9 Lesion #3 abducens nucleus lesion. At rest, eyes deviate to the left [12, 13]

right abducens nucleus, both eyes will have a slow drift to the left at rest (Fig. 11.9).

When you ask them to look right, they will have difficulty with both eyes, which is known as ***lateral gaze paralysis*** (Fig. 11.10).

Lesion 4: Left Medial Longitudinal Fasciculus *Internuclear ophthalmoplegia.* In a patient with a lesion to the left MLF the patient will not have any deficit when the eyes are at rest. Yet when asked to look to the right, their left eye will not be able to look right because the medial rectus is not getting a signal. And their right eye will flutter back and forth, which is known as effort nystagmus. They will not have nystagmus at rest. The nystagmus appears when they make an *effort* to look right. This patient with a lesion to the left MLF will not have any deficit looking to the left. Internuclear ophthalmoplegia is an

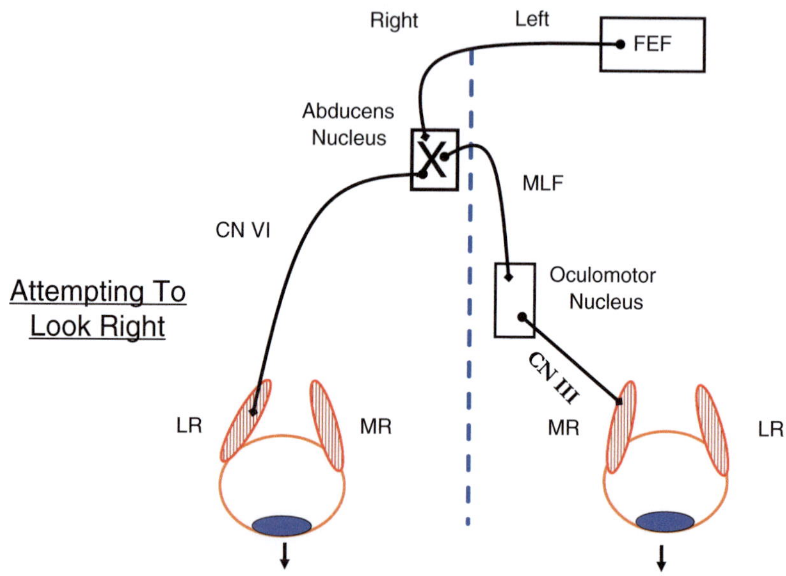

Fig. 11.10 Lesion #3 abducens nucleus lesion. Attempt to look right and best the eyes can do is midline [12, 13]

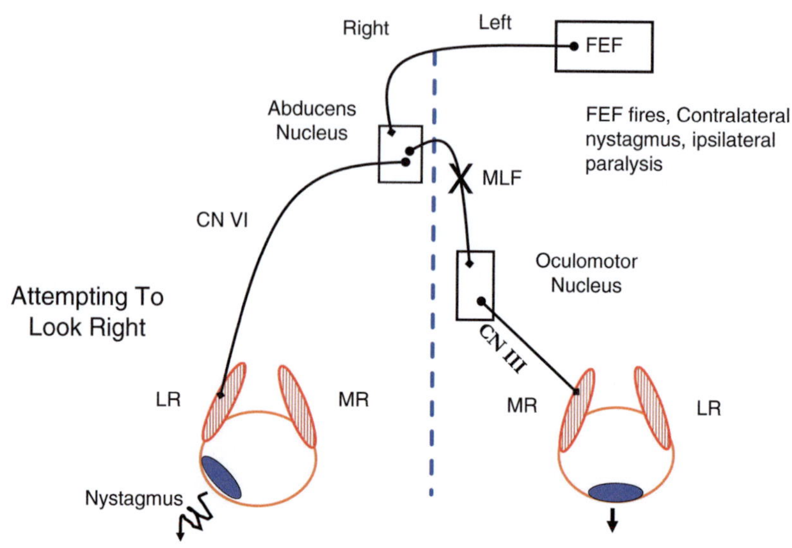

Fig. 11.11 Lesion #4 medial longitudinal fasciculus lesion. Patient attempt to look right, and exhibits contralateral nystagmus, ipsilateral paralysis [12, 13]

early sign of MS. The lesion can be found on one side, like the example given, or it could be bilateral and affect both eyes (Fig. 11.11).

One and a Half Syndrome

In the one and a half syndrome, there is a lesion to the abducens nucleus and the MLF on the same side. If the lesion is on the right side, when the patient is asked to look to the right, the best that both eyes can do is the midline because of

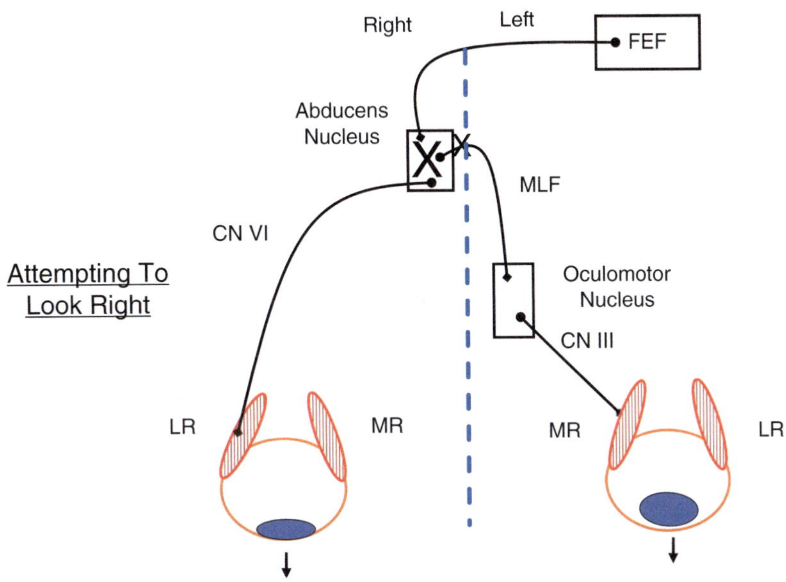

Fig. 11.12 One and a half syndrome. Patient looking right. Horizontal gaze paralysis [12, 13]

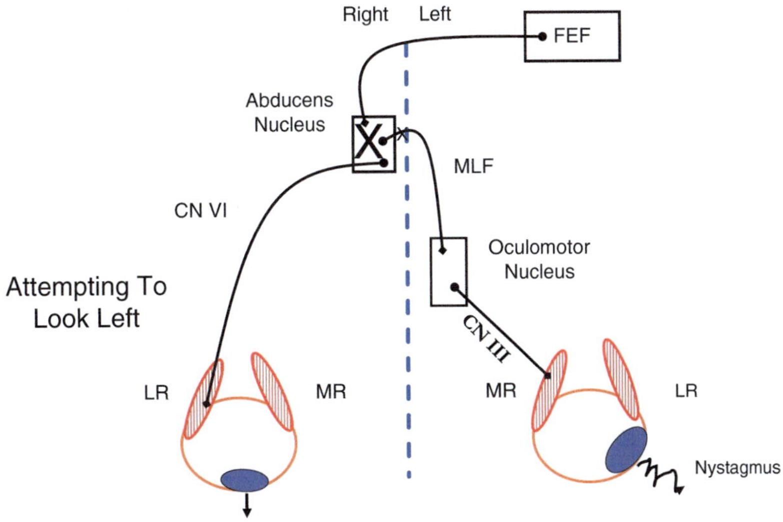

Fig. 11.13 One and a half syndrome. Looking left. Paralysis of right medial rectus. Nystagmus of left eye [12, 13]

lesion to the nucleus (Fig. 11.12). And then when asked to look to the left, the right eye cannot do any better than the midline, and the left eye will have effort nystagmus, because of the lesion to the MLF (Fig. 11.13). *Remember lesions to the MLF will lead to contralateral effort nystagmus.*

Who Are the Neighbors?

The question that usually comes up at this point is, if you are looking at the patient's eyes how do you tell the difference between a FEF lesion (#1 in previous example) and an abducens nucleus lesion (#3 in previous example) since both these patients have the same eye movement deficit? When you are first learning neuroanatomy, you naturally go through the tracts and cranial nerves one by one, such as one lecture on the corticospinal tract, then

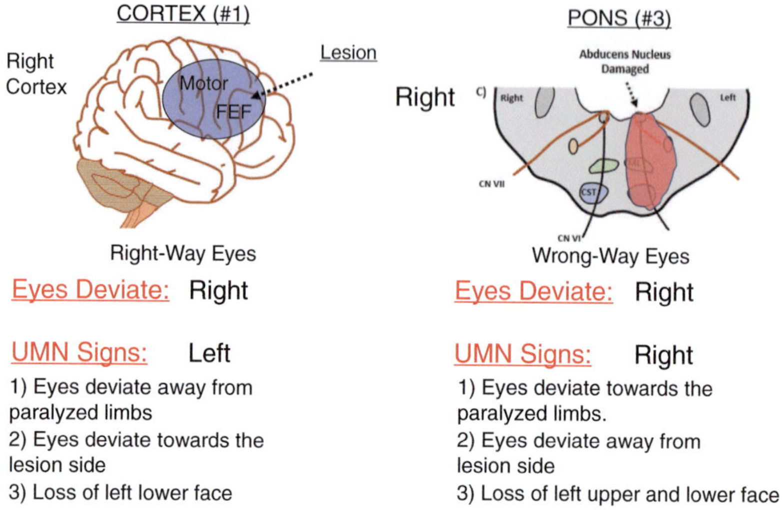

Fig. 11.14 Comparison of lesions to FEF and abducens nucleus and their surrounding structures [12, 13]

another lecture on CN VII, and then another on CN VI, and onwards. But keep in mind, patients do not present with just one tract or one nerve that is affected. Patients present with multiple symptoms. This is why when you learn about damage to a structure you need to pay attention to its neighbors—since they can be compromised also. It is good to know your neighbors, especially in neuroanatomy. You are not just memorizing facts but learning how to synthesize the information so that you can solve the problem.

The way to think about the typical neurology patient or a case study on an exam is that the patient will present with several different signs or symptoms. Your job is to figure out where is the one location in the nervous system where a lesion can account for all the patient's symptoms. In the case of these two patients, consider that more than just the abducens nucleus or more than just the FEF will be compromised. Consider two different lesions and the importance of the neighbors (Fig. 11.14).

In the patient with a lesion to the right frontal eye field, at rest the eyes will slowly drift to the right. In addition, the precentral gyrus is damaged which will lead to UMN signs on the left. Thus, the eye deficit can be related to the UMN deficit by saying: "the patient's eyes drift away from the paralyzed side of the body." You will sometimes hear this referred to as "right-way eyes." In addition, the patient will have a contralateral loss of lower facial muscles (Fig. 11.14). As an aside, imagine you suspect that the right frontal eye field is affected in a patient. During the exam one way to check the FEF is to stand on the patient's paralyzed side of the body—the affected side. As you are standing there simply say "hello" to the patient and see if they look at you. If they look at you then the frontal eye field is intact. If their gaze is away from you then the FEF has been compromised.

In the patient with the lesion to the left abducens nucleus, the eyes will have a slow drift to the right. Because the left corticospinal tract is damaged in the pons, above the decussation, they will have UMN signs on the right side of the body (contralateral). Thus, the patient's eyes will drift towards the paralyzed side of the body—often referred to as "wrong-way eyes." The patient will also have an ipsilateral loss of both upper and lower muscles of the face on the left. (See the chapter on the facial nerve for a more detailed explanation of the face deficits.)

Case #1 A 28 year old female presents to your office complaining of diplopia. She is an immigrant from Norway. Extraocular movements examination reveals failure of the left globe to adduct associated with effort nystagmus of the right globe upon attempted right gaze. Where would you localize the lesion and what is the likely diagnosis?

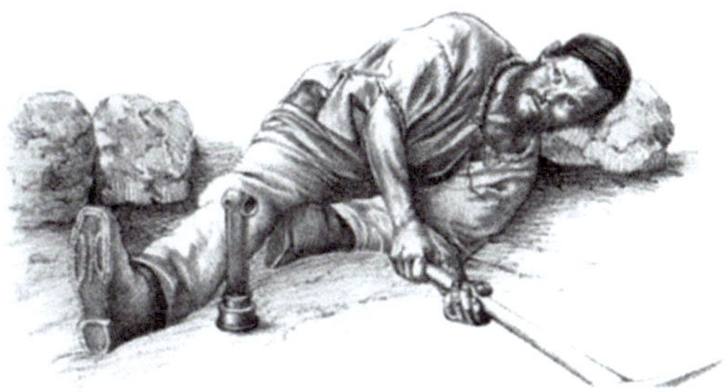

Fig. 11.15 Coal miner's nystagmus. Miners spent long hours on their backs looking at up at a poorly lit coal face. Some of them developed nystagmus. Reprinted from Snell

The patient most likely has MS and there is a lesion to the left MLF.

Historical Snippet: Coal Miner's Nystagmus

One of the fist occupational job injuries documented in the medical literature was the presence of nystagmus in coal miners. *Coal Miner's Nystagmus* as it came to be called was first described in the early 1900s in Britain when it was observed that miners who spent much of the day underground in low light conditions and often on their backs looking up at the ceiling developed nystagmus. As working conditions improved, such as the lighting of the coal face, the condition disappeared. Not surprisingly, at the time, because of workplace injury claims, there was significant amount of debate about the nature of the symptoms (Fig. 11.15).

Further Reading

1. Afifi AK, Bergman RA. Functional neuroanatomy: text and atlas. New York: McGraw-Hill; 1998.
2. Azarmina M, Azarmina H. The six syndromes of the sixth cranial nerve. J Ophthal Vis Res. 2013;8(2):160–71.
3. Brazis PW, Masdeu JC, Biller J. Localization in clinical neurology. Philadelphia: Lippincott Williams & Wilkins; 2016.
4. Blumenfeld H. Neuroanatomy through clinical cases. 2nd ed. New York: Wiley-Blackwell; 2010.
5. Brodal P. The central nervous system. 5th ed. New York: Oxford University Press; 2016.
6. Campbell W, Barohn RJ. Dejong's the neurological examination. Philadelphia: Lippincott Williams & Wilkins; 2019.
7. Carpenter M. Core text of neuroanatomy. New York: Williams and Wilkins; 1991.
8. Fishman RS. Dark as a dungeon: the rise and fall of coal miner's nystagmus. Arch Ophthalmol. 2006;124:1617–44.
9. Fuller G. Neurological examination made easy. 6th ed. Edinburgh: Elsevier; 2019.
10. Goldberg S. Clinical anatomy made ridiculously simple. Miami: MedMaster; 1991.
11. Goldberg S. Clinical neuroanatomy made ridiculously simple. Miami: MedMaster; 2002.
12. Leo J. Medical neuroanatomy for the boards and clinic: finding the lesion. 2nd ed. Cham: Springer; 2024.
13. Leo J. Clinical anatomy and embryology: a guide for the classroom, clinic, and clinic. 2nd ed. Cham: Springer; 2024.
14. Snell S. Fatigue of ocular muscles owing to constrained attitude at work as the main cause of nystagmus. BMJ. 1892;2:838–9.
15. Splittgerber R. Snell's clinical neuroanatomy. 8th ed. Philadelphia: Lippincott, Williams, & Wilkins; 2018.
16. Swanson PD. Signs and symptoms in neurology. Philadelphia: Lippincott Williams & Wilkins; 1984.
17. Woodburne RT, Burkel WE. Essentials of human anatomy. 9th ed. Oxford: Oxford University Press; 1994.
18. Young PA, Young PH, Tolbert D. Basic clinical neuroscience. Philadelphia: Lippincott Williams & Wilkins; 2015.

Vestibulocochlear Nerve Lesions 12

Introduction

The vestibulocochlear nerve includes both an auditory portion responsible for hearing, and a vestibular portion responsible for balance and eye movements. The sensory receptors for both the vestibular and auditory portion of the nerves are hair cells, and it is the mechanical movement of the hair cells which leads to changes in the afferent nerve signal. It is these hair cells that translate information about sound and balance into nerves signals. Interestingly, the hair cells are unique in that the extracellular environment around the hair cells is high in K^+ and low in Na^+ which is the opposite of the usual arrangement for cells.

Equilibrium is sometimes referred to as the sixth sense, and involves three systems: vision, vestibular, and somatosensory. Patients who have a false sense or illusory sense of movement are suffering from *vertigo*. If you turn around several times you may experience this. Vertigo is not a physical diagnosis but is a symptom and it strongly suggests a deficit with the vestibular system. One job for the clinician is to determine if the CN VIII pathology is found on the nerve in the PNS or to structures inside the CNS.

Semicircular Canals and Hair Cells

Starting with the vestibular nerve, when you focus on something in front of you, and then turn your head, your eyes slowly move opposite the head rotation. This is the slow phase of head rotation, which is under control of the vestibular system. The other way to think of this is to imagine walking down the street and trying to focus on a sign. As you walk towards the sign, your head is continuously moving up and down, and side to side, but regardless of these movements, your eyes stay focused on the sign. It is the hair cells in the semicircular canals that are sensing your head movement and through a complicated pathway keeping your eyes focused—the vestibuloocular reflex. With a deficit of this reflex a patient will have blurred vision and feel like everything is jiggling up and down and side to side which is referred to as *oscillopsia*. How do we keep out eyes focused on what is in front of us?

Within the skull is a bony labyrinth of three tunnels filled with perilymph. And within this bony labyrinth is a membranous labyrinth of three tunnels filled with endolymph. This network forms three semicircular canals and within each canal is a dilated chamber referred to as the

J. Leo, *Gross Anatomy, Neuroanatomy, and Embryology for Medical Students*,
https://doi.org/10.1007/978-3-031-87151-1_12

ampullae or crista ampullaris, and within each ampullae are hair cells that project up into a gelatinous mass, the cupula.

Each semicircular canal is responsible for sensing movement of the head in a different plane—either pitch, yaw, or roll. While there are three different planes of movement, we are going to focus on moving the head from side-to-side (the yaw axis), which is detected by the two lateral semicircular canals—one on each side.

As an analogy to the hair cells, think of an empty beaker. Take a feather, and with some epoxy, attach the base of the feather to the beaker, and then fill the beaker with water. The base of the feather is stuck to the beaker, but the feather itself is free to move in the water. When the beaker moves one way, the fluid will move the feather in the opposite direction. If the beaker is suddenly pushed to one side, say to the right as in the accompanying figure, the current will move left, and the hair cells will fall to the left. On each side of your head, you have a semicircular canal with hair cells surrounded by endolymph, analogous to a beaker with a feather surrounded by water. When you turn your head, the semicircular canal on one side is pushed anteriorly, and on the other side is pushed posteriorly (Fig. 12.1).

Take a head turn to the left as an example. The semicircular canal on the left follows your head and moves posterior, forcing the hair cells to fall anteriorly. This leads to a depolarization of the hair cell and a subsequent depolarization of the left vestibular nerve. Meanwhile on the right everything is reversed. The semicircular canal is pushed anteriorly with the hair cells falling posteriorly, hyperpolarizing the right vestibular nerve.

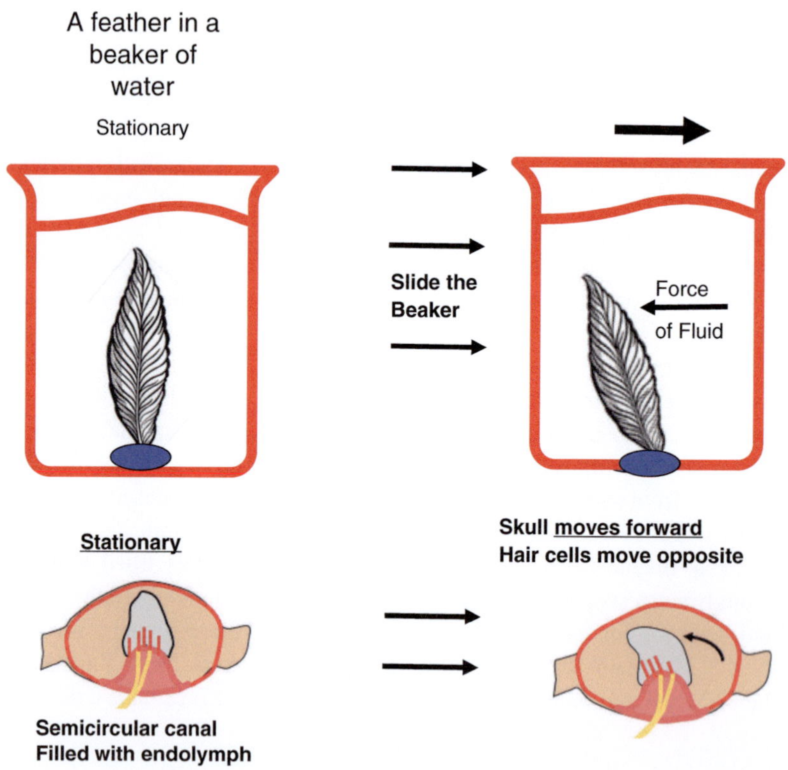

Fig. 12.1 Hair cells as a feather. The feather is equivalent to a hair cell, the beaker to the skull, and the water in beaker to the endolymph. When the beaker, or skull, slides in one direction the fluid pushes the hair cell or feather in the opposite direction. [12, 13]

The hair cells are organized in a stepwise pattern with the smallest stereocilia at one end and then each individual cilia in line being taller and taller. At the end of a row of hair cells is one single large kinocilium. This organization leads to what looks like a staircase. At the tips of each hair cell are K^+ channels. The fluid outside the tips is endolymph and there is a high concentration of K^+ outside the cell. When the K^+ channels on the tips open, the K^+ then runs from the endolymph into the cell at these channels. At the base of the hair cells, abutting the perilymph, there are also K^+ channels. The perilymph has a low concentration of K^+, thus when these channels on the basal surface open, the K^+ runs from inside the cell to the perilymph outside the cell. This also allows Ca^{2+} to enter the cell where it forms intracellular vesicles to be released at the synapse. These hair cells do not have action potentials, but instead they have graded potentials. Thus, they are not "on" or "off," and they do not follow the "all or none" rule of action potentials. Instead, their graded responses allow the cell to become either more positive or more negative.

The hair cell tips with their K^+ channels are the site where mechanical energy is transduced into electrical energy—the mechanotransducer. The high concentration of K^+ in the endolymph is maintained by the dark cells which are located on the apical surface of the hair cells just at the base of the stereocilia. The dark cells have K^+ channels which move the potassium from the intracellular side of the cell into the endolymph. They are like the stria vascularis located on the outer edge of the scala media (Fig. 12.2).

While this entire process is occurring in the hair cells on one side of the head, on the other side there is hyperpolarization (Fig. 12.3).

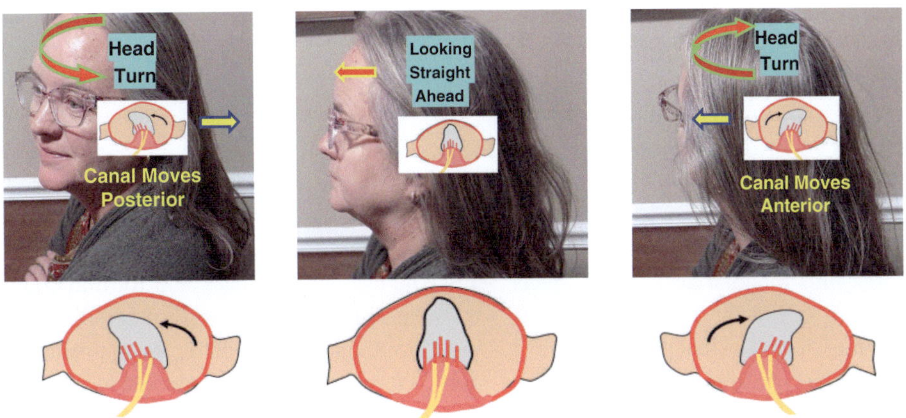

CN VIII is Depolarized

With a head rotation to the left, the left vestibular nerve is **depolarized,** which depolarizes the left vestibular nucleus. This goes to the right abducens nucleus, which then goes to the right lateral rectus. The right abducens nucleus also sends information in the left MLF, which goes to the left oculomotor nucleus and then the left medial rectus. The result is that both eyes turn to the right.

CN VIII is Hyperpolarized

With a head rotation to the right, the left vestibular nerve is **hyperpolarized** which hyperpolarizes the left vestibular nucleus. This goes to the right abducens nucleus, which then goes to the right lateral rectus. The abducens nucleus also sends information in the left MLF, which goes to the left oculomotor nucleus and then the medial rectus. All these structures are being hyperpolarized.
On the other side everything is being depolarized. The result is that both eyes turn to the left.

Fig. 12.2 Head turns and the left vestibular nerve [12, 13]

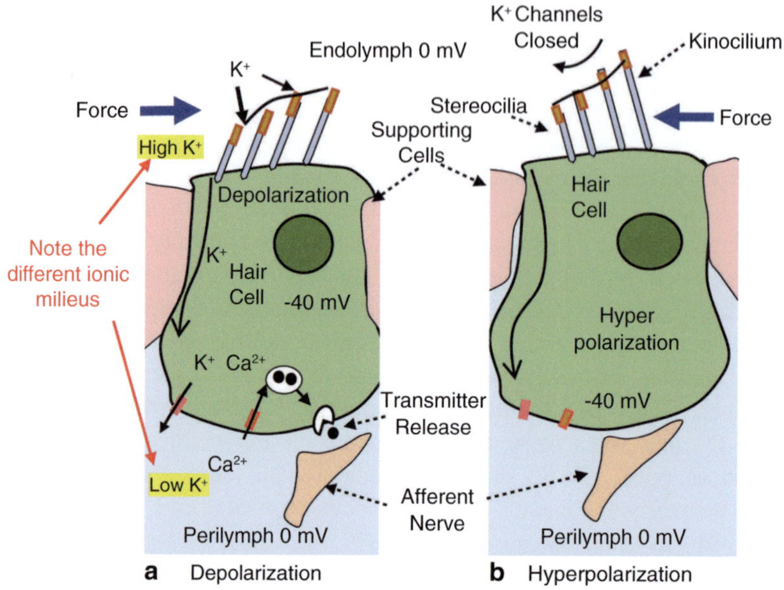

Fig. 12.3 Vestibular hair cells and graded potentials. In panel (**a**) note that there is a high concentration of K^+ in the endolymph surrounding the hair cells. When the hair cells fall towards the kinocilium this opens the K^+ channels (This is the opposite of most cells in the body). The K^+ is moved out of the cell into the perilymph at the basal surface. Ca^{2+} then enters the cell to form vesicles which will eventually be used at the synapse. Panel (**b**) shows the stereocilia falling away from the kinocilium which leads to hyperpolarization [12, 13]

Vestibular Nerve and the Slow Phase of Nystagmus

Continuing with the head turn to the left, the left vestibular nerve fires (depolarizes), and projects into the brainstem to fire the left medial rectus and the right lateral rectus so that both eyes move to the right. This slow phase is strictly under control of the brainstem (Fig. 12.4). Just like a tap on the quadriceps tendon tests the integrity of the spinal cord reflex, you can also test the vestibulocochlear reflex by applying cold (30 °C) or warm water (44 °C) to the ear canal. By adding the water and observing eye movements you are testing the integrity of CN III, VI, and VIII and the associated nuclei that reside in the brainstem (Fig. 12.4).

Cold or warm water in the ear canal sets up a convection current which moves the hair cells, tricking the person into thinking that their head turned. The direction of the convection current depends on the temperature of the water. The cold water in the right ear will cause the eyes to slowly deviate to the right and then quickly go left. The eyes will go back and forth alternating between slow and fast. Warm water will also lead to a slow and fast phase but in the opposite directions. Warm water in the right ear leads to slow deviation to the left and fast deviation to the right (Fig. 12.5).

If you apply cold or warm water and observe a slow phase of eye movements this tells you that the brainstem pathways are intact. Just like a healthy patellar tendon reflex tells you that the spinal cord reflex pathways are intact. If you see a fast phase after the slow phase this tells you that the cortex is intact. In a healthy patient you would observe this slow phase followed by a fast phase after applying either cold or warm water (Fig. 12.5).

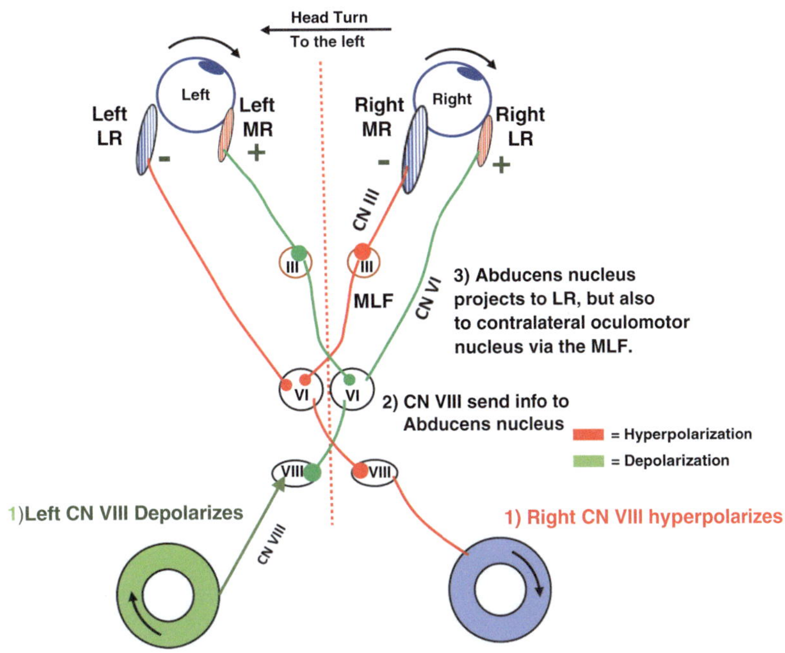

Fig. 12.4 Vestibulo-ocular reflex. With a head turn to the left the eyes slowly move to the right. In the left semicircular canal, the fluid is pushing the hair cells anteriorly which leads to depolarization. On the right, the fluid is pushing the hair cells posterior, which is hyperpolarization. [12, 13]

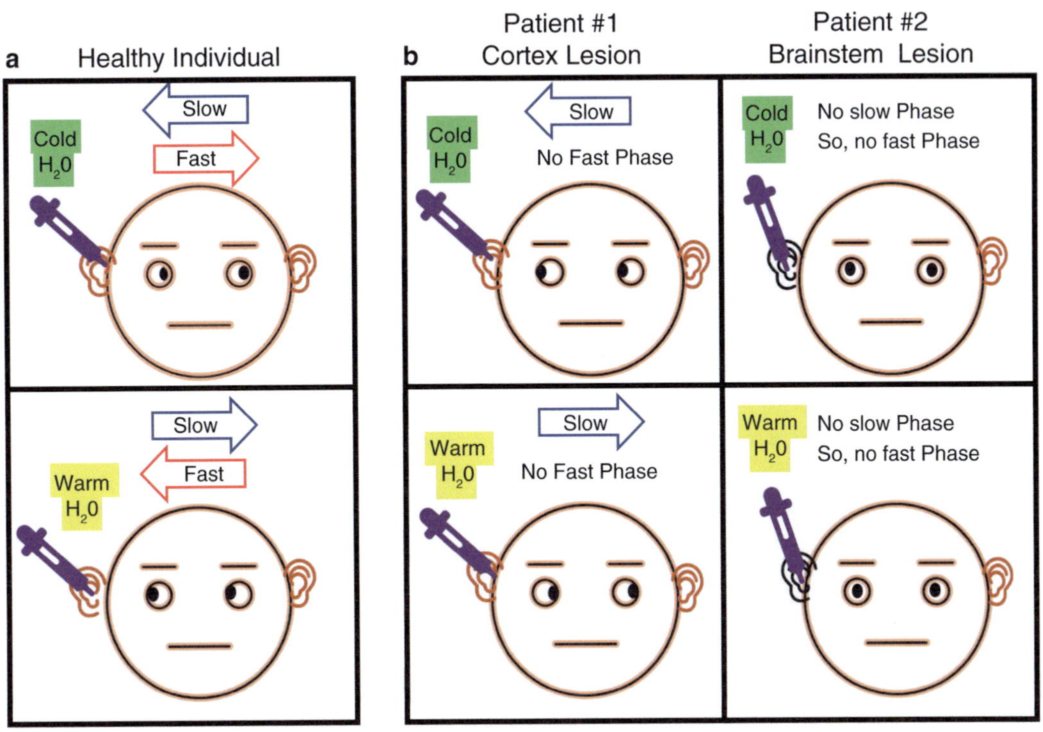

Fig. 12.5 Panel (**a**). In a healthy individual when you add cold water to the right ear there is a slow phase to the right followed by a fast phase to the left (Eyes in the picture show fast phase movement). Warm water leads to the opposite motions. Panel (**b**). With a cortex lesion with cold or warm water there is a slow phase but no corresponding fast phase (normally cortex does fast phase). With a brainstem injury there is no slow phase, and without the initial slow phase there is no corresponding fast phase [12, 13]

COWS Are Fast

At some point in medical school, every student will hear the mnemonic: COWS, which stands for Cold Opposite Warm Same. However, there is an important caveat to this phrasing. You need to remember that it is referring to the fast phase—not the slow phase. In other words, COWS are fast. When you add cold or warm water to the ear there will first be a slow phase and then a fast phase. As an example, cold water in the left ear will lead to a slow phase to the left, followed by a fast phase to the right-cold opposite, as the saying goes. Or take warm water in the left ear, there will first be a slow phase to the right, and then a fast phase to the left. Again, you must remember that the COWS mnemonic refers to the fast phase. In the healthy individual there will be both a fast and slow phase, with the eyes going in opposite directions. If you get confused and think about COWS referring to the slow phase, then your predictions for the head turns will be in the wrong direction.

This test can be used in a comatose patient to determine whether the lesion is in the cortex or the brainstem. Coma is typically due to a bilateral lesion in either the cortex, thalamus, or the brainstem that damages the reticular activating system (RAS). The RAS receives sensory information from many regions of the body and in turn projects to widespread areas of the cortex, thalamus and the basal ganglia and plays a role in maintaining alertness. Damage to it can lead to lethargy, stupor, or coma. With the comatose patient, the pertinent question is what structures are still intact. If the damage is in the cortex, then some of the descending tracts from the brainstem can be intact. But if the damage is lower down, then those descending tracts originating in the brainstem can be destroyed.

Imagine you have two patients in the hospital, and both are in a coma. One has a bilateral brainstem deficit, and one has a bilateral cortical deficit, and you want to differentiate between the two. You can use the water test as one way to determine if the vestibular tracts are involved. If the patient has a slow phase, but then no corresponding fast phase this suggests that the lesion is in the cortex (patient #1 in accompanying image). If you put warm or cold water in either ear and there is no subsequent slow phase, this tells you that there is a lesion in the brainstem (patient #2). In this second patient without an initial slow phase there will be no fast phase (Table 12.1).

In *postrotatory nystagmus* the eye movements are opposite the normal eye movements. If you spin someone around in a swivel chair approximately 10 turns, and then stop them and have them attempt to look straight ahead, you will notice their eyes going back and forth. The lay person will notice the eyes are fluttering, but there is more to the flutter. If you look closely, you will see a slow phase in the direction of the original turn, and a fast phase away from the head turn—in other words the eye movements are opposite what you would notice if the person just turned their head. This is because when you spin in the chair enough times the fluid in your semicircular canals will catch up with your head, just like if you spin a beaker in a circular motion the fluid will start spinning with the beaker. Then when you stop the head turn, or the beaker from spinning, the fluid keeps moving and turns the hair cells opposite the normal head turn.

Table 12.1 Oculovestibular response and comatose patient

	Slow phase	Fast phase	Lesion
Coma patient #1 Add cold or warm H_2O	Present	No fast phase	Cortex
Coma patient #2 Add cold or warm H_2O	No slow phase	NA	Brainstem

The *doll's eye reflex* is another way to test for the location of a lesion in a comatose patient. If the brainstem is intact when you turn the patient's head to either side, the eyes should turn away from the head rotation. If the eyes follow the head rotation this indicates that the brainstem pathways are disrupted (Fig. 12.4).

There are four vestibular nuclei in the brainstem: lateral, medial, inferior and superior. The medial and superior vestibular nuclei project via the medial longitudinal fasciculus (MLF) up to the cranial nerve nuclei involved in eye movements. Lesions to these nuclei will lead to a fast phase of nystagmus to the contralateral side. Let us walk through the reasoning of this. Take your left vestibular system. The left vestibular nerve is responsible for the slow phase to the right—the fast phase will be to the left. If the left system is damaged, then the right side overtakes it, slowly driving the eye to the left and quickly to the right.

The *utricle and saccule* are also part of the vestibular apparatus. Their sensory epithelium is referred to as the macula, which also has hair cells. The macula of the saccule is vertically oriented and senses vertical acceleration. The macula of the utricle is oriented horizontally and senses horizontal acceleration. These hair cells are covered by a gelatinous cap which in turn is covered by the otolithic membrane which has calcium crystals or *canaliths* embedded in it. The weight of the canaliths on the otolithic membrane puts pressure on the hair cells. Just like the semicircular canals, head movements result in shearing forces which bend the hair cells in the utricle and saccule.

Running down the middle, or the axis, of the macula is the *striola*. When the head tilts, the hair cells on one side will tilt toward the striola and depolarize, while the hair cells on the opposite side will tilt away from the striola and hyperpolarize.

Benign paroxysmal position vertigo (BPPV) is a common cause of vertigo—the feeling of spinning while not moving. It results from the canaliths, which normally lie in the utricle coming loose and becoming misplaced. The *Dix-Hallpike test* is a test that can be performed in the office to determine if the otoliths are misplaced. In brief, the patient starts sitting down in an upright position. The physician then turns the patient's head and has them lie down on the table. If the patient exhibits nystagmus or complains of balance problems this suggests that the otoliths are out of position. In some cases, they can be moved back into place with appropriate head movements, referred to as a *canalith repositioning procedure*, also known as the Epley Maneuver.

The hair cells in the vestibular system are extremely sensitive, thus any perturbations in the amount of fluid in the semicircular canals is problematic. *Meniere's disease* is thought to be caused by excessive fluid in the semicircular canals which leads to unwanted movement of the hair cells which leads to dizziness.

Lateral Vestibular Nucleus and Lateral Vestibulospinal Tract

The lateral vestibular nucleus receives input from both the cerebellum and the vestibular apparatus. Specifically, the fastigial nucleus, the Purkinje cells, and the vestibular nerve. Remember that the majority of Purkinje cell dendrites project to the deep cerebellar nuclei, thus they do not leave the cerebellum. However, this projection of Purkinje cells to the lateral vestibular nucleus is an exception. In one sense, given the role of the lateral vestibular nucleus in balance, and its connection via the Purkinje cells to the cerebellum, it is like the deep cerebellar nuclei (Fig. 12.6).

The *lateral vestibulospinal tract* projects from the lateral vestibular nucleus (Dieter's Nucleus) to the ipsilateral antigravity muscles. If you are in a standing position and get pushed on the right shoulder, then the extensor muscles on your left will contract to maintain your upright stance. If you lesion the left nucleus or tract, you will have ipsilateral ataxia. When these patients walk, they will tend to deviate or sway towards the lesioned side (Fig. 12.7).

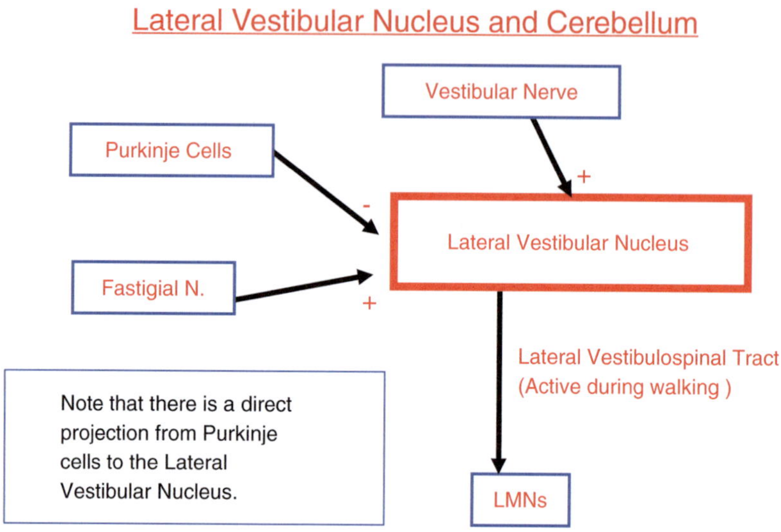

Fig. 12.6 Lateral Vestibular Nucleus. The nucleus receives inputs from multiple regions. It then projects as the lateral vestibulospinal tract (uncrossed) to extensor (antigravity) muscles mediating posture and balance [12, 13]

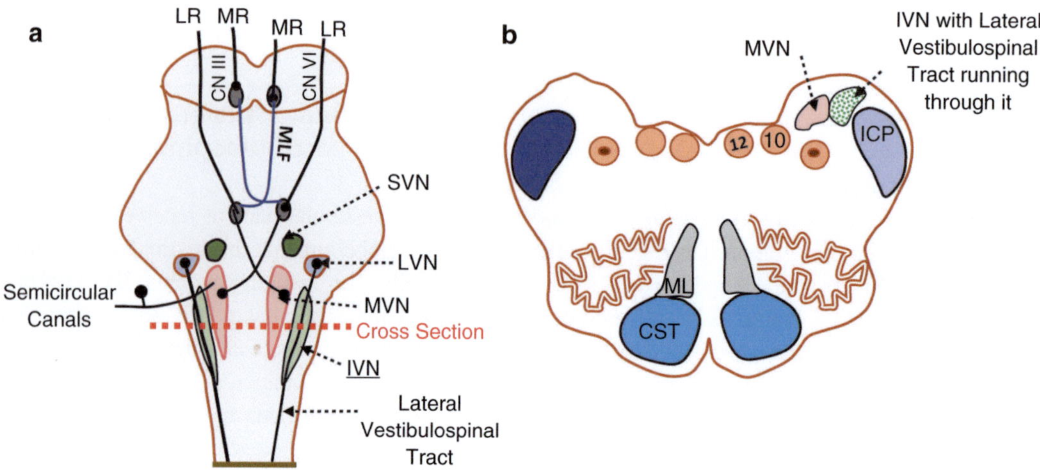

Fig. 12.7 Vestibular system connections. Panel (**a**) note that the lateral vestibulospinal tract runs down through the inferior vestibular nucleus, which gives the IVN a dotted look to it. The LVN also projects to the contralateral abducens nucleus. The cross section in panel (**b**) is through the IVN and the MVN. The IVN is easy to identify because of its dotted look. Once you ID the IVN then you move medial, and you have the MVN. *MVN* medial vestibular nucleus, *LVN* lateral vestibular nucleus, *SVN* superior vestibular nucleus, *IVN* inferior vestibular nucleus [12, 13]

Decorticate and Decerebrate Rigidity

As mentioned above, coma is the result of a bilateral lesion to either the brainstem or the cerebral cortex. In both cases, the lower limbs will be in a similar position—the feet will be plantarflexed. It is the upper limb position that will be different. There are three tracts that come into play with both scenarios: (1) corticospinal, (2) rubrospinal, and (3) lateral vestibulospinal. In decorticate rigidity, the lesion is above the red nucleus so both the rubrospinal and lateral vestibulospinal tracts are intact. Because the rubrospinal tract projects to the flexors of the upper limb, the elbows will be in a flexed position. In addition,

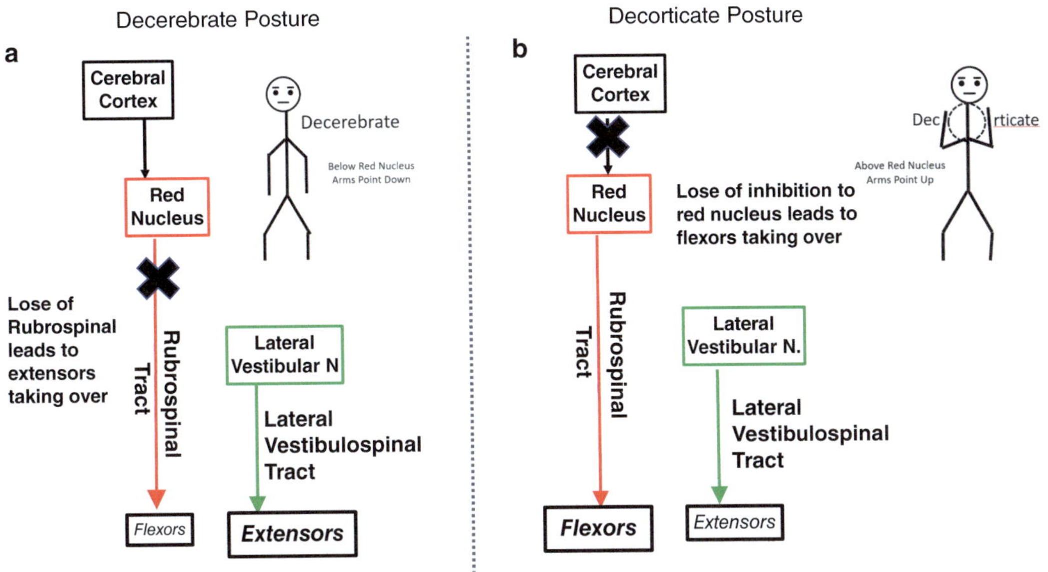

Fig. 12.8 Decerebrate and decorticate pathways. Panel (**a**): In decerebrate posturing there is a lesion below the red nucleus so lateral vestibular tract predominates leading to extensor activity. Panel (**b**): In decorticate posturing there is a lesion above the red nucleus. The uninhibited rubrospinal tract to flexors leads to flexion of the upper limbs. The decorticate patient has their arms pointed up, making an "O" with their upper limbs [12, 13]

the lateral vestibulospinal tract going to the extensors of the lower limb is intact so there will be extension of the patient's leg and foot.

Decerebrate rigidity is a lesion below the red nucleus so the rubrospinal is now cut, which leads to extension of the upper limbs. Just like decorticate posturing, the lateral vestibulospinal tact is intact so the lower limbs are extended.

One way to remember this, is that in decorticate rigidity, with your upper limbs flexed at the elbow you are making an "O" with your upper limbs, and since your hands are pointing up the lesion is up high—above the red nucleus, and in the cortex (Fig. 12.8).

In some patients, as the lesion expands, they can move from a decerebrate to a decorticate posture or vice versa. Because the brainstem is the location for the breathing and respiration centers, decerebrate rigidity is generally considered more problematic than decorticate rigidity. In some cases, the lesion is not symmetrical so the patient may exhibit decorticate rigidity on one side and decerebrate rigidity on the other side.

Chemically Induced Vestibulotoxicity

Several antibiotics such as gentamicin, streptomycin, and tobramycin can build up in the vestibular system and eventually lead to balance deficits and difficulty standing. Besides pharmacologic agents, numerous solvents and other chemicals used in manufacturing plants, such as toluene, xylene, and styrene, can lead to balance problems. In general, chemically induced agents tend to have a bilateral effect on balance.

Auditory

The *cochlea* is a hollow fluid-filled spiral shaped bone resembling a shell. Within the coil are three fluid filled tubes. The middle tube is the *scala media* with the *basilar membrane* as its base or floor, and *Reissner's membrane* as the ceiling. The scala media is bounded on one side by the *scala tympani* and on the other side by the *scala*

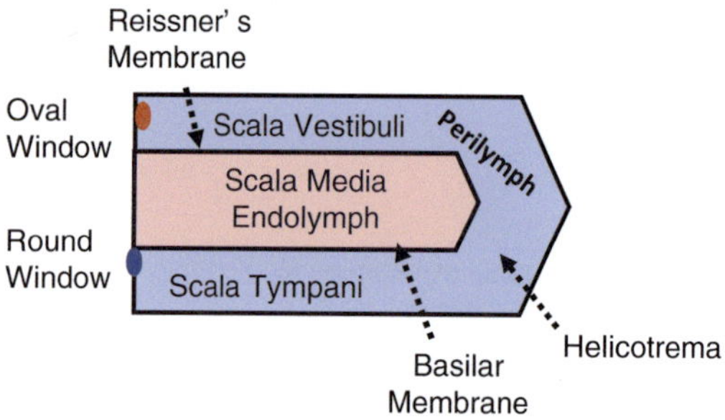

Fig. 12.9 Rolled out cochlea. The middle canal is the scala media with endolymphatic fluid which is high in potassium and low in sodium. The scala media is flanked on either side by the scala vesibuli and scala tympani which communicate with each other at the helicotrema [12, 13]

vestibuli. The scala media is filled with endolymph, while the scala vestibuli and scala tympani are filled with perilymph. The scala vestibuli and scala tympani are really one long tube as they are connected at the apex or *helicotrema*. The organ of Corti is in the scala media atop the basilar membrane (Fig. 12.9).

The basilar membrane runs down the middle of the cochlea from base to apex and is responsible for our ability to differentiate various tones. The key feature of the basilar membrane is that it is not a uniform structure, so that different regions of the membrane will vibrate in response to different tones. At its base, the membrane is narrower, thicker, and stiffer so that it responds to high frequencies; at the apex, the membrane is wider, thinner, and more pliable so that it responds to low frequencies. In other words, distinct parts of the membrane are tuned to different tones. The vibrations on the basilar membrane then lead to movement of the hair cell stereocilia. The tonotopic organization of the basilar membrane in mammals is not the case for all animals. In birds, for example, the ability to detect tones is based on their hair cells being tuned to different tones (Fig. 12.10).

In the auditory system, the base of each hair cell is on the basilar membrane and the hair tips project into the scala media where they are bathed in endolymph which has the high concentration of K^+. This high concentration of K^+ is maintained by the stria vascularis which is located on

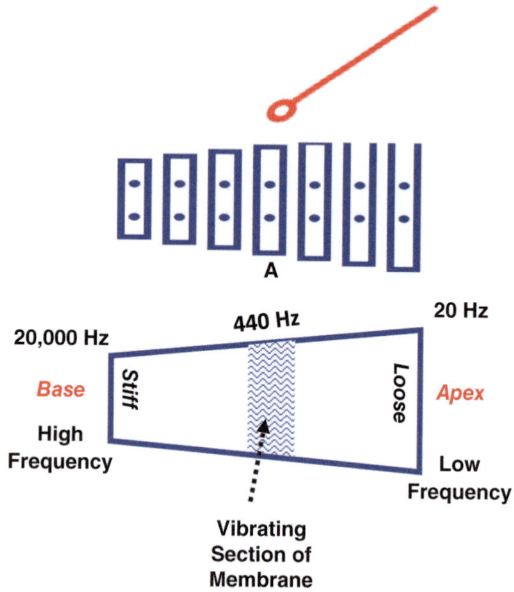

Fig. 12.10 Basilar membrane. The basilar membrane is tonotopically organized. Different parts of the membrane will vibrate to different tones. It is organized something like a xylophone. If you play a note on the instrument, say an "A" which leads to vibrations of 440 Hz in the air then the middle of the membrane will vibrate. Low tones lead to the apex vibrating, while high tones lead to the base vibrating [12, 13]

the outer edge of the scala media. As its name implies, it is a highly vascularized structure. The stria vascularis is equivalent to a battery, as it pumps positive ions into the endolymph. Located in the scala media. In the vestibular system, the Dark Cells maintain the K^+ gradient—also functioning like a battery (Fig. 12.10).

There are two types of hair cells located on the basilar membrane—the inner hair cells and the outer hair cells. Both have *aff*erent fibers projecting into the CNS. In addition, there are *eff*erent fibers projecting to the hair cells. The inner hair cells are lined up in a single row, on the inner part of the organ of Corti. Ninety-five percent of the afferent fibers in the auditory nerve come from the inner hair cells. Most of the efferent fibers in the auditory nerve project to the outer hair cells, which are lined up in three rows. The outer hair cells are unique in that they can change shape. They can go from short and squat, to tall and thin. As they become taller the hair cells reach up

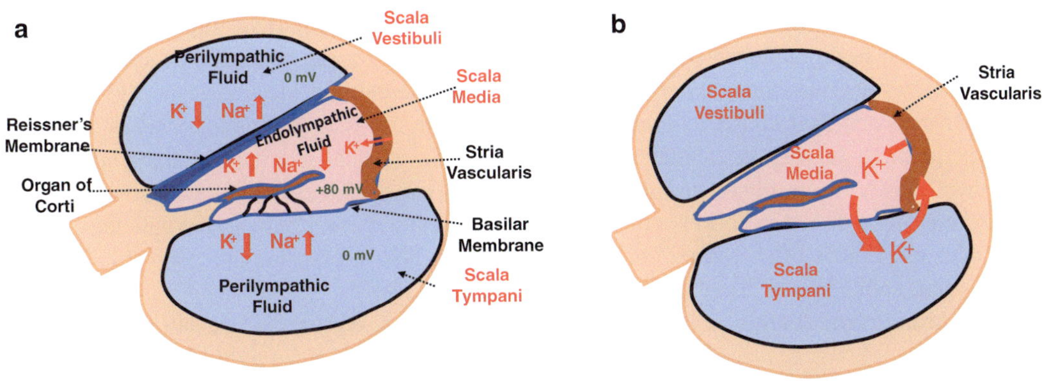

Fig. 12.11 Cochlea. Panel (**a**) The middle canal is the scala media with endolymphatic fluid which is high in potassium and low in sodium. The scala media is flanked on either side by the scala vestibuli and scala tympani, both of which contain perilymphatic fluid which is low in potassium and high in sodium. On the edge of the scala media is the stria vascularis. Panel (**b**) shows the movement of the potassium ions from the stria vascularis to the scala media, to the scala tympani, and back to the stria vascularis [12, 13]

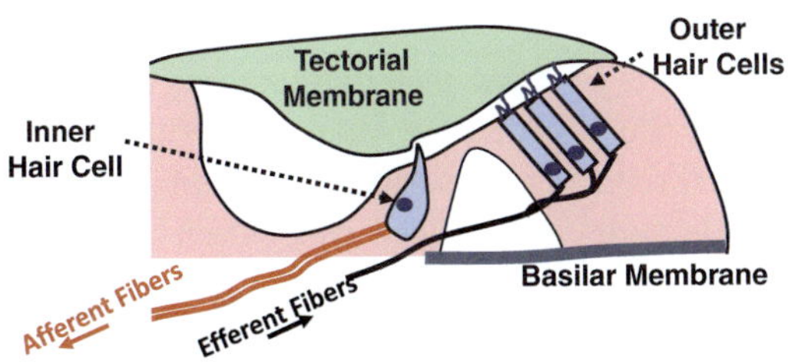

Fig. 12.12 Auditory hair cells the bulk of the auditory nerve is made up of afferent fibers coming from the inner hair cells. The inner hair cells *do not touch* the tectorial membrane. The efferent fibers run to the outer hair cells, which *do touch* the tectorial membrane. Outer hair cell loss leads to sensorineuronal hearing loss [12, 13]

closer to the tectorial membrane (Figs. 12.11 and 12.12).

The tectorial membrane, running parallel to the basilar membrane, overlays the top of the hair cells. When the basilar membrane vibrates there is a shearing force on the hair cells, which in turn leads to either a depolarization or hyperpolarization depending on whether there is upward or downward force on the hair cells. The shearing force transduces this mechanical change into an electrical change. This is sensed by the inner hair cells which lead to depolarization of the afferent fibers, and the sensation of hearing. However, the inner hair cells only account for miniscule movements of the basilar membrane and by themselves cannot account for the sensitivity of human hearing. This is where the outer hair cells, sometimes called *the cochlear amplifier,* come into play. The system functions as a positive feedback loop. The organ of Corti senses movement along the basilar membrane and the information travels along the afferent nerves back to the brainstem. The efferent nerves then carry the information out of the brainstem to the outer hair cells which amplify the movement. This amplifier allows mammals to hear sounds that many animals cannot (Fig. 12.12).

The outer hair cells also reach up and touch the tectorial membrane and, with their ability to change shape, can amplify the movement of the basilar membrane over 100 times. The motor protein in the outer hair cells changes shape in response to the efferent input is *prestin*. Aspirin (salicylate) interferes with the outer hair cell motility. Many sensorineuronal hearing deficits are the result of disruption of the outer hair cells. For instance, short-term exposure to extremely loud noises can break the connection between the outer hair cells and the tectorial membrane, leading to loss of the amplifier and a temporary hearing deficit. Longer term exposure can lead to cell death of the hair cells, and in humans there are only approximately 20,000 of these hair cells and they do not regenerate. Thus, a loss of hair cells can lead to permanent hearing loss.

If you are in a crowded restaurant, your ability to tune out the background noise and hear the person next to you is also thought to be due to the outer hair cells and their ability to change shape and hyperpolarize. As we age, the outer hair cells lose their ability to respond, and hearing is reduced causing a deficit in conversational hearing. Older individuals often have a challenging time hearing softer voices. They do not have a deficit in hearing loud sounds.

Weber's and Rinne Tests

In a patient with hearing loss, you want to determine if there is either a conduction deficit or a sensorineuronal deficit. The conducting portion involves the external and middle ear (malleus, incus, and stapes), while the sensorineuronal portion involves the vibrations of the basilar membrane and the subsequent action potentials in the cochlear nerve. If you tap on your mastoid process, the sound you hear is coming through the bone.

In *Weber's test*, the clinician holds a tuning fork to the center of the forehead. With no deficit, the sound will be heard on both sides equally—there is no localization to one side or the other. Conversely, if there is a conduction deficit, then the sound will localize to the side with the deficit. You can demonstrate this on yourself by putting your finger on your right tragus and humming. You have just given yourself a conduction deficit and the sound will localize to the right ear. The reasoning for why the sound localizes to the ear with the deficit is controversial and experts debate the mechanism, but the mechanism aside the sound will localize to the ear with the conduction deficit, wax in the ear for instance (Table 12.2).

However, Weber's is not definitive, because sound localizing to the right could also be due to a sensorineuronal loss on the left. This is where *Rinne's test* come in. In Rinne's test the clinician starts by holding a vibrating tuning fork just outside the ear and asks the patient to signal when they cannot hear the vibrations. The clinician then touches the fork to the mastoid process. In a healthy person, air conduction should be stronger than bone conduction. If bone conduction is stronger, then this suggests that there is a conduction deficit on that side. With Rinne's test, if there is a sensorineuronal deficit both air conduction and bone conduction will be decreased, with the net result being that air conduction is still superior to bone conduction.

Presbycusis refers to a gradual hearing loss that occurs as we age. It is a form of sensorineuronal deficit that can arise for several distinct reasons, such as: atrophy of the outer hair cells, nerve cells, or stria vascularis, or from stiffening of the basilar membrane.

Table 12.2 Tuning fork interpretation

Test	Normal	Conductive deafness	Sensorineuronal deafness
Rinne	AC > BC	BC > AC	AC > BC
Weber	Not lateralized	Lateralized to weaker ear	Lateralized to better ear

Audiometry and Audiograms

An audiogram is a representation of an individual's hearing ability. On the y-axis, running from top to bottom, we see loudness measured in decibels going from 0 to 120 dB. Running on the x-axis from left to right is pitch going from low to high sounds measured in Hertz—think of a piano keyboard with the high notes on the right and low notes on left. For each frequency, there is a point representing the decibels the person can hear. Hearing will be represented as two lines, one for each ear. The person can hear *everything below the line.* The picture below shows air conduction only. Bone conduction is not shown. The left ear is represented as either an "X" or blue line, while the right ear is either an "O" or a red line. Normal hearing falls into the 0–20 dB for each frequency. Mild hearing loss will be between 20 and 40 dB. Profound hearing loss will be between 90 and 120 dB (Fig. 12.13).

The next figure (Fig. 12.14) separates out each ear into its own audiogram and shows bone conduction as either an < or > symbol (greater than or less than). When you look at an audiogram of a healthy individual you see that both bone conduction and air conduction will be at the same location.

With a conduction deficit, air conduction will be reduced but bone conduction will be normal, so the gap between the two will be greater. In the picture below note the separation between air conduction and bone conduction on the right ear (Fig. 12.15).

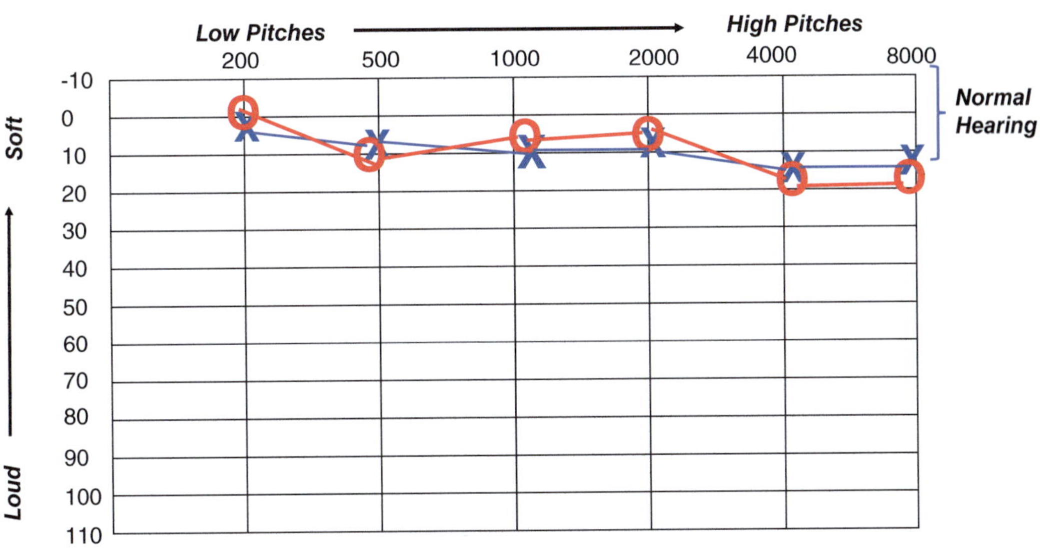

Fig. 12.13 Audiogram showing just air conduction in a healthy individual. Note that this person can hear everything below the line. Red Os are right ear. Blue Xs are left ear [12, 13]

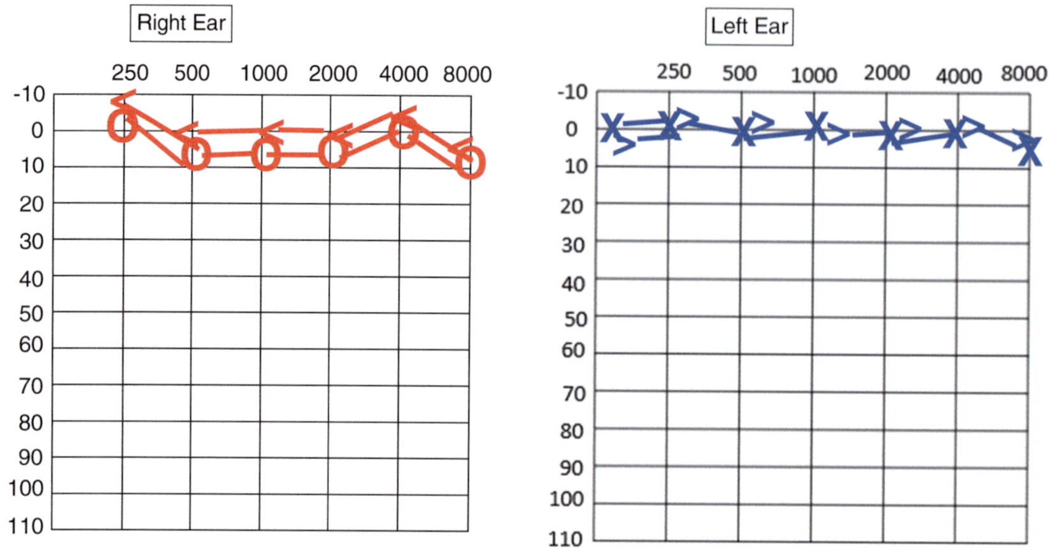

Fig. 12.14 Audiogram showing no hearing deficit in either ear. Bone conduction and air conduction are similar for both ears. O and X represent air conduction. < and > represent bone conduction [12, 13]

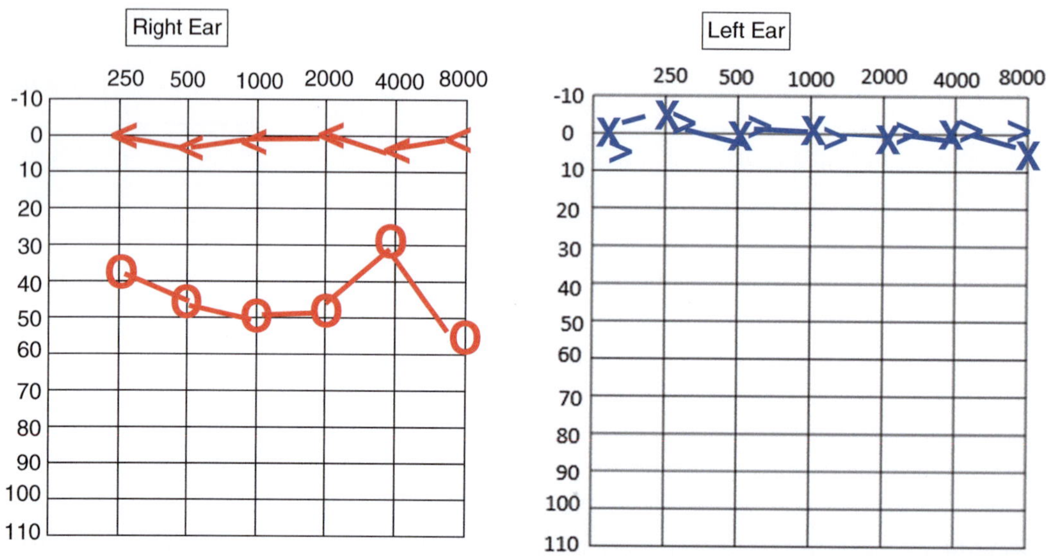

Fig. 12.15 Audiogram. In the right ear, bone conduction is greater than air conduction indicating a conductive hearing loss. There is no deficit in the left ear [12, 13]

With a sensorineuronal deficit, both air and bone conduction will be reduced on the audiogram, meaning that there is no gap between the air conduction line and the bone conduction line. In Fig. 12.16, note that both air and bone conduction are reduced in equal amounts on the left.

Auditory: Central Portion

The auditory portion of CN VIII comes into the pons and projects to both the ventral and dorsal cochlear nuclei (Fig. 12.17). From the cochlear nuclei, approximately 75% of the information projects to the contralateral side through the trap-

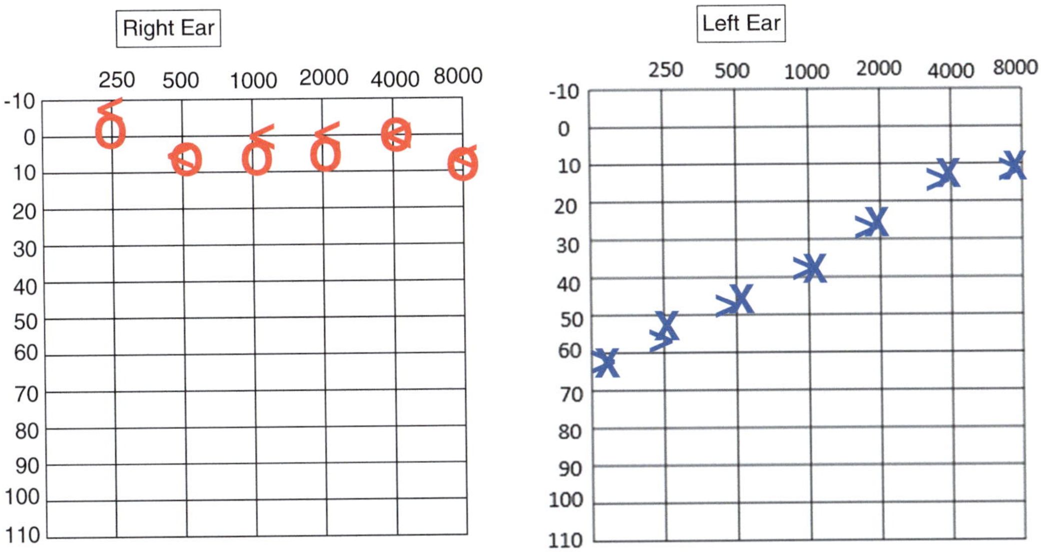

Fig. 12.16 Audiogram. Hearing in the right ear is normal for both bone and air conduction. In the left ear both bone and air conduction are diminished indicating a sensorineuronal deficit [12, 13]

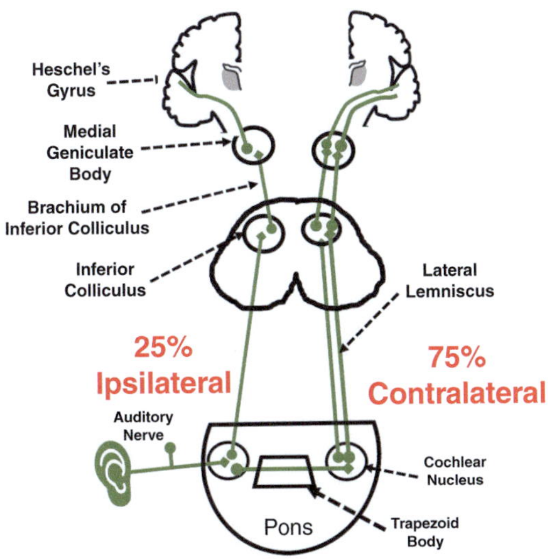

Fig. 12.17 Central auditory pathways. The information from the auditory nerve enters the CNS. 75% of the information decussates to the contralateral side and ascends, while 25% ascends on the ipsilateral side [12, 13]

ezoid body, while 25% stays on the ipsilateral side. On both sides the information ascends in the lateral lemniscus to the inferior colliculus, and then to the medial geniculate body, which then project to the auditory cortex. The auditory cortex, also known as Heschel's gyrus, sits atop the superior temporal gyrus. Because of these bilateral auditory projections, there are two ways to look at lesions here. One, is that a lesion along this pathway will lead to bilateral effects—a bilateral diminution of hearing with the loss greatest on the contralateral side of the body. Two, the lessons here will only have minor deficits because the other side is a backup (Figs. 12.17 and 12.18).

Lesions along this pathway will lead to patients complaining that while they can hear a sound, they have difficulty localizing where the sound is emanating from.

Lesions to the cochlear nerve or the cochlear nucleus will lead to complete 100% deafness from the ipsilateral ear.

An *acoustic neuroma* is a benign schwannoma of CN VIII, typically between where the nerve exits the brainstem and where it enters the internal acoustic meatus. The clinical symptoms will usually start off with an auditory deficit followed by a vestibular deficit. As the tumor expands it can also encroach on other cranial nerves such as the trigeminal and facial nerves. An important aspect is that when you are looking at the signs and symptoms of an acoustic neuroma because there are so many and such varied signs and symptoms, it might be tempting to conclude that

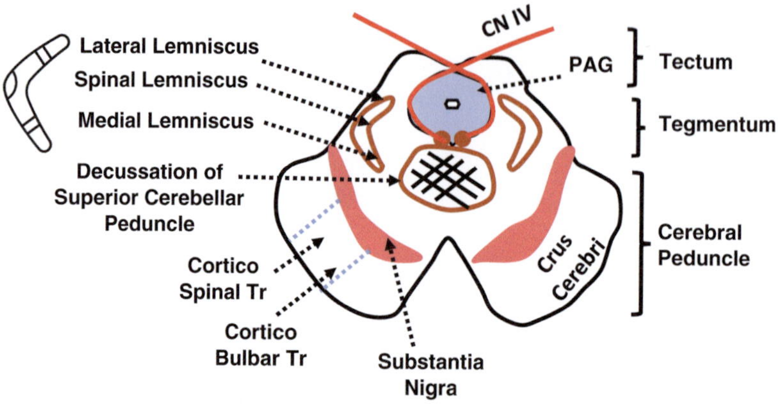

Fig. 12.18 Cross section at level of inferior colliculus. The section is divided up into tectum, tegmentum and cerebral peduncle. The corticospinal and corticobulbar tracts are housed in the middle third of the peduncle. The medial, spinal, and lateral lemnisci are lined up in a row looking like a boomerang. The crus cerebri is the anterior portion of the cerebral peduncle. The decussation of the superior cerebellar peduncle houses the dentatothalamic fibers coming out of the cerebellum and heading towards the contralateral ventral lateral nucleus of the thalamus [12, 13]

the lesion is in the CNS. But this lesion is in the PNS. When you look closely at the symptoms, you see that the deficits involve several cranial nerves but not the long tracts. There is no deficit of the corticospinal, dorsal columns or spinothalamic pathways.

The *labyrinthine artery* is a branch of the anterior inferior cerebellar artery or the basilar artery and perfuses the vestibulocochlear nerve. The facial nerve, the vestibulocochlear nerve, and the labyrinthine artery all travel together through the internal acoustic meatus. A sudden presentation of deafness and vertigo could be the result of a compromised labyrinthine artery.

Lateral Lemniscus and the Inferior Colliculus

In the brainstem the lateral lemniscus carries auditory information up to the inferior colliculus. As the lateral lemniscus moves up the brainstem it lies just lateral to the spinal lemniscus, which in turn is just lateral to the medial lemniscus. The three pathways look like a boomerang. At the level of the inferior colliculus the lateral lemniscus merges with the nucleus of the inferior colliculus. From there, the auditory information will travel along the brachium of the inferior colliculus to the medial geniculate body. Also, at the level of the inferior colliculus one can see the decussation of the superior cerebellar peduncle which are the fibers that left the dentate nucleus and are on their way to the ventral lateral nucleus of the thalamus. The trochlear nucleus can also be seen at this level. Remember that the LMN fibers coming out of the trochlear nucleus decussate before exiting the brainstem (Fig. 12.18).

The HiNTS Exam

In keeping with the idea that your clinical skills are the most important part of making the correct neurological diagnosis, consider the HiNTS Exam, which can be used at the bedside to determine whether vertigo arises from a central issue such as a posterior stroke, or a peripheral issue such as vestibular neuritis. The mnemonic stands for **H**ead **I**mpulse, **N**ystagmus, and **T**est for **S**kew. There are three parts to the exam. All involve the patient sitting in front of the clinician and looking at the clinician. The clinician has the patient do a series of head moves while examining the patient's eye movements. Remember we are not determining if the person has vertigo, but we are starting with a patient with vertigo and attempting to determine if the patient has a peripheral lesion or a central lesion.

1. **HI**-The first part of the exam involves the clinician holding the patient's head under the chin, asking the patient to look at the examiner's nose, and then turning the patient's head sharply side to side. If the eyes do not stay focused on the examiner but instead follow the patient's head and then show a correction, this is a positive, or abnormal finding. If it is positive in one direction only, this is indicative of a peripheral issue. If it is positive in both directions this suggests a central issue.
2. **N**-The next step of the exam is to examine for nystagmus in the primary and lateral gaze. If the patient exhibits fast beating nystagmus to one side regardless of whether they are looking to the right or the left (unilateral nystagmus) this indicates a peripheral issue. A patient with nystagmus when turned to both sides (bilateral nystagmus) most likely has a central issue.
3. **TS**-The test of skew involves covering one of the patient's eyes and determining if that eye moves. An abnormal correction is indicative of a central problem and is a positive result. A negative test is indicative of a peripheral issue.

Again, as I have mentioned before with these types of tests, my goal here is to explain the neuroanatomy involved in each test, so that when you get to that stage in your career when you are learning about the mechanics of a test, and practicing it, the knowledge of the pathways will help you be a better clinician.

Historical Snippet: The Caloric Reflex, the Nobel Prize, and a POW

The use of the water test to check for the integrity of the vestibular ocular reflex was developed by Robert Bárány (1876–1936), an Austrian physician, who noticed that patients with ear infections became dizzy when they had their ear canals irrigated and that their eye movements were dependent on the temperature of the water. He coined the term "caloric response," and subsequently won the Nobel Prize for Medicine in 1914. In the modern era, most people learn about their Nobel Prize via a phone call, but not Bárány. In WWI he was a surgeon in the Austro-Hungarian Army and was captured by the Russian Army. It was while he was a prisoner of war in a Russian prison camp that he learned about his Noble Prize. In 1916, after the intervention of several countries, he was released and was able to accept his Nobel Prize in person (Fig. 12.19).

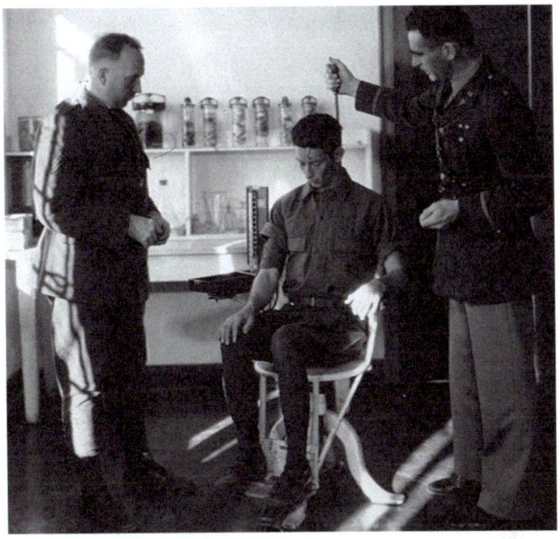

Fig. 12.19 Barany equilibrium chair. Being used by US School for Aviation Medicine to test for balance. *National institutes of Health*

Further Reading

1. Afifi AK, Bergman RA. Functional neuroanatomy: text and atlas. New York: McGraw-Hill; 1998.
2. Ashmore J, Avan P, Brownell WE, Dallos P, Dierkes K, Fettiplace R, et al. The remarkable cochlear amplifier. Hear Res. 2010;266(1–2):1–17.
3. Blumenfeld H. Neuroanatomy through clinical cases. 2nd ed. Hoboken: Wiley-Blackwell; 2010.
4. Bracha A, Tan SY. Robert Bárány (1876–1936): the Nobel prize-winning prisoner of war. Singapore Med J. 2015;56(1):5–6.
5. Brazis PW, Masdeu JC, Biller J. Localization in clinical neurology. Philadelphia: Lippincott Williams & Wilkins; 2016.
6. Burns TE, Baguley DM, Griffiths TD. The functional anatomy of central auditory processing. Pract Neurol. 2015;15:302–205.

7. Campbell W, Barohn RJ. Dejong's the neurological examination. Philadelphia: Lippincott Williams & Wilkins; 2019.
8. Fuller G. Neurological examination made easy. 6th ed. Edinburgh: Elsevier; 2019.
9. Gans RE, Rauterkaus G. Vestibular toxicity. Pharmacol Ototox. 2019;20(20):144–53.
10. Kattah JC, Talkad AV, Wang DZ, Hsieh YH, Newman-Toker DE. HINTS to diagnose stroke in the acute vestibular syndrome. Three-step bedside oculomotor examination more sensitive than early MRI diffusion-weighted imaging. Stroke. 2009;40(11):3504–10.
11. LaPlant W, Parmar M. Vertigo: a hint on the HiNTS exam. NUEM Blog; 2018. Retrieved from: http://www.nuemblog.com/blog/hints
12. Leo J. Medical neuroanatomy for the boards and clinic: finding the lesion. 2nd ed. Cham: Springer; 2024.
13. Leo J. Clinical anatomy and embryology: a guide for the classroom, clinic, and clinic. 2nd ed. Cham: Springer; 2024.
14. McPherson DR. Sensory hair cells: an introduction to structure and physiology. Integ Comp Biol. 2021;58(2):282–300.
15. Oghalai JS. The cochlear amplifier: augmentation of the traveling wave with the inner ear. Curr Opin Otolaryngol Head Neck Surg. 2004;12(5):431–8.
16. Ropper M, Samuels M, Klein J, Prasad S. Adams and Victor's principles of neurology. 12th ed. New York: McGraw Hill; 2023.
17. Splittgerber R. Snell's clinical neuroanatomy. 8th ed. Philadelphia: Lippincott Williams & Wilkins; 2018.
18. Swanson PD. Signs and symptoms in neurology. Philadelphia: Lippincott Williams & Wilkins; 1984.
19. Walker JJ, Cleveland LM, Davis JL, Seales JS. Audiometry and screening. Am Fam Phys. 2013;87(1):41–7.
20. Weatherall MW. The mysterious. BMJ. 2005;325:26.
21. Wong D, Zhou J. The kinocilia of cochlear hair cells: structures, functions, and diseases. Front Cell Develop Biol. 2021;9:Article 715037.

13 Visual Pathway Lesions

Introduction

It is important not to confuse, on the one hand, how we refer to the retina, and, on the other hand, how we refer to the visual fields. The nasal retina sees the temporal visual field; and vice versa, the temporal retina sees the nasal visual fields. If you are looking at the retina through the ophthalmoscope and observe pathology on the temporal retina, realize that the patient will have a nasal field defect.

Information from each nasal retina travels back along the optic nerve and decussates at the optic chiasm. Information from each temporal retina travels back along the optic nerve, but at the chiasm it does not cross over, and instead stays on the same side. From the optic tracts the information goes to the lateral geniculate bodies where it synapses. From the LGB, the information then travels on the optic radiations to the occipital cortex. The fact that the nasal retina fibers decussate while the temporal retina fibers stay ipsilateral allows the right and left visual fields to stay separate and go to one side of the brain. The right visual field thus makes it to the left brain, while the left visual world makes it to the right brain.

It is common during your first course on neuroanatomy to discuss the various lesions by looking at shaded pictures of the visual field. The shaded area shows what the patient *cannot* see during visual field testing. But keep in mind that you need to test each eye individually so the other eye should be closed during the test. This is because of the overlap of the nasal fields, and that we see objects in the nasal fields with both eyes (Fig. 13.1).

Lesion #1 Anopia This is a complete lesion to the optic nerve. This could be due to an occlusion of the ophthalmic artery which is the sole blood supply of the retina. This lesion would lead to complete blindness in this eye.

Lesion #2 Bitemporal Hemianopia This lesion is to the optic chiasm and is due to a pituitary tumor which damages the fibers from the nasal retinas of both eyes which see the temporal visual fields.

Lesion #3 Nasal Hemianopia This is a lesion to just the corner of the optic chiasm and could be the result of an aneurysm of the internal carotid artery. This would block the information coming from the temporal retina which is the nasal visual field of one eye.

Lesion #4 Left Homonymous Hemianopia This is a lesion to the right optic tract which will lead to a loss in the right nasal visual field and the left temporal visual field.

J. Leo, *Gross Anatomy, Neuroanatomy, and Embryology for Medical Students*,
https://doi.org/10.1007/978-3-031-87151-1_13

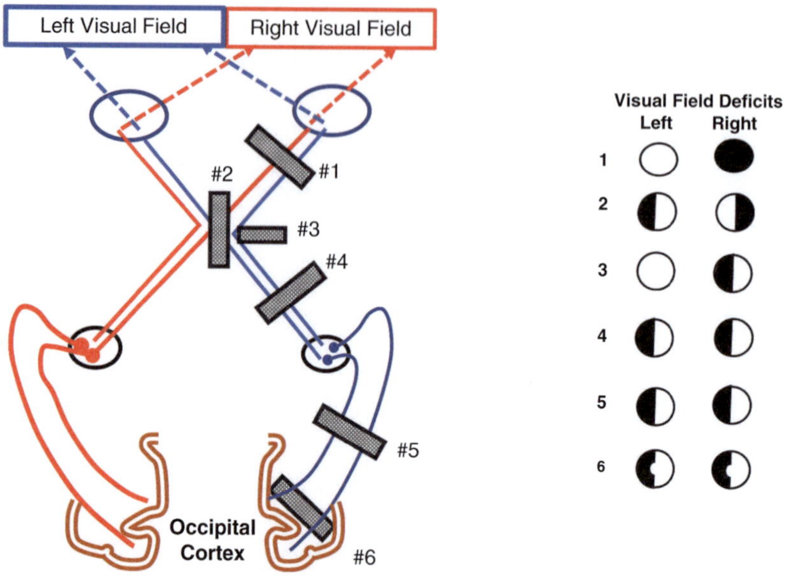

Fig. 13.1 Lesions and Visual Field Deficits [18]

Lesion #5 Left Homonymous Hemianopia This is a lesion to the optic radiations which would lead to the same deficit as the lesion to the optic tract. However, there is a difference in patient presentation. The patient with the lesion to the optic radiations will have an intact pupillary light reflex, while the patient with the optic tract lesion will have a disrupted light reflex.

Lesion #6 Left Homonymous Hemianopia with Macular Sparing This is a lesion to the occipital lobe which will lead to contralateral homonymous hemianopsia. In contrast to a patient with a lesion to the optic tract, this patient will have macular sparing. Macular sparing is thought to be the result of a dual blood supply to the occipital pole which is the cortical region that receives fibers from the macula. The theory postulates that because the macular region of the occipital pole receives blood from both the middle and posterior cerebral arteries, a lesion to just the posterior cerebral artery may not deprive the occipital pole of blood, which in turn spares the fibers from the macula. However, macular sparing is controversial and some ophthalmologists have suggested that the patient can move their eyes ever-so-slightly during the exam and trick the examiner into concluding that macular sparing is present, and that, because of this, macular sparing is not a useful clinical sign that can be used to localize lesions. But regardless of the debate about macular sparing, a patient with macular sparing has a lesion in the occipital lobe that spares the occipital pole.

Macular *splitting*, on the other hand, refers to a visual field defect that is the reverse of macular sparing, and the vision from half the macula on each side is affected. The patient with a lesion to the optic tract exhibits macular splitting. Patients with either macular splitting or macular sparing will have 20/20 vision because all you need is half your visual field to maintain visual acuity. A significant difference between macular splitting and macular sparing is that patients with macular sparing are still able to read, while those with macular splitting have a harder time reading.

Words of warning: While the presence of macular sparing suggests that the lesion is in the occipital lobe, not all lesions to the occipital lobe will lead to macular sparing. Because of variation, some patients with lesions to the occipital lobe will present with a homonymous hemianopia without macular sparing. Thus, while macular sparing is often found with occipital lesions, it is not always the case, so do not automatically rule out the occipital lobe if you see a patient without macular sparing.

Some Advanced Visual Field Defects

Pie in the Sky and Pie on the Floor

Fibers leaving the lateral geniculate nucleus head for the occipital lobe but there is a slightly different path for fibers from the superior retina versus inferior retina (Fig. 13.2). The fibers from the superior retina head straight back to the cuneate gyrus of the occipital lobe, while fibers from the inferior retina take a detour into the temporal lobe, forming a loop before heading to the lingual gyrus of the occipital lobe. The detour of these fibers and the loop they form in the temporal lobe is called ***Meyer's loop***.

Lesions in the temporal lobe will often damage Meyer's loop resulting in a patient with a superior quadrantanopia or "pie in the sky." This is because the fibers in Meyer's loop come from the inferior temporal retinas, which take in information from the superior fields of both eyes.

Lesions in the parietal lobe may lead to "pie on the floor" which is the opposite of the temporal lobe lesion. The patients will lose the fibers from the superior retinas, which take in information from the inferior fields (Fig. 13.2).

Optic Chiasm Details

When you look at a midsagittal section of the optic chiasm you will see that the fibers from the superior retina are located superiorly in the chiasm, while the fibers from the inferior retina are located inferiorly. But again, note that the fibers from the superior retina take in information from the inferior field, while the inferior fibers take in information from the superior field. In its initial stages a craniopharyngioma will compress the superior surface of the chiasm which will lead to an inferior field defect. As the craniopharyngioma expands it will eventually encompass the entire temporal field (Fig. 13.3).

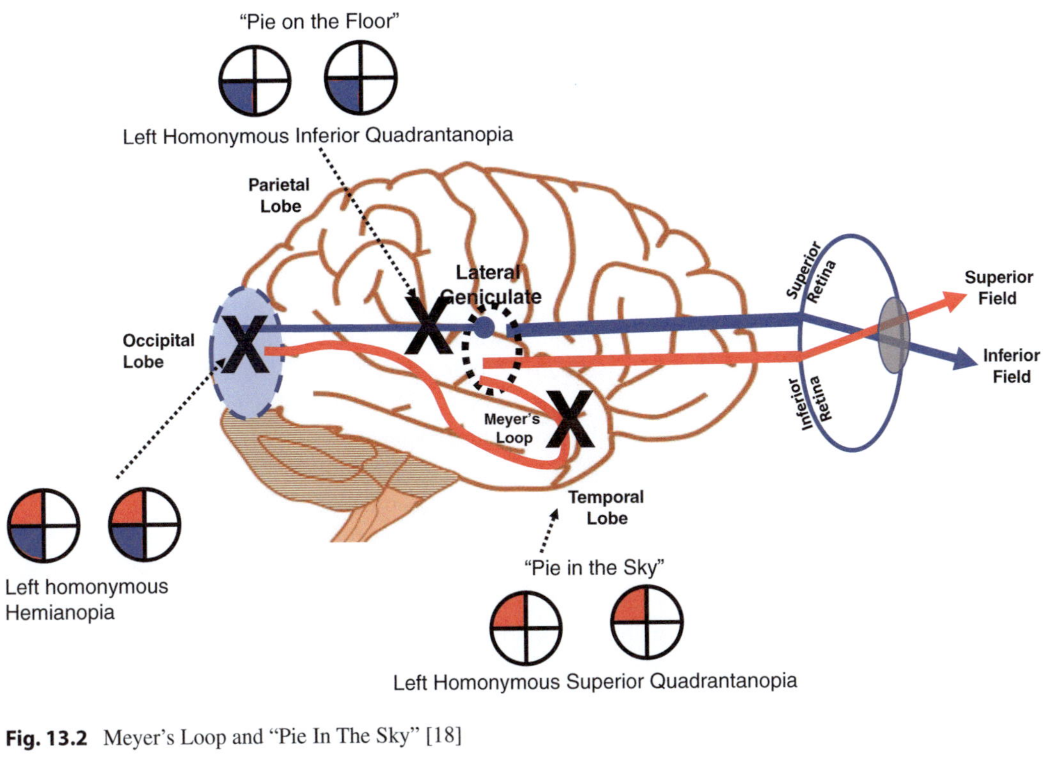

Fig. 13.2 Meyer's Loop and "Pie In The Sky" [18]

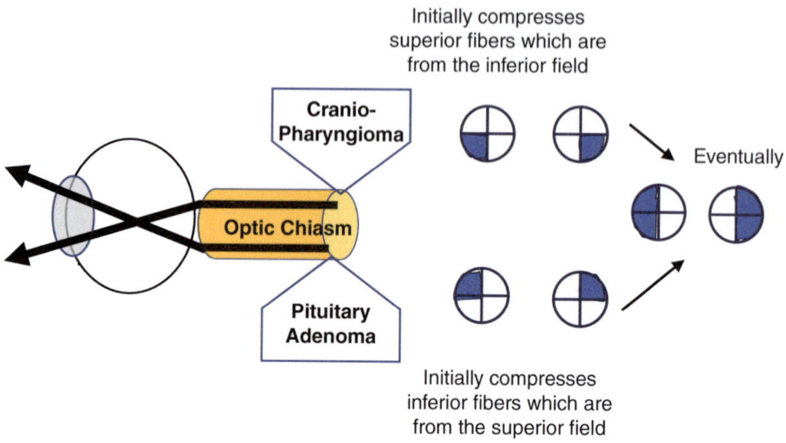

Fig. 13.3 Lesions to the optic chiasm [18]

The opposite of this is a pituitary adenoma which is located inferior to the optic chiasm. Because of this location, it will first impinge on the fibers from the inferior retina which is superior field.

Anterior Communicating Artery Aneurysm

The most common site for an aneurysm in the Circle of Willis is the anterior communicating artery. The aneurysm can compress an optic tract leading to a homonymous hemianopia, or the optic chiasm leading to bitemporal hemianopsia.

Prechiasmal versus Retrochiasmal Lesions

Lesions to the retina or optic nerve can lead to visual acuity deficits and loss of color vision in the ipsilateral eye, and an ipsilateral RAPD. With lesions past the optic chiasm there will be no deficit in visual acuity or the ability to see colors (achromatopsia). Take the optic tract for instance. The optic tract gets information from both eyes, and thus both foveas (foveae). Thus, a lesion to the optic tract will not completely block the information from either eye, as information from both foveae are represented in both optic tracts. A lesion to the optic tract will also lead to a contralateral RAPD, and contralateral bow tie atrophy of the optic disc. These topics are discussed in more detail with the retina.

Cortical Blindness

Lesions to the occipital cortex can lead to cortical blindness, either unilateral or bilateral. In these patients, because CNs II and III are intact, the light reflexes and eye movements are not affected. It can be permanent or temporary, and can result from a compromised posterior cerebral artery, preeclampsia, carbon monoxide poisoning, or the side effects of cyclosporine.

Swinging Flashlight Test

The swinging flashlight test involves starting with a patient in a semi-darkened room and then moving the penlight back and forth from one eye to the other. In a healthy individual the light will cause each eye to constrict. As the examiner goes back and forth from one eye to the other, both eyes will constrict.

This procedure tests the integrity of CNs II and III, along with the brainstem circuits involved in constriction. When light is shown to one eye, the information travels on the optic nerve, to the optic tract, and then prior to the LGB, the fibers peel off from the optic tract to project to the pre-

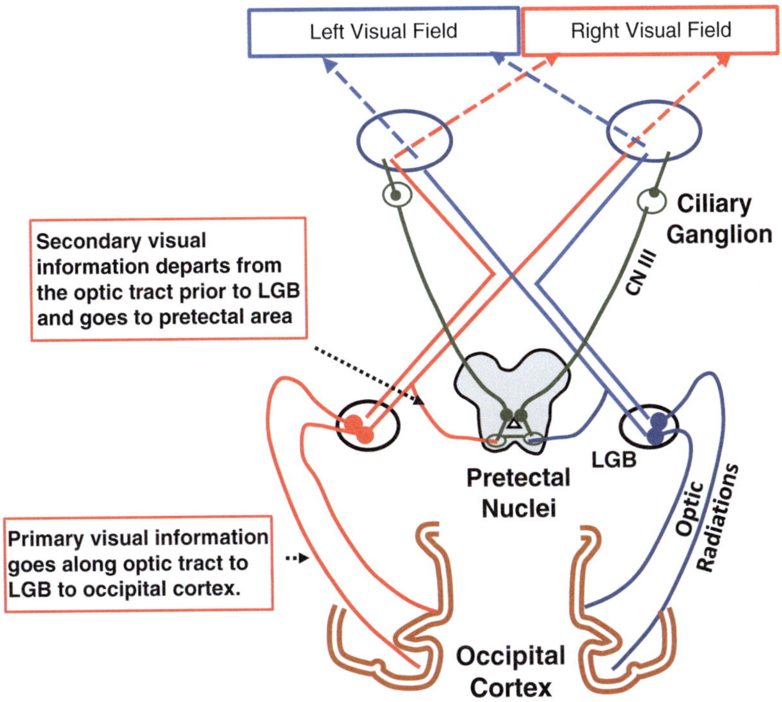

Fig. 13.4 Pupillary Light Reflex. When light is shined in one eye, the information goes down the optic nerve to the optic tract, but then peels off to go to the pretectal nucleus which projects bilaterally to the EW nucleus and from there on to CN III to constrict both eyes [18]

tectal nucleus. The pretectal nucleus is located near the superior colliculus and posterior commissure. The two pretectal nuclei talk to each other via the posterior commissure which allows the pretectal nucleus fibers to send information bilaterally to both Edinger-Westphal nuclei and then from there to the constrictor pupillae muscles to constrict both eyes. The response of the eye that the light is shown to is referred to as the *direct response*, while the response in the opposite eye, which also constricts, is referred to as the *consensual response* (Fig. 13.4).

Relative Afferent Pupillary Defect (RAPD) or a Marcus Gunn Pupil

A patient with a lesion to the retina or the optic nerve will have a relative afferent pupillary defect (RAPD) (Fig. 13.5). In a patient with a deficit in the optic nerve, during the swinging flashlight test, when you shine your penlight into the lesioned eye both eyes dilate. This is often referred to as a paradoxical dilation because you would expect the eye to constrict when you shine the light in the eye. The reasoning for this is shown in the figure below. The patient in this scenario has a lesion to the right optic nerve. When the light is shown in the left eye, the pretectal nucleus receives 100% of the information from that eye. The fibers from the pretectal nucleus project to both eyes and lead to constriction of both eyes. When the light moves to the right eye, which in this example has 50% of its fibers compromised, then the pretectal nucleus senses less light than a moment ago, so both eyes dilate—in other words when the light moves from the healthy eye to the pathological eye, the brain thinks the world got darker, so the eyes dilate.

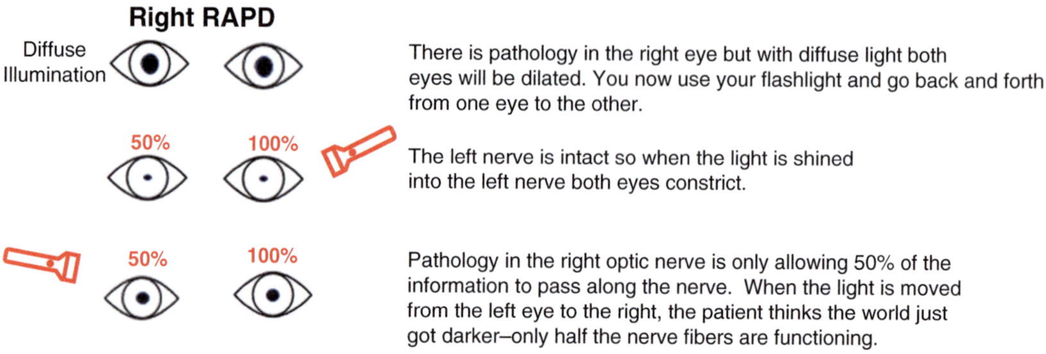

Fig. 13.5 Relative Afferent Pupillary Defect (RAPD). There is a defect in right optic nerve affecting 50% of the fibers. Light in the left eye leads to constriction. Light in the right eye leads to a bilateral dilation [18]

The Accommodation Reflex

Accommodation, or the near reflex, occurs when the individual wants to focus on an object close to them. To test this, the examiner can move their own finger towards the patient's nose. In a healthy individual, several things will occur: the medial rectus on both eyes will fire and bring both eyes in towards the nose; the constrictor pupillae will fire and constrict the eye; and the ciliary body will relax to allow the lens to thicken.

While the light reflex pathway does not include the occipital cortex, the pathway for accommodation does pass through the occipital cortex. When you test the accommodation reflex by moving your finger towards a healthy individual's nose, the signal travels down the optic tract, goes to the LGB, and then travels along the optic radiations *to the occipital cortex.* With their occipital cortex, the individual *consciously* sees the clinician's finger moving towards their nose. From the cortex, the pathway then projects to the Edinger-Westphal nucleus *bypassing the pretectal region* and posterior commissure. From the Edinger-Westphal the signal travels to the third nerve nucleus and then along CN III to the constrictor muscle.

Thus, while both the light reflex and the near reflex have very similar pathways, there is a slight difference between the two which has clinical implications and leads to scenarios where the patient exhibits what is referred to as *light-near dissociation* where the patient loses the light reflex but not the near reflex. (Figs. 13.6 and 13.7).

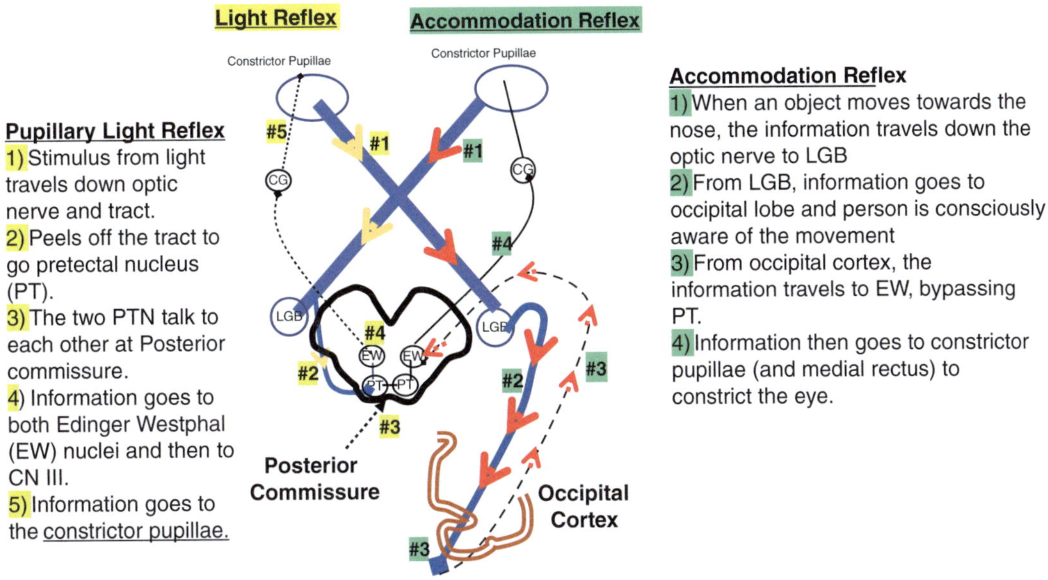

Fig. 13.6 Comparison of the Light and Accommodation Reflexes [18]

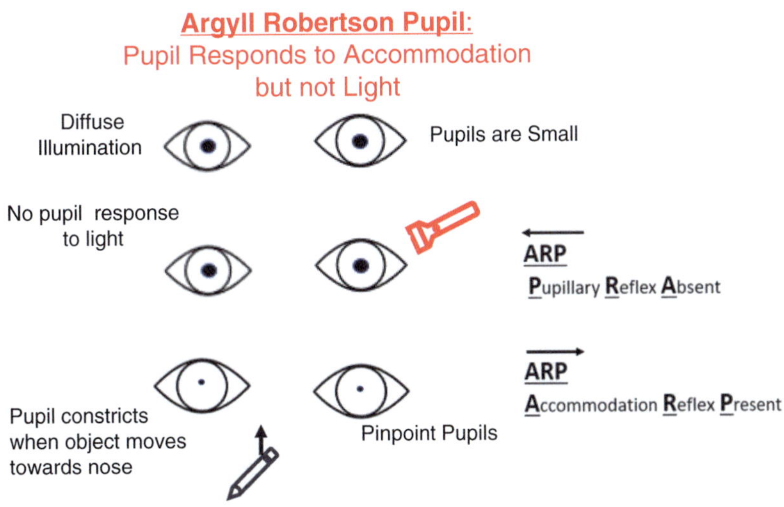

Fig. 13.7 Argyll Robertson Pupil. At rest, the pupil is small. When light is shined in the eye, there is no pupillary response. When an object like the pencil moves towards the nose there is pupillary constriction down to pinpoint size. Pupil goes from small to pinpoint [18]

Argyll Robertson Pupil

The most often mentioned example of a patient with light-near dissociation is an Argyll Robertson Pupil. In a patient with an Argyll Robertson Pupil, the pupil responds to accommodation but not the light reflex. In diffuse light, the pupil is smaller than normal to begin with. When light is shined in the eye there is no response. However, when an object moves towards the nose the pupil goes from small to pinpoint (Fig. 13.7).

Argyll Robertson pupils are found in patients with late-stage syphilis, also known as tertiary syphilis or neurosyphilis.

In this scenario it is thought that the pretectal nuclei and the posterior commissure are damaged which disrupts the light reflex pathway but not the accommodation pathway. The lesion spares the Edinger-Westphal Nucleus which means that the fibers from the occipital cortex carrying information about accommodation are not damaged. (Fig. 13.8).

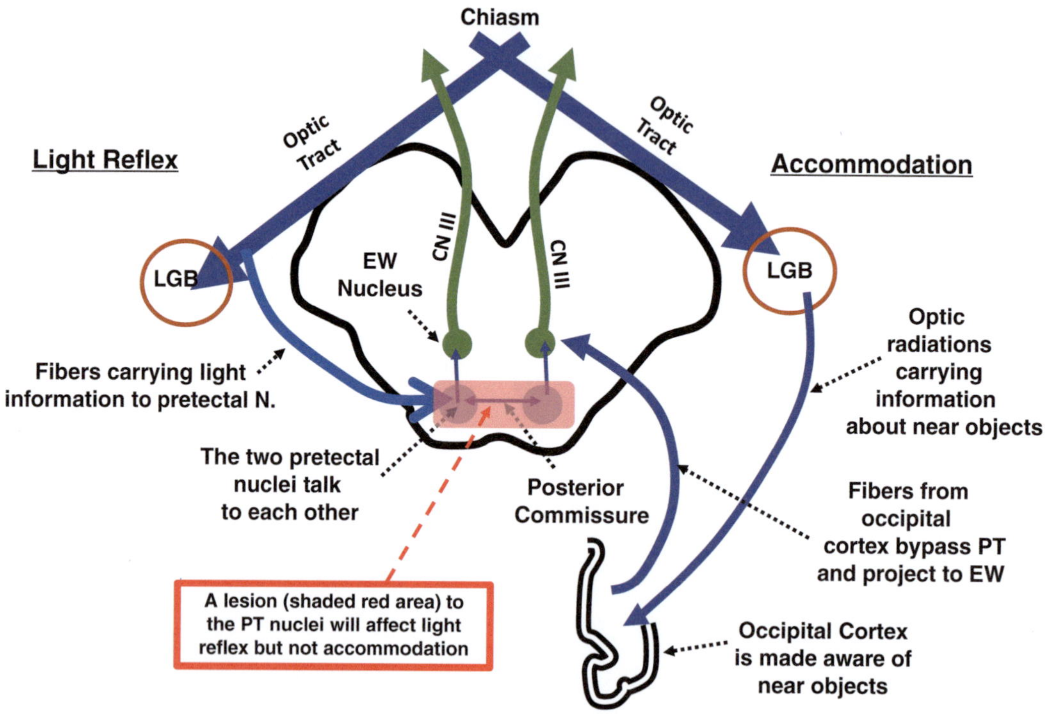

Fig. 13.8 Argyll Robertson Pupil/Light Near Disassociation. On one side is the light reflex pathway and on the other is the accommodation pathway. The lesion at the pretectal nuclei and posterior commissure affects the light reflex but not the accommodation reflex [18]

Parinaud's Syndrome

Another syndrome that leads to a light-near dissociation is Parinaud's syndrome which can result from the pressure of a pineal gland tumor, hydrocephalus, arteriovenous malformation, or an infection in the region of the dorsal midbrain. With hydrocephalus the swollen third ventricle puts downward pressure on the tectum. Besides the light-near dissociation there are several other pupillary findings with Parinaud's syndrome:

Light-Near Dissociation The lesion in the region of the pretectal nucleus will lead to loss of the pupillary light reflex, but because the lesion does not directly impinge on the EW nucleus, accommodation will not be affected. This is sometimes referred to as *Pseudo Argyll Robertson Pupil*. Of note is that in some of these patients, the eye can have a slight response to a bright light source. Again, this is not considered an Argyll Robertson pupil.

Convergence Retraction Nystagmus (CRN) Because the cortical input to the motor nucleus of CN III is damaged the nucleus fires indiscriminately and all the muscles innervated by CN III receive a stimulatory input resulting in a rhythmic movement of retraction and convergence. The medial rectus will pull both eyes medially—convergence, and the simultaneous firing of the superior rectus and inferior rectus will retract the eyeball. This CRN will usually be made worse on the attempted elevation of the eyes.

Collier's Sign The loss of cortical inhibition to the nucleus of CN III and the levator palpebrae superioris can also lead to retraction of the upper eyelid, known as Collier's sign.

Paralysis of Upward Gaze The patient has a challenging time looking up. The eyes will be depressed which is sometimes referred to as the *Setting Sun Sign* because the eyeballs look like they are descending below the horizon.

Ptosis Because of the third nerve palsy, the patient will have a droopy eyelid.

Diplopia and Blurry Vision Because of all the problems with the eyes mentioned above, the patient will have bilateral diplopia. The diplopia in turn will lead to complaints of blurry vision.

Parinauds for the Non-Ophthalmologist

The above explanation for Parinaud's is quite in depth and includes a fair amount of complex neuroanatomy along with subtle eye deficits which brings up the question: How much does a primary care doctor need to know for this? Here is the condensed version of Parinaud's (or a dorsal midbrain lesion): A hallmark of Parinaud's is a paralysis of upward gaze. The paralysis of upward gaze is almost 100% indicative of Parinaud's. If you see a patient, or a patient scenario, that mentions: "the patient has a paralysis of upward gaze" you should think of Parinaud's Syndrome. If present, all the other subtle findings just confirm Parinaud's Syndrome—the icing on the cake. In short:

1. Paralysis of upward Gaze = Parinaud's
2. Light-near Dissociation ≠ Argyll Robertson, necessarily. If the only finding is a light-near dissociation, then it would indicate an Argyll Robertson Pupil. But a Light-Near Dissociation can also go along with other conditions such as Adie's or Parinaud's, in which case it would be called a *Pseudo Argyll Robertson Pupil.*

Adie's Tonic Pupil

Adie's Tonic Pupil is another condition with a light-near dissociation. The pupil does not respond to light, but it does respond to near objects, although it constricts very slowly—known as a tonic response. Adie's results from damage to the ciliary ganglion or the postganglionic parasympathetic fibers traveling to the constrictor pupillae muscle in the iris (the opposite of Horner's). Because the parasympathetic fibers are lost, the sympathetics take over and, at least in the initial stages, the pupil will dilate. Although, over time, (typically years), because of the regeneration of previously damaged nerve fibers, the pupil will become small (little old Adie's). Remember: Adie's = Parasympathetic, and Horner's = Sympathetic.

The etiology of Adie's is unclear, but it is thought to result from either an autoimmune disease or an infection. In some cases, it can arise from neurosyphilis. It is more common in women than men, and it is typically seen in one eye but can progress to the other eye. While initially just the pupil is affected, Adie's pupil often goes along with excessive sweating and the absence of the deep tendon reflexes. The reason for this is speculative, but once the findings go beyond just the pupil, the condition is referred to as *Adie's Syndrome* or *Holmes Adie Syndrome.*

Pilocarpine is a cholinergic agonist that if strong enough will lead to constriction of the pupil. A dilute solution of pilocarpine (0.1%) is normally not strong enough to constrict the pupil—except in the patient with Adie's pupil. The reason for this is that in the Adie's pupil, over time there is a compensatory upregulation of muscarinic cholinergic receptors in the constrictor pupillae. With this increased number of recep-

Table 13.1 Light- Near Dissociation and Three Conditions

	Argyll Robertson	Parinaud's	Adie's
Light and near reflex	Light-near dissociation	Light-near dissociation	Light-near dissociation
Pupil	With near reflex goes from small to pinpoint and back	Normal pupil size but does not respond to light but does to near	Tonically dilated; over time becomes smaller. Usually, unilateral
Other findings	Tabes dorsalis	Paralysis of upward gaze, CRN, collier's sign. Ptosis.	No ptosis or other CN III issues. Responds to low dose pilocarpine. Reduced DTRs.
Etiology	Neurosyphilis	Pineal gland tumor, hydrocephalus	Loss of parasympathetics. From infection, autoimmune, or neurosyphilis

tors, when the affected eye is presented with the dilute solution it is now able to constrict. In the patient's normal eye there will be no response to the dilute solution of pilocarpine. This is referred to as *denervation supersensitivity*.

It can be difficult to distinguish an Adie's Tonic Pupil patient from an Argyll Robertson Pupil. With Adie's, think of the word *tonic*. In a patient with Adie's, at first, the pupil stays tonically large and has a very slow reaction to a near object.

In Argyll Robertson, the pupil starts off small, but it can constrict quickly down to a pinpoint during the near response, and then when the object is moved farther away the pupil quickly dilates—although it will still be small. Remember that with Argyll Robertson the pupil goes from small to pinpoint and then back to small (Table 13.1).

The Retina

The retina can be divided into two main divisions. During development, the two layers of the eye cup are separated by the ventricular space, and it is these two layers which give rise to the two parts of the retina in the adult, one to the neural retina and one to the pigmented epithelial layer (Fig. 13.9).

1. *Inner neural retina.* To start with the neural retina, we are going to first look at the three layers of cells, organized by the mnemonic RBG. The first layer, which is on the outer part of the neural retina is the layer of rods and cones (The R in mnemonic). The rods and cones then project to the bipolar cells (B in the mnemonic) and the bipolar cells project to the ganglion cells (G in mnemonic). If we then look at the connections between each of these cellular layers, we see fiber layers where the cells in one layer communicate with the cells in the adjacent layer. Between the rods and the bipolar cells, we see fibers making up what we call the outer plexiform layer. And between the bipolar cells and ganglion cells we see the inner plexiform layer. And then enwrapping the layer outside the rods and cones we have the pigmented epithelia layer, and then finally the choroid.
2. The outer retinal pigment epithelial layer. The pigmented layer is a single sheet of cells held together by tight junctions. The pigmented layer also supplies a steady source of nutrients such as vitamin A to the neuronal layer, and it absorbs the waste products generated by the constant turnover of the rods and cones.

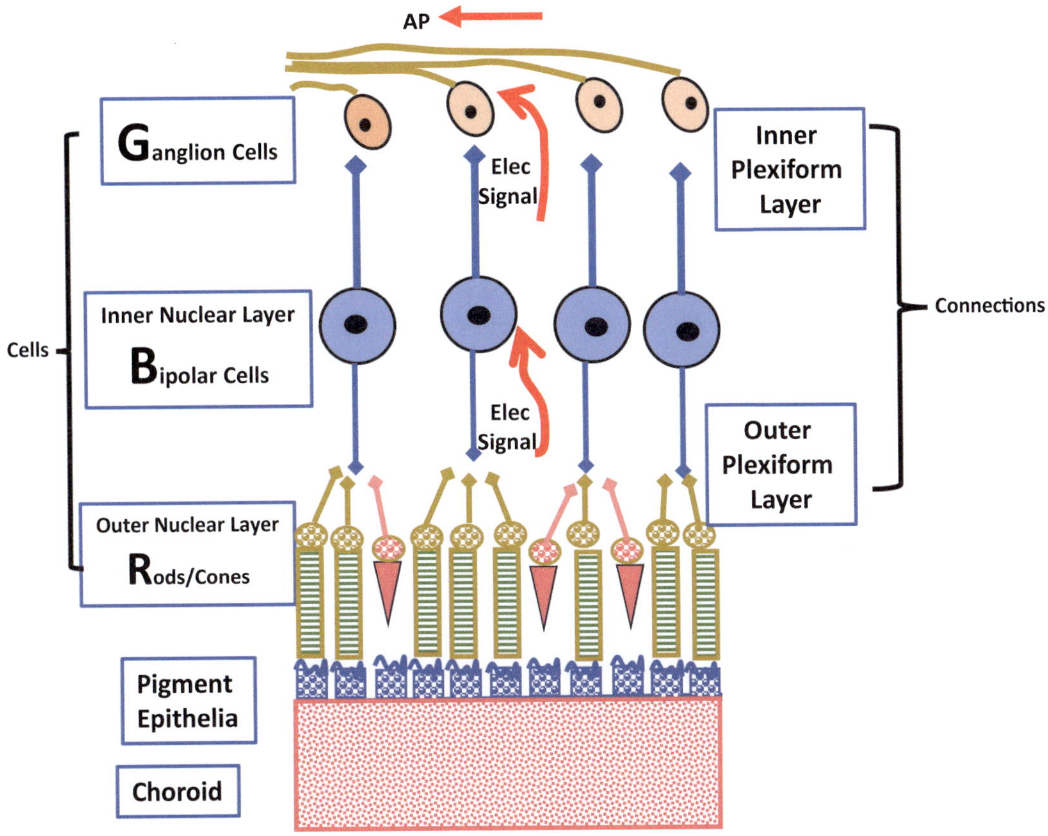

Fig. 13.9 Organization of Retinal Layers. There are three cellular layers: (1) Rods (and Cones) (2) Bipolar Cells, and (3) Ganglion Cells. Where these cells talk to each other we have two more layers. Since these two layers are made up of fibers, we call them outer and inner plexiform layers. Continuing past the rods and cones is the pigment epithelial layer and the choroid [18]

Photoreceptors: Rods and Cones

The most important job of the neural retina is to transform a light wave or a photon into an action potential. It does this job via an elegant but complex pathway. Several steps in the pathway seem counterintuitive, at least when compared to what you already know about transmitters, receptors, and action potentials.

Phototransduction starts in the photoreceptor cells known as rods and cones. Both the rods and cones have an outer segment, an inner segment, and a cell body with a nucleus. The outer segment of cones, which are cone-shaped, are characterized by invagination of the cell membrane that look like shelves, and within the membrane are the pigment molecules. For the purposes of this discussion, we are going to focus on the rods, with their columnar shaped outer segments containing disks of flattened membranous sacs.

Embedded in the membranes of these disks are pigment molecules called rhodopsin which contain a transmembrane protein called *opsin*, and 11-*cis*-retinal which is the chromophore that absorbs light. When a photon of light hits the 11-*cis*-retinal in rhodopsin, the 11-*cis*-retinal is transformed into all-*trans*-retinal which detaches from the opsin. In the dark, 11-*cis*-retinal remains bound to opsin.

Retinitis Pigmentosa is a genetic condition arising from a mutation in one of the genes coding for one the proteins involved in phototransduction, such as rhodopsin. It typically starts in middle age and involves a progressive loss of vision.

The Signaling Pathway

As we follow this signaling pathway from the rods and cones and dive deeper into the interactions of these retinal layers with each other. There are several interactions that seem odd, at least when we think about how other parts of the body function. As a framework for understanding the retina we will focus on these oddities.

Oddity #1

The first oddity, or counterintuitive organizational framework, concerns the overall organization of the retina. The neuronal portion of the retina includes the receptor layer (rods and cones), a relay (bipolar cells), and finally an output layer (ganglion cells). If a human engineer designed the eye, they would model it after a camera and place the receptor, the relay, and the output all in a straight line, with the receptor layer directly facing the light source, but evolution has not followed this model and has instead led to a very distinctive design (Fig. 13.10).

Of the three cellular layers, the receptor layer of rods and cones is the farthest from the light source. This receptor layer then connects to the bipolar cells in the middle layer, and then to the ganglion cells. Thus, the light coming in through the lens passes by the ganglion cells and the bipolar cells before hitting the rods and cones This organization is referred to as the inverted retina, and while it first seems odd, it allows the retinal pigmented epithelial (RPE) layer to be situated behind the rods and cones so that it can catch the back splatter of light while not blocking the incoming light rays. If the retina did not have this inverted arrangement, and the RPE layer was the first layer then it would be like putting window blinds up between the light source and the sensors.

The impulse on its way from the outer retina to the inner retina starts with graded potentials (not action potentials) in the rods and cones, which then stimulate the bipolar cells, which in turn trigger action potentials in the ganglion cells of the retina. Thus, the light rays and electrical potentials are going in opposite directions, like ships passing in the night, with light coming into the retina, and nerve stimuli going out of the retina.

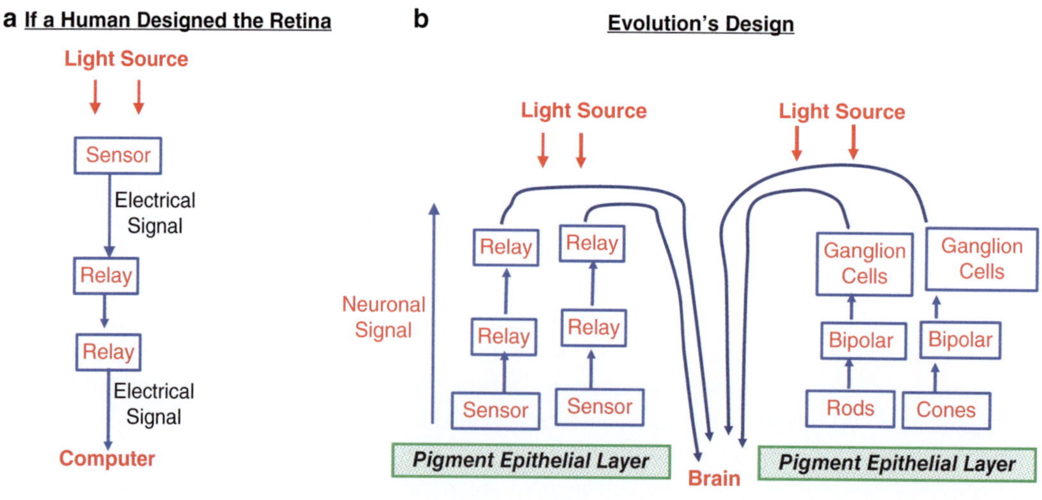

Fig. 13.10 Panel (**a**) is how a human engineer would probably have designed the retina, with the primary sensors in the front of the retina. Panel (**b**) is evolution's design with primary sensors at the back of the retina [18]

Oddity #2 Rods and Cones in the Light and in the Dark

The neurochemistry of vision refers to the interaction of the cells in these three layers, and it is here where we encounter two more counterintuitive processes. The next counterintuitive step is that in the dark, the rods and cones are in a depolarized state. I say counterintuitive because when first thinking about visual processing, one might assume that in the dark, the cells are quiet or hyperpolarized, and that it is photons from the light rays that depolarizes the cells. This is not the case. Again, in the dark the rods and cones are depolarized, and in the presence of light they become hyperpolarized—all of which seems counter intuitive. In the dark, when they are in a depolarized state, 11-*cis*-retinal is bound to opsin which leads to activation of phosphodiesterase which leads to the production of cGMP, which opens sodium channels to allow calcium to enter the cell. In this state, glutamate is released at the terminal of the rods and cones.

When light hits the rods and cones, the 11-*cis*-retinal is transformed into all-*trans*-retinal and separates from opsin. The unbound opsin now activates transducin which in turn binds to phosphodiesterase which inactivates the production of cGMP and blocks the sodium channels. Calcium therefore cannot enter the cell and the cell is in a hyperpolarized state (Figs. 13.11, and 13.12).

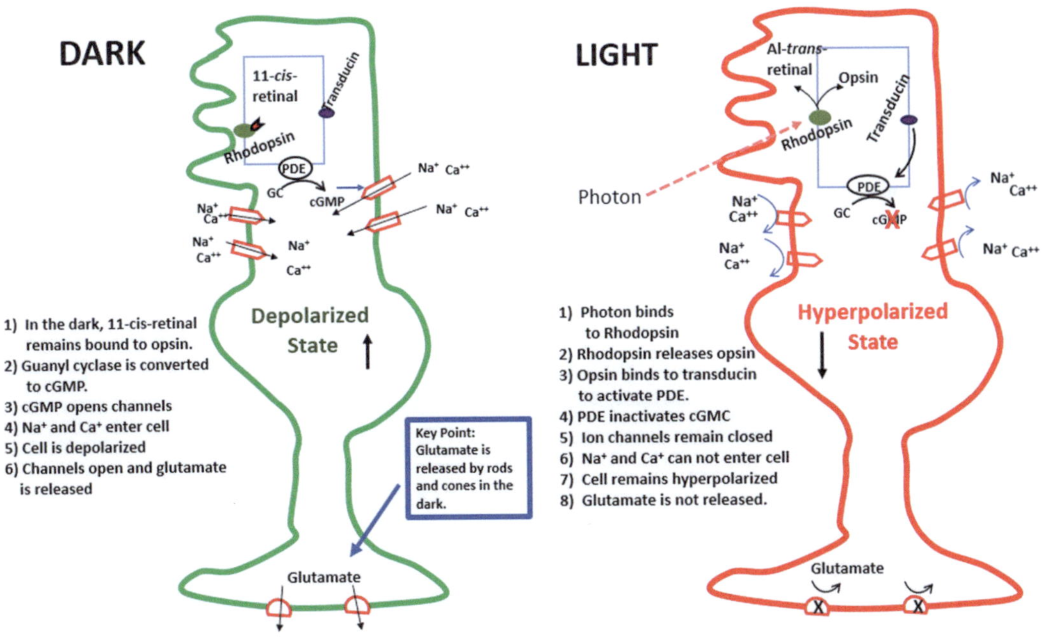

Fig. 13.11 Phototransduction [18]

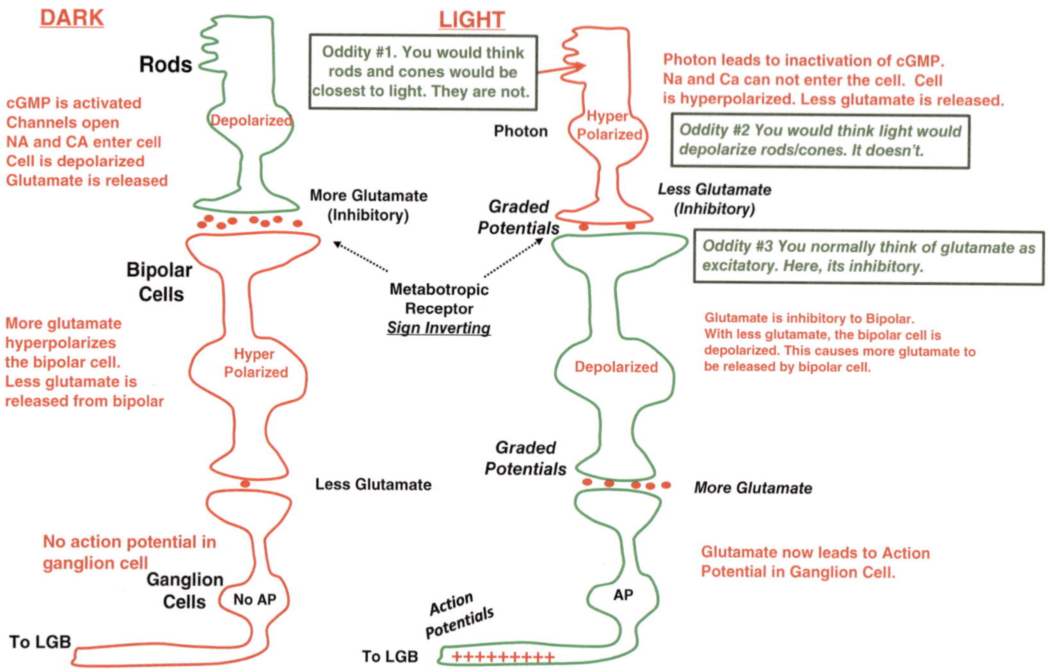

Fig. 13.12 The Quirks of Retinal Processing [18]

Oddity #3 the Bipolar Cells

In the dark, when the rods and cones are depolarized, glutamate travels across the synaptic cleft to meet the receptors on the bipolar cells and it is here where we encounter our second counterintuitive step. The receptors on the bipolar cells are sign inverting. When you first learned about glutamate you learned that it depolarizes the postsynaptic cell, however, at the synapse where the rods meet the bipolar cells, when glutamate binds to the postsynaptic cell it leads to hyperpolarization. Thus, in the dark, when the rods and cones are depolarized, leading to more glutamate being released into the synaptic cleft between the rods and the bipolar cells, it is the sign inversion properties of the bipolar cells which lead to glutamate hyperpolarizing the bipolar cells.

Conversely, in the presence of light the rods are hyperpolarized, which leads to less glutamate in the synaptic cleft between the rods and the bipolar cells, and with the sign inversion, the bipolar cells are now depolarized (Fig. 13.12).

Ganglion Cells

As mentioned, the ganglion cells themselves follow the typical scenario. In the presence of light, the bipolar cells release more glutamate which in turn leads to an action potential in the ganglion cells. And then, vice versa, in the dark, the bipolar cells are now hyperpolarized and release less glutamate which leads to hyperpolarizing the ganglion cells.

One More Way to Think about it

If we look at the *ganglion cells*, they do what seems intuitively correct—in the presence of light they produce an action potential—activity equals action potential. And conversely then, in the dark they are quiet. But if we look back at the rods and cones, in the dark they are depolarized—the opposite of what you think would happen. It is as if the rods make a mistake (which in reality of course they are not doing) and this mistake is corrected by the bipolar cells with their sign inversion. In a sense, the bipolar cells come to the rescue of the rod cell's odd behavior, and the bipolar cells get everything back on track so that the result is that light leads to an action potential in the ganglion cells.

The cones which are responsible for visual acuity are in the fovea, which is the center of the macula. The rods are located on the periphery and sense low levels of light. If you are outside on a clear night, you can sometimes see a star when you look off to the side but not when you look directly at it. This is because when you look directly at the light, you are lining up your cones which are not as sensitive to low light. Whereas, when you look off to the side you can sense the low light with your rods.

The fovea is also the thinnest part of the retina. At the fovea, the nerve fiber layers are pushed off to the side, resembling something like a crater, with the cones in the central part of the fovea referred to as the *fovea pit*. The cone in this area are not covered by the other nerve fiber layers. Where the fibers are pushed off to the side, they come to resemble a sloped mountain, referred to as the *fovea slope*. At the top of the fovea slope is the *fovea rim* (the top of the crater) which are the pushed-aside fibers (Fig. 13.6).

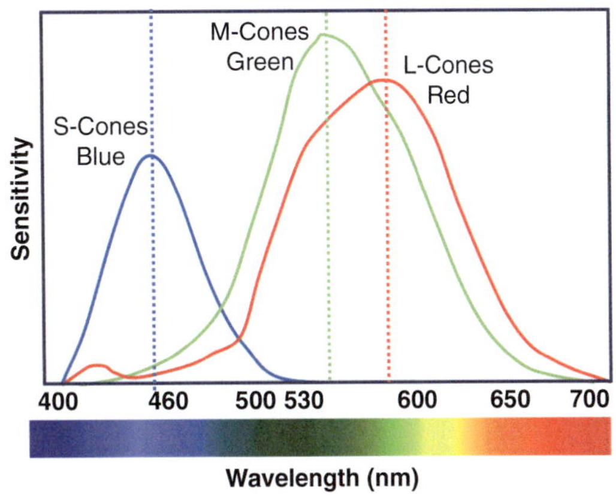

Fig. 13.13 Three Types of Cones. Each type of cone absorbs a different spectrum of light. All three overlap with each so none of the three respond to only one wavelength. Not shown are the rods which absorb light in the 498 nm range which is grey

Color Vision

Humans are *trichromats,* meaning that our ability to detect assorted colors is because we have three distinct types of cones, each of which is tuned to a different wavelength of light, and each of which overlaps. Some species, such as birds and reptiles are tetrachromatic—have four types of cones, and at the extreme end are mantis shrimps with12 types of cones. But back to humans, the L-cones, also called red cones, respond to long wavelengths of light, the M-cones or green cones respond to midrange, and the S-cones or blue cones respond to the shortest wavelength of light. They all overlap with each other, and none of the three cones respond to only one wavelength. If there was no overlap and each cone responded to a separate wavelength, we could only see three colors, but because of the overlap we see different shades of colors.

In an individual who is red-green colorblind, it is thought they have a defect in the L-cones (red ones) with the cones shifting their ability towards the green end of the spectrum—an *anomalous trichromat*. This defect is more common in males than females because the genes for color vision are found on the X chromosome. The extent of the defect depends on how much the spectrum has shifted towards green. Many people have a very mild red-green defect (Fig. 13.13).

As an example of the genetic transmission of the color gene, take a male with a red-green color deficit. We will refer to him as "the patient." Let us start with the patient's grandfather who also had a red-green deficit. The grandfather passed his X chromosome with the problematic color gene to his daughter—the patient's mother—who was then a carrier but did not exhibit the condition, because she also carried a healthy X chromosome from her mother (the patient's grandmother). She then passed the problematic X chromosome with the defect onto her daughters who became carriers. But she also passed the X chromosome carrying the problematic colorblind gene onto fifty percent of her sons—one of which was the patient. Thus, the condition has passed from the grandfather to the grandsons. The mother, between the grandfather and grandson, was just the carrier.

The Optic Disc and Glaucoma

In the center of the optic disc is the *optic cup*. As the ganglion cell fibers travel along the inner part of the retina to reach the *optic disk*, they are unmyelinated. As they penetrate the retina to form the optic nerve, they become myelinated. In a normal healthy nerve with many nerve fibers the cup is noticeably smaller than the disc (Fig. 13.14).

At the convergence of these axons, there are no rods and cones, and this region is referred to as the "blind spot" of the eye. The optic cup is the central part of the optic disc—the cup is smaller than the disc. The cup is usually a whitish color compared to the yellow tone of the disc. The ratio of the cup to the disc can be measured and this ratio can be used to detect and monitor the progression of glaucoma. When pressure rises in the globe, this puts pressure on the region of the optic disc and the cup enlarges. In addition, the nerve cells die and the space around the cup becomes smaller. The normal cup to disc ratio falls between 0.4 and 0.8. Anything higher than 0.8 is indicative of glaucoma (Fig. 13.15).

Open-Angle Glaucoma results from increased pressure in the anterior chamber of the eye. Aqueous humor is produced by the *ciliary body* in the posterior chamber of the eye and then percolates around the iris to the anterior chamber where it drains via the trabecular meshwork into the *canal of Schlemm* (the uveoscleral drainage system). In open-angle glaucoma, there is no change in the angle between the iris and the cornea—it stays open—but the trabecular meshwork is blocked. This leads to a slow build-up of pressure. It is painless and the visual field loss is slow, so that by the time the patient presents with noticeable symptoms the disease progression is

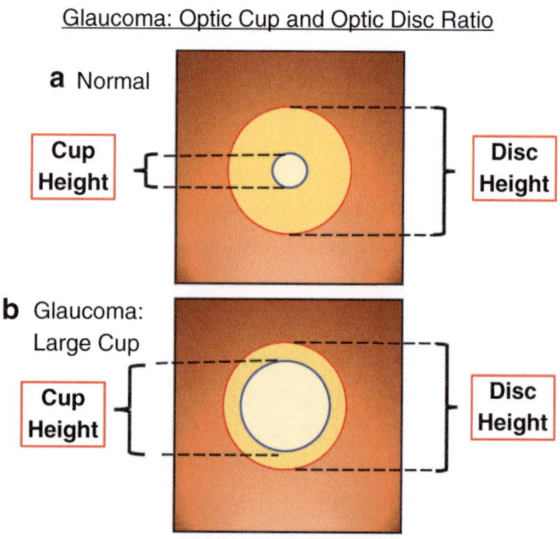

Fig. 13.15 Glaucoma and Optic Nerve. Glaucoma is caused by increased intraocular pressure which puts pressure on the optic nerve. This can be visualized at the optic disc. Panel (**a**) shows normal ratio of cup to disc. Panel (**b**) shows the increase in cup size but not disc size [18]

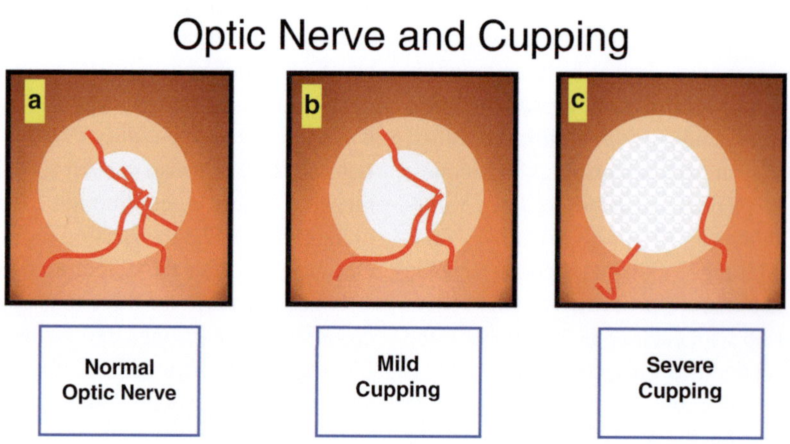

Fig. 13.14 Optic Nerve and Cupping. Panel (**a**) shows a normal optic nerve, Panel (**b**) shows mild cupping, and Panel (**c**) shows severe cupping which leads to blockage of the blood vessels and optic nerve atrophy [18]

significant. There is no cure, which makes early detection important. Once a diagnosis is made, preventive measures to slow the progress can be implemented. Initial treatment usually involves hypotensive drops to reduce the pressure. The situation is improved with constriction of the eye; thus sympathetic agonists or parasympathomimetics can be administered (Fig. 13.15).

Closed-Angle Glaucoma is a sudden, very painful presentation that typically results in a visit to the emergency room. In closed-angle glaucoma, there is a change to the shape of the iris such that it sags and closes off the angle leading to both the canal of Schlemm and the uveoscleral opening. Without treatment, the retina is at risk, and permanent vision loss is a possibility. It will typically involve just one eye. In dim light, the pain will sometimes lessen. This results from the subsequent pupillary constriction which tightens the iris and moves it away from the blockage. The most common treatment for closed-angle glaucoma is a trabeculectomy which involves removing a piece of the trabecular mesh (Fig. 13.16).

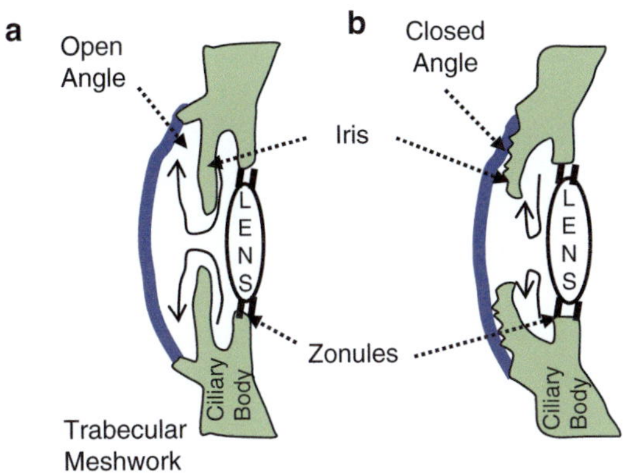

Fig. 13.16 Glaucoma. Panel (**a**) shows open angle glaucoma Aqueous humor (arrows) made in the ciliary body percolates from the posterior chamber to the anterior chamber. Its drainage is impeded. This leads to a slow build up of pressure, is painless, and is not an emergency. Panel (**b**) shows closed-angle glaucoma where the iris blocks the drainage of aqueous humor so pressure builds up very quickly. This is typically sudden, very painful, and an emergency [18]

In patients with glaucoma, the optic cup, but not the optic disc, will become enlarged. If the cupping is severe enough, the retinal vessels emerging from the optic disc will become occluded, which in turn will lead to optic nerve atrophy (Fig. 13.15).

Optic Nerve Sheath

The three membranes that surround the brain—the dura mater, arachnoid, and pia mater - also continue to surround the optic nerve. As these three membranes surround the optic nerve, they are called the optic sheath. Thus, the dural and subarachnoid spaces also continue out onto the optic nerve. In cases of increased intracranial pressure these spaces around the eye will typically enlarge. Ultrasound of the optic nerve at the bedside can be used to diagnose intracranial pressure.

Papilledema Papilledema refers to swelling of the optic nerve. Normally the optic disc is indented slightly. Increased intracranial pressure from either a tumor, infection, abscess, bleeding, meningitis, or encephalitis will lead to pressure on the optic nerve leading to a swollen, or choked look, to the optic disc. Some patients report hearing a "swooshing" sound or machinery-like sound when lying down. It is thought that this results from compression of the dural venous sinuses and subsequent disruption in flow. One test to confirm papilledema is a lumbar puncture to determine CSF pressure.

Rod Shedding

Rods do a tremendous amount of work, and daily they lose about ten percent of their rhodopsin molecules when the outer segment of the rods are sloughed off in a process called rod shedding. New rhodopsin molecules are continuously made on the inner side of the rods and then pushed towards the outer layer, where they are eventually sloughed off and consumed by the pigmented epithelial layer.

Retinal Detachment

As light rays enter the eye and moves towards the rods and cones, the pigmented epithelial layer catches the back spatter of light. This layer also nourishes and maintains the rods and cones by providing nutrients and removing waste products. For instance, the RPE supplies a constant source of Vitamin A, a precursor of rhodopsin, to the rods and cones. This pigmented epithelial layer has a layer of cilia that projects to the rods and cones so that these substances can be shuttled back and forth across the membrane. As we age, the cilia can tear with the rods and cones subsequently pulling away from this layer—retinal detachment. The patient often reports that their vision resembles a room with the shades being pulled down.

Surrounding the retina is the *choroid,* a spongelike structure which has the highest blood flow in the body. The innermost layer of the choroid is *Bruch's membrane*. The retina is one of the most metabolically active parts of the body, thus it produces a significant amount of heat. The choroid is a heat exchanger and allows the heat from the retina to dissipate into the blood stream. As we all know, staring into the sun can burn the retina, but interestingly it is more likely to occur in a cadaver because of the loss of the heat exchanger. Choroidal detachment occurs when the choroid becomes detached from the retina either from a build-up of blood or serous fluid. Serous fluid detachments can occur in cancer patients, as a side effect from certain medications, or following eye surgery. The patient reports an uncomfortable feeling but not severe pain. Hemorrhagic detachment on the other hand is extremely painful. It can also occur following eye surgery particularly in patients taking blood thinners.

Macular Degeneration

Age related macular degeneration is the most common cause of visual defects in the elderly. There are two types, the wet type, and the dry type.

The *wet type of macular degeneration* is the result of a proliferation of blood vessels in the choroid just behind the macula which diminishes the patient's ability to see objects in the central visual field. It spares the peripheral field.

The *dry type* results from disruption at the interface between the retina and the pigment epithelium. As mentioned earlier, one job of the retinal pigment epithelial layer is to absorb the waste products produced by the high metabolic activity in the rods and cones. As we age, the efficiency of what is a garbage disposal mechanism is diminished. Waste products then build up between the retina and Bruch's membrane of the choroid and form what look like small stones or pebbles which are referred to as *drusen*. As of now, there is no treatment or procedures for removal of the accumulating drusen. On an eye exam, drusen appear as small yellowish deposits on the retina.

The Lens, Cornea, and Refraction

As the light rays enter the eye, they pass through two lenses. The first lens is the liquid filled cornea, and the second is the actual lens. As the light rays pass through the less dense air, they then hit the dense fluid filled cornea and the light rays slow down and bend. The light rays then hit the lens, slow down, and bend some more.

As an aside, when you are underwater, the fluid-filled cornea is now surrounded by water, not air. Thus, the light rays passing into the cornea do not slow down or bend like they do above the water. The way to get around this is to wear a diving mask that restores the air layer in front of your cornea.

When the lens and cornea are functioning optimally the light rays converge onto a focal point directly on the retina. In some cases, the light rays converge on a point either in front of or behind the retina.

Myopia (Nearsightedness). In this case the eye is too long, or the cornea is too curved, so that the image is focused in front of the retina. The lens is too strong for the length of the eye. The term "near sighted" means that they can see things right in front of them, but they have a tough time seeing objects in the distance. When they look at objects in the distance, the lens wants to become thinner (the opposite of accommodation), but it is simply too curved. To correct the condition the patient needs a biconcave lens that diverges the light. If you see a young person with glasses, it is usually because of myopia.

Lasik surgery involves using a laser to flatten out the cornea to move the point of focus further back onto the retina.

Hyperopia (Far sightedness). In this case the orbit is too short, and the image is focused on a point behind the retina. The lens is too weak for the length of the eye. The patient can see objects far away but cannot see objects close to them. The lens is all right when looking afar but when it comes to time to look at something closer the lens wants to become thicker, but it cannot. The patient will need convex lenses.

Astigmatism In this case the cornea or the lens is uneven. In the healthy eye the lens and cornea are round, in a patient with astigmatism the surface of the lens or cornea is egg shaped. so that the image does not focus down to a point but projects onto too large an area. The patient needs custom lenses to correct this.

Presbyopia As we age, the lens becomes stiffer and less flexible and thus loses its ability to respond to near vision. It usually starts around 40 years of age. Reading glasses to correct presbyopia are often used.

Memory Tricks An aide to remembering the terminology for myopia versus hyperopia is the length of each word. Myopia is the *shorter word* of the two words, and it is the one where the focus point is too short. You can also think of the word myopic pertaining to the person who is too concerned or focused with matters right in front of them and not the big picture—they are nearsighted. Hyperopia on the other hand is the *long word* and the focus point is too far. When it comes to presbyopia, think older people, and this occurs as we age. The word "presby" in Latin means "old man." As an aside, the term "presbycusis" refers to a gradual hearing loss that occurs as we age (Fig. 13.17).

Goldmann Visual Fields When you first took neuroanatomy, you worked through the visual field defects with the type of pictures used in the examples above. In those pictures, the visual field defects are represented by the shaded portion of the pie. Goldmann visual field defects represent

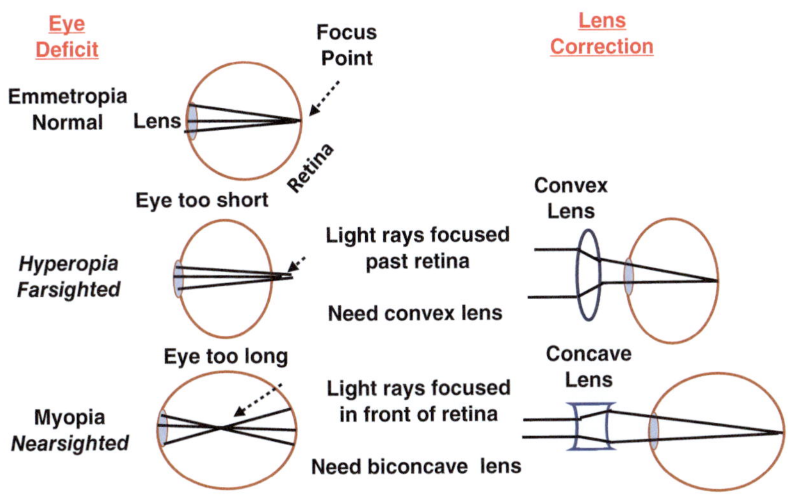

Fig. 13.17 Normal and Problematic Image Projection on Retina. With hyperopia, the image is focused past the retina and convex lenses bring the image back to the retina. With myopia, the image is focused in front of the retina, and concave lenses bring the image back to the retina [18]

the visual fields from a different point of view. Rather than show what the patient *cannot* see, they show what the patient *can* see. A Goldmann field is generated by perimetry bowl testing, which involves the patient's chin resting on brace and looking forward into a bowl-shaped structure.

With their head stationary, they are then shown various small lights in the periphery of the bowl. When they see a light, they respond by clicking a button. This generates a line (isopter) representing the perimeter of the patient's visual field. As we get older our visual field gets smaller. When you look at a picture of the Goldmann field, such as the one below, note that it is from the patient's point of view (Fig. 13.18).

On the other hand, in the fundoscopic view, the clinician is looking into the patient's eye, towards their brain. A couple of things stand out on a normal Goldmann field: (1) our inferior fields cover more territory than our superior visual fields, (2) our temporal fields encompass more territory than our nasal fields, and (3) the physiological blind spot is located temporally. Remember the nasal retina sees the temporal field. The picture below (Fig. 13.19) shows the Goldmann fields of both eyes.

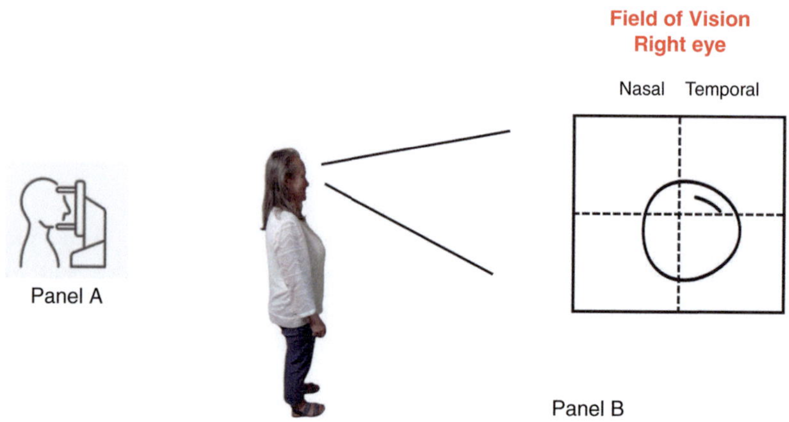

Fig. 13.18 Panel (**a**) shows the patient being tested in the perimetry bowl. Anel (**b**) depicts the visual field of the standing woman. Note that inferior field covers more area than the superior field. And the temporal field covers more area than the nasal field [18]

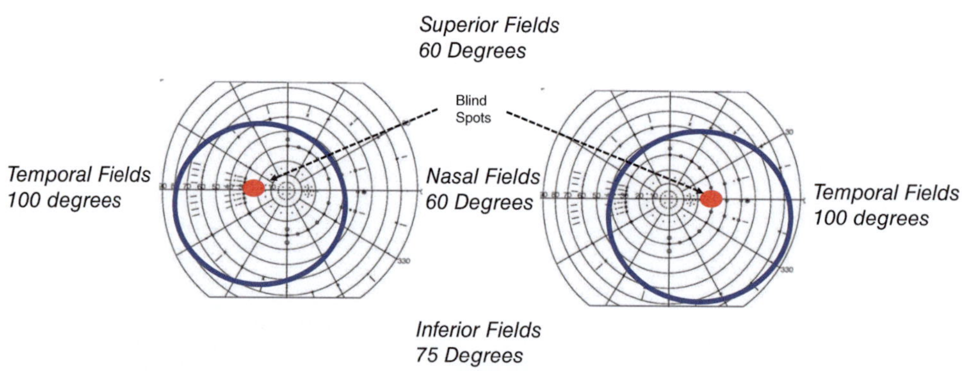

Fig. 13.19 Goldmann Visual fields of healthy individual for each eye. Note this is not drawn exactly to scale and is strictly for teaching purposes. The optic discs are in the nasal half of each retina, which equates to physiological blind spots in the temporal fields [18]

Again, you want to be able to differentiate from the view of the fundoscopic exam (Fig. 13.20) when you are looking inward towards the patient's eye, versus the Goldmann field depiction which is from the patient's point of view looking outward.

Make sure you understand the pictorial representations of both the Goldmann fields and the shaded visual field defects (Fig. 13.21). They both represent a pituitary tumor and a subsequent bitemporal hemianopia. The picture on the left shows what the patient *can* see as depicted by a Goldmann field test, and the picture on the right shows the visual field defects -what the patient *cannot* see.

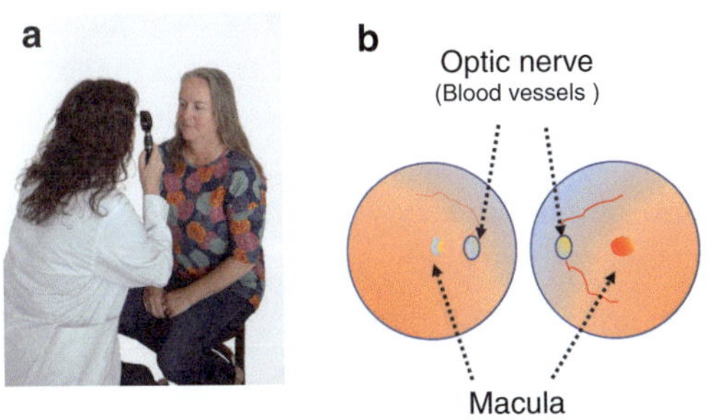

Fig. 13.20 Fundoscopic Exam. Panel (**a**) is of the doctor looking into the patient's eye. Panel (**b**) shows what the doctor is seeing through the ophthalmoscope. Note the optic nerve is located medially which translates into the blind spot being in the temporal field [18]

Case #1 A 63-year old professor was brought to the Emergency Department by a fellow professor who found him wandering around the hallway. He had no recollection of how he came to be there. The last thing he remembered was that he was driving to work when he smelled something burning. A neurological examination also reveals a left superior homonymous quadrantanopia. Where is the lesion?

The combination of the memory deficit and the superior quadrantopia suggests a lesion to the right temporal lobe.

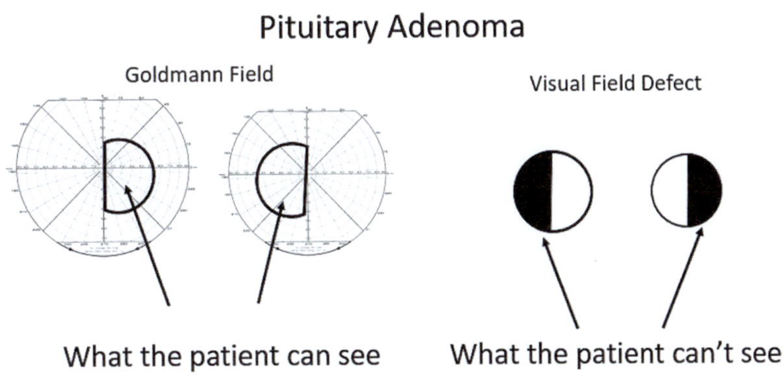

Fig. 13.21 Goldmann Field versus Visual Field Defect. The two representations are from the same patient [18]

More Complex Neuroophthalmolgy

The following sections on the eye go beyond what some students will get in a first-year anatomy class. However, you will be exposed to this information as you move into your second year and learn the basics of ophthalmology.

Blood Supply to Retina

The blood supply to the retina comes from two sources, both of which are branches of the ophthalmic artery, which in turn are branches of the internal carotid artery. The central artery of the retina pierces the optic nerve, travels down the nerve, and emerges onto the retina at the optic disk. From here the artery branches out into superior and inferior divisions, and then temporal and nasal divisions, all of which perfuse the inner half of the retina. The second source of blood to the retina comes from a set of 3 to 5 posterior ciliary arteries which travel on the periphery of the nerve and perfuse the outer half of the choroid and outer half of the retina. You can think of this second set as arteries to the choroid which in turn supply blood to the outer half of the retina (Fig. 13.22). The two sets of arteries meet at a watershed zone in the region of the bipolar cells.

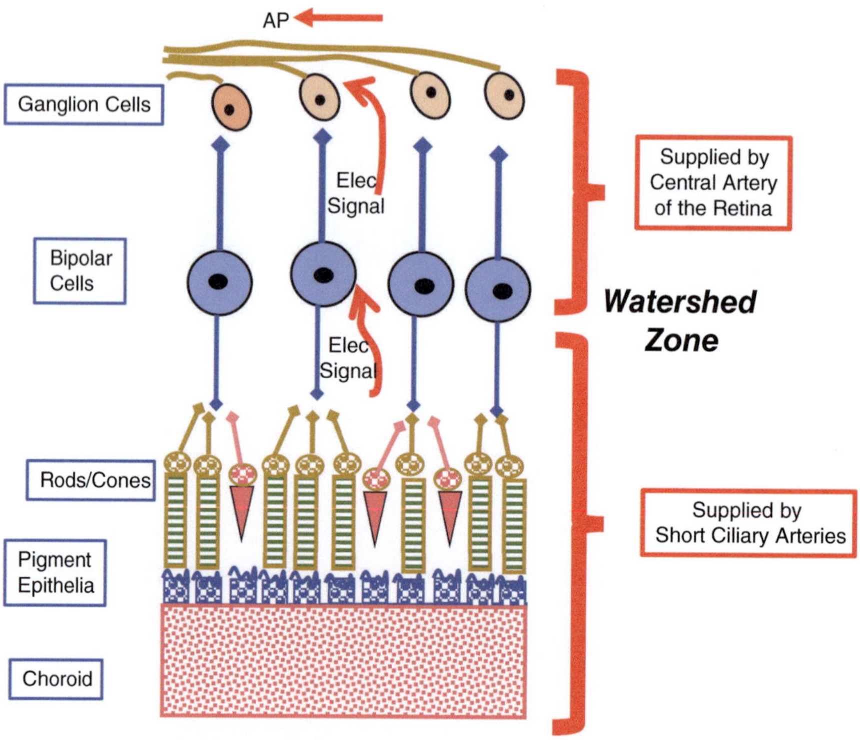

Fig. 13.22 Blood Supply of Retinal Layers. The inner layers are supplied by the branches of the central artery of the retina. The outer layers and choroid are supplied by the short ciliary arteries [18]

Occlusions to the Central Artery of the Retina

The central artery to the retina can become occluded, potentially leading to sudden, painless, temporary blindness referred to as *amaurosis fugax*. A hallmark feature of a *central retinal artery occlusion* (CRAO) is a *cherry red spot* on a fundoscopic exam. Keep in mind that cherry red spots can also be found in other conditions such as lysosomal storage diseases. To understand the cherry red spot in this case we need to focus on the blood supply to the retina mentioned earlier. The inner part of the retina is supplied by the central artery of the retina, while the outer layer, made up of the rods and cones, is supplied by the short ciliary arteries. With an occlusion of the central artery of the retina, there will be a loss of the inner retina, but the outer retina and choroid will be spared (Fig. 13.23).

A CRAO is often caused by an embolus in a hypertensive patient breaking loose from the heart or carotid artery and should be considered an emergency. In the initial stages, on a fundoscopic exam you might see segmentation or "box-caring" (the segmentation of the blood looks like train cars) of the blood in the branches of the central artery. Most of the retina will have a pale or opaque look to it since its inner portion has lost its blood supply. However, at the fovea there is a red spot because the nerve fiber layer is so thin here that you can see the underlying blood supply from the posterior ciliary arteries (choroidal arteries) going to the choroid.

The term *amaurosis fugax* (amaurosis = darkening, and fugax = temporary) refers to a temporary loss of vision that is present when blood flow to the retina is compromised. The CRAO mentioned above is just one example that can lead to this condition, others include: subclavian steal syndrome, atherosclerotic disease of the carotid artery, cardiac emboli, malignant hypertension, or several other conditions.

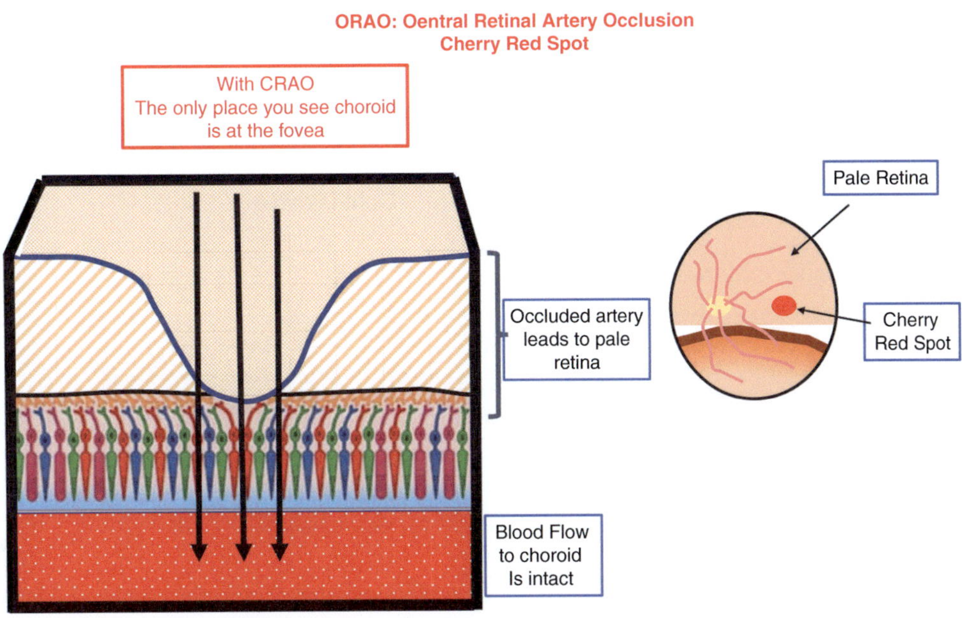

Fig. 13.23 Cherry Red Spot. The outer part of retina is perfused by the central artery. When it is occluded the retina becomes pale on the ophthalmoscope view. However, at the fovea, one can still see the underlying layers which appear as a cherry red spot [18]

Ischemic Optic Neuropathy

In contrast to strokes of the retina, there can also be strokes of the optic nerve. Strokes to the optic nerve are referred to as Ischemic Optic Neuropathy (ION), and can be categorized with two different headings, based on the presence or absence of inflammation, or on the location of the pathology along the nerve—either anterior (AION) or posterior (PION) (Fig. 13.24).

Location: Lesions to the anterior part of the nerve, where the nerve meets the retina, are referred to as *anterior ischemic neuropathy* and occur to the small area of the optic nerve right at the optic disc. Posterior lesions refer to the much larger and remaining part of the nerve—really all the nerve except for the optic disc. Damage to either division, either anterior or posterior, is due to the difference in blood supply to the two divisions. The anterior part of the nerve, right at the optic disc, is perfused by the posterior ciliary arteries). The various branches) of the posterior ciliary arteries anastomose at the beginning of the optic nerve at a point called the *circle of Zinn*. The posterior part of the nerve is perfused by several branches but mainly by the arteries on the surface of the pia that descend into the nerve. Because of these different perfusion patterns, anterior lesions, but not posterior lesions, lead to swelling of the optic nerve head. Both anterior and posterior ischemic optic neuropathy can also occur following surgery, particularly cardiac and spine surgery.

Etiology: IONs can be further subdivided by etiology, into either (Fig. 13.25):

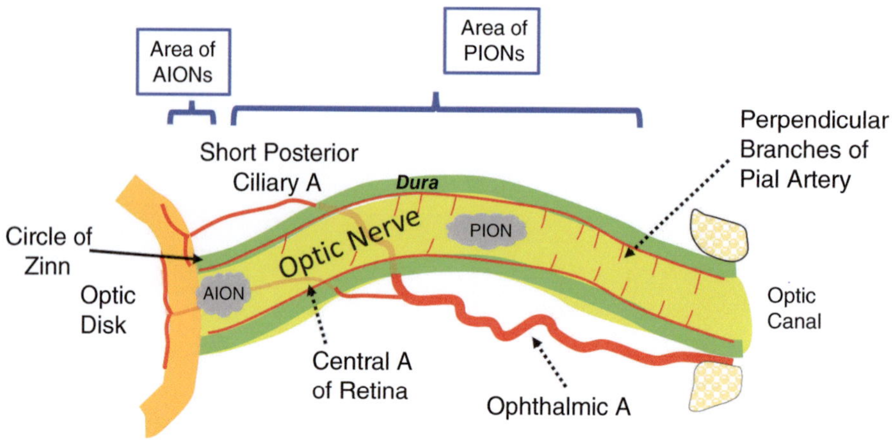

Fig. 13.24 Ischemic Optic Neuritis Locations [18]

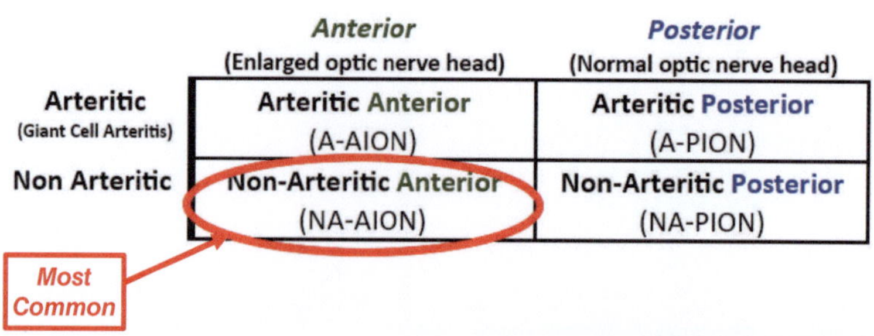

Fig. 13.25 Ischemic Optic Neuritis (ION). Ischemic optic neuritis is caused by reduced blood flow to the optic nerve. There are two types: (1) Nonarteritic, which is caused by reduced blood flow without inflammation, and (2) Arteritic which includes inflammation. Each of these two categories has two subdivisions referring to location. It can occur either to the anterior part of the nerve—where the nerve meets the retina, or to the posterior part of the nerve. The most common one is, non-arteritic anterior ischemic optic neuritis (NAION). Most arteritic ION is caused by giant cell arteritis [18]

1. *Arteritic* refers to vascular insufficiency *with* inflammation. Arteritic ION whether either anterior (A-AION) or posterior (A-PION) is usually due to giant cell arteritis (GCA). With the arteritic version, inflammation will typically be present in other arteries, such as the superficial temporal artery.
2. *Non-arteritic* (NA) refers to vascular insufficiency *without* inflammation. For these two etiological divisions, the non arteritic is much more common. And for the locational division, the anterior is much more common. This makes the NA-AION the most common ION. Non-Arteritic Anterior Ischemic Optic Neuropathy (NA-AION) (some books will abbreviate this as NAION) is thought to be due to a lack of blood flow from the posterior ciliary arteries to the optic disc—the anterior portion of the optic nerve. The subsequent ischemia leads to swelling of the nerve as it passes) through the scleral canal at the back of the orbit, resulting in compartment syndrome. Patients with NA-AION often have risk factors such as hyperlipidemia, diabetes, smoking, and hypertension. During the exam, the opposite eye is often examined for a "disc at risk.

The term "disc at risk" is based on the presence of normal human variation, meaning that the size of the disc can vary from one individual to the next. While having a small disk is not pathological itself, it does mean that those individuals who have a small disc are more likely to suffer the consequences of ION. In these individuals, the bony) structure of the orbit leads to a narrower disc area. The fibers here are crowded into this smaller than typical space which makes these fibers more prone to nerve damage with ION. But how would you examine this in a pathological eye? In a patient with ION in one eye, the disc in the healthy eye can be observed to see if they have a "disc at risk." Patients with ION can spontaneously recover, but the prognosis for those with a "disk at risk" is not as optimistic.

It can be difficult to distinguish patients having a stroke of the retina (CRAO) versus having a stroke of the optic nerve such as NA-AION. Both patients will present with similar symptoms: acute unilateral painless loss of vision, and an ipsilateral RAPD. On fundoscopic examination), the CRAO patient will have a cherry red spot, while the NA-AION patient will present with a swollen optic nerve. It is the CRAO patient who has an emergency condition and needs to be admitted and treated immediately.

Running with the central artery of the retina in the optic nerve is the *central vein of the retina* heading towards the cavernous sinus. Like the artery, it can also become occluded leading to *central retinal vein occlusion* (CRVO). Elevated cholesterol, diabetes, and high blood pressure are all predisposing conditions that can result in CRVO. The patient starts off complaining of blurry eyes which can progress to loss of vision. A central retinal vein occlusion will affect the entire retina, while a *branch retinal vein occlusion* will affect just one sector of the retina.

Optic neuritis is inflammation of the optic nerve that leads to pain and a loss of vision. The most common cause of optic neuritis is multiple sclerosis. MS leads to inflammation and damage to the myelin sheath of the optic nerve.

Retinal Fiber Organization

The fibers coming out of the ganglion cells all head towards the optic nerve (optic disc) and in turn project to the lateral geniculate body. Normally the optic disc is indented slightly. If we look closely at the optic nerve head, there are four quadrants—four pieces of the pie—and this organization is clinically significant. Fibers from the ganglion cells in the temporal retina project to the superior and inferior quadrants. Fibers from the macula project towards the lateral quadrant. We call these fibers the *papillomacular bundle*. Fibers from the nasal retina head towards the medial quadrant. This has important clinical implications. Keep in mind that temporal fibers are responsible for the nasal field and vice versa.

Bow-Tie Atrophy

Lesions of the optic nerve, chiasm, or tract will lead to degeneration of the ganglion cell fibers which can be followed back to the optic disc

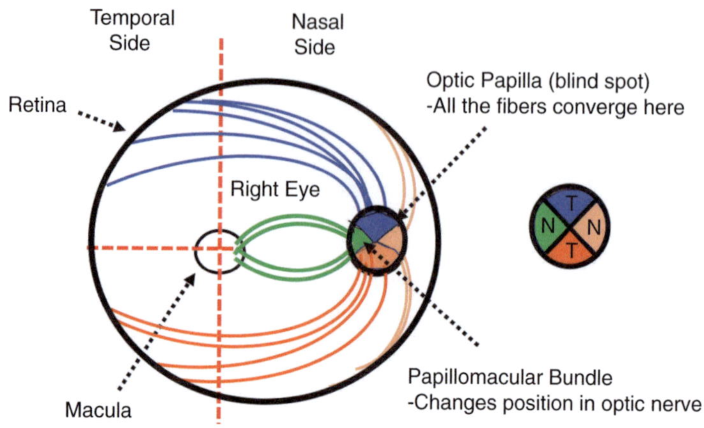

Fig. 13.26 Nerve fibers Entering the Optic Tract. Temporal fibers come into superior and inferior quadrants, papillomacular fibers to the lateral quadrant, nasal fibers to medial quadrant [18]

resulting in optic atrophy. In the case of a lesion to the optic tract or chiasm there will be a pattern of nerve cell degeneration at the disc that resembles a bow tie, which can be visible on a fundoscopic exam.

Let us walk through the logic of "bowtie atrophy." Take a lesion to the optic chiasm: A lesion to the middle of the chiasm will damage fibers coming from the nasal half of the eye, while the temporal retinal fibers located on the periphery of the chiasm are unaffected. This will lead to atrophy of the fibers coming into the medial and lateral quadrants of each optic disc; it will spare the superior and inferior quadrants. The subsequent degeneration of the fibers leads to an image resembling a bow tie (Fig. 13.26).

Lesions to the optic tract will also lead to bow tie atrophy but only on the contralateral side. The logic is as follows: (1) A lesion to the right optic tract will damage fibers coming from the left nasal retina, whose fibers in turn are going to the lateral and medial quadrants of the optic nerve.

Optic Tract Pathology

Lesions to either the optic tract or the optic radiations can lead to contralateral homonymous hemianopsia. To determine if the lesion is in the nerve or the tract, we must look at other signs. Besides the visual field defect, optic tract lesions will also lead to a contralateral RAPD and a contralateral bow tie atrophy.

The contralateral RAPD occurs because at the chiasm it is not a 50/50 cross over of fibers. When the optic nerves converge at the chiasm, 60% of the fibers will cross and 40% will stay on the ipsilateral side. Thus, in either one of the optic tracts, more of the fibers are from the contralateral eye, so a lesion at the tract leads to a greater loss on the contralateral side, which leads to the contralateral RAPD. A lesion to the optic radiations will not have any effect on the pupillary light reflex.

Central Scotoma

In some conditions, such as multiple sclerosis, hypertension, methanol poisoning, or nutritional deficiencies, patients will lose just one small piece in the central part of the visual field—a central scotoma. In these conditions, because the pathology is occurring globally these patients would have a bilateral central scotoma. If the central scotoma is only on one side, you would suspect a more localized issue such as a vascular insult.

The reason for the scotoma is that the central part of the visual field is the fovea in the macula. The fibers coming out of the macula are the busiest players in the retina—the most metabolically active—and thus the most susceptible to insult. In addition, these fibers converge on the lateral quadrant of the optic disc, and then move into the optic nerve and head towards the chiasm. As the fibers move along the optic nerve, they assume a position in the center of the optic nerve.

Red Glass Test

The red glass test can be used to test for diplopia. Consider the fact that the center of our visual field is detected by both eyes—even if the right eye cannot detect an image from the central field, the image is still detected by the left eye. So how can we separate the central fields of the two eyes? One way to do thi, and its ingenious, is with colored filters. If we put a red filter over the right eye and a green filter over the left eye we are now separating the two eyes such that if we shine a red light in the center then it will only be seen by the right eye, and if we shine a green light in the center it will only be seen by the left eye. The red and green filters are the most complete way to do this, but we can also use a red glass on one eye and still separate the two fields with just a penlight. By convention, clinicains use the red glass over the right eye when performing this test.

With a healthy person, when you put the red glass over the right eye and then shine a light in front of them, the individual will see one pink light in front of them. In this case, the images from the red light and the white light are sitting right on top of each other and merging together, thus the patient reports seeing one pinkish light. If the eyes are misaligned, as in diplopia, the two images are now separated and the patient will see one white light and one red light along the horizontal plane. Furthermore, some patients will see the red light on the right side and others will see it on the left side—it all depends on the pathology. With the red glass test you can determine which eye is affected and the nature of the pathology.

During testing of the eye movements, the relationship of the red light and the bright white light will also change depending on the deficit. To understand the concepts behind this red glass test, the explanation below is limited to just medial and lateral deficits and subsequent side to side movements.

Esotropia or Exotropia of *Right* Eye

In these first two cases, the pathology is in the right eye. By placing the red glass over the pathological eye (the right eye) we are moving the red image in relation to the image from the bright light source. In other words, we are holding the bright light steady (the healthy left eye) and we are manipulating the red image seen by pathological eye (right eye) (Fig. 13.27).

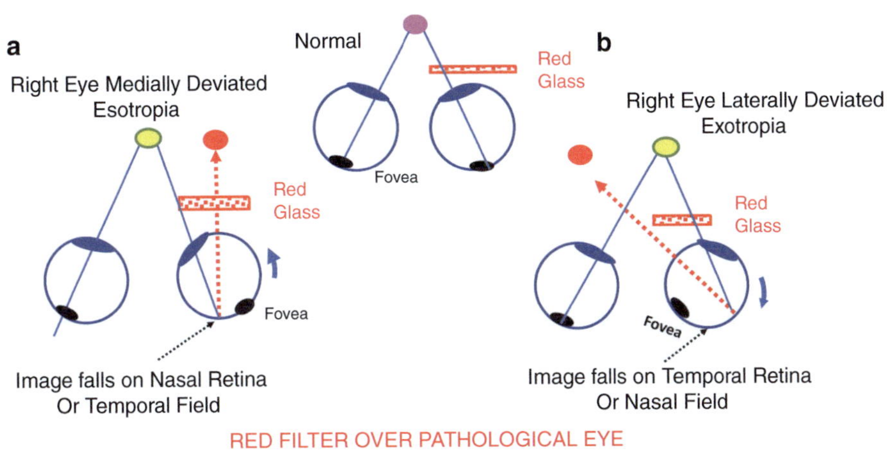

Fig. 13.27 Red Glass Test: Red glass is on the pathological eye. The healthy individual sees one pink light in front of them. The pink color comes from the fusion of the red light and bright light images sitting on top of each other. Panel (**a**) In the patient with esotropia, the image on the right eye is falling on the nasal retina, which is temporal field, thus the red image has moved to the right. Panel (**b**) With a right exotropia the image has moved the opposite direction. Note that in both these cases, with the glass over the eye with the deficit, it is the red light moving on the patient's visual field

Esotropia of Right Eye In this patient, the right eye is medially deviated. The red glass is placed in front of the right eye. With the eye medially deviated, the fovea has moved laterally so the red light is now falling on the nasal retina which is temporal visual field so the red light has moved to the right of the light source.

Exotropia of Right Eye In this patient, the right eye is laterally deviated. The red glass is still in front of the right eye. With the eye laterally deviated, the fovea has moved medially so the red light is now falling on the temporal retina which is the nasal field so the red light has moved to the left of the light source.

Esoptropia or Exotropia of the *Left* Eye

In the next two cases the pathology is on the left eye, but we are keeping the red glass over the healthy right eye. In these cases we are now moving the bright light seen by the light source relative to the red light. In other words we are holding the red image steady in the healthy eye and moving the bright light seen by the pathological eye (Fig. 13.28).

Exotropia of Left Eye In this patient, the left eye is laterally deviated so the fovea has shifted medially. The image from the light source is falling on the temporal retina which is nasal field and the image from the light source is now moved to the right of the red light.

Esotropia of the Left Eye In this patient the left eye is medially deviated and the red glass is over the right eye. On the left eye the fovea has moved laterally so the image from the light is falling on the nasal retina which is temporal field so the white light has moved to the left of red light.

Besides just looking straight ahead as in the examples above, there are more details involved with the mechanics of the test, such as having the patient look side-to-side, and then and up and down. And there is another version of the test called the Maddox Rod test, but if you understand the basics described in the scenarios above, then other variations of the test should make sense.

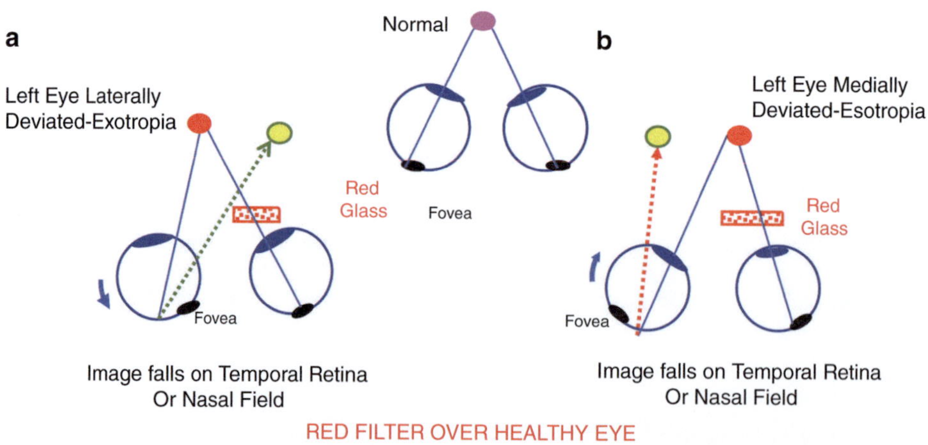

Fig. 13.28 Red Glass Test: Red glass is on the healthy eye. The healthy individual sees one red light in front of them. Panel (**a**) In the patient with exotropia of left eye, the image on the left eye is falling on the temporal retina, which is nasal field, thus the light source has moved to the right. Panel (**b**) With a left esotropia the image has moved the opposite direction. Note that in both these cases, with the glass over the healthy eye, it is the image from the light moving on the patient's visual field

Historical Snippet: Lesion Analysis of the Visual System

Much of what we know about the nervous system comes from an earlier era of very observant clinicains. Prior to the advent of MRIs and other high tech visualization tools, these clinicains took extensive notes about their patients' various signs and symptoms while they were alive, and then at autopsy they observed the locations of the lesions. They could then correlate the lesions with the symptoms. After many cases, they could then draw conclusions about the function of specific regions of the nervous system.

The mapping of the visual pathways is a perfect example of this lesion analysis. During the 1904–1905 war between the Russians and the Japanese, the Russian military used the Mosin-Nagant Model 91 rifle. Because of its unusually high-velocity, in many cases a bullet wound to the skull did not always kill the victim but would leave them with a well-demarcated and circumscribed penetrating wound to the brain. The Japanese ophthalmologist Tatsuji Inouye (1881–1976) studied the survivors of these injuries, many of whom had visual field deficits. He was a able to correlate the visual deficits with the location of the damaged regions in the nervous system. Innouye studied 29 patients and was a pioneer in efforts to map out the visual pathway. Along the way he was also the first person to write about macular sparing.

Further Reading

1. Brazis PW, Masdeu JC, Biller J. Localization in clinical neurology. LWW; 2016.
2. Blumenfeld H. Neuroanatomy through clinical cases. 2nd ed. Wiley-Blackwell; 2010.
3. Broadway DC. How to test for a relative afferent pupillary defect (RAPD). Community Eye Health J. 2016;29(96):68–9.
4. Brodal P. The central nervous system. 5th ed. New York: Oxford University Press; 2016.
5. Campbell, W., And Barohn, R.J. Dejong's the neurological examination, LWW; 2019.
6. Carpenter M. Core text of neuroanatomy. New York: Williams and Wilkins; 1991.
7. Cooper, Talmage, Neuro-ophthalmology illustrated Chap. 13—diplopia 2 -assessment. Available at: Neuro-ophthalmology Illustrated Chapter 13 Diplopia 13 – Localization of Findings & Treatment of Diplopia – Syndromes — Neuro-Ophthalmology (stanford.edu)
8. Dersu I, Wiggins MN, Luther A, Harper R, Chacko J. (2006) understanding visual fields, part 1: Goldmann perimetry. J Ophthal Med Tech. 2006;2(2):1–10.
9. Fuller G. Neurological examination made easy. 6th ed. Elsevier; 2019.
10. Glickstein M. The discovery of the visual cortex, Scientif Amer; 1988. p. 118–27.
11. Fite DJ, Walker HK. Chapter 60 Cranial nerves III, IV, and VI: The oculomotor, trochlear, and abducens nerves. In: Walker HK, Dall WD, Hurst JW, editors. Clinical methods: the history, physical, and laboratory examinations. 3rd ed. Boston: Butterworths; 1990.
12. Havreh SS. Management of ischemic optic neuropathies. Indian J Ophthalmol. 2011;59(2):123–36.
13. Horton JC, Economides JR, Adams DL. The mechanism of macular sparing. Ann Rev. Vis Science. 2021;7:155–79.
14. Kandel E, Koester JD, Mack SH, Siegelbaum SA. Principles of neural science. McGraw Hill; 2021.
15. Kardon RH, Longmuir RA, Lee AG, Anderson S. Smaller optic disc area correlates with greater permanent damage following non-arteritic ischemic optic neuropathy (NAION). Investig Ophthalmol Vis Sci. 2010;51(13):653.
16. King A. Glaucoma. BMJ. 2013;346:f3518.
17. Kolb H. How the retina works. Amer Scient. 2003;91:28–35.
18. Leo J. Medical neuroanatomy for the boards and clinic: finding the lesion. 2nd ed. Switzerland: Springer; 2024.
19. Leo J. Clinical anatomy and embryology: a guide for the classroom, clinic, and clinic. 2nd ed. Springer; 2024.
20. Lindegger DJ, Pless. The discovery of the visual field representation in the brain. J Ophthalmol Science. 2019;1(1):6–12.
21. Miller N. Walsh & Hoyt's clinical neuro-ophthalmology: the essentials. 4th ed. Williams, and Wilkins: Lippincott; 2020.
22. Ortiz JF, Eissa-Garces A, Ruxmohan S, Cuenca V, et al. Understanding parinauds syndrome. Brain Sciences. 2021;11:1469.
23. Prasad S, Galetta SL. Anatomy and physiology of the afferent visual system. Handbook Clin Neurol. 2011;102(3rd Series):1–19.
24. Splittgerber R. Snell's clinical neuroanatomy. 8th ed. Lippincott, Williams, and Wilkins; 2018.

25. Stein JD, Khawaja AP, Weizer JS. Glaucoma in adults-screening, Diagnosis, and Management. JAMA Review. 2021;325(2):164–74.
26. Stevenson M. Diagnosing and managing ischemic optic neuropathy. Review Ophthalmol. 2010;
27. Swanson PD. Signs and symptoms in neurology. Lippincott Williams and Wilkins; 1984.
28. Woodburne RT, Burkel WE. Essentials of human anatomy. 9th ed. Oxford University Press; 1994.
29. Wong S, Plant GT. How to interpret visual fields. Prac Neurol. 2015;15:374–81.
30. Young PA, Young PH. and Tolbert, D. Basic clinical neuroscience: LLW; 2015.

14 Autonomics, Lesions, and Cell Bodies of Origin

Introduction

Before getting into the details, it is important to clarify the difference between autonomic ganglia and sensory ganglia (Fig. 14.1).

The dividing line between the CNS and PNS is the pia mater (Fig. 14.1). All the efferent motor neurons have their cell bodies of origin in the CNS. If we are talking about the cord, the somatic motor fibers come from the ventral horn. If we are talking about the brainstem, the somatic motor fibers come from cranial nerve nuclei. Somatosensory fibers on the other hand have their cell bodies in the periphery, either in the DRG, or a specifically named ganglion, such as the trigeminal or geniculate ganglia. These ganglia have a cell body *but no synapse*.

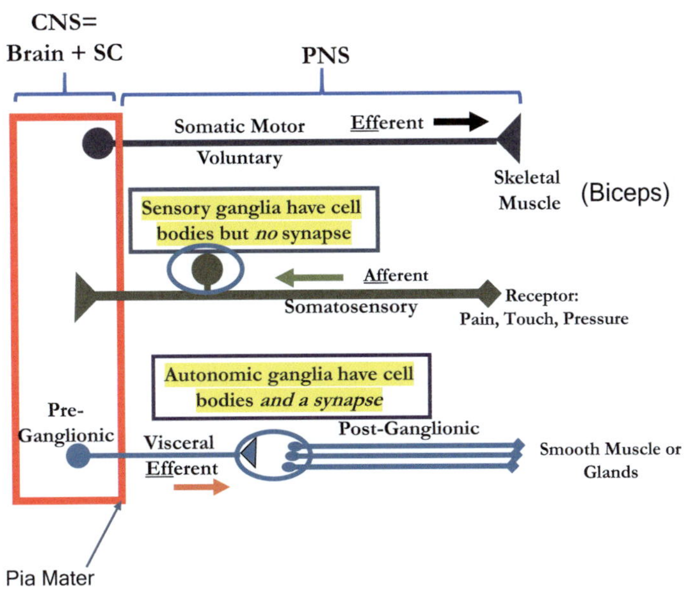

Fig. 14.1 Comparison of Autonomic and Sensory Ganglia [11]

J. Leo, *Gross Anatomy, Neuroanatomy, and Embryology for Medical Students*,
https://doi.org/10.1007/978-3-031-87151-1_14

Sensory Ganglia in the Head

In the head, the sensory ganglia have individual names such as geniculate ganglion or trigeminal ganglion. As an example, take the trigeminal ganglion which sits in Meckel's cave in the middle cranial fossa. Its branches V1, V2, and V3 all have fibers carrying sensation from the face. These sensory fibers all have cell bodies in the trigeminal ganglion (pseudounipolar neurons). They then continue into the brainstem to synapse in the spinal nucleus of V. Meanwhile, V3 has motor fibers with cell bodies of origin in the motor nucleus of V. These fibers travel through the trigeminal ganglion without synapsing to innervate the muscles of mastication. So if you pointed to say, the inferior alveolar nerve and asked the question: "where are the cell bodies of origin?" The answer would be the trigeminal ganglion (sensation) in the PNS and the motor nucleus of V (motor) in the CNS (Fig. 14.2).

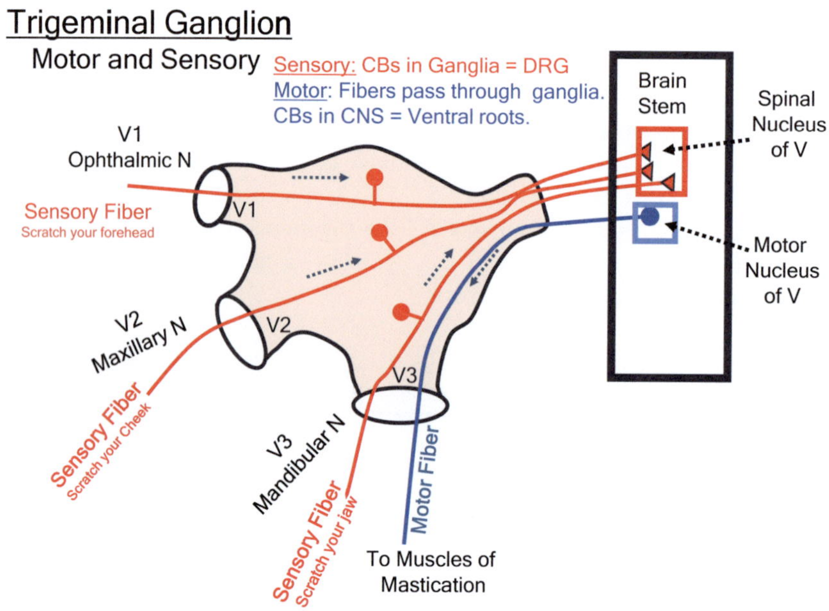

Fig. 14.2 Trigeminal Ganglion

The Parasympathetics to the Head

When we discuss parasympathetic fibers, we need to differentiate preganglionic from postganglionic. The preganglionic fibers on cranial nerves come out of nuclei and travel to and synapse in the peripherally located autonomic ganglia which will have a *cell body and a synapse*. These parasympathetic preganglionic fibers are cholinergic and synapse on nicotinic cholinergic receptors on the postganglionic cells. The post ganglionic fibers which are also cholinergic will then travel to the target, such as a gland or smooth muscle, and synapse on a muscarinic receptor (Fig. 14.3).

You need to remember this list forever: CNs III, VII, IX, and X. These are the four cranial nerves with parasympathetic fibers emerging from the brain (Fig. 14.3). Note that CN V is not on this list, however while no parasympathetic fibers originate on CN V, three of the cranial nerves with parasympathetics, III, VII, and IX all take advantage of CN V by hitching a ride on CN V to reach their targets.

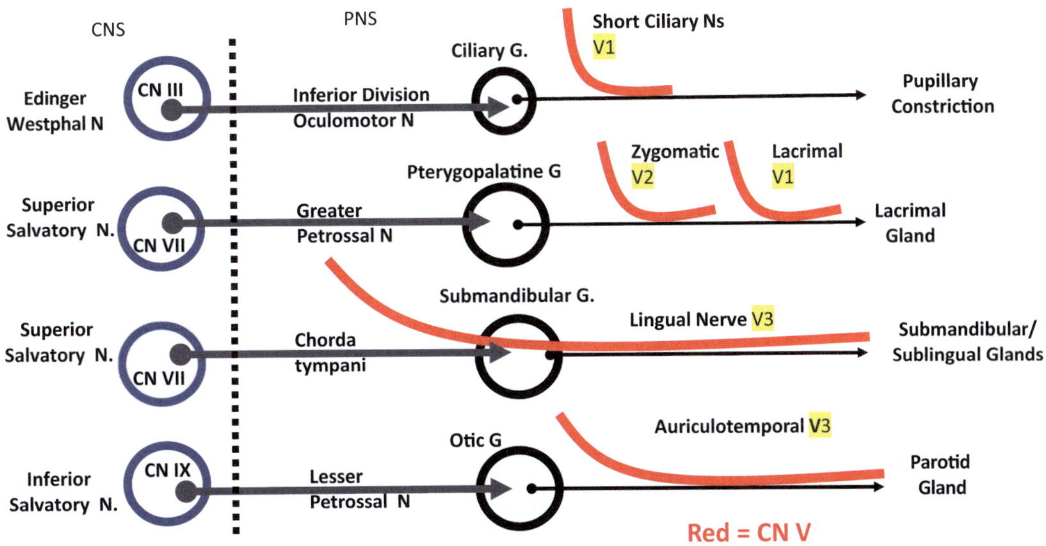

Fig. 14.3 Cranial Nerve Parasympathetic Hitchhikers. Fibers from CN III, VII, and IX hitch a ride on CN V. [11]

Cranial Nerve III

Cranial nerve III's parasympathetic fibers come out of the Edinger Westphal nucleus in the midbrain, travel through the midbrain, and then exit the brainstem at the interpeduncular fossa to eventually reach the orbit. In the orbit the parasympathetics travel on the inferior division of the oculomotor on their way to the ciliary ganglion. After synapsing at the ciliary ganglion, the fibers travel on the short ciliary nerves to the ciliaris muscle and the sphincter pupillae in the eye.

Cranial Nerve VII and Cell Bodies

Because CN VII has motor, sensory, and parasympathetic fibers it is also a suitable time to revisit cell bodies. When you look at the *motor* fibers of CN VII, they have their cell bodies in the motor nucleus of CN VII which is inside the pons—these are functionally equivalent to the motor nerves to the limbs coming out of the anterior horn cells. The *sensory* fibers for general sense, which come from a small area by the external ear, have their cell bodies in the geniculate ganglion (cell bodies, no synapse) inside the facial canal. These fibers are functionally equivalent to the sensory fibers from limbs that have their cell bodies in the dorsal root ganglion. The taste fibers also have their primary cell body in the geniculate ganglion. These fibers enter the pons and project to the nucleus solitarus. The parasympathetic fibers come from the superior salvatory nucleus and project to the pterygopalatine, submandibular, and sublingual ganglion (synapse and cell body). From the ganglion, the post ganglionic fibers travel to the glands—lacrimal, submandibular, and sublingual (Fig. 14.4).

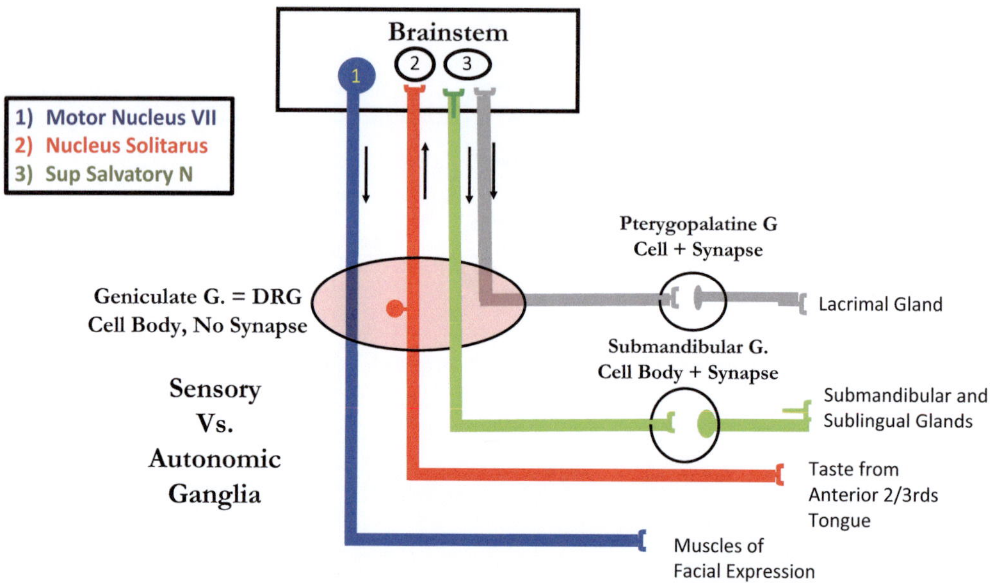

Fig. 14.4 Comparison of Autonomic and Sensory Ganglion of Facial Nerve. The geniculate ganglion is the location of the ganglia for the sensory fibers. At the geniculate ganglion, the other fibers just pass through it [11]

Cranial Nerve VII Branches

Cranial nerve VII has two parasympathetic branches. The first is the greater petrosal nerve that projects to the pterygopalatine ganglion in the pterygopalatine fossa. The postganglionic fibers then jump onto the zygomatic temporal branch of the infraorbital nerve, which is a branch of V2; they then make another jump onto the lacrimal nerve which is a branch of V1 to make their way to the lacrimal gland. The other group of parasympathetics of CN VII leave in the chorda tympani, travel through the middle ear between the incus and malleus, exit the skull through the petrotympanic fissure, enter the infratemporal fossa to join the lingual nerve, and project to the submandibular ganglion. The postganglionic fibers then travel to the submandibular and sublingual glands. Keep in mind that the lingual nerve is a branch of V3 which carries temperature, pain, and touch sensations back along the trigeminal nerve (Fig. 14.5).

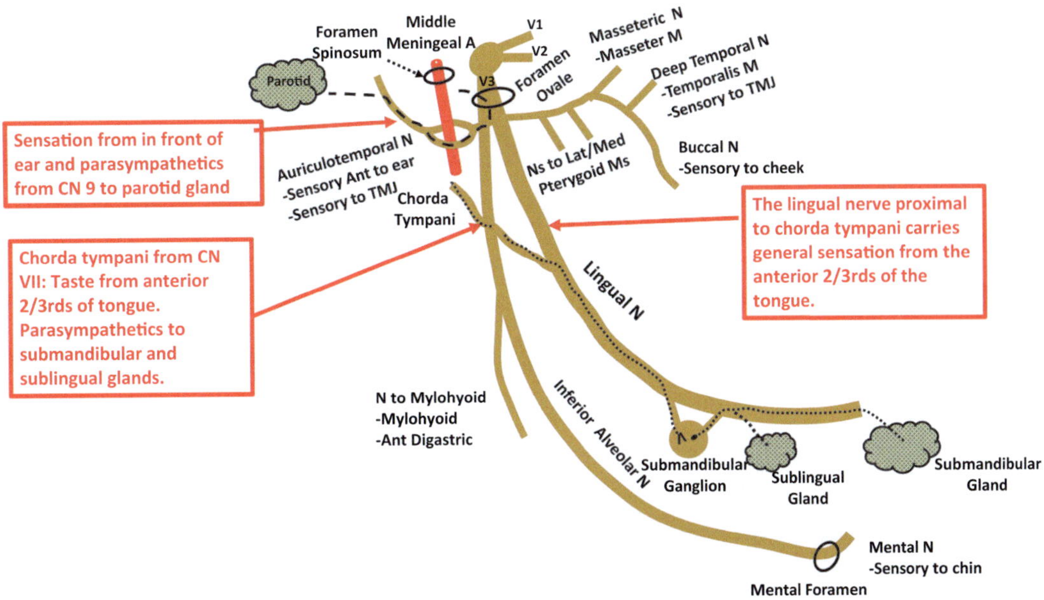

Fig. 14.5 Mandibular Nerve (V3). V3 is seen entering the infratemporal fossa through the foramen ovale. The chorda tympani is a branch of the facial nerve hitchhiking on the lingual nerve that carries taste from anterior 2/3rds of the tongue and parasympathetic fibers (dotted black line) to the submandibular ganglion. The parasympathetics from CN IX (dashed black line) hitchhike on the auriculotemporal nerve to reach the parotid gland [11]

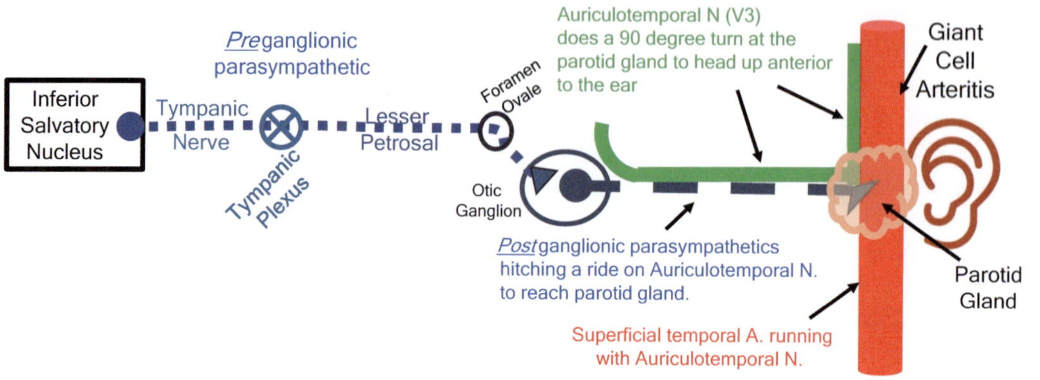

Fig. 14.6 Cranial Nerve IX Parasympathetics. Tympanic nerve turns into lesser petrosal N, which jumps through foramen ovale to reach the otic ganglion. The postganglionic fibers then travel on the auriculotemporal N. to the parotid gland. Giant cell arteritis is often foundin the superficial temporal artery

Cranial Nerve Nine

Cranial nerve IX's preganglionic fibers originate from the tympanic plexus as the lesser petrosal nerve and travel along the base of the skull, exiting the skull through the foramen ovale and finally projecting to the otic ganglion (Fig. 14.6). From the otic ganglion the postganglionic fibers jump on the auriculotemporal nerve, a branch of V3, and hitch a ride to the parotid gland.

Sympathetic Fibers and White and Grey Rami

The preganglionic sympathetic fibers all originate from the lateral horn which runs from T1 (maybe C8) to L2, but from this lateral horn, the sympathetic information travels to virtually every nerve and blood vessel in the body. How does it manage this?

After emerging from the lateral horn, the preganglionic fibers travel on the ventral rami to the spinal nerve. From the spinal nerve they jump onto the white rami and travel to the sympathetic chain where they have three options. (1) At the ganglia, the preganglionic fibers synapse with the post ganglionic cell body. The postganglionic fibers then travel back to the spinal nerve via a grey ramus to follow out the nerve at that level. (2) some fibers will emerge via the white rami but instead of synapsing right away, will travel up or down the chain to synapse at a higher or lower level, and then jump via a grey ramus onto a spinal nerve. (3) Some preganglionic fibers will travel along the white rami, enter the chain ganglia, and then keep on going without synapsing, and then meet a ganglion located farther out in the body. An example of this would be fibers making up the greater splanchnic nerve coming from the lateral horn of T5–9, joining the spinal nerve, coming off on the white ramus, entering the chain ganglia, but then just passing through the chain without synapsing to eventually synapse in the celiac ganglia. Note that the greater splanchnic nerve is a myelinated preganglionic sympathetic nerve, thus, while it has its own name, it is functionally equivalent to a white ramus.

Sympathetic Nerves to the Face

The sympathetic projection to the face is a three-neuron pathway. When taking gross anatomy, you probably thought of this sympathetic pathway as just a two-neuron pathway, because in the gross anatomy lab you would have focused on the pre- and postganglionic fibers. The preganglionic fibers come out of the lateral horn at T1, travel on the ventral root, join the spinal nerve, jump off the spinal nerve via white rami, travel up the sympathetic chain, and synapse in the superior cervical ganglion (SCG). The postganglionic fibers travel from the SCG to the eye. During gross anatomy you didn't know about or focus on the CNS. However, later when you took neuroanatomy, you learned about the descending sympathetic fibers in the CNS coming down from the hypothalamus and projecting to the lateral horn at the T1 level of the spinal cord. (Fig. 14.7).

This first neuron in the pathway projects out of the hypothalamus and descends on the dorsolateral fasciculus (DLF) to the lateral horn at T1.

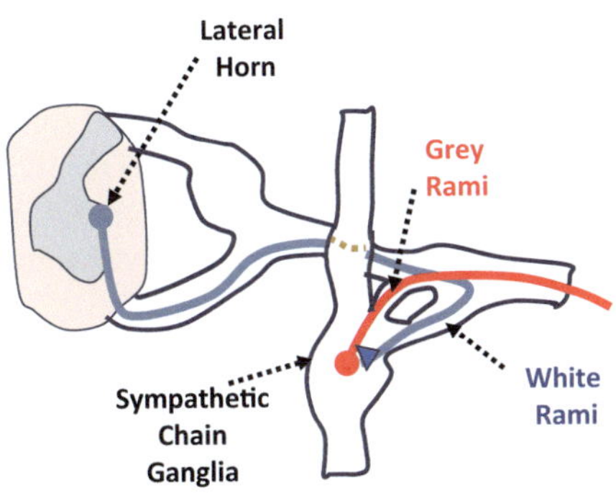

Fig. 14.7 White and Grey Rami. Preganglionic sympathetic fibers (blue) come from the lateral horn. They travel on the spinal nerve but then jump off via a white rami. They meet postganglionic sympathetic fibers (red) in the chain ganglia and then travel back to the spinal nerve via a grey rami [11]

From the lateral horn at T1, the cholinergic preganglionic neurons (neuron #2) jump onto the sympathetic chain and travel up to the superior cervical ganglion (SCG). After synapsing in the ganglion, the postganglionic neurons (neuron #3), which use norepinephrine, run on blood vessels and nerves to reach their targets on the face, most importantly the eye. These postganglionic neurons synapse on adrenergic receptors. An exception is the post ganglionic sympathetics to the sweat glands which are cholinergic. The postganglionic sympathetic fibers dilate the eye.

Damage to the sympathetic fibers anywhere along the three neuron pathway from hypothalamus to the face will lead to Horner's syndrome which consists of a constricted pupil, a slight droopy eye, and a red face. Tumors of the lung, lower brachial plexus injuries, aneurysms of the carotid artery, and several other lesions can lead to Horner's syndrome (Fig. 14.8).

There are seven lesions depicted in Fig. 14.8 of the sympathetic pathway above, all these lesions will result in Horner's syndrome. As the first order neurons descend from the hypothalamus through the brain stem, they are located on the lateral side of the brainstem, so they are typically compromised in both lateral pontine syndrome (Lesion 1) and lateral medullary syndrome (Lesion 2). Realize that a hemisection of the cord

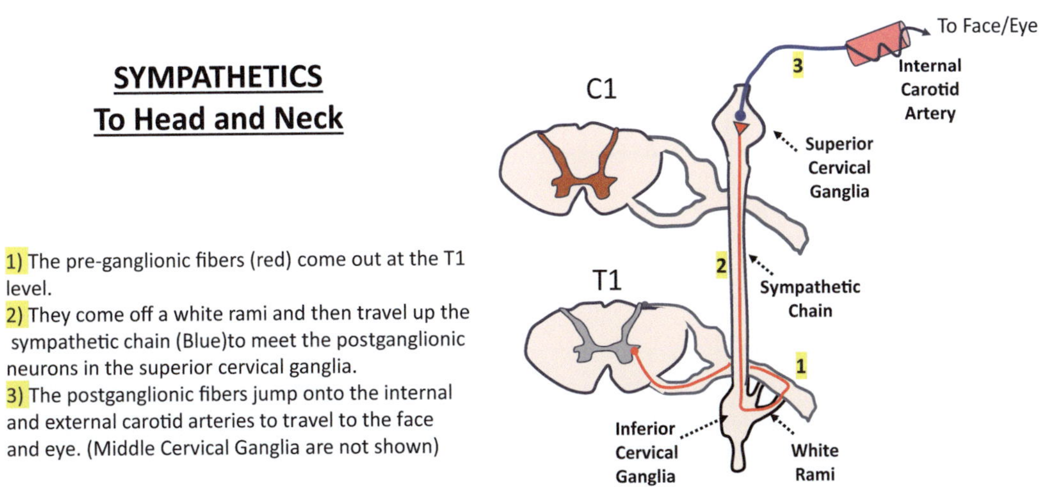

Fig. 14.8 Sympathetics to Head and Neck [11]

above T1 will also result in Horner's syndrome (Lesion 3). As the preganglionic fibers emerge through the roots at T1 they can be injured in a lower brachial plexus injury (Lesion 4). As the pre-ganglionic fibers travel across the root of the lung they can be injured by a lung tumor (Lesion 5). As they travel up to the SCG on the carotid artery they can be compromised by an aneurysm of the carotid artery (Lesion 6). And as the post-ganglionic fibers travel through the cavernous sinus (Lesion 7) they can also be injured. One caveat with the lesion to the sympathetics in the cavernous sinus is that the parasympathetics on CN III are also traveling through here so the effect on the autonomics to the eye is variable.

Lesion 6 in the image above could also result from a *carotid artery dissection*. The patient could present with ipsilateral neck pain, and ipsilateral Horner's syndrome because of the compromised preganglionic sympathetic fibers traveling alongside the carotid. Because the blood supply to the cerebral cortex could be compromised, they could also present with contralateral long tract findings.

Coma, the Autonomics, and the Eyes

For a patient in a coma, depending on where the lesion is, the pupils will assume a characteristic shape. The picture below is a perfect example of the importance of understanding scenarios, rather than just memorizing the plain facts. If you look at the picture it can seem daunting to just memorize what the pupil does when certain regions are lesioned. It makes sense to walk through this logically (Fig. 14.9).

The thin dashed (red) line represents the descending sympathetic fibers projecting from the hypothalamus down to T1. The thick (blue) horizontal line represents the preganglionic parasympathetic fibers projecting from the Edinger-Westphal nucleus to the eye. The lesions compromise either the sympathetics, the parasympathetics, or both. Location is everything.

Lesion #1 is to the hypothalamus which will damage the sympathetics. With the parasympathetics taking over, the pupil will be constricted.

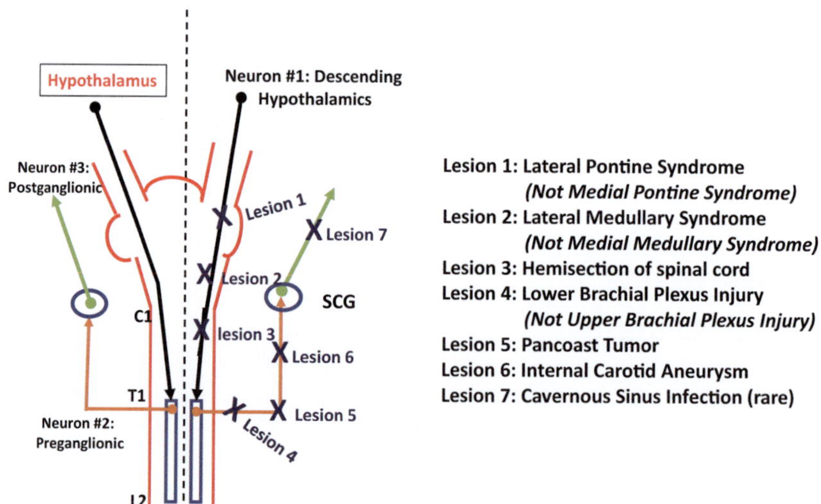

Fig. 14.9 Sympathetic Pathway and Horner's Syndrome. The descending fibers from hypothalamus project to the lateral horn at T1 in the spinal cord. Preganglionics then project to the superior cervical ganglion. Postganglionics then project to targets in face and particularly the eye [11]

Lesion # 2 is to the tectum which will damage the parasympathetics. With the sympathetics taking over, the pupil will be dilated.

Lesion #3 is to the tegmentum of the midbrain which will damage both sympathetics and parasympathetics leading to the eye being stuck in the mid-position.

Lesion #4 is to either the lateral pons, lateral medulla, or spinal cord above T1 which will damage the descending sympathetics causing Horner's syndrome.

Lesion #5 is an uncal herniation which damages the preganglionic parasympathetic fibers on CN III which will lead to an ipsilateral dilated (blown) pupil.

Lesion #6 is the result of drug-induced pinpoint pupils.

Reynaud's Disease

In Reynaud's disease the sympathetic nervous system to the arteries of the upper limbs is overactive leading to cyanosis and pain in the fingers. In severe cases a stellate ganglion sympathectomy (this is a controversial surgery) may be performed to relieve the symptoms, however many complication of the surgery are possible, one of which is Horner's syndrome.

Overview of Autonomics to GI Tract

The parasympathetic fibers to the GI tract are responsible for both peristalsis of the tract and the opening of the various sphincters of the tract. There is a helpful mnemonic to remember the function of the parasympathetic nervous system called SLU**DD** mnemonic which stands for salvation, lacrimation, urination, digestion, and defecation– think of the DD part - **D**igestion and **D**efecation for the discussion below.

Go back in time to when you took gross anatomy, and you were dissecting the region around the celiac trunk and found a nerve plexus. This is the celiac plexus, and in this plexus, we have a celiac ganglion. Around the superior mesenteric artery is a superior mesenteric ganglion, and around the inferior mesenteric artery is the inferior mesenteric ganglion. These three ganglia: celiac, superior mesenteric and inferior mesenteric *are all sympathetic ganglia*—they are not parasympathetic ganglia. To understand this, we need to start with a simple picture of the gut tube divided into foregut, midgut, and hindgut. In the picture, one side of the tube shows the parasympathetics, and one side shows the sympathetics (Fig. 14.9).

On the parasympathetic side, we have the vagus nerve sending preganglionic fibers to the foregut and midgut. And the pelvic splanchnic nerves sending preganglionics to the hindgut. These preganglionics fibers meet the terminal ganglia, invisible to the naked eye, which are in the walls of the GI tract. The terminal ganglia are cell bodies of the postganglionic parasympathetic fibers.

The splanchnic nerves carrying sympathetic fibers to the GI tract, arise from spinal cord segments T5–12. The preganglionic fibers come out of the lateral horn, enter the ventral root, join the spinal nerve, jump off via white rami, but instead of coming back to the spinal nerve on gray rami, the preganglionic fibers continue straight on through the ganglia and leave the ganglia as splanchnic nerves. These splanchnic nerves then travel through the diaphragm and head to either the celiac or superior mesenteric ganglia. After synapsing at the ganglia, the postganglionic fibers travel on branches of either the celiac trunk or superior mesenteric arteries to reach their targets (Fig. 14.17).

These sympathetic ganglia are located on the abdominal aorta. You can see these ganglia with the naked eye when you are dissecting. From the ganglia, the postganglionics then travel on the branches of the celiac trunk and superior mesenteric artery to the foregut and midgut. The lumbar splanchnic nerves coming from L1 and L2 and project to the inferior mesenteric ganglia, synapse, and then the postganglionics jump onto branches of the inferior mesenteric artery to the

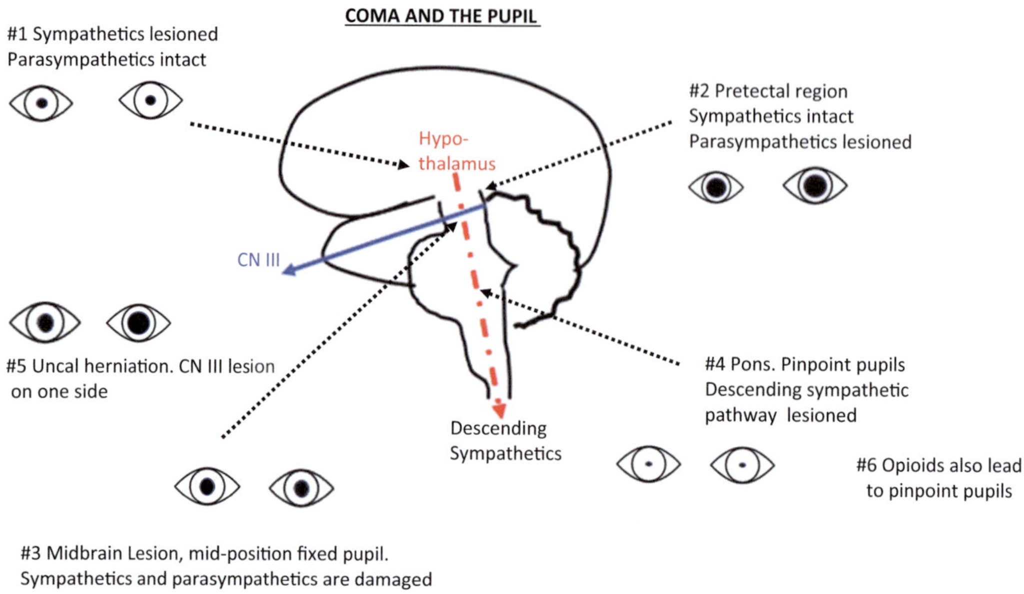

Fig. 14.10 Dashed red vertical line represents the sympathetics. Solid blue horizontal line represents the parasympathetics [11]

hindgut structures. Keep in mind, thoracic and lumbar splanchnic nerves are preganglionic *sympathetic* fibers, while the pelvic splanchnic nerves are preganglionic *parasympathetic* fibers (Fig. 14.10).

Going into greater detail. There are three thoracic splanchnic (sympathetic) nerves:

Greater Splanchnic Nerves from T5–9 projecting to the celiac ganglion.

Lesser Splanchnic Nerves from T10-T11 projecting to the superior mesenteric ganglion.

Least Splanchnic Nerve from T12 projecting to the aorticorenal ganglion (often considered a subdivision of the superior mesenteric ganglion).

The pain fibers from the GI tract follow back along the sympathetic fibers and are responsible for visceral pain sensations. Pain from the foregut travels along the greater splanchnic nerves and is referred to the epigastric region; from the midgut along the lesser splanchnic and is referred to the umbilical area; and from the hindgut along the least splanchnic nerves and is referred to the hypogastric region.

Hirschsprung's disease results from a failure of neural crest cells to migrate into the hindgut, which means that there is no development of the parasympathetic nerves in the hindgut. With no pelvic splanchnic nerves or peristalsis in the hindgut, the descending colon and sigmoid colon become constricted resulting in fecal material backing up in the transverse colon.

Bladder Control

The term neurogenic bladder is a non-specific term that refers to any type of bladder dysfunction. A neurogenic bladder can result from damage to either the CNS, spinal cord for instance, or PNS, pudendal nerve for instance. Nervous system damage can result in an overactive or underactive bladder. Control of the bladder and bowel operate on similar mechanisms. The names of the various sphincters change whether you are talking about the bowel or bladder, but the nerve control of the two is similar. We will look at bladder control first. The bladder has internal and external urethral sphincters, plus the detrusor muscle. The internal urethral sphincter is smooth muscle under control of the autonomic system via the pelvic splanchnic nerves coming from S 2, 3, and 4. It surrounds the urethra just above the prostate. The external urethral sphincter is skeletal muscle under control of the somatic nervous system via the pudendal nerve (Fig. 14.8), and it sits below the prostate within the deep perineal space. The pudendal nerve arises from the ventral horn of S 2, 3, 4 (Onuf's Nucleus).

The first diagram shows the process of normal voiding—also called the *Urge-to-Purge*. When contents come into the bladder, the pressure stimulates the afferent nerve fibers that travel into S 2, 3, and 4 of the spinal cord. The information goes on to make a reflex loop with the efferent parasympathetic pathway, but the information also goes up the spinal cord to tell the cerebral cortex that the bladder is full. The efferent fibers of the reflex loop then tell the internal urethral sphincter to relax. In an adult, when urine moves into the bladder and the internal urethral sphincter relaxes, the adult can now voluntarily fire their pudendal nerve to contract the external urethral sphincter. The adult will then look for the bathroom, and, when the time is right, relax their external urethral sphincter and contract the detrusor to void (Fig. 14.11).

When it comes to the anal canal, instead of the internal and external urethral sphincters, there are the internal and external *anal* sphincters. As fecal material moves into the anal canal, the internal anal sphincter is contracted, and the external is relaxed. During voiding the external anal sphincter relaxes. This explains the anal sphincter reflex, however voiding also involves the abdominal muscles raising abdominal pressure. A lesion in the thoracic cord could lead to an automatic anal reflex because the abdominal muscles are paralyzed, and subsequently, fecal material will build up in the anal canal.

Upper Motor Neuron—Spastic bladder

In this first scenario, there is a lesion in the cervical or thoracic cord which will lead to blockage of the corticospinal pathway. The sacral regions are still functioning, they are just cut off from cortical control. This person's bladder reflex is still intact, they just have no voluntary control over their bladder so they will have spontaneous voiding. The bladder fills up, sensory fibers tell the sacral cord that the bladder is full, the reflex loop is active, and the efferent fibers relax the external anal sphincter. The reflex loop operates on its own and has no cortical involvement (Fig. 14.12). However, keep in mind that spinal shock also comes into play here. Right after an injury, in the acute phase, the patient could have a flaccid bladder or LMN type symptoms. Several days later, after spinal shock, the patient will exhibit UMN symptoms.

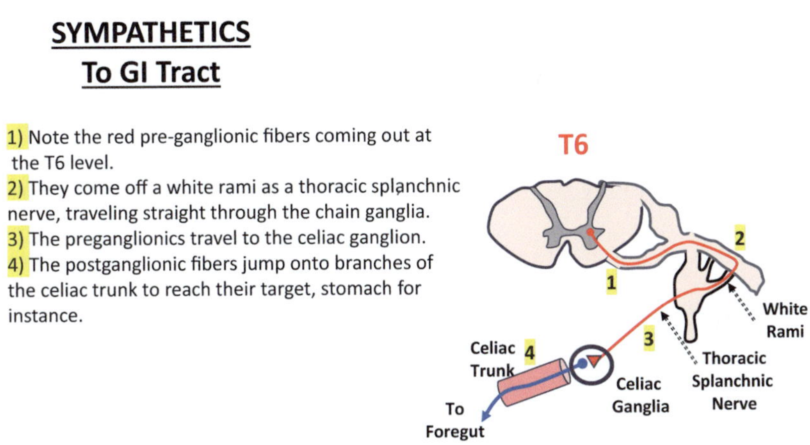

Fig. 14.11 Sympathetics to Gi Tract [11]

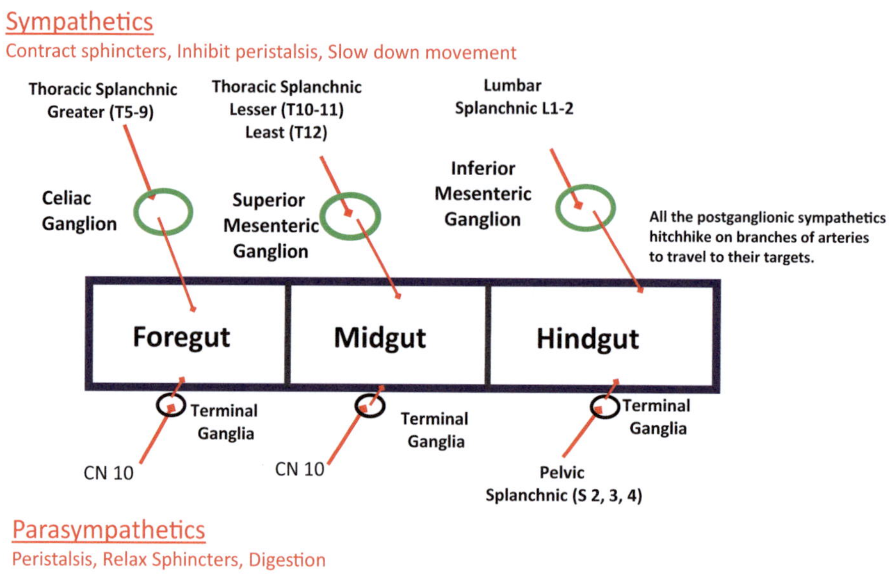

Fig. 14.12 Overview of Autonomic Projections to the GI Tract [11]

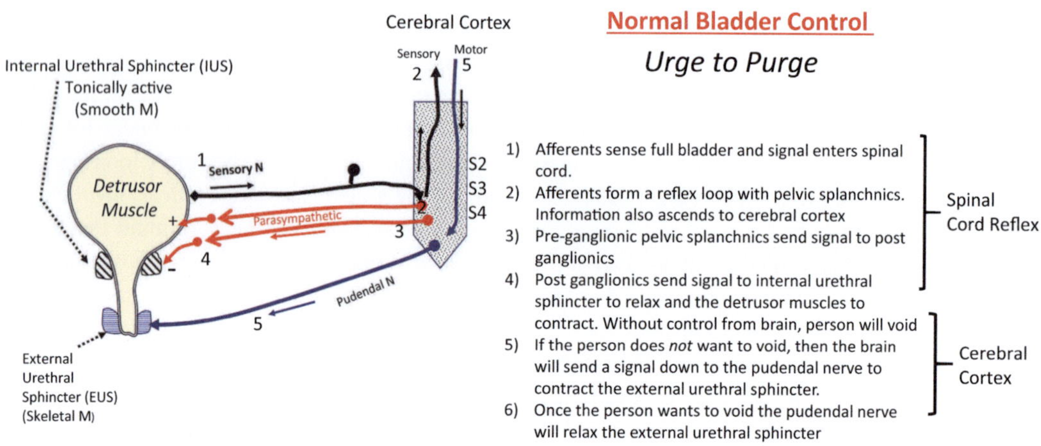

Fig. 14.13 Autonomic and Somatic Nerve Control of Bladder [11]

In some cases of spinal cord injury, where the sacral segments are spared, a reflexogenic erection is possible, however in most of these cases, ejaculation is not possible.

Lower Motor Neuron—Flaccid Bladder

In this second scenario, there is major trauma to the sacral region and the lower motor neurons are lost. In this case, the internal urethral sphincter remains tonically active, and the individual does not have the ability to relax the muscle. Without the ability to contract the detrusor the patient's bladder will fill up with urine and there will be a slow seepage of contents out of the urethra—overflow incontinence (Fig. 14.13).

Parasympathetic Ganglia in the Head

Another way to test yourself on these pathways is to simply take one of the nerves and ask: where are the cell bodies of origin? See Fig. 14.14 which is a self-test. Figure 14.15 is the key.

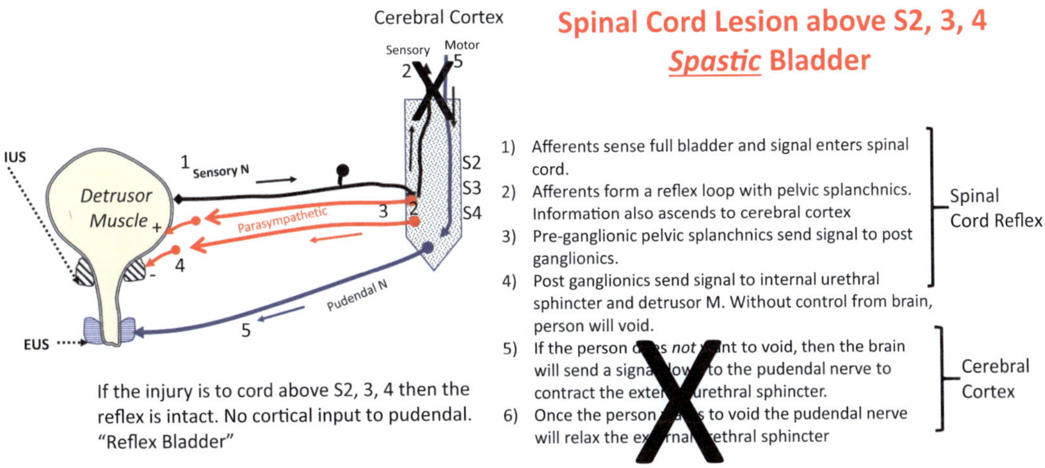

Fig. 14.14 With a lesion to the cord above S 2, 3, 4 then the reflex arc is still present and the internal urethral sphincter will relax. Because the patient has no control over pudendal nerve the bladder is only operating at the reflex level. "Upper Motor Neuron Deficit" "Spastic Bladder." [11]

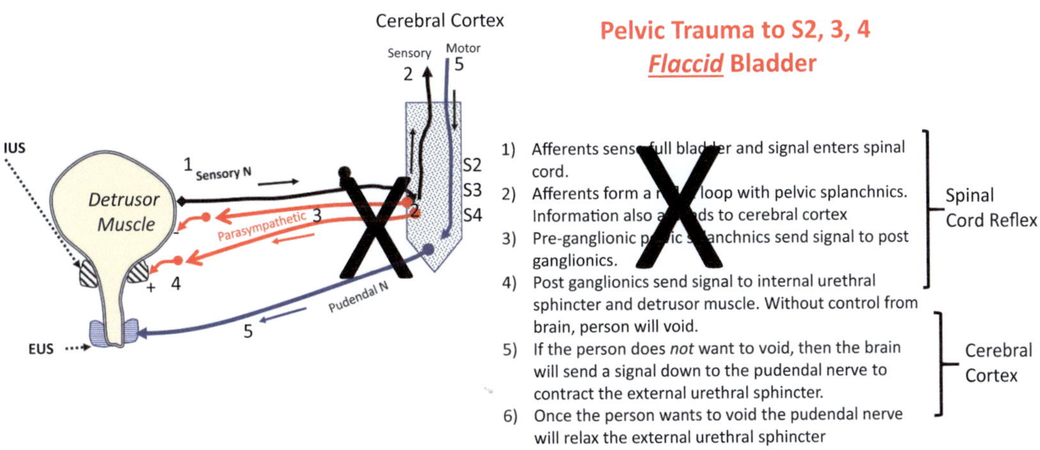

Fig. 14.15 Bladder Control and LMN Injury. With trauma to the pelvis that damages the conus medullaris (S 2, 3, 4) there is no reflex arc or cortical control. The internal urethral sphincter remains tonically active, and person cannot void. Urine will build up until it eventually seeps out. "Lower Motor Neuron Deficit" or "Flaccid Bladder" [11]

How the Sympathetic Fibers from L2 get into the L5 Nerve

To understand why we find grey rami at every level but white rami only from C8-L2, let us take a specific example. Take the L5 nerve. If there are no sympathetics that emerge from the L5 cord level how do the sympathetics get onto the L5 nerve? Note that the sympathetics also get into the S1—S5 nerves, but we are just picking L5 as one example. The preganglionic fibers will emerge from the L2 lateral horn, travel on the ventral rami, the spinal nerve, and the white rami all at the level of L2. However, once these preganglionic fibers enter the sympathetic chain, instead of synapsing at that level they travel down the chain and then synapse at the L5 sympathetic chain ganglia. From here the postganglionic fibers jump to the L5 nerve via a grey ramus and are distributed along the L5 nerve. Thus, at the L5 level there is no white ramus. This is because at the L5 level, because there is no lateral horn, there are no preganglionic fibers emerging at the L5 level to form a white ramus. However, grey rami are found at every level from C1 to S5. This is because at L5 there are some preganglionic fibers that came from L2, traveled down the sympathetic chain, synapsed, and then the post ganglionic fibers merged onto the L5 nerve via the grey rami (Figs. 14.16 and 14.17).

<u>Where are the Cell Bodies of origin for fibers in the?</u>

1) Greater Petrosal N
2) Deep Petrosal N
3) Nerve of Pterygoid Canal
4) Chorda Tympani
5) Lingual nerve proximal to chorda tympani
6) Lesser Petrosal Nerve
7) Auriculotemporal Nerve
8) Lacrimal nerve
9) Greater Palatine Nerve

<u>Key</u>

1) Superior Salvatory N
2) Superior Cervical G
3) Superior Salvatory N, Superior Cervical G
4) Geniculate G, Superior Salvatory N
5) Trigeminal G
6) Inferior Salvatory N
7) Trigeminal G, Otic G
8) Trigeminal G, Pterygopalatine G
9) Trigeminal G, Pterygopalatine G

Fig. 14.16 Self Test for Understanding Parasympathetic Fibers to the Head. The questions are on the left. The answers are on the right. Use the following figure (Fig. 14.14) to visualize the answers

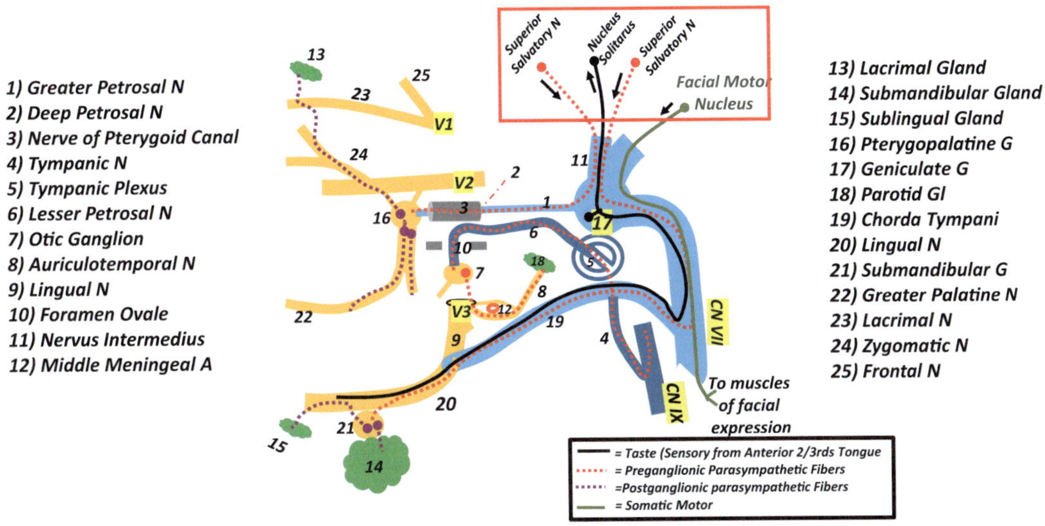

Fig. 14.17 Parasympathetics to Glands. Both CN VII and CN IX have parasympathetic f fibers that use CN V to travel to their targets. CN VII has the greater petrosal nerve (parasympathetic) that meets the deep petrosal nerve (sympathetic) to form the nerve of the pterygoid canal (parasympathetic and sympathetic) that travels to meet the pterygopalatine ganglion in the pterygopalatine fossa. After synapsing in the PT ganglion, the post ganglionic parasympathetic fibers jump on the zygomatic nerve (V2) and then jump onto the lacrimal nerve (V1) to reach the lacrimal gland. They also travel on the greater and lesser petrosal nerves to the glands on the palate. In addition, CN VII has the chorda tympani with preganglionic fibers that joint the lingual nerve (V3) to reach the submandibular ganglion. In addition, the chorda tympani has taste fibers from the anterior 2/3rds of the tongue. CN IX has the tympanic nerve, which meets the tympanic plexus, which gives off the lesser petrosal nerve that exits the skull through foramen ovale to meet the otic ganglion. The post ganglionic parasympathetic fibers then jump on auriculotemporal to reach the parotid gland

Cushing's Triad

Cushing's Triad of hypertension, decreased heart rate, and irregular respiration should not be confused with Cushing's Syndrome. One way to think of Cushing's Triad is that it results from the sympathetic and parasympathetic nervous systems becoming confused. In cases of increased intracranial pressure, usually from severe head trauma, the body can respond with the three characteristic findings of Cushing's. Trauma that leads to a subdural or epidural bleed can lead to increased intracranial pressure, which in turn blocks blood coming into the brain. To get blood into the brain, the sympathetic nervous system responds with vasoconstriction of the systemic vessels. This leads to an increase in MAP with the goal of overcoming the high-pressure present in the arteries to the brain. But things are not so simple and in one sense the body gets confused. This increase in pressure as part of the sympathetic response leads to a paradoxical parasympathetic response.

As the MAP rises, the baroreceptors in the carotid arteries and aorta sense the increased pressure which in turn triggers the parasympathetics to respond by initiating a reduction in heart rate and respiration. The reduction in respiration is referred to as Cheyne-Stokes respiration. The patient exhibiting Cushing's Reflex is in a dire situation which is most likely irreversible. At this point, the patient is at risk of a brain herniation (Figs. 14.18 and 14.19).

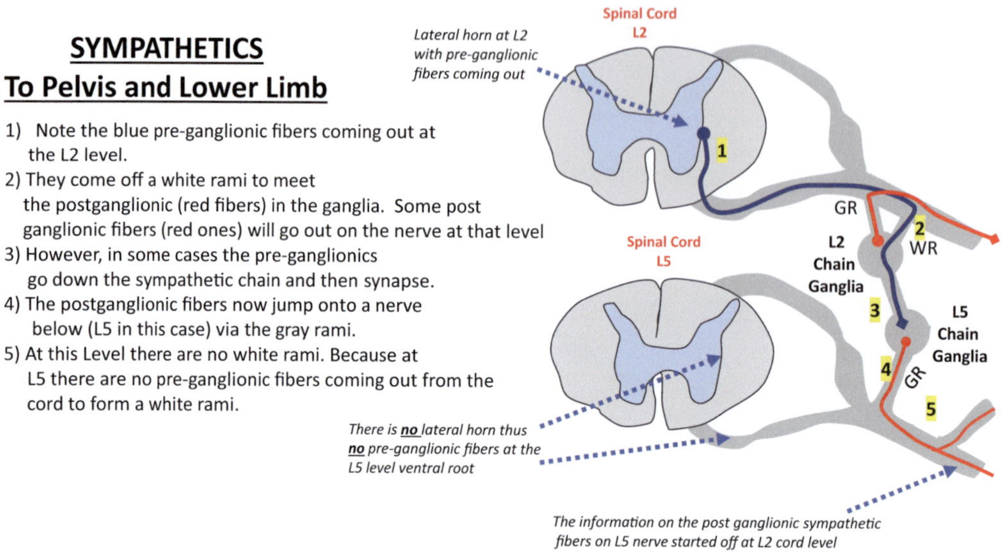

Fig. 14.18 Sympathetics to Lower Limb [11]

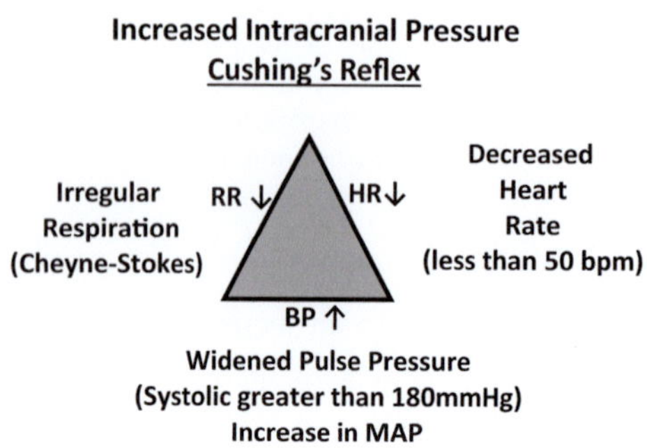

Fig. 14.19 Cushing's Reflex. In cases of increased intracranial pressure, the MAP is not high enough to send blood to the brain. The sympathetic nervous system responds by systemic vasoconstriction to increase MAP *(Hypertension).* This in turn leads to a parasympathetic response triggered by the carotid and aortic baroreceptors resulting in a slower heart rate *(bradycardia),* and slower respiratory rate *(bradypnea).* The patient is at risk for brain herniation [11]

Further Reading

1. Afifi AK, Bergman RA. Functional neuroanatomy: text and atlas. McGraw-Hill; 1998.
2. Brazis, P.W., Masdeu, J.C., and Biller, J. Localization in clinical neurology, LWW; 2016.
3. Blumenfeld H. Neuroanatomy through clinical cases. 2nd ed. Wiley-Blackwell; 2010.
4. Callaghan B, Furness JB, Pustovit RV. Neural pathways for anorectal control, relevance to spinal cord injury and treatment: a narrative review. Spinal Cord. 2018;56:199–205.
5. Campbell, W., and Barohn, R.J. Dejong's the neurological examination, LWW; 2019.
6. Carpenter M. Core text of neuroanatomy. New York: Williams and Wilkins; 1991.
7. Fuller G. Neurological examination made easy. 6th ed. Elsevier; 2019.
8. Goldberg S. Clinical anatomy made ridiculously simple. MedMaster; 1991.

9. Goldberg S. Clinical neuroanatomy made ridiculously simple. MedMaster; 2002.
10. Leo J. Medical Neuroanatomy for the boards and clinic: Finding the Lesion. 2nd ed. Switzerland: Springer; 2024.
11. Leo J. Clinical anatomy and embryology: A guide for the classroom, clinic, and clinic. 2nd ed. Springer; 2024.
12. Maamouri R, Ferchichi M, Houmane Y, Gharbi Z, Cheour M. Neuro-Ophthalmological manifestations of Horner's syndrome: current perspective. Eye and Brain. 2023;15, 5
13. Posner J, Saper C, Schiff ND, Classen J. Plum and Posner's diagnosis and treatment of stupor and coma. 5th ed. Oxford: Oxford University Press; 2019.
14. Ropper M, Samuels M, Klein J, Prasad S. Adams and Victor's principles of neurology. 12th ed. New York: McGraw Hill; 2023.
15. Splittgerber R. Snell's clinical neuroanatomy. 8th ed. Lippincott, Williams, and Wilkins; 2018.
16. Swanson PD. Signs and symptoms in neurology. Lippincott Williams and Wilkins; 1984.
17. Woodburne RT, Burkel WE. Essentials of human anatomy. 9th ed. New York: Oxford University Press; 1994.
18. Wu F, Zhao Y, Zhang H. Ocular autonomic nervous system: an update from anatomy and to physiological functions. Vision. 2022;6. Available at: https://doi.org/10.3390/vision6010006
19. Young, P. A., Young, P.H., and Tolbert, D. Basic clinical neuroscience, LLW; 2015.

15 Cerebellar Lesions

Introduction

The cerebellum sits between the cerebral cortex and the spinal cord and is referred to as a "comparator." It compares one stream of information coming down from the cortex, and another stream of information coming up from the spinal cord. The cortex is sending commands—the plan of action—down to your muscles via the corticospinal and corticobulbar pathways and the cerebellum is getting a sample of those commands. Meanwhile as your limb is moving, there is information about proprioception coming into the CNS and traveling up to the cerebellum. The cerebellum then compares what you *plan to do* with *what is really happening* and then adjusts or fine tunes the movement by projecting back to the thalamus and cerebral cortex. Lesions to the cerebellum do not result in paralysis, or loss of strength, but result in an intention tremor.

Lobes, Zones, and Divisions

There are three ways that scientists have divided up the cerebellum. The first is on an anatomic basis by lobes. If you take a midsagittal cut through the cerebellum, you notice two prominent fissures: (1) the primary fissure, which gives us the large anterior and posterior lobes, and (2) the posterolateral fissure, which gives us the small flocculonodular lobe. We can also talk about zones, which moving medial to lateral gives us the vermis, intermediate zone, and lateral hemispheres. Or we can talk about functional divisions, which are based on connections, giving us the cerebrocerebellum, spinocerebellum, and vestibulocerebellum. The central inferior part of the vermis is referred to as the tonsil, which in the presence of increased intracranial pressure can herniate through the foramen magnum.

The Big Picture Corticospinal and Corticopontocerebellar

Take the circuits involved in picking up a piece of paper on the street in front of you. But to complicate it there is a slight breeze in the air, causing the paper to move every now and then. On Fig. 8.1 you can see the corticospinal tract projecting down from the left cerebral cortex to the right cord to tell the hand to move towards the paper. As the signal travels through the pons on its way to the spinal cord, it sends a sample of the information to the pontine nuclei, which in turn sends information into the contralateral cerebellum via the middle cerebellar peduncle. It is via this corticopontocerebellar pathway that the cerebellum listens into your plan to move your arm and pick up the paper. Note that this is an **afferent** pathway into the cerebellum (Fig. 15.1).

J. Leo, *Gross Anatomy, Neuroanatomy, and Embryology for Medical Students*,
https://doi.org/10.1007/978-3-031-87151-1_15

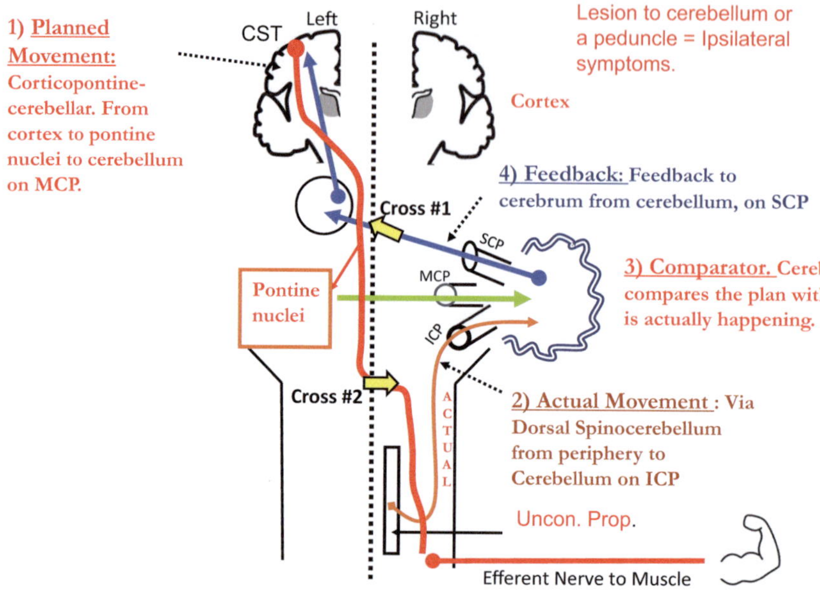

Fig. 15.1 Cerebellar Inputs and Outputs. It is a double-crossed pathway. *Decussation #1 is the dentatothalamic pathway*

Dorsal Spinocerebellar and Cuneocerebellar

As your right arm is moving towards the piece of paper, there is all sorts of proprioceptive information about the relationship of your arm to the paper coming into your cerebellum, especially important since the wind is moving the paper. As the paper is moving, your initial plan will need to be modified mid-course. The proprioceptive information from the limbs comes into the spinal cord and synapses in the dorsal nucleus of Clark which runs from T1 to L2. After synapsing, the fibers jump onto the dorsal spinocerebellar tract. The equivalent nucleus and tract for the neck is the lateral cuneate nucleus and the cuneocerebellar tract, which also travel through the inferior cerebellar peduncle. The dorsal spinocerebellar and cuneocerebellar are both *afferent* pathways into the cerebellum carrying information about what is happening with your limb (Fig. 15.2).

There is also a ventral spinocerebellar pathway projecting from the spinal cord to the cerebellum, which crosses twice. When it enters the spinal cord, it crosses immediately to the contralateral side, it travels up the spinal cord, and then in the brainstem it crosses back to the original side before entering the cerebellum. When you think about the lesions to the spinal cord, the dorsal spinocerebellar tract is more important (Fig. 15.3).

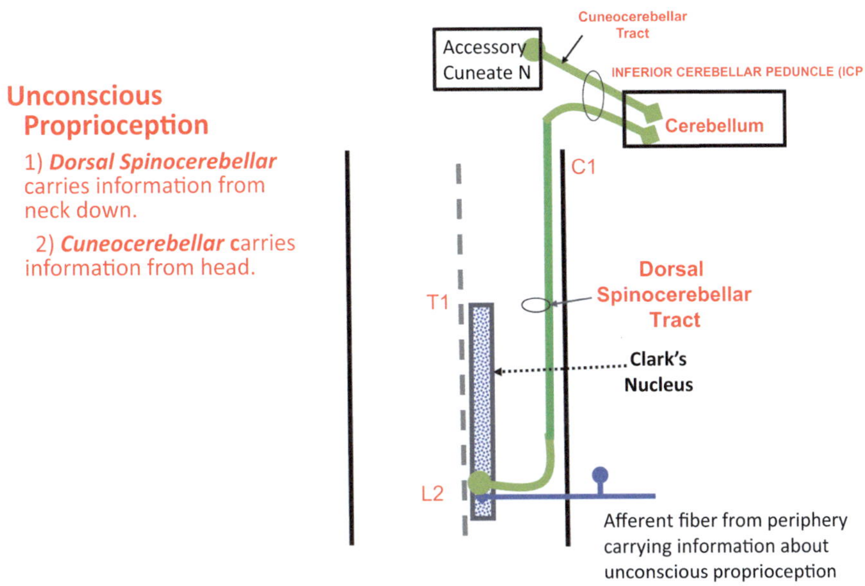

Fig. 15.2 Dorsal Spinocerebellar and Cuneocerebellar Pathways. Information from both tracts goes to the cerebellum via the inferior cerebellar peduncle (ICP). They carry proprioceptive information, and are uncrossed. Decussation #2 is the corticospinal tract [12]

Inferior Cerebellar Peduncle	**Afferents into Cerebellum** 1) Dorsal Spinocerebellum 2) Cuneocerebellum 3) Olivocerebellar
Middle Cerebellar Peduncle	**Afferents into Cerebellum** 1) Pontocerebellar
Superior Cerebellar Peduncle	**Efferents out of Cerebellum** 1) Dentatothalamic 2) Dentatorubrothalamic

Fig. 15.3 Three Cerebellar Peduncles. The inferior cerebellar peduncle is carrying information from the spinal cord *into* the cerebellum. The middle cerebellar peduncle is carrying information from the pons *into* the cerebellum. The superior peduncle is carrying Information *out of* the cerebellum onto the thalamus and red nucleus [12]

Dentatothalamic

The right cerebellum gets information about your plan of action via the middle cerebellar peduncle, while the proprioceptive information comes in through the inferior peduncle. To fine tune the movement, so that you can pick up the paper, the right cerebellum sends its information out of the cerebellum on the superior cerebellar peduncle via the dentatothalamic pathway to the contralateral thalamus, which in turn goes to the left cerebral cortex. And originating in the left cerebral cortex is the corticospinal tract sending information to the right forearm (remember, corticospinal decussates).

This circuit explains why a lesion to the cerebellum or one of its peduncles will lead to signs and symptoms on the ipsilateral side. This is because the circuit has two crossing points. Take a lesion to the right cerebellum. The output from the right cerebellum decussates (cross #1) to project to the left thalamus, which in turn goes to the left cerebral cortex, but the left cerebral cortex sends information down the corticospinal tract which decussates at the pyramidal decussation (cross #2) to go to the right cord, and then to right upper limb. Thus, a lesion to the right cerebellum will disrupt movements on the right side of the body.

Cerebellar patients will have an "intention tremor" which refers to the fact that in most cases if a cerebellar patient is sitting in your office, you will not see a tremor at rest. The tremor will not appear until the patient intends to move. For instance, if the patient is asked to touch their nose, they can move their finger towards their nose, but they will have a tremor. And as their finger approaches the target, the tremor will worsen.

A common lesion that leads to cerebellar signs is lateral medullary syndrome which damages the dorsal spinocerebellar tracts, leading to ipsilateral ataxia. These are addressed in more detail in the brainstem chapter.

Red Nucleus

The red nucleus receives a projection from the cerebellum and projects to the contralateral flexors of the upper limb via the rubrospinal tract. Lesions of the red nucleus will lead to a contralateral tremor. For the purposes of human clinical neuroanatomy, lesions to the rubrospinal tract in the spinal cord are not often discussed because the rubrospinal tract sits on top of the corticospinal tract, so that a lesion to the rubrospinal tract would also lead to a lesion of the corticospinal tract and the patient would exhibit UMN signs. The rubrospinal tract is also discussed in the section of decerebrate and decorticate rigidity.

Inputs

Another way to look at the cerebellum is that there are inputs into the cerebellum and outputs out of the cerebellum. On the inferior cerebellar peduncle, there are three major inputs into the cerebellum:

1. The **dorsal spinocerebellar tract** carries information from the spinal cord about unconscious proprioception.
2. The **cuneocerebellar tract** carries information from the head region about unconscious proprioception.
3. The **olivocerebellar tract** carries information from the inferior olive via the climbing fibers through the inferior cerebellar peduncle.

There is also a major input into the cerebellum through the middle cerebellar peduncle:

1. The **pontocerebellar tract** (which could also be referred to as the corticopontocerebellar tract) into the pons.

The major outputs from the cerebellum are the:

1. **Dentatothalamic tract** from the dentate nucleus to the VL of the contralateral thalamus. This is the pathway involved with voluntary movement (corticospinal tract).
2. The **globose and emboliform** nuclei (interposed together) project to the red nucleus and the thalamus. Coming out of the red nucleus is the rubrospinal tract.
3. The **fastigial nucleus** projects to the vestibular nuclei and is involved with balance.

Internal Cerebellar Circuitry

In the previous section we looked at those tracts coming into and out of the cerebellum with the idea that the cerebellum compares the plan with the actual movement and then fine tunes the ongoing movement. On the picture of the schematic, you will see a question mark located in the cerebellum. We are now going to zoom in with a microscope and look at some of the internal circuitry.

Just like the cerebral cortex, the outer surface of the cerebellum consists of gray matter, however, unlike the cerebrum with its six layers, the cerebellum has three layers. Deep to the gray matter is the white matter, with the four deep cerebellar nuclei embedded in the white matter on each side. From outside to inside, the layers of the gray matter are: (1) Molecular, (2) Purkinje, and (3) Granule (Figs. 15.4 and 15.5).

The Purkinje Layer gets its name from the flask-shaped Purkinje cells which are lined up in rows, or monolayers. Their dendrites project out into the molecular layer, and their axons project down through the granule cell layer to synapse on

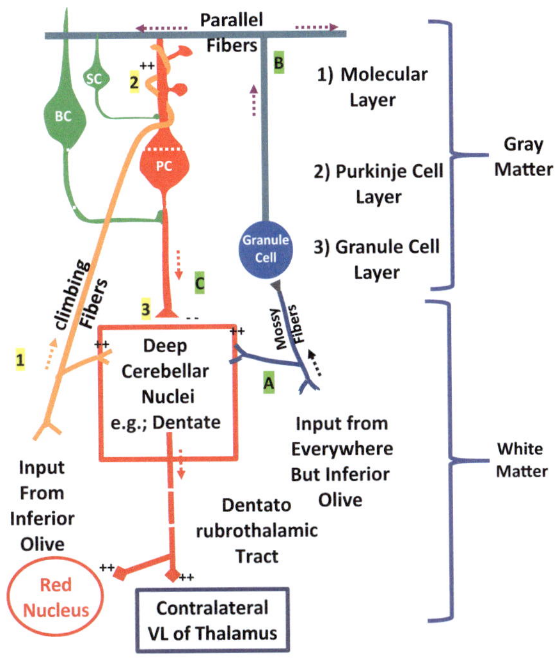

Climbing Fibers	Mossy Fibers
1) Climbing fibers (CF) send a collateral to the deep cerebellar nuclei (DCN)	A) Mossy fibers (MF) send a collateral to the DCN
2) Each CF synapses with one PC dendrite	B) MFs project to the granule cells which send PFs to PCs
3) PC axons project to the DCN	C) PCs project to the DCN

Fig. 15.4 Cerebellar Circuitry. A climbing fiber enters the cerebellum, sends a collateral to a DCN, and then synapses with one Purkinje cell (PC) dendrite. The PCs then synapse with the deep cerebellar nuclei (DCN). The mossy fibers send a collateral to the DCN, and then synapse with the granule cells (GC). The GCs then send parallel fibers to synapse with thousands of PC dendrites. The DCN project out of the cerebellum as the dentatorubrothalamic on the superior cerebellar peduncle to thalamus and red nucleus. Note that the DCN are getting a barrage of inhibitory and excitatory inputs, which will affect the output to thalamus and red nucleus [12]

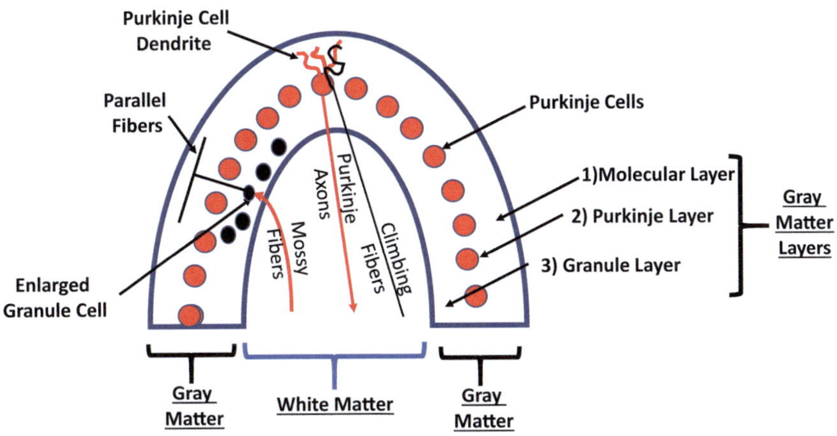

Fig. 15.5 The Three Layers of the Cerebellar Gray Matter. Note the grey matter surrounds the white matter [12]

the deep cerebellar nuclei, which are embedded in the white matter. The Purkinje cell projections are such that the cells in the midline or vermis project to the midline located deep cerebellar nuclei—the fastigial nucleus. Moving out from the midline the Purkinje cells project to the globose and emboliform nuclei (together referred to as the interposed nucleus). And the Purkinje cells in the lateral hemisphere project to the dentate nucleus (Fig. 15.6).

Fig. 15.6 Purkinje Cell Projections to the Deep Cerebellar Nuclei [12]

Input	Nucleus	Output Via:	Projection To	Function
Purkinje Cells: Vermis	Fastigial	ICP	Vestibular Nucleus	Balance
Purkinje Cells: Intermediate Hemisphere	Globose Emboliform	SCP	Red Nucleus	Limbs
Purkinje Cells: Lateral Hemisphere	Dentate	SCP	VL of Thalamus	Voluntary Movement
		SCP	Red Nucleus	Gait

Cell	Neurotransmitter (Charge)
Granule Cell	Glutamate (Excitatory)++
Purkinje Cell	Gaba (Inhibitory) --
Basket/Stellate Cell	Gaba (Inhibitory) --
Golgi Cell	Gaba (Inhibitory) --
Inferior Olive (Climbing Fibers)	Aspartate (Excitatory) ++

Fig. 15.7 Cerebellar Cells and their Neurotransmitters [12]

The Granule Cells are much more numerous than the Purkinje cells and cover a wider area. The granule cells have axons that project up into the molecular layer and bifurcate to form a T, referred to as parallel fibers. The parallel fibers travel across the molecular layer synapsing on rows of Purkinje cells (and Basket and stellate cells).

The Molecular Layer is made up of the dendrites of Purkinje cells, climbing fibers, parallel fibers, and basket and stellate cells. The basket and stellate cells are involved in lateral inhibition.

Most of the cells within the cerebellum are GABAergic and thus inhibitory (Fig. 15.7). The only internal excitatory cell is the granule cell. The climbing fibers from the inferior olive are also excitatory, however keep in mind that while their axons enter the cerebellum, their cell bodies are located outside the cerebellum.

Cerebellar Inputs

There are numerous inputs to the cerebellum, but they can be subdivided into two classes: (1) Climbing Fibers, (2) Mossy Fibers (Fig. 15.8).

The *climbing fibers* only come from the inferior olivary nucleus (ION). As they enter the cerebellum, they send a collateral to the deep cerebellar nuclei and then continue to the Purkinje cell dendrites where they resemble a vine wrapping itself around a trellis—thus the name "climbing fiber." There is a one-to-one connection between climbing fibers and Purkinje cells. They are excitatory neurons and are thought to be involved with error correction.

All the other inputs to the cerebellum are characterized as *mossy fibers*. As they enter the cerebellum, each mossy fiber sends collaterals to the deep cerebellar nuclei and then continues onto the granule cells which in turn project into the molecular layer as parallel fibers. In contrast to the one-to-one relationship of climbing fibers to Purkinje cells, each parallel fiber synapses on thousands of Purkinje cells (Fig. 15.9).

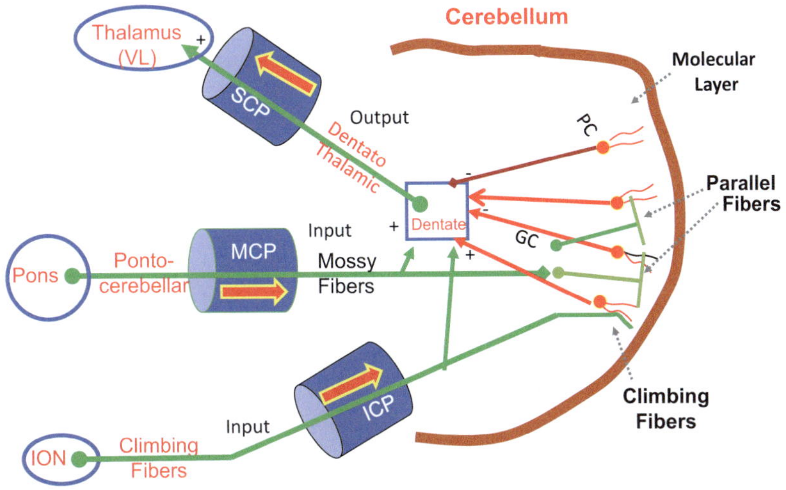

Fig. 15.8 The Three Cerebellar Peduncles. Climbing fibers come from the inferior olive (IO), parallel fibers come from the granule cells, and mossy fibers come from all the extrinsic nuclei except IO. *PC* Purkinje cell, *GC* Granule cell [12]

Origin	Via Fibers	Projection To
Inferior Olive	Climbing Fibers	One Purkinje Cell Dendrite
Granule Cells	Parallel Fibers	Many Purkinje Cell Dendrites
Numerous Nuclei	Mossy Fibers	Granule Cell Bodies

Fig. 15.9 Three Types of Cerebellar Fibers. The climbing fibers come out of the inferior olive and wrap around one Purkinje cell dendrite. The parallel fibers run from the granule cells to many Purkinje cell dendrites. The mossy fibers run from various nuclei to the cell bodies of granule cells [12]

Deep Cerebellar Nuclei

The four deep nuclei are the *fastigial, globose, emboliform*, and *dentate* (**D**on't **E**at **G**reasy **F**oods). Each of these nuclei receives an excitatory input from either the climbing or mossy fibers, and an inhibitory input from the Purkinje cells. Like a computer, the deep cerebellar nuclei are monitoring and responding to the differential barrages of excitatory and inhibitory inputs.

The deep nuclei do not project directly to the lower motor neurons, but instead, exert their influence by projecting to areas of the extrapyramidal and pyramidal system by projecting to the thalamus and red nucleus via the dentatothalamic or dentatorubrothalamic tract.

The fastigial nucleus projects to vestibular nuclei and reticular nuclei which give off vestibulospinal and reticulospinal tracts, respectively. The dentate nucleus projects mainly to the thalamus and then to the cerebral cortex. The globose and emboliform project mainly to the red nucleus, and the red nucleus in turn gives rise to the rubrospinal tract. In this manner, the cerebellum can affect corticospinal and rubrospinal output.

The somatotopic organization of the cerebellum is not as precise as in the cerebral cortex, and we can only make rough generalizations about it. The trunk afferents project to the vermis and paravermal cortex, and their efferent output is primarily concerned with posture, muscle tone, and stabilization of the proximal limb musculature. The lateral cerebellar hemispheres reciprocally interact with cerebral cortex for fine control of distal muscles.

Basket Cells, Stellate Cells, and Lateral Inhibition

Lateral inhibition is a one method to increase contrast in the nervous system by firing one group of neurons, while simultaneously inhibiting the neighboring neurons. The cerebellum is one of several structures that uses lateral

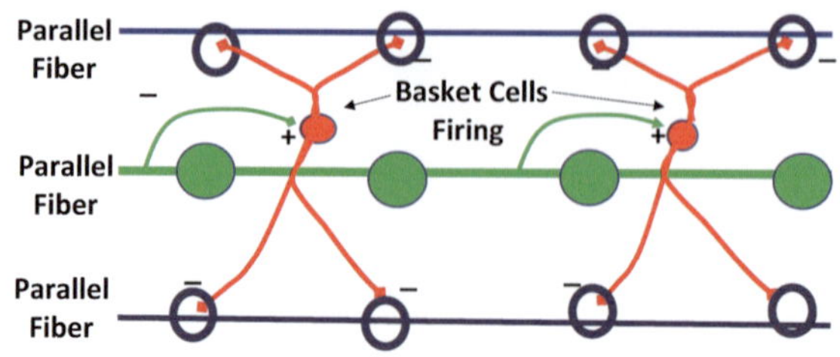

Fig. 15.10 Lateral Inhibition in Cerebellum [12]

inhibition. In the cerebellar cortex, Purkinje cells and their dendrites are lined up in rows. Parallel fibers from the granule cells then run down these rows of Purkinje cell dendrites. A single parallel fiber can then synapse with hundreds of thousands of Purkinje cells. When a parallel fiber depolarizes it "turns on" a row of Purkinje cells. At the same time, the collaterals from these same parallel fibers will contact basket and stellate cells which are inhibitory to the neighboring rows of Purkinje cells and will inhibit or "turn off" these neighboring rows. Various other areas of the nervous system such as the visual cortex and auditory cortex also use lateral inhibition to increase the contrast of whatever modality is being monitored (Fig. 15.10).

Clinical Symptoms of Cerebellar Lesions

There are several ways to divide up the cerebellum to talk about clinical signs and symptoms but the most straightforward way is to divide it into the lateral lobes, flocculonodular, and anterior lobe.

Lesions to the lateral lobe will result in limb ataxia, especially with the upper limbs. Hypotonia will also be present. Lesions to the intermediate zone will result in truncal ataxia—drunken gait. Lesions to the anterior lobe will lead to dysfunction with tandem walking.

Lesions to the cerebellum will result in various signs and symptoms. The mnemonic.

DANISH will help remember them.

Dysmetria: the inability to stop a movement at the intended target. For example, in the cerebellar patient if you ask the patient to touch their nose, they have a tremor. Notably, the tremor becomes more severe the closer the finger gets to the target. The heel to shin test is also a sign of cerebellar pathology. ***Dysdiadochokinesia***: the inability to perform alternating rapid movements such as pronation-supination of the hands.

Ataxia: a disturbance in posture and gait. Lesions of the midline region of the cerebellum cause difficulty in maintaining an upright stance, and the gait is staggering like that seen in drunkenness. Lesions to one side of the cerebellar hemisphere lead to an ipsilateral limb ataxia.

Nystagmus: is present with cerebellar lesions due to disruption of the vestibular fibers or vestibular nuclei.

Intention Tremor: often present during purposeful movements. It is not present at rest.

Slurred or Scanning Speech

Hypotonia: decreased muscle tone.

We are going to look at three different lesions, each one involving a cerebral peduncle.

Superior Cerebellar Peduncle The superior cerebellar peduncle (SCP) carries the dentatothalamic fibers from the dentate nucleus to the contralateral thalamus. When the superior peduncle carrying these fibers is injured, there will be an ipsilateral intention tremor. Also in the vicinity of the SCP are the descending hypothalamic fibers so there will be an ipsilateral Horner's Syndrome. Because the spinothalamic and the ventral trigeminothalamic tracts are lesioned there will be a contralateral loss of pain and temperature. And

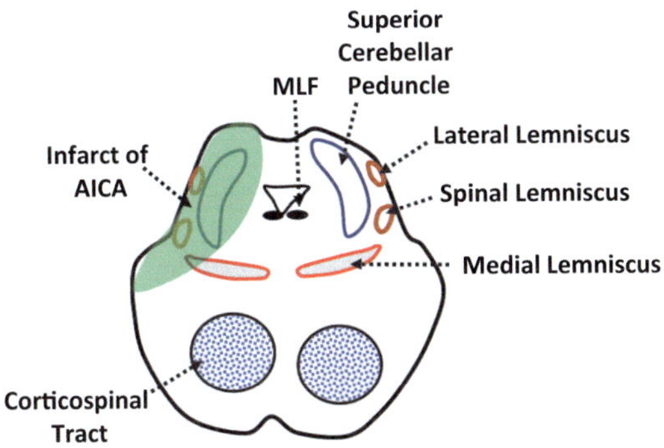

Fig. 15.11 Lesion to Superior Cerebellar Peduncle. Patient has an infarct of the AICA leading to bilateral diminution of hearing, contralateral loss of pain and temperature, plus ataxia [12]

because the lateral lemniscus is damaged, there will be a bilateral diminution of hearing with the loss greatest on the contralateral side of the body. The superior cerebellar artery peruses this territory (Fig. 15.11).

Middle Cerebellar Peduncle The middle cerebellar peduncle (MCP) is damaged in lateral pontine syndrome. The MCP is carrying the pontocerebellar fibers from the pontine nuclei to the contralateral cerebellum. The patient will have ipsilateral ataxia, nystagmus, and most likely a facial nerve deficit. Because the vestibulocochlear nerve is injured, they will lose hearing in the ipsilateral ear. They will also have an ipsilateral Horner's Syndrome. The anterior inferior cerebellar artery perfuses this territory.

Inferior Cerebellar Peduncle The inferior cerebellar peduncle (ICP) is damaged in lateral medullary syndrome. The patient will have ipsilateral loss of pain and temperature to the face, and contralateral loss of pain and temperature to the body. They will also have an ipsilateral Horner's Syndrome, ipsilateral ataxia, and nystagmus. Plus, because of nucleus ambiguus, dysarthria and dysphagia will be present. The artery posterior inferior cerebellar artery (or in some cases the vertebral artery) perfuses this territory.

Central Pontine Myelinolysis occurs in patients with hyponatremia who have had their low sodium levels treated too quickly which leads to a pathological response resulting in demyelination of the corticospinal and corticobulbar tracts in the pons. The patients present with quadriparesis, cranial nerve deficits, and emotional lability.

Olivopontocerebellar Atrophy is characterized by degeneration in the cerebellum, pons, and inferior olive resulting in deficits with balance, coordination, posture, voluntary movements, and bladder control. Symptoms usually begin in the lower limbs, progress to the upper limbs, and then onto the cranial nerves. The initial symptom is usually a broad-based gait.

Medulloblastomas arises from neuroectoderm, are found in the cerebellum close to the fourth ventricle and are one of the most common tumors in children. Increased intracranial pressure can lead to blockage of the fourth ventricle. Patients present with a wide-based gait, and truncal ataxia (drunken sailor gait) affecting the midline muscles such as shoulder and hip.

Dandy-Walker Syndrome is a congenital malformation of the fourth ventricle and the cerebellum. The vermis of the cerebellum is either absent or smaller than normal. Most patients will present with hydrocephalus due to blockage of the foramen of Magendie.

Progressive Supranuclear Palsy (PSP) is due to degeneration of the substantia nigra, midbrain, and the dentate nucleus of the cerebellum. PSP patients and Parkinson's patients have similar motor deficits. However, PSP patients tend to stand upright with their head bent backwards and they tend to fall backward (axial rigidity), which contrasts to Parkinson's patients who tend to lean forward and fall forward. The PSP patients will have eye movement deficits and trouble shifting their gaze, leading to blurred vision. They also have deficits with opening their eyes and they tend to blink excessively. PSP patients tend to have a wide-eyed stare, furrowing of the forehead, and a permanent frown. Sagittal MRIs of a PSP patient can show a *hummingbird sign*, which is due to the degeneration of the brain stem.

In PSP patients, in several regions of the brain that are involved in motor control, there is often an abundance of the microtubule associated protein *tau* that congregates in neurofibrillary tangles. Regions such as the subthalamic nucleus, red nucleus, substantia nigra, and striatum are sites for these accumulations of tangles.

Chiari Malformations

There are two types of Chiari malformations. In a *Type I Chiari Malformation*, there is a downward displacement of the cerebellar tonsils on the brainstem at the foramen magnum. It is often not diagnosed until adolescence or adulthood, and the patient may be asymptomatic. It may go along with syringomyelia. *Type II* is usually diagnosed in young children and there is a herniation of the cerebellum and the brainstem through the foramen magnum. These patients are also often diagnosed with a myelomeningocele. The term “Arnold Chiari Malformation” refers to the Type II form. The most common treatment for a Chiari malformation is decompression of the posterior cranial fossa.

Ataxic Hemiparesis

A lesion in the basis pontis can lead to the syndrome of *ataxic hemiparesis*. In this scenario, the lesion damages the corticospinal tract which leads to contralateral UMN signs. The lesion also damages the pontocerebellar fibers projecting to the contralateral cerebellum that leads to contralateral ataxia. At first glance a patient with UMN signs and ataxia on the same side sounds counterintuitive. In most patients, in the initial stages of the condition, the UMN signs will predominate, however as time goes on, the ataxia will be revealed. It is also unclear why there is no evidence of ipsilateral ataxia. One would think that because the pontocerebellar fibers projecting to the ipsilateral cerebellum area should also be damaged then there would be an ipsilateral deficit however this is typically not seen—we do not know everything about the brain.

Summary of Cerebellar Lesions and Two Homunculi

While anatomists divide the cerebellum up into various subdivisions, lesions in the cerebellum don’t always follow these clear cut divisions—its not as simple as it is in some other areas of the nervous system where a specific lesion equates to a specific deficit. To start the discussion, there are two homunculi or topographical maps that can be used to think of clinical scenarios that involve the cerebellum. In the first map, there are two people, each in a position of touching their toes, with their backs against each other mapped out onto the cerebellum. Think of this map in terms of ataxia. Lesions anywhere in the cerebellum can lead to ataxia, but there are subtle differences in what type of ataxia is present depending on where the lesion is located. Lesions in the midline affect the trunk and can lead to bilateral truncal ataxia. While lesions located on the more lateral hemispheres can lead to ipsilateral appendicular ataxia. Lesions in the midline can also lead to problems with posture and eye movements.

The other homunculus map is an upside down person with their lower limbs in the anterior lobe (more superior) and their upper limbs in the posterior lobe (more inferior). Long-term use of alcohol tends to preferentially damage the anterior lobe and leads to problems with the lower limb. Thus gate and balance are affected. Posterior lobe syndrome on the other hand tends to preferentially affect the upper limb. For example, planned movements with the forearm and hand (Fig. 15.12).

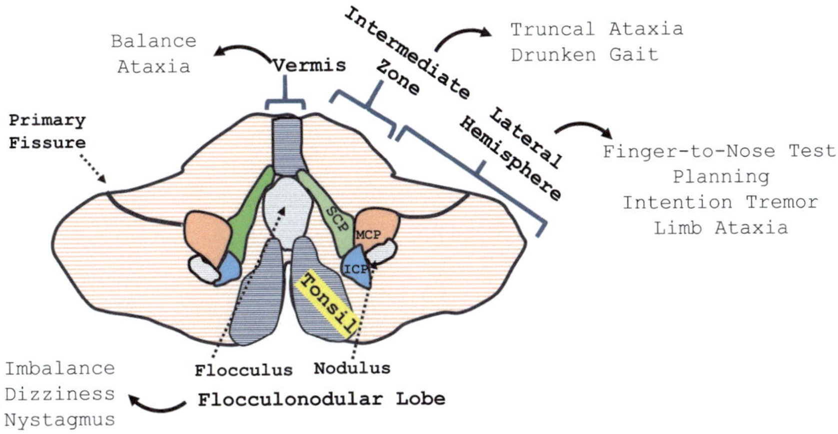

Fig. 15.12 Cerebellar Lesions and Symptoms

Further Reading

1. Afifi AK, Bergman RA. Functional neuroanatomy: text and atlas. McGraw-Hill; 1998.
2. Bally J, Megevan P, Nguyen D, Landis T, Granziera C. Crossed ataxia. Stroke. 2011;42(11):e571–3.
3. Brazis PW, Masdeu JC, Biller J. Localization in clinical neurology. LWW; 2016.
4. Blumenfeld H. Neuroanatomy through clinical cases. 2nd ed. Wiley-Blackwell; 2010.
5. Campbell, W., and Barohn, R.J. Dejong's the neurological examination, LWW; 2019.
6. Carpenter M. Core text of neuroanatomy. New York: Williams and Wilkins; 1991.
7. Choi SM. Movement disorders following cerebrovascular lesions in cerebellar circuits. J Move Disorders. 2016;9(2):80–8.
8. Fuller G. Neurological examination made easy. 6th ed. Elsevier; 2019.
9. Goldberg S. Clinical anatomy made ridiculously simple. MedMaster; 1991.
10. Goldberg S. Clinical neuroanatomy made ridiculously simple. MedMaster; 2002.
11. Gruol DL, Koibuchi N, Manto M, Molinari M, Schmahmann JD, Seng Y. Essentials of cerebellum and cerebellar disorders: a primer for graduate students. Springer; 2016.
12. Leo J. Medical Neuroanatomy for the boards and clinic: Finding the Lesion. 6th ed. Switzerland; 2024.
13. Leo J. Clinical anatomy and embryology: a guide for the classroom, clinic, and clinic. 2nd ed; 2024.
14. Splittgerber R. Snell's clinical neuroanatomy. 8th ed. Lippincott, Williams, and Wilkins; 2018.
15. Swanson PD. Signs and symptoms in neurology. Lippincott Williams and Wilkins; 1984.
16. Walker K. The Cerebellum. In: Walker HK, Hall WD, Hurst JW, editors. Clinical methods: the history, physical, and laboratory examinations. 3rd ed. Boston: Butterworths; 1990. p. 356–9.
17. Yaknitsa V, Barmack NH. Topsy turvy: functions of climbing and mossy fibers in the Vestibulo-Cerebellum. Neuroscientist. 2011;17(2):221–36.
18. Young PA, Young PH, Tolbert D. Basic clinical neuroscience. LLW; 2015.

Basal Ganglia Lesions 16

Introduction

The term "basal ganglia" refers to a group of subcortical structures that have long been known to be involved with movement. In the past two decades they have also been implicated in several psychiatric conditions. Before looking at the circuits it is helpful to look at the location of the nuclei and some of the terminology involved.

The term "striatum" refers to the caudate and putamen together. The two caudate nuclei have a large anteriorly located head which sits just lateral to the lateral ventricles. As you move posteriorly, the caudate becomes smaller such that the terminology changes a bit. As we move posteriorly, the head becomes the body, and the body then becomes the tail. The tail of the caudate loops down and around into the temporal lobe where it lies just superior to the inferior horn of the lateral ventricle (Fig. 16.1).

The putamen and globus together are referred to as the lenticular nucleus as they resemble a lens. Of the two, the putamen is more lateral, and the globus pallidus is more medial. The globus pallidus in turn can be subdivided into internal and external sections (sometimes referred to as medial and lateral). The putamen and globus pallidus together also look like something like a funnel with the wide part of the funnel being the putamen, and the point of the funnel being the medial globus pallidus which is nestled in at the genu of the internal capsule. The subthalamic nucleus sits just below the thalamus, and the substantia nigra is in the midbrain.

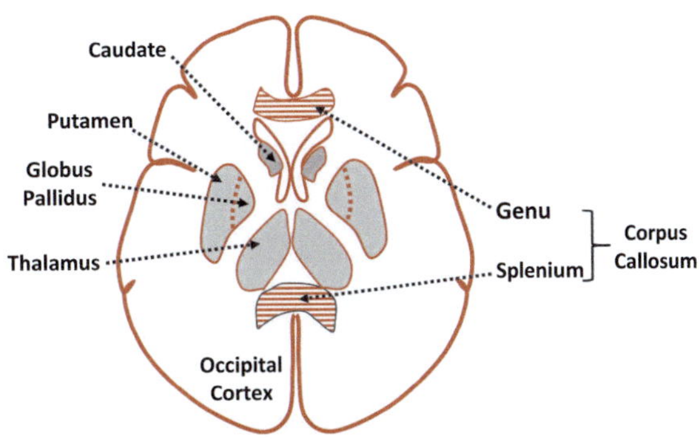

Fig. 16.1 Cross Section through Cerebral Cortex In this cross section one can see the caudate pushing into the lateral ventricle. You can also see the putamen and globus pallidus pushing in towards the genu of the internal capsule. Both the anterior and posterior limbs of the internal capsule can also be seen here [10]

J. Leo, *Gross Anatomy, Neuroanatomy, and Embryology for Medical Students*,
https://doi.org/10.1007/978-3-031-87151-1_16

Function

To move your hand, your corticospinal tract fires—like stepping on the car's gas pedal. However, when your hand is at rest and not moving, think of a parking brake which is "On" and keeping your hand at rest. The basal ganglia is the parking brake. When it comes time to move your hand, milliseconds before the movement, you need to turn the brake "Off." The following schematics focus on how we turn the brake on or off. Lesions in the basal ganglia can disrupt the break and lead to tremors (Fig. 16.2).

The picture above (Fig. 16.2) is a simplistic picture showing the two main categories of basal ganglia diseases. Think of a movement on a spectrum, with normal movement in the midline. At the far-right end there are hyperkinetic disorders, such as Huntington's Chorea. These patients have too much movement. At the other end, to the left, are hypokinetic disorders such as Parkinson's. These patients have a paucity of movement—either bradykinesia (slower movements) or akinesia (fewer movements).

To think about the braking action of the basal ganglia it is useful to start with symptoms and work back to the basal ganglia. Take a Huntington's patient who has a tremor at rest, they are hyperkinetic and have too much movement. This means that their cortex is overactive, and since the cortex is controlled by the thalamus, the thalamus is also overactive. This means that the brake, or the basal ganglia is underactive—it is "Off."

On the other end of the spectrum, take the Parkinson's patient with not enough movement, who is stuck, or frozen. It makes sense that their cortex is underactive, which in turn means that their thalamus is underactive, which then means that their brake—the basal ganglia—is stuck in the "On" position and cannot be relaxed. There are three neurotransmitters that play a role in normal and pathological functioning of the basal ganglia: *Glutamate, GABA, and Dopamine*.

We can divide the basal ganglia circuit up into inputs and outputs. The input nuclei are the caudate and putamen (together they are referred to as the striatum), which receive information from the cerebral cortex. The output nuclei which are really "the brake" are the internal globus pallidus and substantia nigra pars reticularis.

The major excitatory transmitter in this schematic is glutamate, and the major inhibitory transmitter is GABA. Between the input nuclei and the output nuclei are several internal loops, which is where the basal ganglia becomes complicated. The input nuclei talk to the output nuclei via two pathways, the direct and indirect.

The terms direct pathway and indirect pathways refer to the information coming out of the striatum (caudate and putamen) and projecting to "the brake"- the internal globus pallidus and the substantia nigra pars reticularis. The information coming out of striatum either goes "directly" to the brake, or "indirectly" via the external globus pallidus, to subthalamic nucleus, and then to the brake. If we look at the brake, we can see that the two pathways coming into it give us an "Off" switch and an "On" switch (Fig. 16.3).

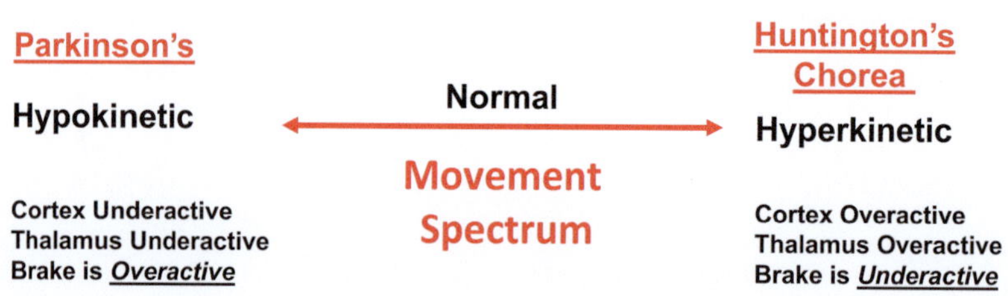

Fig. 16.2 Contrast of Parkinson's to Huntington's Chorea. Parkinson's is a hypokinetic disorder, while Huntington's Chorea is a hyperkinetic disorder. The "Brake" is both the globus pallidus internal and the substantia nigra pars reticulata. In the Parkinson's patient the brake is overactive or "on." In a Huntington's Chorea patient, the brake is underactive or "off" [10]

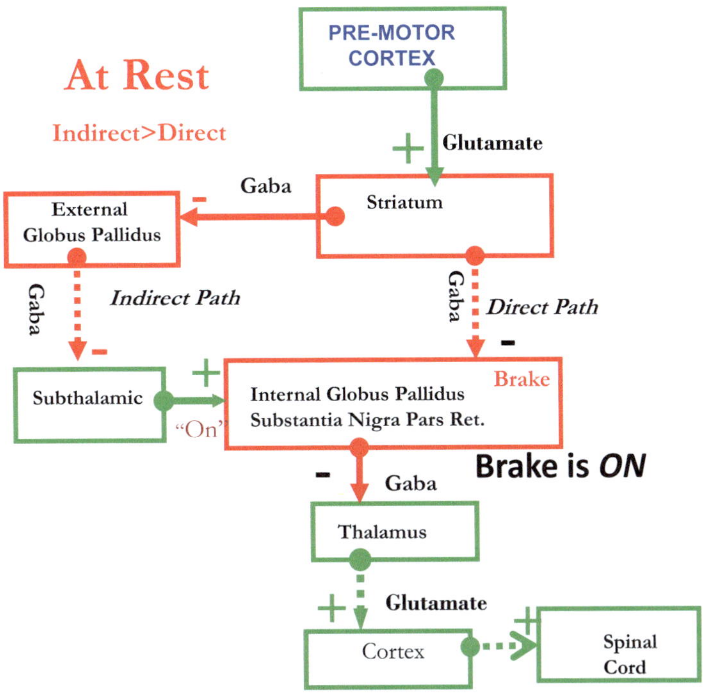

Fig. 16.3 Basal Ganglia Schematic. Shows the activity in the structures while the person is inactive [10]

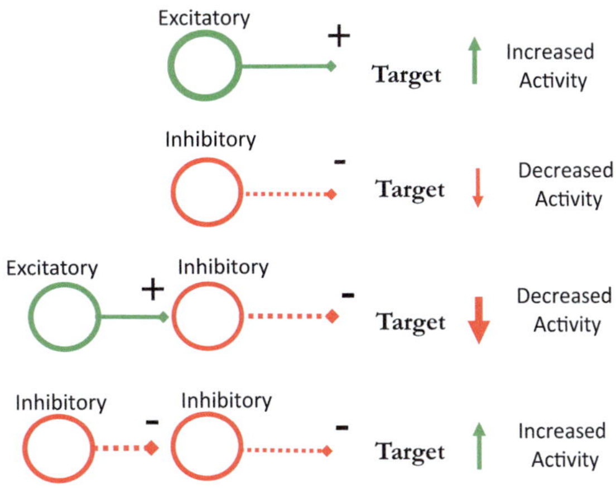

Fig. 16.4 Disinhibition. An excitatory neuron will increase activity in a target, an inhibitory neuron will decrease activity. An excitatory coming into an inhibitory neuron will decrease target activity. An inhibitory neuron projecting to an inhibitory results in an increase (disinhibition) in target activity [10]

Before proceeding, we need to digress for a moment and think about disinhibition, because there are several sites of disinhibition in these circuits. If we look at the image below, we can see that an excitatory input to a target, whether a gland or another neuron, will increase the activity in the target, while an inhibitory neuron will decrease the activity—this is all obvious. If we now add an excitatory coming to an inhibitory, then activity in the first neuron will also decrease the target activity. But with an inhibitory neuron projecting to another inhibitory neuron, it is not as obvious. When we increase the activity in the preganglionic inhibitory neuron, then we increase the inhibition on the postganglionic neuron, but this is an inhibitory neuron, so we increase the activity in the target (Fig. 16.4).

Start with the schematic of the basal ganglia when your hand is at rest. If we look at the brake, we clearly want that to be in the "On" position. Coming into the brake is an "On" switch from the indirect pathway—glutamate release from the subthalamic nucleus, and an "Off" switch from the direct side—a GABAergic projection from the caudate. In the case of the hand at rest, we want the "On" switch from the subthalamic to be active. Glutamate coming from the subthalamic will increase the activity of the internal globus pallidus/substantia nigra reticularis, which in turn is inhibitory (GABA) to the thalamus which reigns in the cortex, and corticospinal tract remains at rest.

When it comes time to move, the pathways flip-flop and the indirect side will prevail over the direct which will inhibit the brake and allow for movement.

Hemiballismus

The simplest lesion to discuss here is hemiballismus which is a wild flinging motion of the limbs due to a lesion—typically a stroke—of the subthalamic nucleus. If you take the subthalamic nucleus out of the equation, then the brake is "Off," the direct side is now overactive, and there is too much movement (Fig. 16.5).

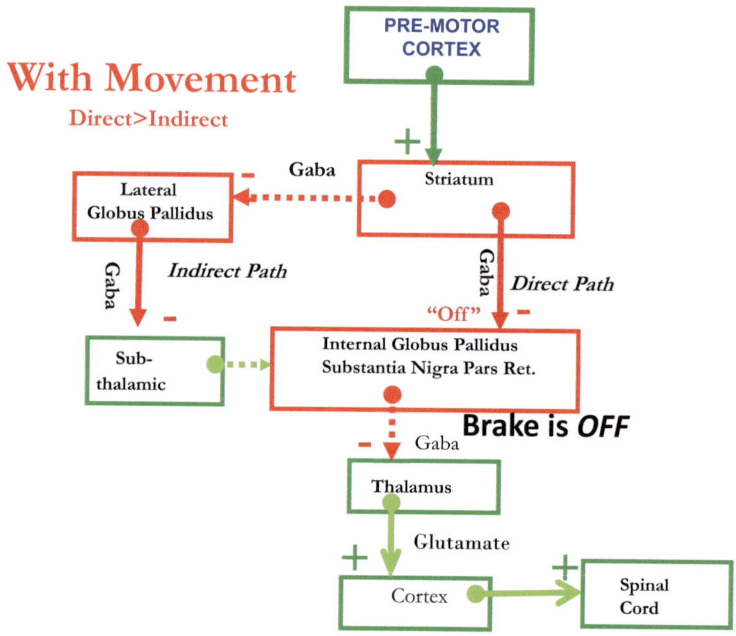

Fig. 16.5 Basal Ganglia Schematic. Shows the activity in the structures while the person is active [10]

Huntington's Chorea

In Huntington's there is a degeneration of the caudate nucleus that leads to a reduced output to the external globus pallidus. Thus, like hemiballismus, without the indirect pathwayx, the direct pathway takes over and there is too much movement—a hyperkinetic disorder (Figs. 16.6 and 16.7).

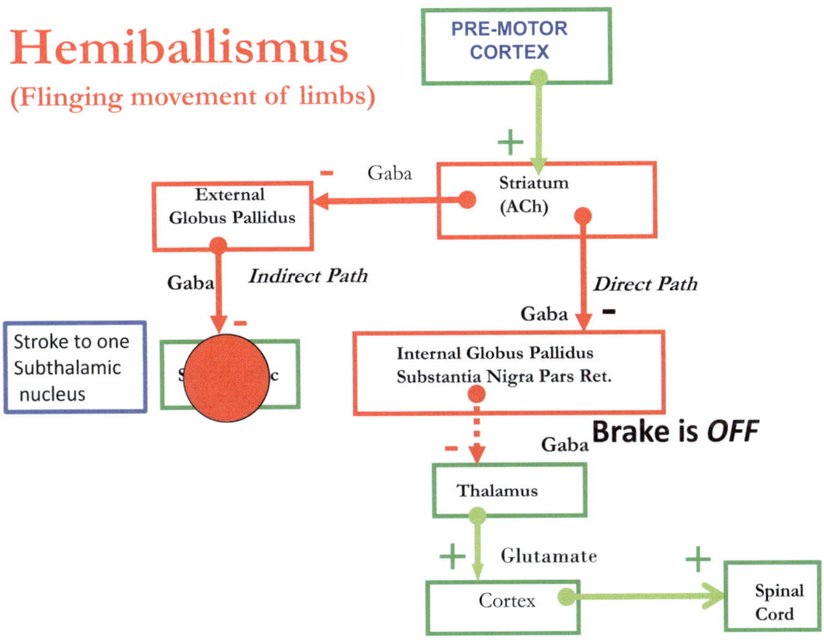

Fig. 16.6 Basal Ganglia Activity in Hyperkinetic Disorders. Shows the activity in various structures. In a patient with Hemiballismus following a stroke to the subthalamic nucleus

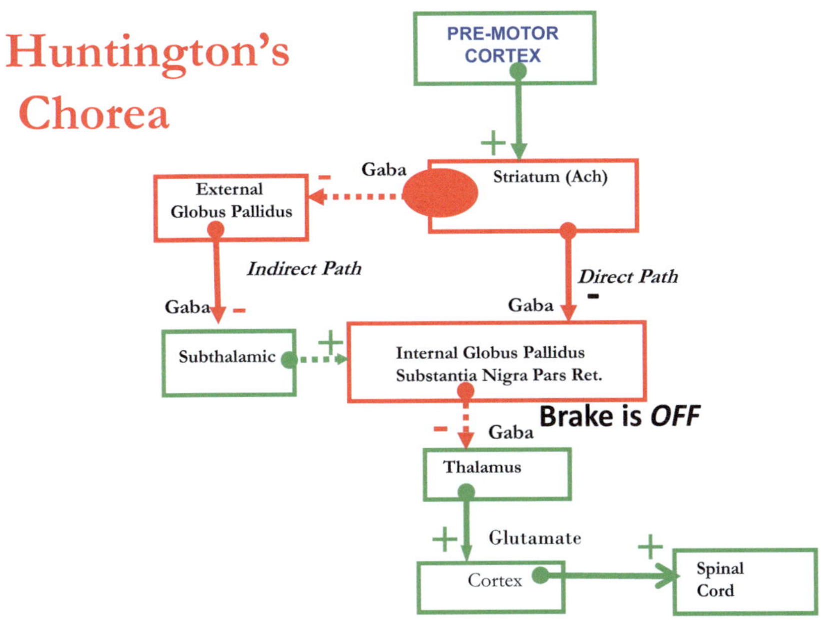

Fig. 16.7 Huntington's Chorea. Shows the activity in structures of a patient diagnosed with Huntington's chorea

Parkinson's Disease

To discuss Parkinson's disease, we need to introduce one other actor to the schematic—the substantia nigra pars compacta (SNpc). The SNpc has a dopaminergic projection to the striatum. Dopamine has two receptors—D1 and D2. The D2 receptors are located on the neuronal cell bodies of the cells in the striatum projecting as the indirect pathway. These D2 receptors are inhibitory. The D1 receptors on the other hand are located on the cell bodies of the neurons projecting out of the striatum as the direct pathway. These D1 receptors are excitatory (Figs. 16.6 and 16.8).

A loss of dopamine results in the indirect pathway being more active than the direct pathway so that the brake is stuck in the "on" position. This leads to the patient being frozen with a blank facial expression. The terminology can be confusing here. You will often here statements such as "dopamine drives movement" or that "dopamine increases the direct pathway." The wording here is confusing and needs an important clarification. While dopamine increases activity of the direct pathway, the direct pathway is inhibitory so when the activity in the direct path is increased, we are really increasing the inhibition. Or put another way, dopamine drives movement, but it does this by leading to more inhibition coming out of the direct pathway (Fig. 16.9).

The ideas presented in the schematic above for Parkinson's disease form the basis for neurosurgical attempts to reduce the motor symptoms in Parkinson's patients. If we start with the idea that cortical activity is reduced in Parkinson's, then the goal is to increase the cortical activity. Looking at the schematic, we see that the brake is overactive, making the internal globus pallidus the most likely culprit. A *medial pallidotomy*

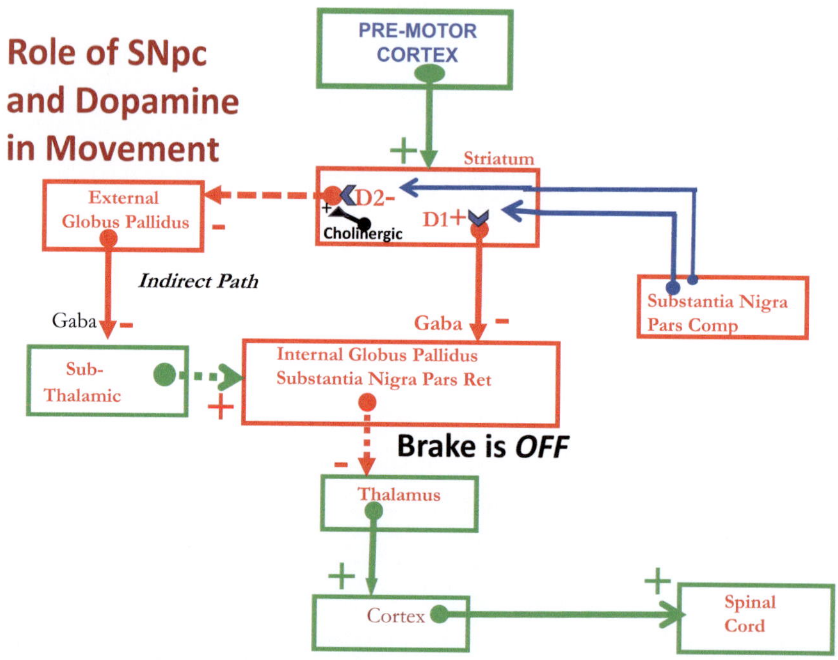

Fig. 16.8 Role of Substantia Nigra Pars Compacta in Movement. Cells of the striatum have 2 types of dopamine receptors: D1 and D2. The D1 receptors are excitatory while the D2 receptors are inhibitory. Cholinergics are excitatory [10]

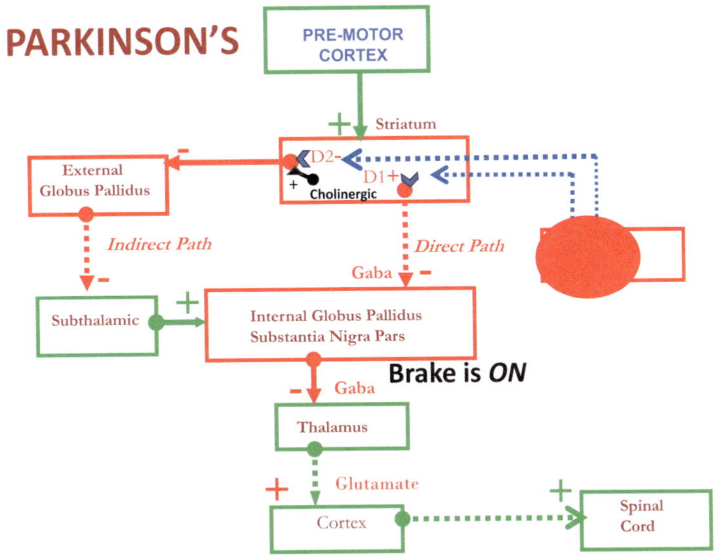

Fig. 16.9 Parkinson's symptoms result from lose of dopamine in substantia nigra pars compacta. (Based on Delong, 1990 [10])

involves ablation of the internal (medial) section of the globus pallidus to reduce the output of the brake and increase cortical activity. Besides ablation of the internal globus pallidus, deep brain stimulation of the subthalamic nucleus is also being used to increase cortical activity. The subthalamic nucleus projects to the internal globus pallidus and functions as "on switch" for the brake. By removing the "on switch" this leads to the brake decreasing its activity which in turn leads to an increase in cortical activity. The term deep brain stimulation can be confusing because the word "stimulation" seems to imply increasing the activity in the subthalamic nucleus when in fact, stimulation of the nucleus leads to a reduced output from the nucleus.

Acetylcholine and Parkinson's

Besides dopamine, when we talk about Parkinson's we need to look at acetylcholine. Within the caudate there are cholinergic interneurons that along with the dopaminergic cells synapse with the projection neurons coming out of the caudate. These cholinergics are excitatory so they have the opposite effects of dopamine. If dopamine is depleted, then the cholinergics in the system will exacerbate the Parkinson's symptoms. Thus, in addition to trying to increase dopamine levels, another line of pharmacotherapy is to block acetylcholine (Fig. 16.10).

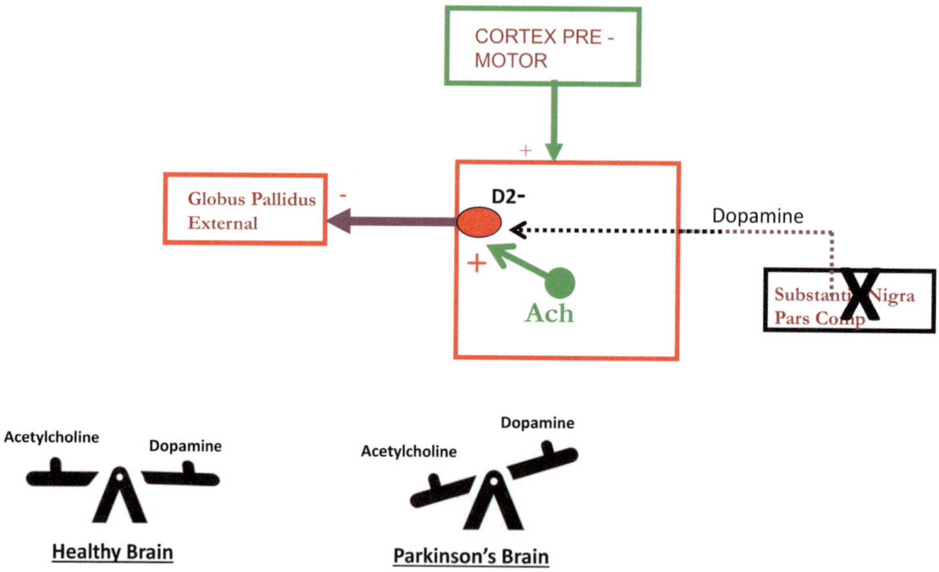

Fig. 16.10 Relationship of Acetylcholine and Dopamine in Caudate. In Parkinson's patients there is a deficit in dopamine coming from SNpC leading to an imbalance with acetylcholine [10]

Basal Ganglia and Cerebellum Together

Both the basal ganglia and the cerebellum project to the thalamus but there are some details and nuances that are important for understanding clinical scenarios.

Taking the basal ganglia first, the big picture is that the basal ganglia projects to the ipsilateral thalamus so a lesion to a single basal ganglia nucleus, a stroke to one caudate nucleus for instance, will lead to contralateral symptoms. Looking at the details of the basal ganglia output, the medial section of globus pallidus has two pathways coming out of it: (1) the ansa lenticularis, and (2) the lenticular fasciculus, both of when head to the ipsilateral ventral anterior nucleus of the thalamus.

Looking at the big picture of the cerebellum, it projects to the contralateral thalamus, so a lesion to the cerebellum or one of its peduncles will lead to symptoms on the ipsilateral side of the body. The details of this pathway are that the output of the cerebellum is from the dentate nucleus to the contralateral ventral lateral nucleus of the thalamus—the dentatothalamic tract.

Both the output of the cerebellum and the basal ganglia come together as the thalamic fasciculus on their way to the thalamus (Fig. 16.11).

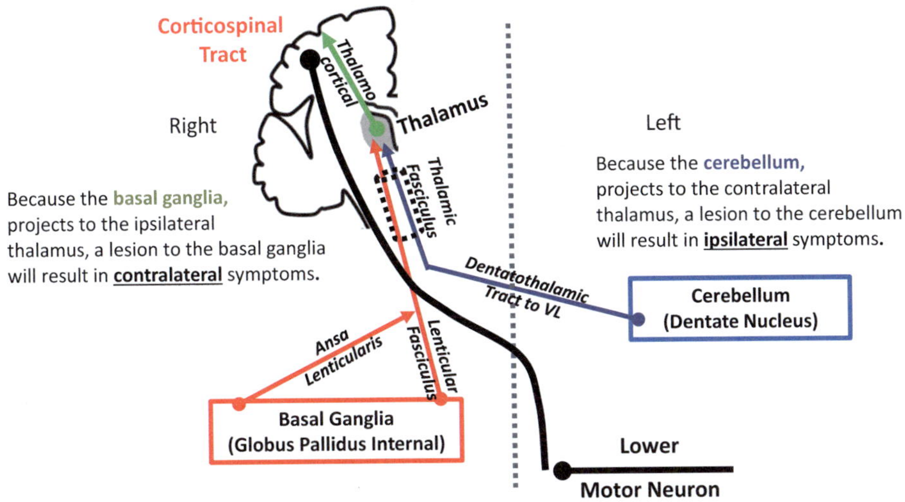

Fig. 16.11 Cerebellum and Basal Ganglia Lesions. The internal globose pallidus has two projections: the ansa lenticularis and the lenticular fasciculus which together join the thalamic fasciculus. Also joining the thalamic fasciculus is the dentatothalamic path from the dentate to the thalamus. Note the cerebellum projects to the contralateral thalamus (VL Nucleus), and the basal ganglia projects to the ipsilateral thalamus (VA Nucleus) [10]

Glabellar Reflex

Parkinson's patients may have a positive glabellar reflex (Myerson's Sign). When their glabella is tapped, they continue to blink their eyes. Healthy individuals will blink their eyes several times and then stop, while the Parkinson's patient will keep blinking for a much longer time.

Wilson's Disease

Wilson's disease, also known as hepatolenticular degeneration, is due to a genetic defect that leads to a pathological build-up of copper in the body. It usually presents in the mid-twenties to thirties. In the liver the copper build-up leads to cirrhosis; in the eye it leads to a build-up on the inner surface of the cornea and results in Kayser-Fleischer rings; and in the brain excess copper produces lesions in the putamen and globous pallidus. Wilson's patients have a characteristic wing-beating tremor, rigidity, and mental deterioration.

Various Basal Ganglia Pathology

Methanol poisoning attacks the putamen, optic nerves, and retina. Carbon monoxide poisoning is thought to damage the globus pallidus (although this is controversial). A stroke to one caudate nucleus will lead to chorea symptoms on the contralateral side of the body. Tourette's syndrome which is characterized as excessive speech and wild flinging movements of the limbs is thought to related to a hyperkinetic disorder with pathology in the indirect pathway—the brake is off.

The Table 16.1 shows the changes in various structures in Huntington's and Parkinson's patients. Words of warning: Do not panic at the sight of this table. There are certain facts in neuroanatomy that you should remember for the rest of your career, such as the meaning of Babinski's sign. If I tap you on the shoulder twenty years from now and ask you the meaning of Babinski's sign, then you should be able to rattle it off without thinking about it. This summary table of the basal ganglia table is not like that. No one expects you thirty years from now to remember what

Table 16.1 Summary of changes to Basal Ganglia structures in Parkinson's and Huntington's patients

	Parkinson's	Huntington's
Clinical presentation	Hypokinetic (Overstabilization)	Hyperkinetic (tremor)
Cortex	Underactive	Overactive
Thalamus	Underactive	Overactive
GPI and SNpr (brake)	Overactive, more inhibition	Underactive, less inhibition
Subthalamic (turns brake on	Overactive	Underactive
GP external	Underactive, less inhibition	Overactive, more inhibition
Caudate/putamen	Decreased activity	Deficit (weakened projection to GP external)
SNpc	Dopamine deficit	

exactly happens to the internal section of globus pallidus in Huntington's patients—unless you are a neurologist. Rather, I would look at the direct and indirect pathways with the table in front of you and compare what happens in these two patients. Make sure everything makes sense.

Further Reading

1. Adam EM, Brown EN, McCarthy M. Deep brain stimulation in the subthalamic nucleus for Parkinson's disease can restore dynamics of striatal networks. PNAS. 2022;119(19):e2120808119.
2. Afifi AK, Bergman RA. Functional neuroanatomy: text and atlas. McGraw-Hill; 1998.
3. Blumenfeld H. Neuroanatomy through clinical cases. 2nd ed. Wiley-Blackwell; 2010.
4. Brazis PW, Masdeu JC, Biller J. Localization in clinical neurology. LWW; 2016.
5. Calabresi P, Picconi B, Tozzi A, Ghiglieri V, Filippo DM. Direct and indirect pathways of basal ganglia: a critical appraisal. Nat Neuro. 2014;17(8):1022–30.
6. Campbell W, Barohn RJ. Dejong's The neurological examination. LWW; 2019.
7. Delon MR. Primate models of movement disorders of basal ganglia disorders. Trends Neuro. 1990;13(7):281–5.
8. Delong MR, Wichmann T. Circuits and circuit disorders of the basal ganglia. Arch Neurol. 2007;64(1):20–4.
9. Fuller G. Neurological examination made easy. 6th ed. Elsevier; 2019.
10. Leo J. Medical neuroanatomy for the boards and clinic: finding the lesion. 2nd ed. Switzerland: Springer; 2024.
11. Leo J. Clinical anatomy and embryology: a guide for the classroom, clinic, and clinic. 2nd ed. Springer; 2024.
12. Splittgerber R. Snell's clinical neuroanatomy. 8th ed. Lippincott, Williams, and Wilkins; 2018.
13. Swanson PD. Signs and symptoms in neurology. Lippincott Williams and Wilkins; 1984.
14. Utter A, Basso W. The basal ganglia: an overview of circuits and function. Neuroscience Behavioral Rev. 2008;32(3):333–42.
15. Wichmann T, DeLong M. Deep brain stimulation for movement disorders of basal ganglia origin: restoring function of functionality. Neurotherapeutics. 2016;13:264–83.
16. Young, P. A., Young, P.H., And Tolbert, D. Basic clinical neuroscience, LLW; 2015.

Thalamus and Hypothalamus

17

Organization

The thalamus is an almond shaped structure sitting atop the brain stem and nestled in at the center of the cerebrum. It is often referred to as the doorway to the cortex as everything traveling up to the cortex, except olfaction, goes through the thalamus. Think of the thalamus as acting like a flashlight which allows you to focus on notable events in the environment, while ignoring non-important events. Imagine sitting in a coffee shop reading this book. There are all sorts of sensory inputs coming into your thalamus competing for the book's attention. There is the sound of people ordering; there is a cold breeze that comes and goes as someone opens the door; there is the smell of the coffee and other odors in the air; and there are all types of interesting people coming and going into and out of your visual fields. All this information is flooding your thalamus, but you want to pay attention to what you are reading. Your thalamus, like a flashlight, focuses on the page in front of you and tries to ignore all the other sensory inputs. If someone comes rushing into the front door yelling, then your thalamus, or flashlight, is going to change its focus and shift its focus to the person yelling in the doorway.

Circuits

To diagram the thalamus, in the accompanying figure we are going to pull out the thalamus from the cerebral cortex and enlarge it. Running down the middle of the thalamus is a white-matter-bundle called the internal medullary lamina. It forms a Y shape at its anterior portion. Tucked in at the Y is the anterior nucleus of the thalamus which is involved with the limbic system. Along the medial side is the **Dorsomedial (DM) Nucleus**, on the lateral side we have several nuclei. Going from anterior to posterior we have **Ventral Anterior (VA), Ventral Lateral (VL), Ventral Posterior** divided into **Ventral Posterior Medial (VPM)** and **Ventral Posterior Lateral (VPL)**, and **Pulvinar (PUV).** Hanging off the back of the pulvinar are two knobs, the **Lateral Geniculate Body (LGB)** and the **Medial Geniculate Body (MGB)** (Fig. 17.1).

Each of these nuclei has an input coming from a different region of the nervous system, and a corresponding projection to a specific region of the cerebral cortex (Fig. 17.1). Starting with the ventral tier, the first nucleus is the ventral anterior nucleus (VA). The VA receives information from the basal ganglia, and projects to the premotor

J. Leo, *Gross Anatomy, Neuroanatomy, and Embryology for Medical Students*,
https://doi.org/10.1007/978-3-031-87151-1_17

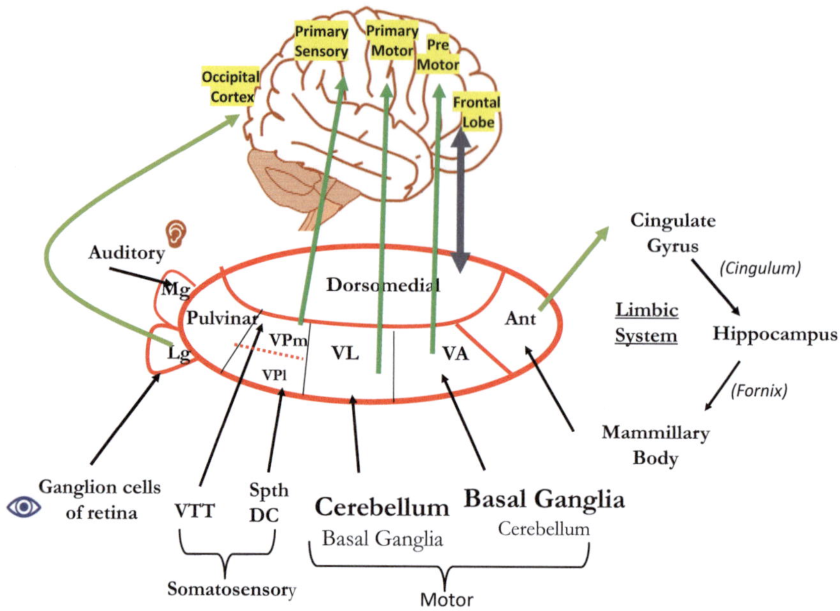

Fig. 17.1 Overview of Thalamic Connections [13]

cortex. Right next to the VA is the ventral lateral nucleus (VL) which receives information from the cerebellum and projects to the primary motor cortex—the precentral gyrus. It makes sense for the basal ganglia to project via the VA to the premotor cortex, when you consider that the VA is involved with taking the brake "Off" several milliseconds before you move. Likewise, it makes sense that the cerebellum via the VL projects to the precentral gyrus since it is involved with ongoing movement. Together, the VA and VL are often referred to as the motor thalamus. Note that while the VA receives most of its information from the basal ganglia, it also receives some information from the cerebellum. Likewise, the VL receives most of its information from the cerebellum, but it also receives some of its information from the basal ganglia.

Next in line are the VPM and VPL which receive the somatosensory information from the face and limbs. The spinothalamic and dorsal column/medial lemniscus pathways project to the VPL, while the ventral trigeminothalamic tract (VTT), coming from the trigeminal system, projects to the VPM. The VPL and VPM in turn project to the limb and face areas of the primary sensory cortex—postcentral gyrus. At the front of the thalamus is the anterior nucleus which is part of Papez's circuit and is discussed in the chapter on the limbic system.

The pulvinar nucleus is a catch-all nucleus for receiving information from various association areas. Not to downplay its function but it does not play a prominent role when it comes to understanding the various lesions. The lateral geniculate body (LGB) receives information from the retina, or more specifically the ganglion cells of the retina, and in turn projects to the occipital cortex. The medial geniculate body (MGB) receives information from the lateral lemniscus and is discussed with the auditory pathways. The dorsal medial nucleus is the largest thalamic nucleus, and it talks to the frontal and limbic lobes. It is also discussed more in those two chapters.

Thalamic Pain Syndrome

The most important clinical scenario with the thalamus involves a lesion to the VPL and VPM. Both these nuclei receive blood from the thalamogeniculate arteries. The thalamogeniculate arteries come off the P2 segment of the posterior cerebral. The thalamoperforating come off the P1 segment. A stroke in this region will lead to *Thalamic Pain Syndrome*, also called *Dejeurne-Rossy Syndrome*. The initial symptom will be a loss of somatosensory sensation to the contralateral side of the body. However, after several days the patient will report excruciating pain emanating from the contralateral side of the body. Pain relievers will typically not relieve the patient's symptoms.

Reticular Nucleus

The reticular nucleus is a thin layer of cells surrounding the thalamus and running from anterior to posterior. If you think of the thalamus as an egg, the reticular nucleus is something like the eggshell surrounding the egg—although the eggshell only goes around one half of the egg. Some scientists have suggested that the function of the reticular nucleus is like a security guard selectively allowing information to go onto the cerebral cortex. Because it is so thin it is hard to study the reticular nucleus, and it is hard to relate it to a distinct clinical scenario, but it has been implicated in ADHD (Fig. 17.2).

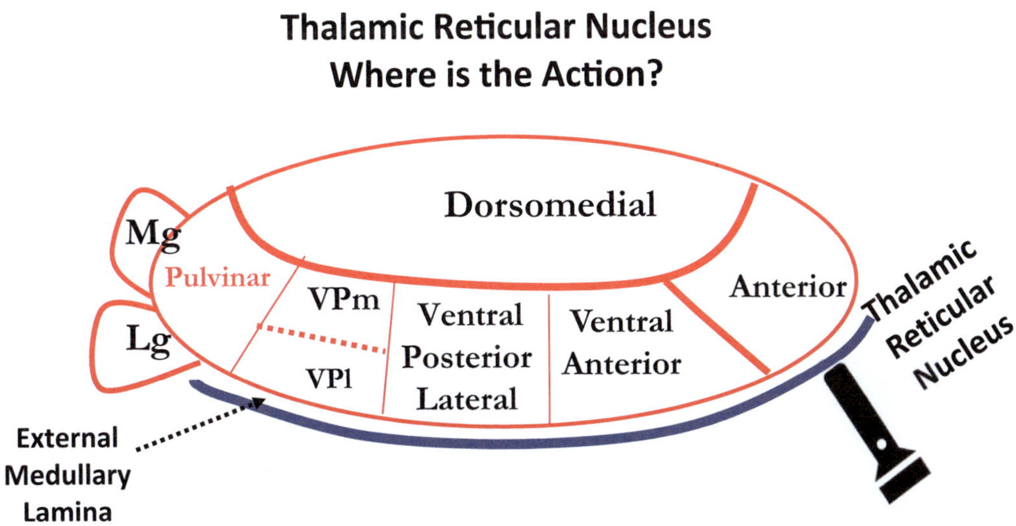

Fig. 17.2 Thalamic Reticular Nucleus. The thalamic reticular nucleus runs from anterior to posterior on the lateral side of the thalamus resembling an eggshell. Some have suggested that it functions like a flashlight allowing an individual to focus on the most important sensory information coming into the thalamus [13]

Internal Capsule and Lacunar Infarcts

Sitting just medial to the thalamus is the internal capsule. The ascending and descending fibers to and from the cerebral cortex travel through the internal capsule which on horizontal section is V-shaped. The most important parts are the genu and posterior limb. The genu carries corticobulbar fibers destined for the cranial nerve nuclei, while the posterior limb carries corticospinal fibers (Fig. 17.3).

The easiest way to talk about the organization of the genu and posterior limb of the internal capsule is to draw a stick figure with the head at the genu and the upper and lower limbs coming back into the posterior limb. Nestled in, medial to the posterior limb, is the thalamus. At the back of the thalamus are the medial and lateral geniculate bodies. The medial geniculate body has fibers that head to the temporal lobe by going deep to the internal capsule—sublenticular. Lesions to this sublenticular portion can lead to auditory deficits. The lateral geniculate body has fibers that go behind (posterior) to the internal capsule—retrolenticular. Lesions here can lead to a homonymous hemianopia or quadrantanopia.

The anterior limb of the internal capsule contains connections from the frontal lobe to the pontine nuclei. Lesions to the anterior limb can result in deficits with higher cortical processing such as abulia, confusion, and agitation.

The internal capsule is especially susceptible to lacunar infarcts. The small vessels perfusing this region come off much wider arteries. In a hypertensive patient, these small arteries are under enormous pressure—imagine turning on a garden hose and winding down the spray nozzle to a pinhole so that the water coming out is a high-pressure jet. Strokes in this area will lead to small areas of pathology—resembling a small lake—right around the compromised vessel.

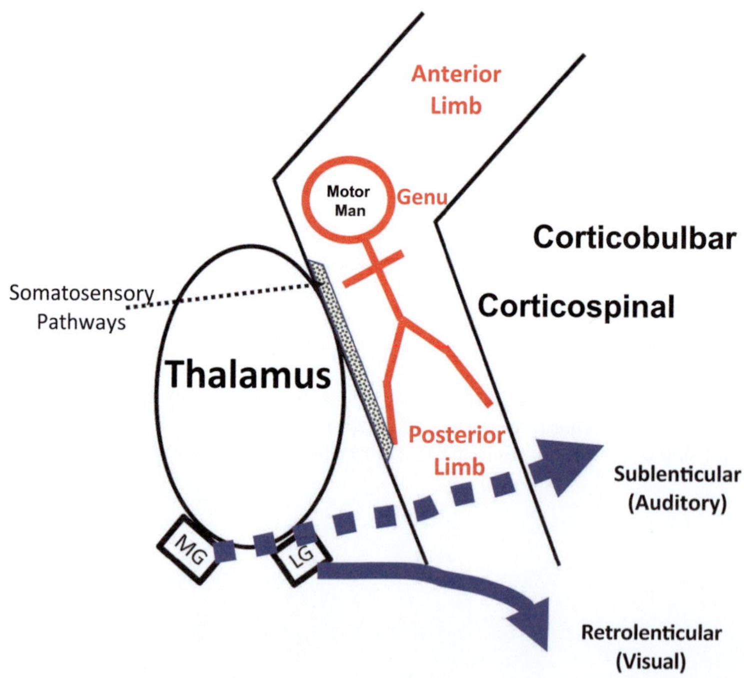

Fig. 17.3 Internal Capsule. The posterior limb of the internal capsule sits just lateral to the thalamus. Note that the corticobulbar fibers are in the genu, while the corticospinal fibers (Motor Man) are in the posterior limb. The sensory tracts are a small strip located just lateral to the thalamus [13]

Lateral Striate Arteries

There are several potential lesions in the internal capsule and thalamus which can lead to various syndromes (Fig. 17.4). Lesions limited to the posterior limb can lead to "pure motor deficits" which are characterized by only motor symptoms, usually due to small infarcts in hypertensive individuals of the lateral striate arteries. The initial stroke might only lead to symptoms in one part of the body, say the upper limbs. But over time it is quite possible that more of these small arteries become involved with more parts of the body affected. Note that bilateral lesions to the thalamus can result in coma. Lesions to the genu can sometimes result in dysarthria-clumsy hand syndrome which results from damage to the corticobulbar tract leading to weakness of the facial, laryngeal, and pharyngeal muscles (dysarthria and dysphagia), plus corticospinal input to the cervical cord which leads to weakness of the hands.

A lesion in the internal capsule will damage the UMNs, but it will spare tracts in the spinal cord that are more involved with involuntary movements—such as the reticulospinal and vestibulospinal tracts. These patients with "capsular degeneration" will have some rudimentary movements. With their shoulder muscles, they can maneuver their upper limbs towards a kitchen shelf, but they cannot grab the can. When they walk, they will have a hemiplegic gait, where the lower limb on the affected side swings out to the side in a circumduction movement so that the toes clear the ground. The upper limb is crossed over the body (Fig. 17.5).

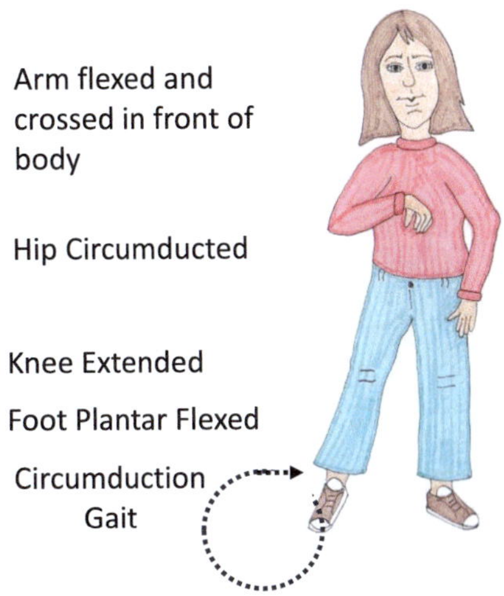

Fig. 17.5 Hemiplegia from Internal Capsule Lesion. Regarding the limbs, the deficit is more severe the farther out on the limb one goes. The hands and feet are more severely affected than the shoulder and hip regions. She will swing her right lower limb when she walks (a circumduction gate). (Strube 2024)

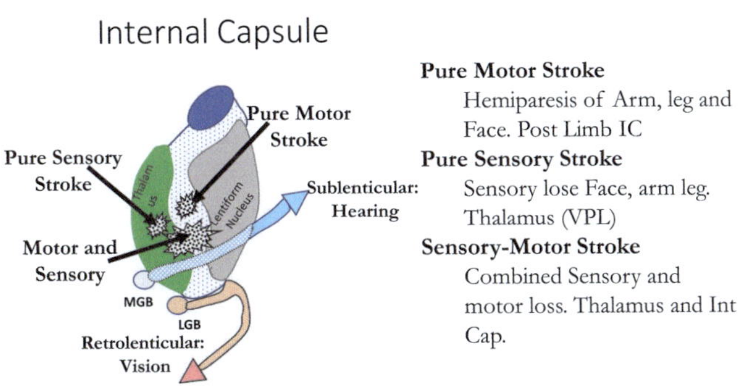

Fig. 17.4 Lacunar Infarcts. There are three common scenarios for lacunar infarcts in the vicinity of the internal capsule. (1) Pure motor stroke = posterior limb of internal capsule, (2) Pure sensory stroke = thalamus and adjacent sensory fibers, (3) Sensory-Motor Stroke = posterior limb of internal capsule and thalamus [13]

Thalamogeniculate Arteries

In a patient with a pure sensory deficit, such as thalamic pain syndrome, one location is in the thalamus, which would typically be due to deficits of the thalamogeniculate arteries. The lesion might also be to the thin strip of sensory fibers on the lateral edge of the thalamus (Fig. 17.6 and Table 17.1).

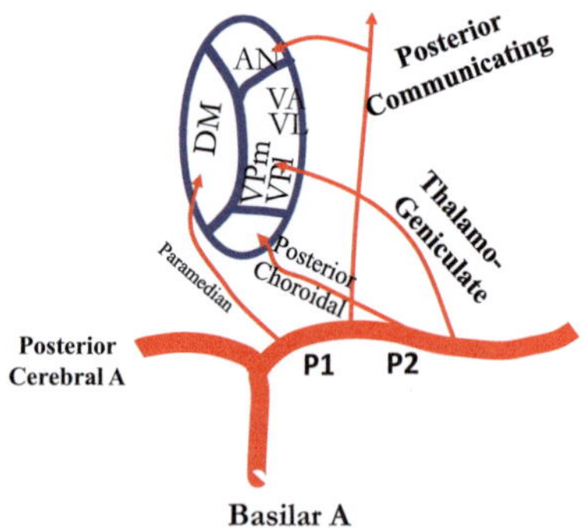

Fig. 17.6 Blood Supply to Thalamus. The thalamogeniculate arteries arise from the posterior cerebral artery and supply the ventral posterior medial (VPM) and the ventral posterior lateral (VPL) nuclei of the thalamus [13]

Artery of Percheron and Coma

Bilateral lesions to the thalamus are rare, but one cause for this scenario is a stroke to the artery of Percheron. In some individuals, the artery to the posterior median portion of the thalamus comes off as a single branch of P1. This single branch called the artery of Percheron quickly divides so that it perfuses both sides of the posterior median section of the thalamus. An infarct in this artery can result in a comatose patient.

Anterior Choroidal Arteries

Although it is rare, and the symptoms can vary from one patient to another, strokes to the anterior choroidal artery can compromise blood flow to the cerebral peduncle and the optic tract. Thus, the patient can have contralateral hemiplegia, and contralateral homonymous hemianopia. In some scenarios the thalamus can also be involved in which case the patients would have contralateral sensory deficits (Table 17.1).

Table 17.1 Lacunar Infarcts: subtypes

Syndrome	Artery	Symptoms
Pure motor hemiparesis Posterior limb IC	Lateral striate A.	Hemiparesis of upper and lower limb and face
Pure sensory syndrome VPL and VPM of thalamus	Thalamogeniculate A.	Sensory loss on face, arm leg
Sensory-motor stroke Both IC and thalamus	Anterior choroidal A	Sensory and motor deficits on contralateral side

Hypothalamus and Pituitary

The hypothalamus is part of the diencephalon and is situated on either side of the third ventricle, with the hypothalamic sulcus above it, and the optic chiasm just below it. The hypothalamus is divided into several different nuclei that play roles in maintaining homeostasis, such as temperature regulation, and various behaviors, such as eating. In some cases, the nuclei tend to blend in with each other and there are no perfect landmarks for dividing it up. However, when neuroanatomists talk about the divisions, they are referring to either an anterior to posterior organization or a medial to lateral organization.

Starting with a coronal cut through the anterior portion, known as the supraoptic region, the obvious landmark is the optic chiasm. Sitting above the chiasm are the appropriately named supraoptic and suprachiasmatic nuclei. Moving posterior, to about the midline of the hypothalamus, is the tuberal region, containing the dorsomedial and ventromedial nuclei, also appropriately named. And along the floor of the third ventricle is the arcuate nucleus. Continuing posteriorly is the mamillary region with the mamillary bodies.

Note the fornix is the outflow tract of the hippocampus and it is visible in cuts through the middle and the posterior sections—the fornix is a landmark for diving the thalamus into medial and lateral regions. The base of the hypothalamus is the median eminence which sits just above the first capillary bed of the hypophyseal portal system (Fig. 17.7).

Hanging off the base of the hypothalamus is the pituitary gland which is divided into the anterior lobe (adenohypophysis) and posterior lobe (neurohypophysis). Both the anterior and posterior lobes arise from ectoderm, but they come from different regions of the ectoderm. The posterior lobe arises from the neural ectoderm, and the anterior lobe arises from the ectodermal tissue at the top of the oral cavity, which is referred to as Rathke's pouch. Knowing the different embryological origins of the two lobes helps to explain how the hypothalamus communicates with each lobe.

The pituitary stalk is formed by contributions from both the anterior and posterior lobes. The pars tuberalis comes from the anterior lobe and partially engulfs the pars infundibularis which comes from the posterior lobe. Running through the pars infundibularis are the axons from the supraoptic and paraventricular nuclei running from the hypothalamus down into the posterior pituitary.

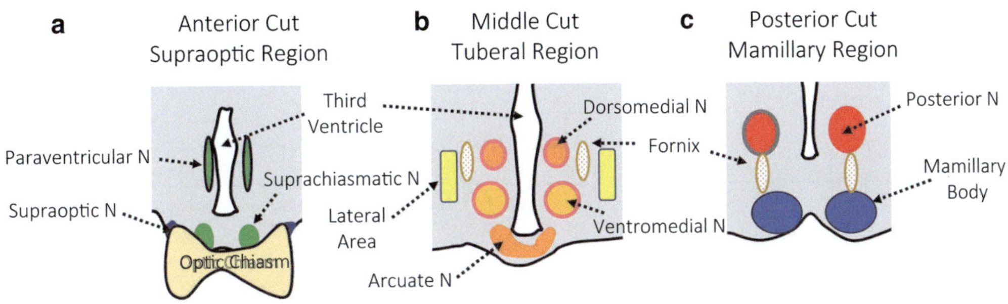

Fig. 17.7 Anterior/Posterior View of Hypothalamus. There are three coronal cuts moving anterior to posterior through the hypothalamus. Panel **(a)** is through the supraoptic region with the supraoptic and suprachiasmatic nuclei sitting above the optic chiasm. Panel **(b)** is through the tuberal region with the arcuate, dorsomedial, and ventromedial nuclei, plus the fornix. Lateral to the fornix is the lateral area. Panel **(c)** is through the mamillary bodies and the posterior nucleus. Entering the mamillary bodies is the fornix carrying fibers from the hippocampus [13]

The Anterior Pituitary and Hypophyseal Portal System

The hypophyseal portal system is a portal system, thus there are two in-line capillary beds. The system starts with the superior hypophyseal artery which enters the median eminence and breaks up into the first capillary bed. Right above this capillary bed are the neurosecretory cells which release inhibiting or releasing hormones into the blood system at this first capillary bed. From here the hormones travel on the portal veins to the second capillary bed which is in the anterior pituitary. In the anterior pituitary, there are cells (chromophils) that respond to these releasing and inhibiting hormones which in turn secrete several different hormones themselves such as: adrenocorticotropic hormone (ACTH), thyroid stimulating hormone (TSH), growth hormone (GH), follicle-stimulating hormone (FSH), and luteinizing hormone (LH). Note that the cells that secrete these hormones do not receive a direct neuronal input; instead, they are triggered by inhibiting or releasing hormones in the blood stream (Fig. 17.8).

Posterior Pituitary

The posterior pituitary is noticeably different. There are cells in the hypothalamus with large nuclei, referred to as *magnocellular neurons*, which send fibers from the hypothalamus directly down into the posterior pituitary. These neurons store their hormones in *herring bodies*. They release their contents in response to various stimuli directly into the blood stream. There are two nuclei that send fibers down into the posterior lobe: (1) the *supraoptic nucleus* secretes ADH which playsa role in the regulation or water content and thus blood pressure, and (2) the *paraventricular nucleus* secretes oxytocin which causes contractions in the myoepithelial cells in the mammary tissue and contractions of the uterus (Fig. 17.8).

Pathology of the posterior pituitary, such as a pituitary adenoma or a craniopharyngioma, can lead to diabetes insipidus and the syndrome of inappropriate ADH secretion.

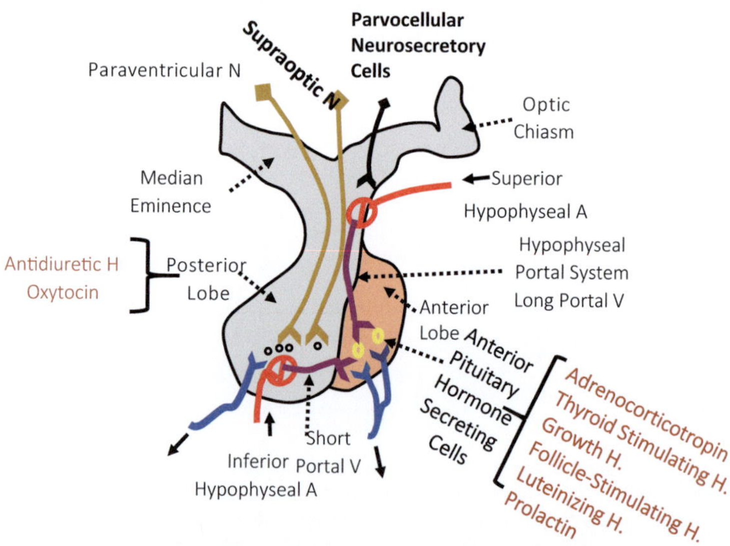

Fig. 17.8 Pituitary. The hypophyseal portal system starts with the superior hypophyseal artery which has a capillary bed in the median eminence. From there the portal veins continue to the anterior lobe. Neurosecretory cells release inhibiting or releasing hormones into the portal system which then travel to the cells (acidophiles and basophiles) in the anterior pituitary to release hormones into the blood stream [13]

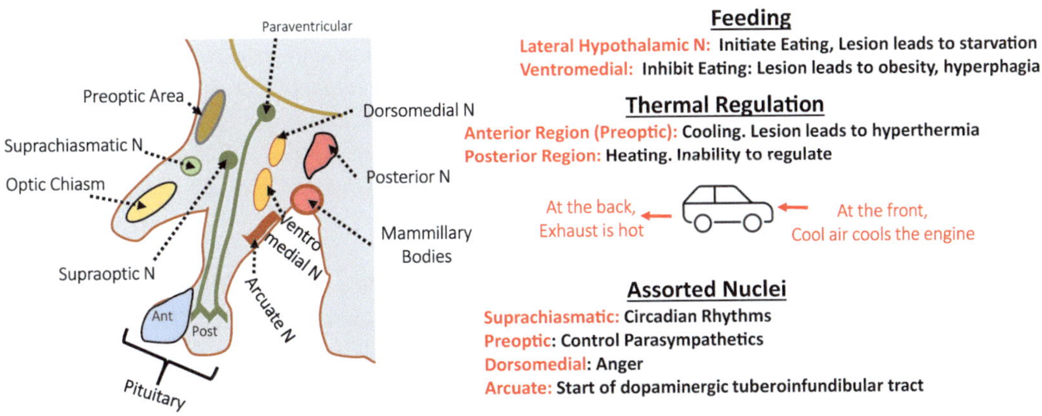

Fig. 17.9 Hypothalamus. The figure and table shows the main hypothalamic nuclei and their functions. The car icon is to jog your memory for temperature regulation. The front of the car is driving into the wind and getting cooler, while the hot exhaust is coming out the rear of the car [13]

Thermal Regulation

The hypothalamus plays an important role in heating and cooling the body. The preoptic nucleus, located in the anterior region of the hypothalamus, senses the internal temperature, and then sends a signal to the posterior hypothalamus via the median forebrain bundle. The posterior hypothalamus then sends signals to elicit the appropriate response such as either vasodilation or vasoconstriction. The preoptic nucleus is thought to be the "thermoregulatory center." Injuries to the hypothalamus from trauma or surgery can lead to hyperthermia or hypothermia in the patient (Fig. 17.9).

Appetite Control

Several hypothalamic nuclei are involved in appetite control. The *ventromedial nucleus,* (some books will call it the anteromedial) known as the satiety center, is thought to be responsible for inhibiting appetite—thus the saying, "stimulate the ven, get thin." It is responsible for parasympathetic control. Lesions in this nucleus lead can lead to excessive appetite and weight gain. On the other hand, the *lateral hypothalamic nucleus*, known as the hunger center, is thought to be involved with increased food consumption –thus the saying "stimulate the lat get fat." Lesions in this region lead to reduced intake. The lateral hypothalamus produces *orexin*, a peptide that is involved in both alertness and appetite. Deficits in orexin can lead to severe narcolepsy where the patient has drop attacks. The patient will suddenly lose muscle tone but not consciousness- like a possum faking death.

The *arcuate nucleus* is a control switch for appetite. Signals that the host is full or needs to eat are sent to the arcuate nucleus which in turn sends a signal to the appropriate hypothalamic nucleus to either eat or stop eating.

The suprachiasmatic nucleus has also been implicated in feeding behaviors because of its role in circadian rhythms and thus our eating patterns. The suprachiasmatic nucleus receives a direct input from the retina and is thought to be disrupted when we move from one time zone to another leading to jet lag.

Hypothalamus and Sympathetic Control

Hypothalamic activation of the sympathetic nervous system—such as rapid heart rate, sweating and rapid breathing—comes primarily from the dorsomedial nucleus and the parvocellular neurons of the paraventricular nucleus via descending fibers through the dorsal longitudinal fasciculus. The lateral hypothalamic area which is responsible for food intact, increase sympathetic activity.

Diabetes Insipidus

Patients with diabetes insipidus excrete copious amounts of dilute urine (polyuria), which in turn leads to a large increase in drinking fluids (polydipsia). In contrast to diabetes mellitus, the patient with diabetes insipidus has normal values for glucose in blood and urine. Diabetes insipidus results from disruptions, a lesion for instance, to the paraventricular and supraoptic nuclei, or to the neurons coming out of these nuclei.

Syndrome of Inappropriate Secretion of ADHD

This syndrome results from lesions to the supraoptic and paraventricular nuclei that lead to increased production of ADH, which leads to the patient increasing water retention. Symptoms include concentrated urine and a reduction of sodium in the blood. It can lead to hallucinations, seizures, or coma. It is sometimes associated with cancer, notably small cell lung cancer.

Case Studies

Case #1 A 65-year-old female presented to the emergency department with excreting pain emanating from the right side of her body. She reports that several days ago she had a loss of pain, temperature, and touch to the right side of her body but that this has turned into severe pain. She takes insulin for his diabetes, and atorvastatin for his hyperlipidemia. The pain is now disabling. Where is the lesion most likely located? The pain temperature and touch pathways are projecting to which thalamic nuclei?

The patient has diabetes and arteriosclerotic disease. She has suffered a stroke to the left VPL/VPM of the thalamus. The initial stroke led to a loss of sensation from the contralateral side (right side) of the body. Within several days it progressed to the typical thalamic pain syndrome presentation.

Case #2 A 70-year-old female with a history of hypertension presents to the ED complaining of difficulty walking. On the physical exam you note a left dense hemiplegia. She has no deficits with pain and temperature. When she is asked to smile, her left lower face is immobile. She understands questions, and her speech is articulate. Her pupils are equal, round, and reactive. Where is the lesion?

She has suffered from a lacunar infarct of the lateral striate arteries to the posterior limb of the internal capsule and genu on the right side. She has a pure motor deficit.

Further Reading

1. Afifi AK, Bergman RA. Functional neuroanatomy: text and atlas. McGraw-Hill; 1998.
2. Brazis PW, Masdeu JC, Biller J. Localization in clinical neurology. LWW; 2016.
3. Blumenfeld H. Neuroanatomy through clinical cases. 2nd ed. Wiley-Blackwell; 2010.
4. Bordes S, Werner C, Mathkour M, McCormack E, Iwanaga J, Loukas M, Lammle M, Dumont AS, Tubbs R. Arterial supply of the thalamus: a comprehensive review. World Neurosurg. 2020;137:310–8.
5. Brodal P. The central nervous system. 5th ed. New York: Oxford University Press; 2016.
6. Campbell, W., And Barohn, R.J. Dejong's the neurological examination, LWW; 2019.
7. Carpenter M. Core text of neuroanatomy. New York: Williams and Wilkins; 1991.
8. Cotman CW, McGaugh JL. The thalamus: partner to the cortex. In: Cotman CW, McGaugh JL, editors. Behavioral neuroscience. Elsevier; 1980.
9. Crick F. Function of the thalamic reticular complex: the searchlight hypothesis. Proc Natl Acad Sci. 1994;81:4586–90.

10. Fuller G. Neurological examination made easy. 6th ed. Elsevier; 2019.
11. Kultas-Ilinsky K, Ilinsky IA. Basal ganglia and thalamus in health and movement disorders. Kluwer Academic; 2001.
12. Leo J. Medical neuroanatomy for the boards and clinic: finding the lesion. 2nd ed. Switzerland: Springer; 2024.
13. Leo J. Clinical anatomy and embryology: a guide for the classroom, clinic, and clinic. 2nd ed. Springer; 2024.
14. Ropper M, Samuels M, Klein J, Prasad S. Adams and victor's principles of neurology. 12th ed. New York: McGraw Hill; 2023.
15. Schmahmann JD. Vascular syndromes of the thalamus. Stroke. 2003;34:2264–78.
16. Smith AB, Smirniotopoulis JG, Rushing EJ, Goldstein SJ. Bilateral thalamic lesions. Neuroradiology/head and neck. Imaging. 2009;192:W53–62.
17. Splittgerber R. Snell's clinical neuroanatomy. 8th ed. Lippincott, Williams, and Wilkins; 2018.
18. Swanson PD. Signs and symptoms in neurology. Lippincott Williams and Wilkins; 1984.
19. Young PA, Young PH, Tolbert D. Basic clinical neuroscience. LLW; 2015.

18 The Limbic Circuit, Learning, Memory, and How the Brain Works

Introduction

There are two main categories of memory: long term, and short term. Short term or working memory is what we use daily. Long term memory is divided into implicit and explicit memory. Implicit or procedural memory includes activities such as playing a sport or typing. While trying to memorize the names of drugs for an exam is an example of explicit memory, singing a song is an example of implicit memory.

Limbic Circuit

The limbic circuit, or Papez circuit, is a loop involving several sub cortical structures that are involved in memory and emotions. In 1937, James Papez proposed the idea that information from the hippocampus projects via the fornix to the mammillary bodies, then to the anterior nucleus of the thalamus via the mammillothalamic tract, then to the cingulate gyrus, and then back to the hippocampus (Fig. 18.1). In recent years, several authors have proposed additions to the circuit but for the purposes of the discussion we will stick with his original proposal as it serves as a starting point to discuss these structures. The following discussion is overly simplistic, and you should keep in mind that we have an extremely limited understanding of learning and memory.

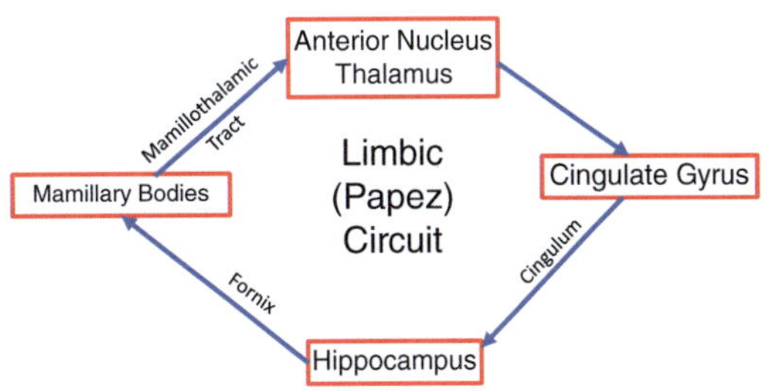

Fig. 18.1 Overview of Limbic Circuit [9]

J. Leo, *Gross Anatomy, Neuroanatomy, and Embryology for Medical Students*,
https://doi.org/10.1007/978-3-031-87151-1_18

Hippocampus

The most important structure in the limbic circuit is the hippocampus, which resembles a seahorse. It is located just caudal to the amygdala and forms the floor of the inferior horn of the lateral ventricle. It is thought that the hippocampus is neither the site nor the location of memories but is involved with generating memory circuits. In other words, the hippocampus transfers short term to long term memory circuits. The hippocampus includes the dentate gyrus and the cornu ammonis (CA) fields (CA1-CA3). The CA1 region or *Sommer's sector* is the most sensitive region of the hippocampus to anoxia and other insults.

One of the more famous patients in neurology is Henry Molaison, usually referred to as HM. HM had intractable temporal lobe epilepsy, and in 1953, when he was 27-years old, his surgeon William Scoville removed HMs medial temporal lobes on both sides. Following the surgery, HM had profound anterograde amnesia and could never make new memories. He did not have retrograde amnesia and he could remember facets of his life before the surgery. For instance, he knew that Richard Nixon was the president at the time of his surgery, but he could never learn the name of the current president. Much of what we know about memory has come from HM. Brenda Milner, his psychologist, extensively documented his condition. HM lived until he was 82 years old.

In Alzheimer's disease, plaques and tangles first appear in the hippocampus. In the initial stages of the disease the patients have difficulty with anterograde memory—they cannot make new memories. However, memories from their past tend to be intact. For instance, a 70-year-old patient cannot tell you what they had for breakfast earlier in the day, but they can list their first grade classmates. It is the explicit memories that these patients lose. An elderly patient with Alzheimer's might not be able to tell you about last Christmas (explicit memory), but they have no problem singing Christmas carols they learned as a child (implicit memories). As an example, Tony Bennet suffered from Alzheimer's but at 96 he had no problem singing his famous songs.

Both late-stage Parkinson's and Alzheimer's patients share some characteristics. Both can have memory problems and motor deficits. One way to think about the progression for each condition is that Alzheimer's is a descending disease. It starts in the cerebral cortex with subtle memory deficits. As the disease progresses, the pathology moves into other structures, and the patient starts to exhibit motor deficits. Parkinson's on the other hand is an ascending disease meaning that it starts off in the midbrain with subtle motor deficits. As the disease progresses, the pathology is evident in higher brain centers, and the patient exhibits memory and cognitive deficits.

Fornix

The fornix is the outflow tract of the hippocampus. It starts as the fimbria, which is a white band of myelinated axons emerging from the cell bodies of the hippocampus. These axons go on to form a band of fibers called the *crus*. The right and left crus are situated on the roof of the lateral ventricles (posteriorly) and come together as the body of each fornix which moves medially to sit side-by-side over the thalamus. The body of the fornix then descends and separates into the *columns of the fornix*, which are located caudal to the anterior commissure. They then curve back through the hypothalamus to project to several locations, the most prominent of which is the mamillary bodies.

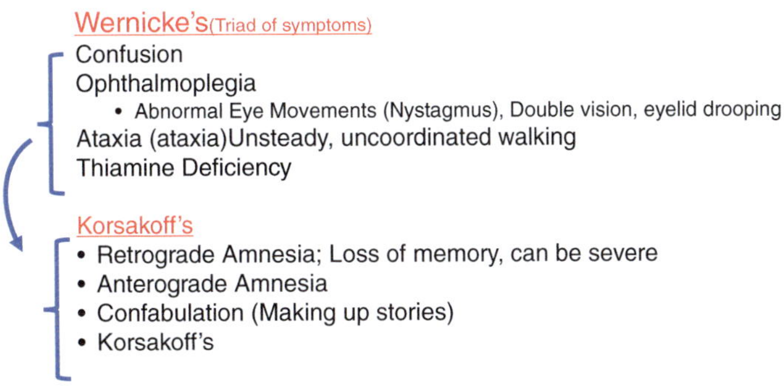

Fig. 18.2 Wernicke-Korsakoff's. In the typical scenario the patient starts off with Wernicke's, which is potentially treatable. Left untreated, patient moves to Korsakoff's

Wernicke Korsakoff's

Wernicke Korsakoff's results from a thiamine (Vitamin B1) deficiency that leads to degeneration of the mammillary bodies, the mammillothalamic tract, and the anterior and dorsomedial nucleus of the thalamus. Think of this as a two-step disease. Wernicke's is the first stage of the condition and consists of a triad of symptoms: ophthalmoplegia, ataxia, and confusion. If Wernicke's is left untreated it will often move onto the next stage, which is Korsakoff's. Korsakoff's patients exhibit anterograde and retrograde amnesia and tend to confabulate or make-up stories. To remember it, think of a coat rack (Fig. 18.2).

Kluver-Bucy Syndrome

Kluver-Bucy syndrome, which exists mostly in textbooks, or neuroanatomy exams, results from a bilateral lesion to the medial temporal lobe. It is extremely rare in humans. The patients exhibit hypersexuality, with no preference for gender; they are placid; show little fear response; and they tend to put objects into their mouth—hyperorality.

Amygdala

The amygdala is a major player in how we respond to emotions, mainly fear. Imagine walking down a path and you see a snake on the trail right in front of you. Your fear response will kick in, you will step back, maybe scream, and possibly run in the other direction. Several seconds later you might logically conclude that it was only a garter snake, which really poses no threat. You owe your immediate fear response to your amygdala, which sent information directly to your cerebral cortex, bypassing your thalamus. This was your fast response. But then several seconds later, your cortex rationally decided that the snake was not a real threat, and you relaxed. This was the more rational, yet slower response.

The amygdala is one of the major structures thought to be involved in PTSD. An overactive amygdala is also thought to be responsible for many of the behaviors in patients with anxiety disorders. The term "amygdala hijack" refers to how in certain stressful situations the amygdala takes over. Imagine driving through town and you get cut off and make an unwanted gesture to the driver. However, a minute or two later you immediately regret your response—maybe it was your grandmother, or one of your professors, who cut you off. Your amygdala was responsible for the sudden, impulsive outburst, while the delayed, more contemplative response came from your prefrontal cortex.

The amygdala is a solid mass of gray matter—think of a soccer ball—and lies in the temporal lobe, deep to the uncus, and just rostral to the hippocampus. Some have said the hippocampus looks like a cat's paw. To identify these two structures on a coronal section, think of a foot (the hippocampus) kicking a soccer ball (the amygdala). In coronal sections you might get a brain slice through just the amygdala (the ball), or a cut through just the hippocampus (the foot), or possibly a cut through both. If the cut happens to be through both, it will be through the point where the foot is kicking the ball, with the posterior edge of the amygdala, and anterior part of the hippocampus in the same slice. Fibers from part of the amygdala project via the stria terminalis to the anterior hypothalamus, preoptic area, and the hypothalamus. The stria terminalis lies medial to the caudate nucleus.

Hippocampus, Amygdala, and Orbitofrontal Cortex and Memories

When you see an apple, there are all kinds of memories that can be evoked. On a superficial level you remember how the shiny skin of the apple feels; you remember what it smells like; and you remember the slightly crunchy feeling of biting into it. But the apple might also elicit more emotional memories: like sitting on your grandmother's porch eating apples when you were a child. Or fall days drinking cider, or eating Applejack cereal for breakfast, or you might even think about your cell phone or your computer (marketers are smart). It is thought that the sensory information about "the apple" entered your prefrontal cortex, and then projected to the hippocampus which packaged all these memories into circuits and sent the circuits back to the frontal lobe and other regions for storage. The amygdala comes into play for the emotional part of the memories and seems to be especially important in warning us about dangers in the environment (Fig. 18.3).

Long Term Potentiation and Learning, AKA How the Brain Works

In 1949, four years before Watson and Crick's discovery of the double-helix model of DNA, and before we had any high-tech technology, the concepts of molecular biology, or knowledge of the workings of the brain, Hebb proposed that learning takes place at the synapse. It seems like a simple and obvious suggestion now, but at the time it was profound. He proposed that when our mind makes associations, it was because certain neurons were firing together, and that this synchronization leads to strengthened synapses.

When Hebb proposed the idea that the strengthening synapses is the key to learning and memory, the mechanisms of this were unclear, but he and others postulated that there could be (1) presynaptic changes—possibly more glutamate released from presynaptic cell, (2) postsynaptic changes– possibly more receptors moved to the postsynaptic membrane, or (3) extrasynaptic changes—maybe alterations in the ability of cells such as astrocytes to reuptake neurotransmitter from the synaptic cleft. Most importantly, he also pointed out that for presynaptic changes to occur the postsynaptic cell would have to be able to send a signal back to the presynaptic cell. He referred to this proposed molecule as a *retrograde messenger*. At the time, scientists did not know what that retrograde messenger might be, but they knew that whatever it was, it had to act extremely fast (Fig. 18.4).

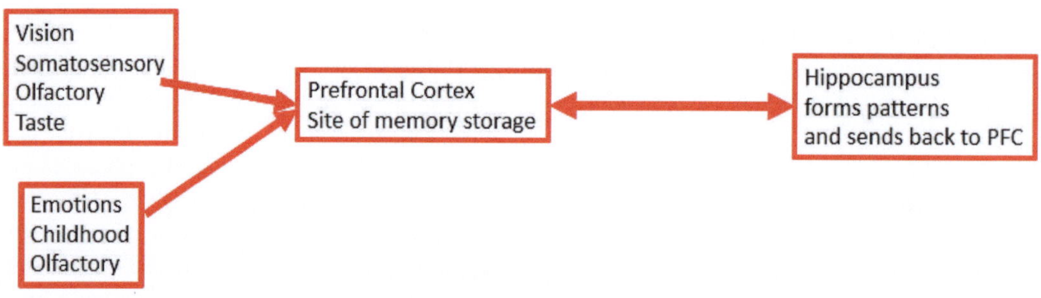

Fig. 18.3 Simplified Overview of Structures Involved with Memory [9]

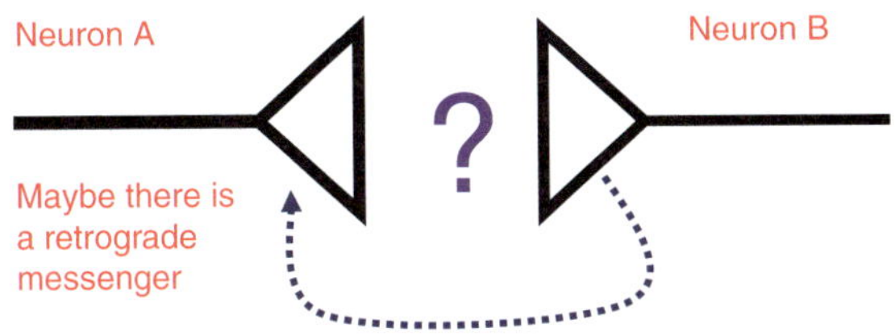

Fig. 18.4 Hebb's Theory: "When an axon of cell A is near enough to excite a cell B and repeatedly or persistently takes part in firing it, some growth process or metabolic change takes place in one or both cells such that A's efficiency, as one of the cells firing B is increased." Hebb proposed that the site of learning was the synapse. The question mark represents the fact that what exactly was happening in the synapse was still unknown. But the theory suggests that there is a retrograde messenger. Hebb, 1849

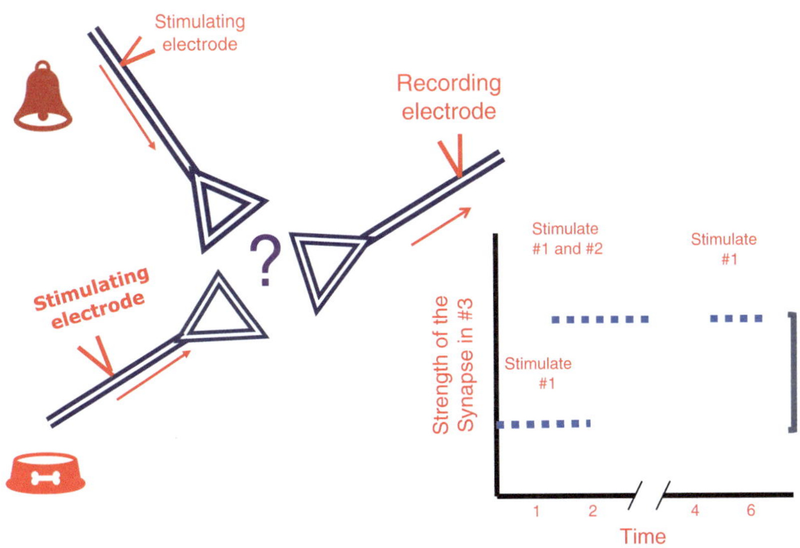

Fig. 18.5 Simplified Version of LTP. As an analogy to Pavlov's dogs. Stimulating electrodes are placed in neuron #1 and #2, while recordings are measured in neuron #3 [9]

In the 1970's an experimental model of isolated rabbit hippocampal slices in a petri dish was developed as a model for learning and memory. As an analogy, one can relate this to Pavlov's dogs. Remember that with Palov's dogs, when a bell is fired the dog typically does not react. If, however, the bell is paired with food, the dog will react. After repeating this pairing of the bell and the food, the dog associates the bell with the food so that just ringing the bell triggers a response.

Figure 18.5 shows three neurons involved in the model—two presynaptic neurons and one postsynaptic neuron. In each of the two presynaptic cells (imagine one being the bell and one being the food) they placed stimulating electrodes, and in the single postganglionic cell they placed a recording electrode. Over several hours they fired one of the stimulating electrodes (neuron #1, the bell) and established a baseline of activity in the postsynaptic cell. They then fired neuron #1 and #2 (bell and food) together and increased the activity in the recording electrode. They then waited several hours and fired neuron #1 and observed that there was increased activity in the recoding electrode. In other words, by pairing the two neurons together they had increased the strength of the synapse. At this point it was still not clear how the synapse was strengthened.

NMDA and AMPA Receptors

In the 1980s, an unusual aspect of glutamate and its receptors was discovered that is thought to play a role in LTP. There are two types of the glutamate receptor: (1) NMDA, and (2) non-NMDA (or AMPA receptor). The non-NMDA receptor is ligand gated meaning that glutamate binds to it, the channel opens, and Na^+ enters the cell. The NMDA receptor is ligand and voltage-gated meaning that it needs the combination of ligand binding, plus a large enough membrane voltage change, to open the channel. At rest, Mg^{2+} blocks the channel. A large enough voltage change moves the Mg^{2+} out of the channel. When the NMDA receptor opens, it allows Ca^{2+} to enter the cell.

In the petri dish example above, when neuron #1 fires just the AMPA receptor opens. Because there is an insufficient voltage change the NMDA receptor does not open. When Neuron #1 and #2 fire together, the voltage change is sufficient to also open the NMDA receptor and allow calcium to enter the cell.

If we look closely at the postsynaptic cell membrane, we can see that when just the bell fires, then neuron #1 is firing while neuron #2 is quiet (Fig. 18.6). This leads to glutamate binding to only half the non-NMDA receptors. With only half the non-NMDA receptors occupied, there is not enough voltage change to open the NMDA receptor.

When both neuron #1 and neuron #2 fire together, then all the non-NMDA receptors are occupied and there is a voltage change in the membrane. This voltage change leads to the Mg^{2+} blocker moving off the receptor which allows calcium to enter the cell. This increase in intracellular calcium can lead to multiple effects in the postsynaptic cell. After many experiments, it was determined that the next critical step in the pathway is the activation of nitric oxide synthase (NOS) which produces nitric oxide (NO). Because nitric oxide is a gas, it can diffuse back very quickly to the presynaptic cell, making it the perfect candidate for the long-postulated and sought-after retrograde messenger (Fig. 18.7).

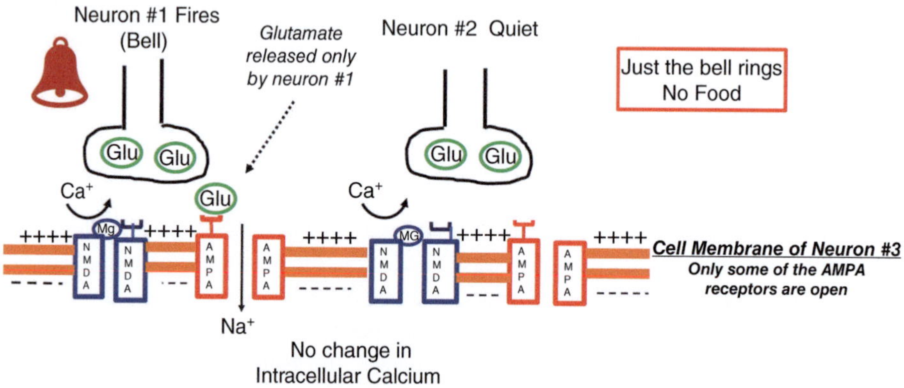

Fig. 18.6 Low Level Stimulus. When only neuron #1 (the bell) fires there is not enough voltage change to move Mg^{2+} out of the NMDA channel on the postsynaptic cell. The open AMPA receptor allows Na^+ to enter the cell but Ca^{++} is blocked [9]

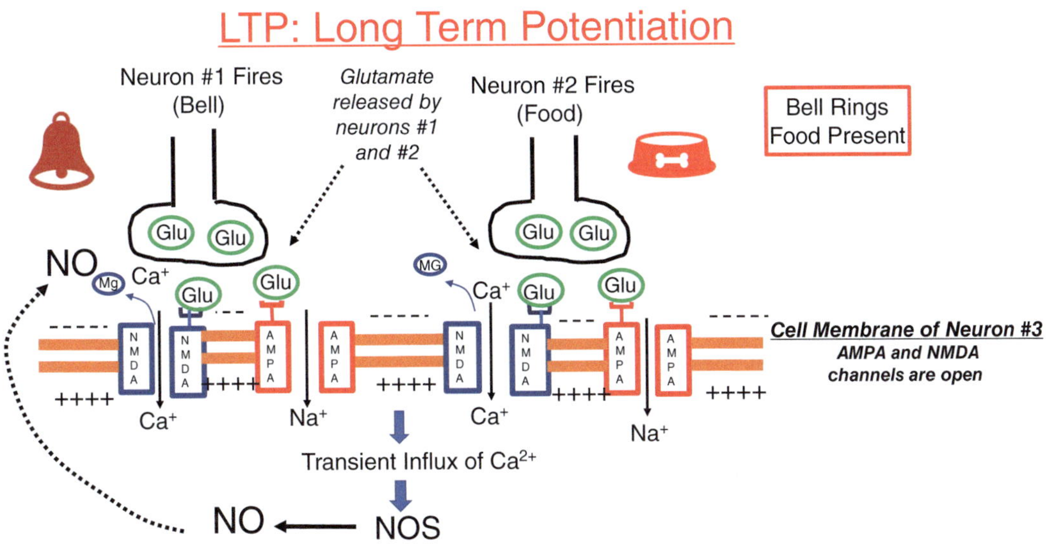

Fig. 18.7 More stimulus. When Neuron #1 and #2 (bell and food) fire together the voltage change moves Mg^{2+} out of the NMDA channel on the postsynaptic cell. This along with glutamate binding to the NMDA receptors allows Ca^{2+} to move through the channel, increasing intracellular Ca^{2+} concentration, which can bind to NOS to produce NO which acts as retrograde messenger [9]

Nitric Oxide: The Good, The Bad, and the Ugly

The other side to the beneficial side of nitric oxide in learning is that too much NO can lead to cell death. When it comes to neuronal damage, you will hear the terms: glutamate toxicity, calcium toxicity, excitotoxicity, or free radical induced damage. They all relate to the idea that too much NO is harmful to cells. Immediately after a stroke there is a pocket of initial neuronal damage, but over time there is a wave of cell death that spreads out from this initial damage. As the cells die, they release their contents and flood the microenvironment with glutamate. This excess glutamate then overloads the neighboring cells which leads to calcium flooding the cell and a spreading wave of cell death. This is all thought to result from activation of NOS, and in turn overproduction of NO. This is one reason that stroke patients brought to the ED are given Mg^{2+}. The Mg^{2+} is thought to block the NMDA receptor.

Naturally, pharmaceutical companies are trying to develop treatments to block this wave of cell death following a stroke. The use of NMDA channel blockers for stroke patients is an active area of research. Unfortunately, these efforts have so far been unsuccessful.

Because disruption of the NMDA/NO pathway has been implicated in so many pathologies there are already several medications in use. For instance, memantine, an NMDA receptor blocker, is given to Alzheimer's patients to balance glutamate levels. Ketamine is an NMDA agonist and is used as sedative, or off-label antidepressant, or in some cases as a hallucinogenic drug.

Historical Snippet: Endothelial Derived Relaxing Factor = NO

The following explanation ties neuroscience with cardiology. Before scientists coined the name nitric oxide, the molecule went by another name which was endothelial derived relaxing factor, or EDRF for short. The name EDRF comes from the fact that in preparations of capillaries in a petri dish when acetylcholine was added to the preparation, it would lead to vasodilation. However, the important caveat to this experimental finding was that endothelial cells also had to be present. If the endothelial cells were removed, then acetylcholine loses its ability to vasodilate the muscle cells in the capillaries. In other words, scientists knew there was something—but they did not know what—that was derived from endothelial cells that led to vasodilation, thus the name EDRF.

It was eventually shown that this hypothesized EDRF molecule was indeed NO. Robert Furchgott, Louis Ignarro, and Ferid Murad won the Nobel Prize for working all this out, a finding that eventually led to the development of sildenafil (Viagra). Viagra acts on the NO pathway to lead to vasodilation of the arteries in the corpus cavernosum. NO has also been implicated as an important molecule during development of neuronal pathways.

Further Reading

1. Blum K, Cull JG, Braverman ER, Comings DE. Reward deficiency syndrome. Am Sci. 1996;84(2):132–45.
2. Bonnet L, Comte A, Tatu L, Millot JL, Moulin T, de Bustos E. The role of the amygdala in the perception of positive emotions: A “intensity detector”. Front Behav Neurosc. 2015;9:117.
3. Brodal P. The central nervous system. 5th ed. New York: Oxford University Press; 2016.
4. Burnett AL, Lowenstein CJ, Bredt DS, Chang TS, Snyder SH. Nitric oxide: a physiologic mediator of penile erection. Science. 1992;257:401–3.
5. Dawson VL, Dawson TM, London ED, Bredt DS, Snyder SH. Nitric oxide mediates glutamate neurotoxicity in primary cortical cultures. PNAS. 1991;88:6368–637.
6. Garthwaite J. Nitric oxide as a multimodal brain transmitter. Brain Neurosc Adv. 2018;2:1–5.
7. Hebb DO. Organization of behavior. Psychology Press; 1949.
8. Leo J. Medical Neuroanatomy for the boards and clinic: Finding the Lesion. 2nd ed. Switzerland: Springer; 2024.
9. Leo J. Clinical anatomy and embryology: A guide for the classroom, clinic, and clinic. 2nd ed. Springer; 2024.
10. Leo J, Sugerman R. In: Keltner N, Folks DG, editors. Psychotropic drugs. Mosby; 2001.
11. Luscher C, Malenka RC. NMDA-receptor-dependent long-term potentiation and long-term depression. Cold Spring Harbor Perspect Biol. 2012;4(6)
12. Malinow R, Mainen ZF, Hayashi Y. LTP Mechanisms: From Silence to Four-Lane Traffic. Curr Opin Neurobiol. 2000;10:352–7.
13. Nabavi S, Fox R, Proulx CD, Lin JY, Tsien RY, Malinow R. Engineering a memory with LTD and LTP. Nature. 2014;511(7509):348–52.
14. Nestler EJ, Hyman SE, Malenka RC. Molec++ular neuropharmacology: a foundation for clinical neuroscience. 2nd ed. McGraw-Hill; 2008.
15. Nichols DE. Psychedelics Pharmacolog Rev. 2016;68:264–355.
16. Nicoli RA. A brief history of long-term potentiation. Neuron. 2017;93:281–90.
17. Scoville WB, Milner B. Loss of recent memory after bilateral hippocampal lesions. J Neurol Neurosurg Psych. 1957;20(1):11–21.
18. Squire L. The Legacy of patient HM for neuroscience. Neuron. 2009;61(1):6–9.

19 Chemical Neuroanatomy

Introduction

The gap or space between two neurons is referred to as the synaptic cleft. As an action potential travels down a presynaptic axon, it allows sodium ions to rush into the cell leading to depolarization. This wave of depolarization moves in a one-way direction away from the cell body towards the synapse. When the action potential reaches the presynaptic terminal, it allows an influx of calcium into the preganglionic cell which in turn leads to the neurotransmitter vesicles fusing with the presynaptic membrane so that the neurotransmitter is released into the synaptic cleft. The transmitter then migrates across the cleft and binds to a postsynaptic receptor.

The stimulus of the postsynaptic receptor then allows an ion to enter the cell, which in turn triggers the action potential in the postsynaptic cell. The action potential then continues down its axon. After the neurotransmitter has done its job, it is metabolized by enzymes or taken back up by reuptake transporters on the presynaptic cell. The goal of this chapter is not to go into all the details of neurotransmitter chemistry, but to integrate the biochemistry of the transmitters and the neuroanatomy to understand the various classes of medications. Hopefully, when you delve into the details of neurochemistry you will be able to relate it to neuroanatomy.

Deep to the cortical grey matter, there are several small subcortical structures, each of which use a different neurotransmitter. Despite their small size, because of their widespread connections to the entire cerebral cortex and many subcortical structures, they play an extremely vital role in behavior.

The *locus coeruleus* is in the pons near the floor of the fourth ventricle and produces *norepinephrine*. It is thought to be involved in arousal, alertness attention, and the stress response. It has been suggested that it is involved in the etiology of Attention Deficit Hyperactivity Disorder (ADHD).

The *Nucleus Basalis of Meynert* sits in the basal forebrain and has cholinergic fibers projecting to the prefrontal cortex, thalamus, and hypothalamus. It is involved in the later stages of Alzheimer's and Parkinson's dementia.

The *dorsal raphe* is a subdivision of the reticular formation and is a major source of *serotonin* in the CNS and is thought to be involved in clinical depression (Fig. 19.1).

When a neurotransmitter is released from the presynaptic cell and crosses the cleft to bind with a receptor on the postsynaptic cell, ion channels open or close allowing ions to move across the postsynaptic membrane. These ion fluxes result in either excitatory or inhibitory changes to the RMP. Receptors can be subdivided into two groups.

J. Leo, *Gross Anatomy, Neuroanatomy, and Embryology for Medical Students*,
https://doi.org/10.1007/978-3-031-87151-1_19

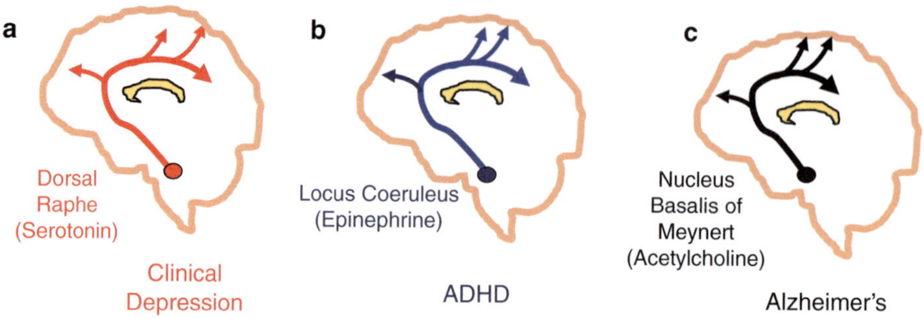

Fig. 19.1 Three subcortical structures and their neurotransmitters. Panel (**a**): dorsal raphe and serotonin. Panel (**b**): locus coeruleus and epinephrine. Panel (**c**): nucleus basalis of Meynert and acetylcholine. They all have widespread connections to cortical and subcortical structures. All use

1. *Ionotropic receptors,* also referred to as ligand-gated channels, open when neurotransmitter binds to the receptor. The term ionotropic refers to the fact that the receptor itself is the ion channel. An influx of sodium will depolarize the cell, while an influx of the chloride ion will hyperpolarize the cell. This type of communication involves changes to the membrane potential that occur within milliseconds.
2. M*etabotropic receptors*, also referred to as G protein-coupled receptors, are not the actual ion channels. In this case, the neurotransmitter binds to a receptor which then triggers a cascade of molecular events so that the signal passes from the receptor through a second messenger system to activate the ion channel. Thus, unlike the ionotropic receptor which has a direct effect, the metabotropic receptor has an indirect effect on ion flux. With the metabotropic receptor the membrane changes are slower compared to the ionotropic receptors.

Second Messenger Systems

The neurotransmitter binding to the receptor is the first message, and it typically does not cross the cell membrane. Second messengers are the ions or small molecules that send a message from the now activated receptor to other proteins. They can also lead to changes in gene expression. Three types of second messengers are discussed below (Fig. 19.2):

1. *Cyclic adenosine 3',5-monophosphate (cAMP),* or cyclic AMP. When a neurotransmitter such as epinephrine binds to its receptor there is a structural change in the receptor which causes a G protein to associate with the transmembrane protein adenylate cyclase. The adenylate cyclase then synthesizes cAMP which activates protein kinase A which in turn leads to phosphorylation of proteins within the cell.
2. *Inositol triphosphate/Diacylglycerol pathway*. When neurotransmitter binds to the G protein coupled receptor it leads to the activation of phospholipase C which produces IP_3. The IP_3 binds to IP_3 receptors on the endoplasmic reticulum. When these receptors open, this allows calcium to move from the ER into the cell. The activation of phospholipase C also activates diacylglycerol (DAG) which in turn activates protein kinase C.
3. *Calcium/Calmodulin Complex.* Beyond just changing the RMP, ions can also function as messengers. One common pathway is the *Ca^{2+}calmodulin complex*. When a neurotransmitter binds to a receptor, calcium channels open and intracellular calcium rises. The calcium then binds with calmodulin which in turn activates a protein kinase that leads to phosphorylation of intracellular proteins.

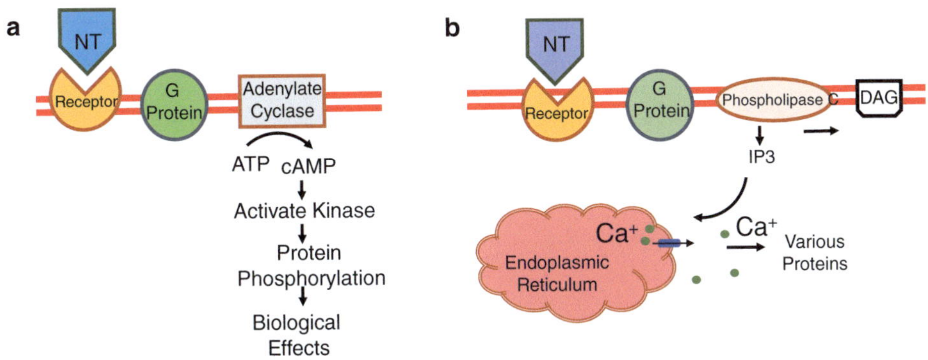

Fig. 19.2 G protein second messenger system. Panel (**a**) Cyclic adenosine 3′,5-monophosphate (cAMP). When neurotransmitter binds to the receptor, this causes the G-protein to bind to the adenylate cyclase, which produces cAMP from adenosine triphosphate (ATP). This in turn activates a kinase, phosphorylates proteins, and leads to biological effects. Panel (**b**) Inositol Triphosphate (IP_3). The neurotransmitter binds to the G protein coupled receptor which activates phospholipase C which produces IP_3. The IP_3 then leads to release of Ca^{2+} from the endoplasmic reticulum. In addition, diacylglycerol (DAG) is activated, and DAG (found in the membrane) activates protein kinase C

Monoamine Systems

The monoamines contain one amine group and include the catecholamines (dopamine, norepinephrine, and epinephrine), serotonin, and histamine. The term *adrenergic* refers to the neurons activated by the catecholamines which are adrenalin like substances also derived from the adrenal gland.

The synthesis of the catecholamines starts with the uptake of tyrosine into the neuronal cell body where it is converted to L-dihydroxyphenylalanine (L-dopa) by tyrosine hydroxylase. L-dopa is then decarboxylated by dopa decarboxylase (DDC) to dopamine. Dopamine is then converted to norepinephrine by dopamine-B-hydroxylase. In some neurons, norepinephrine is converted to epinephrine by phenyl ethanolamine-N-methyl transferase.

Dopamine, epinephrine, and norepinephrine can be broken down by catechol-0-methyltransferase (COMT) and monoamine oxidase (MAO) or taken back up in the nerve terminal by their respective reuptake transporter. COMT is located principally in the cytoplasm of postsynaptic terminals. There are two forms of MAO, both of which are in the outer membrane of mitochondria of nerve terminals and glia. MAO-A is in noradrenergic and dopaminergic terminals, and MAO-B is in serotonergic terminals. In the periphery, L-dopa is degraded by (COMT), which can be inhibited by COMT inhibitors such as Tolcapone. Selegiline is an inhibitor of MAO-B. Carbidopa inhibits DOPA decarboxylase in the periphery to maintain elevated levels of L Dopa. Tolcapone is a COMT inhibitor (Fig. 19.3).

Dopamine

There are four dopaminergic pathways in the brain:

1. The *nigrostriatal pathway* was discussed in detail in the basal ganglia chapter.
2. The *tuberoinfundibular tract* projects from the arcuate nucleus of the hypothalamus to the median eminence. Dopamine inhibits prolactin secretion by the anterior pituitary. Some antipsychotic drugs block the D2 receptor and will lead to an increase in prolactin levels and thus abnormal lactation in women and men.
3. The *mesocortical pathway* projects from the ventral tegmental area to the prefrontal cortex.
4. The *mesolimbic pathway* is discussed below in detail.

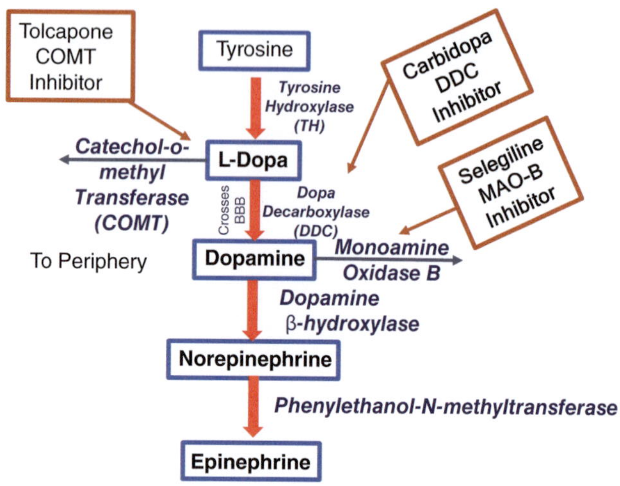

Fig. 19.3 Catecholamine synthesis. Tyrosine hydroxylase is the rate limiting step. L Dopa is broken down in the blood stream by COMT. L Dopa also crosses the BBB where it is broken down by DDC. Carbidopa inhibits DDC. Dopamine is broken down in the synaptic cleft by MAO-B which in turn can be inhibited by Selegiline

Mesolimbic Pathway

The mesolimbic pathway includes several nuclei but the most important one is the ventral tegmental area (VTA) located in the midbrain. The VTA has a prominent dopaminergic projection to the nucleus accumbens in the basal forebrain. This is the hypothesized "Reward Pathway" and is thought to be essential for monitoring pleasurable activities. In one sense, during a normal day we are continually doing our best to accommodate this pathway. We start off with our coffee, which increases dopamine; we then drive to work with the music on, which increases dopamine; we have a midmorning chocolate bar snack, which increases dopamine; we have a beer later that night, which increases dopamine, and the list goes on. Life is all about dopamine, but too much dopamine can be problematic and lead to various addictions. Cocaine and amphetamine block the dopamine reuptake transporter, and amphetamine also causes the release of dopamine. And opioids and cannabis can inhibit the GABAergic interneurons that normally inhibit the VTA projections. With the quieting of the GABA interneurons, the VTA can now release more dopamine (Fig. 19.4).

Dopaminergic Medications and Schizophrenia

Long term use of either illicit drugs, such as cocaine or amphetamine, or licit drugs such as antipsychotic medications, all of which increase dopamine levels in the mesolimbic pathway, can also lead to psychosis. On the other hand, drugs that block dopamine receptors in the mesolimbic system decrease psychotic symptoms,

The *Dopamine Hypothesis of Schizophrenia* is the theory that schizophrenia results from excessive dopaminergic activity. This is the opposite of Parkinson's patients who have too little dopamine. However, it is not just the dopamine *levels* that are important, it is *where* in the brain the dopamine levels are altered. The dopamine depletion in Parkinson's is found in the substantia nigra and the nigrostriatal pathway, while the hypothesized excess of dopamine in schizophrenia is in the mesolimbic pathway (Fig. 19.5).

The first generation of antipsychotics, such as chlorpromazine (Thorazine), block D2 dopaminergic receptors and reduce psychotic symptoms in patients diagnosed with schizophrenia. Their efficacy is presumed to be due to a reduction in dopamine in the mesolimbic pathway, However

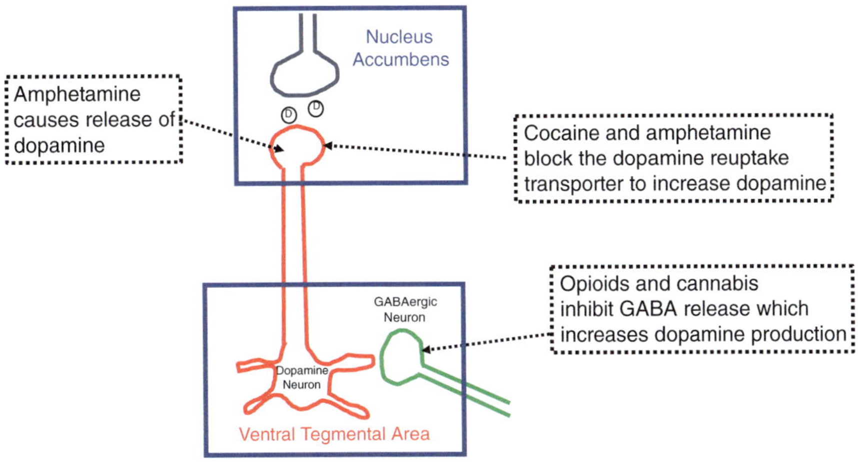

Fig. 19.4 Mesolimbic pathway or the reward pathway. Dopaminergic neurons project from the ventral tegmental area to the nucleus accumbens. GABAergic terminals on the dopaminergic cells are inhibitory

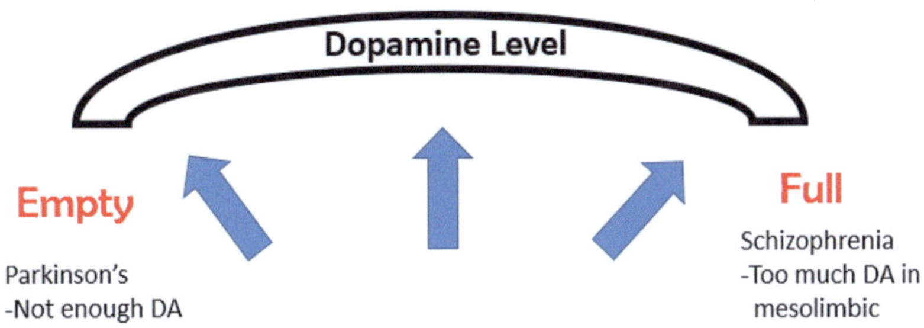

Fig. 19.5 Simplified overview of dopamine. Parkinson's patients lose dopamine in the substantia nigra. On the other hand, the dopamine theory of schizophrenia attributes the condition to an excess of dopamine in the mesolimbic pathway

these medications have problematic motor side effects, which are thought to be due to their action on the nigrostriatal pathway where it also decreased dopamine levels. Thus, there is this dilemma with the use of the first-generation antipsychotics: Namely, that the medication-induced dopamine decrease is responsible for both the efficacy and the side effects seen in the patients. The natural question this raises is: What if there was a drug that could decrease dopamine in the mesolimbic pathway but at the same time increase it in the nigrostriatal pathway? The next generation of drugs, the atypical antipsychotics, are thought to be able to do this. At least this is one idea.

The idea behind the newer atypical antipsychotics, such as Risperidone (Risperdal), Zyprexa (olanzapine), Seroquel (Quetiapine), or Abilify (Aripiprazole), can be summed up in an advertisement from the early 2000s for one of the more popular atypicals. The company's advertisement pictured an image of the cerebral cortex overlaid with a line drawing of a sine wave with peaks and valleys representing neurotransmitter levels. The image suggests that the medication is like a thermostat with the ability to reduce the problematic transmitter in one part of the brain, while simultaneously increasing it another part of the brain, with the result being a leveling out of the problematic transmitter. But how does one drug manage this dual action of decreasing dopamine in one part of the brain but increasing it in another? The answer lies in the receptors. Besides acting on the dopamine receptor which reduces dopamine, the atypicals also act on the 5-HT_{2A} receptor which increases dopamine.

To explain the mechanism of these drugs we need to look at both the D2 and the 5-HT_{2A} receptors along with the serotonergic projection of the dorsal raphe to the substantia nigra. The main target of the dorsal raphe is the caudate nucleus but along the way it sends collaterals to the substantia nigra. This collateral projection to the substantia nigra acts on the 5-HT_{2A} receptors which are inhibitory to the substantia nigra, thus the dorsal raphe is acting like a brake on the substantia nigra's projection to the striatum. When the dorsal raphe releases serotonin at its synapse with the substantia nigra, it inhibits the cell and leads to a reduction in dopamine at the synapse between the substantia nigra and the caudate (Fig. 19.6).

The atypicals act on two synapses: (1) they block the 5-HT_{2A} receptor on the substantia nigra; thus, they release the brake to increase dopamine levels, and (2) they block the dopamine receptor at the synapse between the substantia nigra and the caudate. The natural question then is: How can a medication which increases the dopamine output at one receptor, while decreasing dopamine output at another receptor have a net overall change? After all, the two actions would balance each other out with no net impact on overall dopamine levels. However, what is thought to happen, or hypothesized, is that in different regions of the brain there are different ratios of these two receptors, allowing the same drug to have different effects in different regions. If the D2 receptor is in abundance then the medication will reduce dopamine's effect, but if the 5-HT_{2A} receptor is in abundance then dopamine levels will be increased (Fig. 19.6).

In summary, the first-generation antipsychotics act on the D2 receptor, which leads to decreased dopamine in the mesolimbic pathway—responsible for the medication's efficacy, but the medication also leads to decreased dopaminergic activity in the nigrostriatal pathway—responsible for the side effects. The efficacy of the atypicals is thought to result by increasing the activity in the mesolimbic pathway through their action on the 5-HT_{2A} receptor, while also decreasing the activity in nigrostriatal pathway by acting on D2, and thus minimizing the side effects. Keep in mind this is an overly simplistic notion but provides the basis for understanding the ideas behind how neuroanatomy, neurophysiology, neuropathology, and neuropharmacology work together. This is at least one explanation for the mechanisms of the atypical antipsychotics.

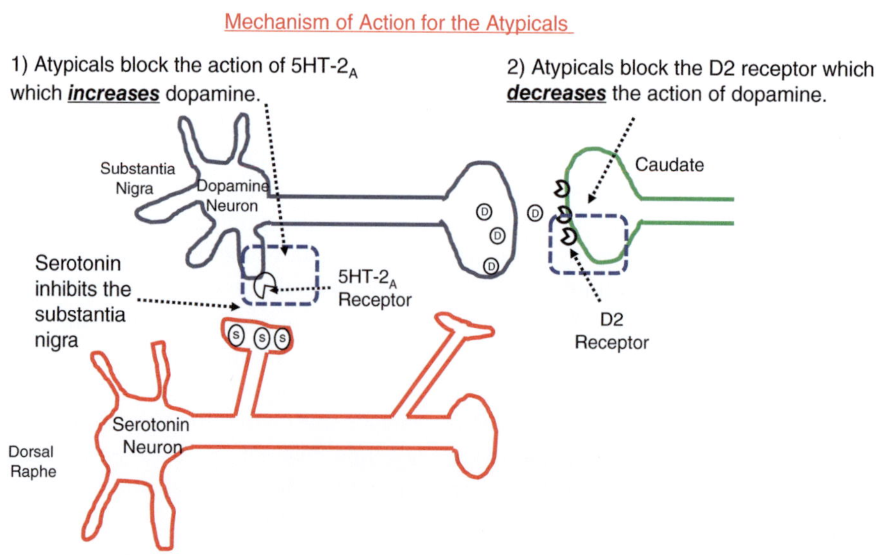

Fig. 19.6 Dorsal raphe to substantia nigra

Parkinson's Medications

The goal of the medications for Parkinson's disease is to either increase dopamine or decrease acetylcholine. A helpful mnemonic for these is *C*arrot ***SALAD*** (Fig. 19.7).

COMT Inhibitor (Entacoponel, tolcapone) COMT is one of the enzymes that breaks down dopamine, so naturally blocking it would lead to more dopamine present in the synapse.

Selegiline inhibits monoamine oxidase-B (MAO-B).

Anticholinergics (trihexphenidyl) The anticholinergics block the cholinergic activity.

L-Dopa (Carbidopa) inhibit the peripheral breakdown of L-Dopa so that more L-Dopa can cross the blood-brain barrier to enter the CNS.

Amantadine.

Dopamine agonists (Bromocriptine) increase dopaminergic activity.

Chemical Imbalance Theory of Depression

The Chemical Imbalance Theory of Depression postulates that depression is due to low levels of catecholamines. It was first formulated in 1965, by Joseph Schildkraut, and was based on two sets of observations. The first was that various drugs had the ability to alter mood, either up or down. The second set of observations, which came later, was the mechanisms of action of these drugs and their effect on catecholamine levels. It was Schildkraut who put all this together and noted that the medications that had a sedating affect decreased monoamine transmission, and that those with an energizing effect were the drugs that increased monoamine transmission. Observations on the three drugs below formed the keystone of the theory (Fig. 19.8):

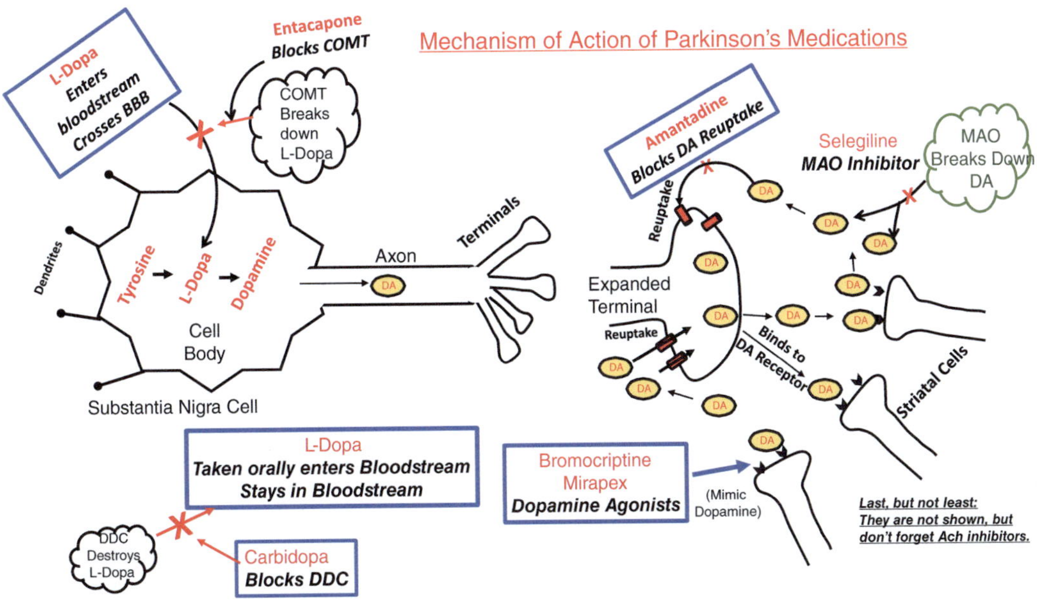

Fig. 19.7 Mechanisms of Parkinson's medications

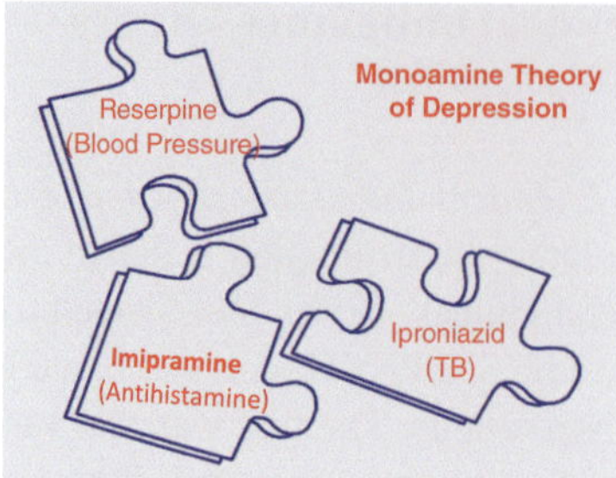

Drug	Affect on Mood	Monoamine Effect
Reserpine	Depress	Decrease
Iproniazid	Elevate	Increase
Imipramine	Elevate	Increase

Fig. 19.8 The monoamine theory of depression. The theory came out of observations of various drugs on mood. Piece #1 was that reserpine given for high blood pressure depressed mood. Piece #2 was that Iproniazid given for tuberculosis (TB) elevated mood. Piece #3 was that imipramine elevated mood. In turn, reserpine lowered monoamines (5HT, NE), while Impramine and iproniazid raised monoamine levels

1. *Iproniazid* was first used to treat TB patients, but it was also noted that it had a calming effect. At the time, the mechanism was not known, but it was eventually discovered that Iproniazid blocked MAO.
2. *Imipramine* was the first tricyclic. It was first given to patients as an antihistamine, and it was discovered that it had an energizing effect. Subsequent studies showed that it blocked the norepinephrine reuptake transporter leading to increased levels of catecholamines.
3. *Reserpine* comes from the snakeroot plant and was first given for hypertension in India where it was noted to have a sedating effect. The sedating effect came from increasing serotonin levels in the synapse by binding to VMAT and blocking the reuptake of serotonin into the vesicles.

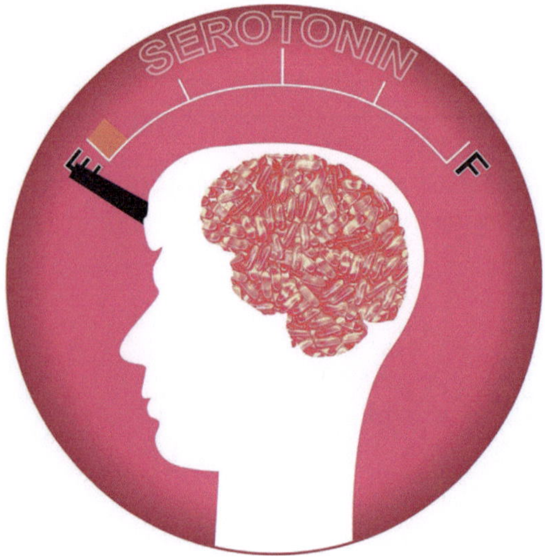

Fig. 19.9 The chemical imbalance theory of depression. The original chemical imbalance theory postulated that depression was the result of a monoamine deficit. This was later revised to be the result of a serotonin shortage [3]

The catecholamine theory was eventually refined to the idea that the most important transmitter was serotonin. Pharmaceutical advertisements portrayed the serotonin theory of depression as a simplistic model that depression was caused by low levels of serotonin (Fig. 19.9). More recent advertisements have backed away from this oversimplification.

The synthesis of serotonin starts with tryptophan being taken up by the cell and metabolized to 5-hydroxytryptohan by tryptophan hydroxylase. and then serotonin by 5-hydroxytryptohan decarboxylase. Serotonin is then taken back up in the presynaptic cell by the serotonin reuptake transporter (SERT). In the presynaptic cells, serotonin is transported into vesicles by the vesicular monoamine transporter (VMAT) and stored until needed (Fig. 19.10).

The first generation of antidepressants acted on several transporters thus they were not considered

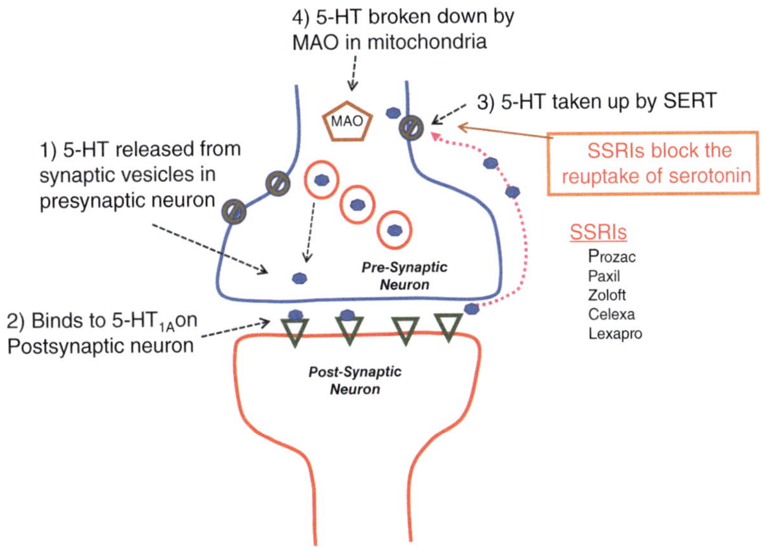

Fig. 19.10 Overview of the serotonergic synapse. Monoamine oxidase breaks down serotonin, dopamine, and norepinephrine. The SSRIs are inhibitors of the serotonin reuptake transporters. *SERT* Serotonin reuptake transporter

selective. For many years, a goal was to find a selective reuptake inhibitor that only acted on one transporter. The first selective serotonin reuptake inhibitor was Prozac, which was soon followed by several others such as: Paxil (paroxetine), Celexa (citalopram), and Zoloft (sertraline). Celexa was eventually refined even further and replaced by Lexapro (escitalopram), which is just the (s)-stereoisomer of the racemate citalopram.

Reuptake Transporters

When it comes to medications, the three neurotransmitters dopamine, serotonin, and norepinephrine are intimately related, largely due to their reuptake transporters. Each transmitter has a specific transporter: Norepinephrine—NERT, Dopamine—DAT, or Serotonin—SERT. However, there are no strict lines of demarcation between conditions and mechanisms, instead there is significant overlap. For instance: Wellbutrin (bupropion) inhibits the NERT and DAT and is used as an antidepressant but is also prescribed for smoking cessation; Reboxetine inhibits NERT and is also used as an antidepressant; Duloxetine (Cymbalta) is another antidepressant that blocks NERT but is also prescribed for urinary incontinence; Venlafaxine (Effexor) is an antidepressant that blocks NERT and SERT but is also prescribed for ADHD; and Strattera which blocks NERT is prescribed for ADHD—it was not effective in clinical trials for depression (Table 19.1).

And some of the antidepressants act via other mechanisms. Located on the presynaptic terminals of serotonergic synapse are α-2 adrenergic receptors which lead to a reduction in serotonin at the synapse. One of the mechanisms of the antidepressant Remeron is to block this receptor which in turn leads to an increased release of serotonin (Fig. 19.11).

Table 19.1 Summary of medications acting on reuptake transporters

Medication	Reuptake transporter	Medicinal use
Imipramine (Tofranil)	NERT, SERT	Antidepressant
Wellbutrin (Bupropion)	NERT, DAT	Antidepressant Smoking cessation
Reboxetine (Deronda)	NERT	Antidepressant
Duloxetine (Cymbalta)	NERT, SERT	Antidepressant Urinary incontinence
Venlafaxine (Effexor)	NERT, SERT	Antidepressant ADHD
Prozac, Paxil, Zoloft, Lexapro	SERT	Antidepressant
Atomoxetine (Strattera)	NERT	ADHD

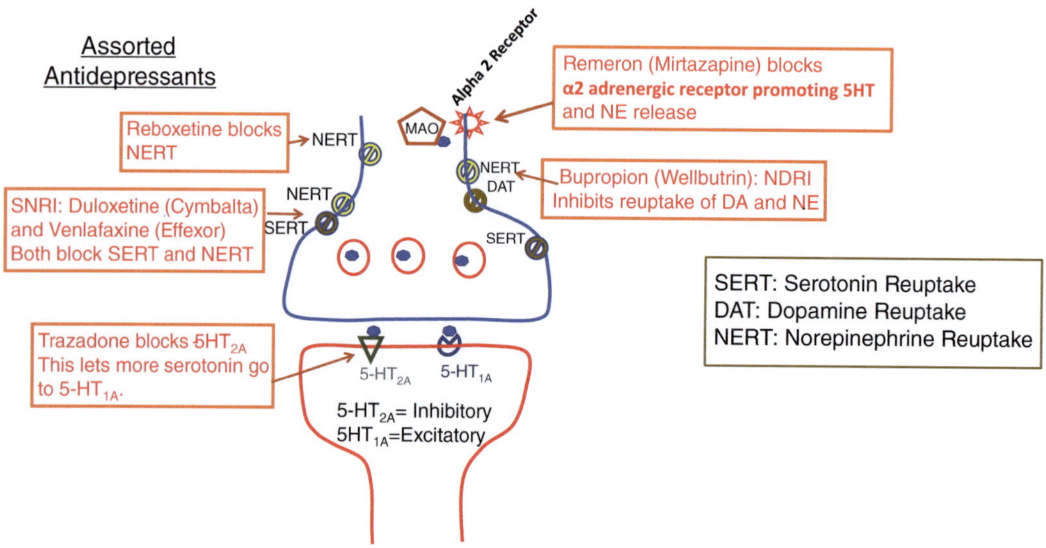

Fig. 19.11 Overview of various antidepressants. Besides inhibiting transmitter reuptake several antidepressants act on other receptors. Remeron blocks the α2-adrenergic receptor which promotes release of serotonin and norepinephrine

Psychedelics and the Serotonin 5-HT$_{2A}$ Receptor

The psychedelics or hallucinogens are mood-altering drugs that act to increase serotonin levels in the brain by agonist activity at the 5-HT$_{2A}$ receptor on the postsynaptic cell at serotonergic synapses. The 5-HT$_{2A}$ receptor is found in several regions of the brain, but the main action of the psychedelics is thought to be the pyramidal cells in layer V of the prefrontal cortex. The psychedelics are commonly used as recreational drugs, while their legitimate use for medical conditions is debated.

LSD (lysergic acid diethylamide) became famous in the 1950s as one of the first hallucinogenic drugs. It was originally investigated by the CIA, and the US Army.

Psilocybin is a recreational hallucinogen found in certain mushrooms that increase serotonin levels. It has been tested for medical use in depression and anxiety, but it is not approved at this time.

MDMA (3,4-methylenedioxy-methamphetamine, Ecstasy, Molly) acts to increase levels of serotonin, dopamine, and norepinephrine, giving it the effect of both psychostimulants and hallucinogens. The dopamine increase is thought to be responsible for increased energy; norepinephrine for increased heart rate and blood pressure; and serotonin for the increased sexual arousal and emotional closeness. It is currently licensed for limited use in psychotherapy. Among psychopharmacologists, there is debate about whether MDMA should be classified as psychedelic or not.

Serotonin syndrome results from overactivation of the serotonin receptors leading to tremors, hyperreflexia, rigidity, tachycardia, and hypertension.

Cholinergics

Acetylcholine is found at the myoneural junction of skeletal muscle, autonomic ganglia, and parasympathetic postganglionic-effector synapses. It is found in both the peripheral nervous system and in the central nervous system, including the spinal cord, basal ganglia, and cerebral cortex. Acetylcholine is synthesized from choline and acetyl-coenzyme A (Acetyl-CoA) by choline acetyltransferase (CHat). It is then transferred to and stored in synaptic vesicles. When intracellular Ca^{2+} increases, the vesicles fuse with the postsynaptic membrane and release their contents. The acetylcholine then binds to its receptors to propagate the action potential in the postsynaptic cell. Acetylcholine is then broken down by cholinesterase (AChE) into choline and acetate to be recycled and used again. The choline is brought back into the cell by the choline transporter (Fig. 19.12 and Table. 19.1).

There are two types of cholinergic receptors:

1. *Nicotinic receptors* are found on skeletal muscle, postganglionic neurons, and adrenal medulla cells. They are ionotropic receptors that are stimulated by nicotine. Curare is an example of a skeletal muscle relaxant.
2. *Muscarinic receptors* are found on parasympathetic target organs and some sympathetic targets (sweat glands for instance). They are metabotropic receptors that are stimulated by

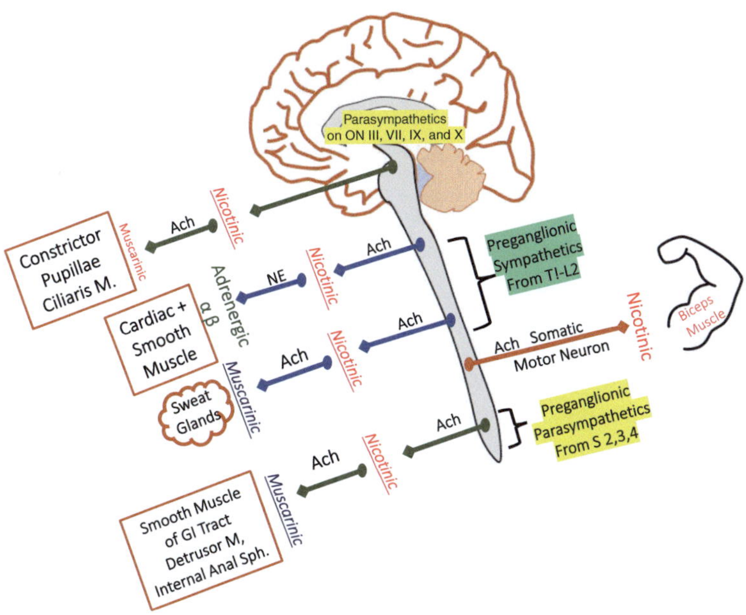

Fig. 19.12 Neurotransmitters and receptors

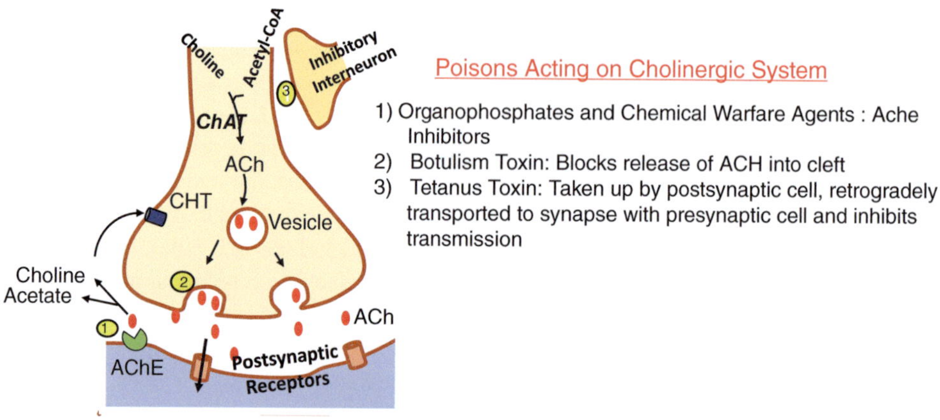

Fig. 19.13 Cholinergic synapse. Acetylcholine (ACh) is synthesized from acetyl coenzyme A (Acetyl CoA) and choline by choline acetyltransferase (ChAT). ACh is transferred to the vesicles to be released at the cleft. Acetylcholinesterase (AChE) breaks down Ach into choline and acetate. Choline then travels back into the cell at the choline transporter (CHT)

muscarine. Atropine and antihistamines are examples of antimuscarinic agents. Pilocarpine is a muscarinic receptor agonist. Scopolamine is a muscarinic anticholinergic that acts by blocking the action of acetylcholine.

Acetylcholine released from the presynaptic neurons binds to nicotinic receptors on the postganglionic neurons. The postganglionic neurons in turn bind to muscarinic receptors on either a gland or smooth muscle. Direct acting cholinergic agonists mimic the effect of acetylcholine. Indirect acting agonists inhibit the acetylcholinesterase, thus producing cholinergic effects (Fig. 19.12).

Various agents can perturb cholinergic transmission: (1) *Organophosphates* and various biochemical warfare agents such as sarin gas, which was used in the 1995 Tokyo subway attack, are AChE inhibitors, (2) *Botulism toxin* blocks the release of ACH at the synaptic cleft, (3) *Tetanus toxin* is brought into the cell at the site of the synaptic cleft and retrogradely transported back to the point where the inhibitory interneuron meets the cell. Tetanus toxin then blocks transmission at that site which leads to overstimulation at the post synaptic cell, (4) *Strychnine* blocks the uptake of glycine in the presynaptic inhibitory neuron which leads to an increase in the cholinergic motor nerve and excessive impulses and severe painful spasms (Fig. 19.13).

Myasthenia gravis is an autoimmune disorder in which antibodies destroy the neuromuscular junction by binding to acetylcholine receptors (AChR). It leads to muscle weakness, difficulty walking, droopy eyelids, and double vision. It is treated with acetylcholinesterase inhibitors.

A helpful mnemonic for remembering the parasympathetics is SLUDD, which stands for **S**alvation, **L**acrimation, **U**rination, **D**igestion and **D**efecation. Note that the S and L part or the mnemonic refers to the head—salvation and lacrimation. And the U, D, D refers to the abdomen and pelvic regions—urination, digestion, and defecation. In terms of the head, the picture below shows the salvation and lacrimation effects of parasympathetics.

Another version of the mnemonic is ***SLUDGE***, which refers to cholinergic toxicity, and stands for **S**alvation, **L**acrimation, **U**rinary incontinence, **D**efecation, gastrointestinal **D**istress, and **E**mesis. Cholinergic toxicity can result from: ingestion of certain chemicals such as organophosphates, complications of general anesthesia, or excess cholinesterase inhibitors.

The reticular activating system (RAS) projects to the cortex, thalamus, and hypothalamus. It is a mixture of cholinergic and adrenergic neurons and is involved in maintaining alertness. Bilateral lesions result in a coma.

The *pedunculopontine nucleus*, along with the Nucleus Basalis of Meynert, is a source of cholinergic projections to higher cortical areas and is thought to be involved in both Alzheimer's and Parkinson's disease. Aricept (Donepezil) is an acetylcholinesterase blocker that is given to Alzheimer's patients to restore cholinergic levels.

GABA, Barbiturates, and Benzodiazepines

Gabe is the main inhibitory neurotransmitter in the nervous system and is involved in numerous medical conditions. Many medications and drugs of abuse act on the GABAergic system. GABA receptors are designated A and B. Type A receptors function by first messenger transmission, whereas Type B use indirect secondary messenger transmission. When activated both receptors result in an influx of chloride ions into the neuron which causes hyperpolarization (inhibition) of the membrane potential. Roughly fifty percent of the inhibitory interneurons in the spinal cord use GABA; the other half use glycine as their neurotransmitter. There are two GABA receptors.

1. *$GABA_A$ receptors* are ionotropic receptors that allow Cl^- to enter the cell when they are open leading to neuronal inhibition. They are found on post synaptic cells in the CNS. They are stimulated by barbiturates, ethanol, and anesthetics. Activation can lead to sedation, euphoria, amnesia, and muscle relaxation.
2. *$GABA_B$ receptors* are metabotropic receptors that are found on pre and post synaptic neurons in the spinal cord. On the postsynaptic cell they lead to inhibition by increasing the permeability of K^+. In the presynaptic cell they lead to inhibition by decreasing the permeability to Ca^{2+}. Activation leads to muscle relaxation, and cognitive impairment.

Both the barbiturates and benzodiazepines stimulate the $GABA_A$ receptor, however there are slight differences. The barbiturates increase the open time of the Cl^-channel activated by GABA, while the benzodiazepines augment the frequency of CL^- channel opening when GABA is present, but not in the absence of GABA. This difference is one reason that the barbiturates are so problematic and why they were eventually replaced in the 1950s, by the benzodiazepines. Gabapentin (Neurontin) is a GABA analogue which is used as a pain reliever for shingles and as an anticonvulsant but is widely used off-label for many conditions such as bipolar disorder and posttraumatic stress disorder just to name a few. Its exact mechanism is unknown but it is thought that Gabapentin increases GABA levels and inhibits the voltage-gated calcium channels in the dorsal horn of the spinal cord.

The Opioids

The use of opioids as a drug go back as far as the ninth century B.C. Besides the exogenous opioids such as morphine and heroin, there are also endogenous opioids, such as enkephalin and β-endorphins that are synthesized in our bodies and used by various neuroanatomical pathways to modulate pain. In 1975, when scientists first discovered the existence of opioid receptors in the nervous system, they did not know about the existence of endogenous opioids. But with the discovery of the opioid receptors, it was assumed that the body itself must also produce its own opioid like chemicals and the search was on for these endogenous opioids. After all, evolution did not result in receptors for synthetic drugs; we have receptors for neurotransmitters and other compounds made by our own bodies.

The descending pain system and the existence of endogenous opioids such as enkephalins were soon discovered, and ever since, there has been a significant effort by pharmaceutical companies to find medications that act on the opioid receptors. As we know, subsequent discoveries have produced some of most dangerous and addictive drugs available.

There are three subtypes of opioid receptors: μ (mu), κ (kappa), and δ (delta). The receptors are in the spinal cord, PAG, locus coeruleus, and peripheral sensory nerves. The most recognized drugs acting on the mu receptors are heroin, morphine, codeine, oxycodone, and fentanyl. Oxycodone is a strong opioid that binds to mu, kappa, and delta receptors. It is also an active ingredient in many narcotic pain medications. OxyContin, an extended-release version of Oxycodone, was introduced in the mid 1990s, as safer and less addictive. Methadone is a long-acting opioid agonist that blocks the effects of opioids to reduce craving and withdrawal symptoms and along with therapy is part of the treatment program for opioid addicts. *Buprenorphine (Suboxone)* is a partial opioid agonist that also reduces cravings. The combination of both medication and therapy for opioid addiction is considered the "whole patient" approach and is referred to as Medication Assisted Treatment (MAT).

Historical Snippet: Opioid Epidemic in a Nutshell

In 1864, Adolph von Bayer (1835–1917) synthesized barbital which subsequently went on to be prescribed for conditions such as insomnia, anxiety, neurosis, psychosis, and epilepsy. By the 1970s, it was also increasingly being used as a recreational drug. Marilyn Monroe died from an overdose of barbiturates. In 1997, the Heaven's Gate Cult committed mass suicide in California by drinking a mixture of phenobarbital and alcohol.

The barbiturates were replaced by benzodiazepines such as diazepam (valium) and alprazolam (Xanax) which are prescribed for various conditions such as panic disorder, anxiety disorders, and insomnia. The benzodiazepines also act on the GABA receptor. Valium was synthesized in 1963, and by the 1970s, it was one of the most prescribed medications in the country. Ten years later, it became clear that benzodiazepines, like barbiturates, also had serious side effects and were widely abused.

The benzodiazepines were replaced by new classes of medications such as the D2 blockers (chlorpromazine), the tricyclics, and eventually the SSRIs. The serious abuse problems, and evidence that large numbers of people became addicted to barbiturates and benzodiazepines, all led to congressional committees, lawsuits, investigative reports, and subsequent changes to medical education. Fast forward to the current time-period and we are repeating history with the opioid epidemic, complete with congressional committees, investigative reports, enormous lawsuits, and subsequent changes to medical education.

The term "Oxy Express" refers to Interstate Highway 75, the north/south corridor running from Florida to Maine. The oxycontin disaster started in the late 2000s, in FL, where lax state laws allowed clinics to pop up overnight. One clinic started in an empty photobooth sitting in the middle of a parking lot and eventually relocated to a large abandoned old bank building with off-site parking, a shuttle service, security guards, and the ability to treat hundreds of people a day. Plus, the owners of the clinic were not even physicians.

With little oversight, dealers in states such as Kentucky and Tennessee would hire individuals and then drive them in caravans to these "Florida Pill Mills." The "patients" would then go to the pill mill and see a doctor, where they could easily get a diagnosis, a prescription, and a bottle of oxycontin—all for about $1000. Upon walking out of the clinic, they would immediately turn the pills over to the dealer. After paying the "patients" a token amount, the dealer could then sell the pills on the street for upwards of $4000 per bottle. A van load of ten people would be a profit of about $30,000 per trip, all for a day or two of work. Because of the lax laws, the police had no recourse to enter the medical building because "technically" the dealers were not breaking the law. The legal system eventually caught up, and new laws put a stop to these once legal clinics. But new drugs were on the way.

Fentanyl is a synthetic opioid that is 50–100 times more potent than morphine. It was first synthesized in 1963 (the year JFK was assassinated, and the Beatles had their first album released in the US). In the 1970s and 1980s, it was first used as an intravenous analgesic during cardiac surgery. In the early 2000s, it began to be manufactured for illicit use, and by the mid 2000s, its illegal use was common in the northeast but then soon spread to other parts of the country. It is now often mixed with other drugs. In some cases, buyers believe they are purchasing heroin, when in fact it is really fentanyl. In an emergency, for patients amid a narcotic overdose the nasal spray Narcan (Naloxone) can be administered. Narcan is an opioid antagonist that has a strong affinity for the mu receptor, so that illicit drugs, such as fentanyl, are blocked from the receptor.

Further Reading

1. Brownstein MJ. A brief history of opiates, opiate peptides, and opioid receptors. Proc Natl Acad Sci. 1993;90:5391–3.
2. Goldstein DS, Eisenhofer G, Kopin IJ. Clinical catecholamine neurochemistry: a legacy of Julius Axelrod. Cell Mol Neurobiol. 2006;122(5):509–22.
3. Lacasse J, Leo J. Serotonin and depression PLOS Medicine. 2005. Available at: https://doi.org/10.1371/journal.pmed.0020392.
4. Leo J. Medical neuroanatomy for the boards and clinic: finding the lesion. 2nd ed. Cham: Springer; 2024.
5. Leo J. Clinical anatomy and embryology: a guide for the classroom, clinic, and clinic. 2nd ed. Cham: Springer; 2024.
6. Löscher W, Rogawski MA. How theories evolved concerning the mechanism of action of barbiturates. Epilepsia. 2012;53(Suppl. 8):12–25.
7. Pletscher A, Shore PA, Brodie BB. Serotonin as a mediator of reserpine action in the brain. Pharmacol Exp Ther. 1956;116(1):84–9.
8. Schildkraut JJ. The catecholamine hypothesis of affective disorders. Am J Psychol. 1965;122(5):509–22.
9. Seeman P. Dopamine receptors and the dopamine hypothesis of schizophrenia. Synapse. 1987;1(2):133–52.
10. Stahl S. Stahl's essential psychopharmacology. 4th ed. Cambridge: Cambridge University Press; 2013.
11. Temple J. American pain. How a young felon and his ring of doctors unleashed America's deadliest drug epidemic. New York: Lyons Press; 2016.
12. Todman D. Henry dale and the discovery of chemical synaptic transmission. Eur Neurol. 2007;60:162–4.
13. Valenstein E. The war of the soups and the sparks. New York: Columbia University Press; 2005.

20 Brain Stem Lesions

Introduction

Now that we have talked in depth about cranial nerves and several other pathways, we are going to go back to the brainstem to look at some details. For the brainstem lesions you want to understand: (1) why the patient exhibits various signs and symptoms, (2) which artery might be affected, and (3) the specific circuit for each compromised tract. A key to understanding lesions is to know a given structure's neighbors. Not every syndrome is a textbook scenario. Tumors, for instance, can start off small and expand over time to compress neighboring structures.

Alternating Hemiplegia

If you see a patient with alternating motor deficits, such as hemiplegia on one side and a cranial nerve motor deficit on the opposite side, then you think about the brain stem as a site for the lesion. To explain this, we need to relate the UMNs in the corticospinal and corticobulbar tracts to the LMNs of the cranial nerves. As the corticobulbar and corticospinal tracts descend through the brainstem, they cross the LMNs coming out of the various nuclei.

Think of the cranial nerve nuclei and their LMNs as being stacked up on a ladder. At the bottom of the ladder, which is the medulla, is the LMN of CN XII. In the middle of the ladder, which is the pons, are the LMNs of CN VI and CN VII. And on top of the ladder, which is the midbrain, is the LMN of CN III. Also running down the brainstem, is the corticospinal tract sending information to the spinal cord, and this tract runs right next to the LMNs of these cranial nerves. In the picture below you can see the UMN fibers of the corticobulbar tract crossing the LMNs of CNs III, VI, and XII (Fig. 20.1).

J. Leo, *Gross Anatomy, Neuroanatomy, and Embryology for Medical Students*,
https://doi.org/10.1007/978-3-031-87151-1_20

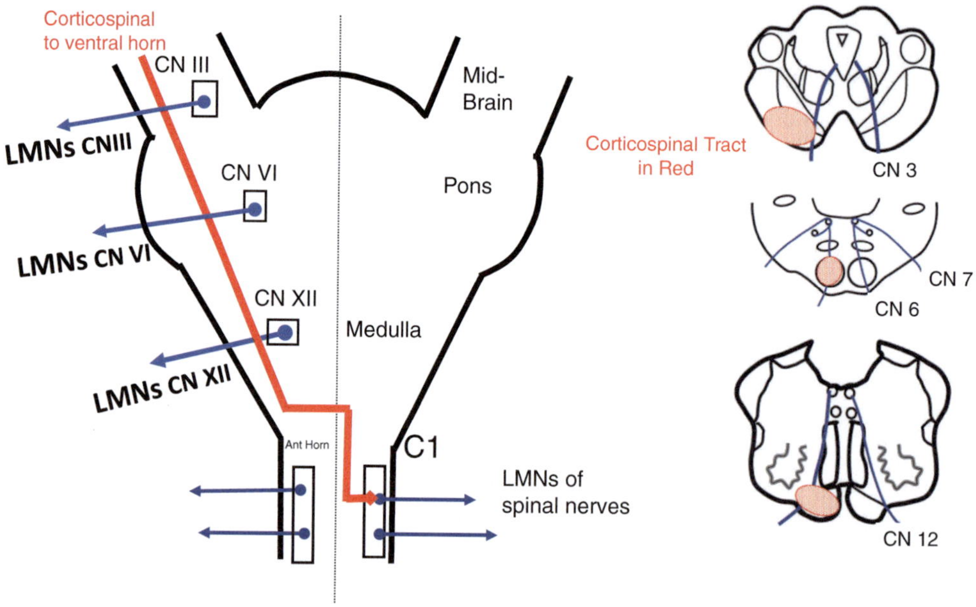

Fig. 20.1 Relationship of corticobulbar and corticospinal pathways to LMNs of CNs III, VI, and XII [12, 13]

Inferior Alternating Hemiplegia

Let us start with a lesion in the medullary pyramid. A lesion to the pyramid will result in contralateral UMN signs to the limbs since the lesion is above the motor decussation. But running immediately lateral to the pyramid are the LMNs of the hypoglossal nerve which came out of the hypoglossal nucleus. And the same lesion will lead to an ipsilateral loss of CN XII. Consider the patient's presentation and your thought process. If you see a patient with a dense hemiplegia to the limbs on one side you might be tempted to think of the cervical cord as a potential site of the lesion, but if you see a tongue deficit on the opposite of the hemiplegia, then you immediately think of the brainstem. How high up on the ladder are you? You are at the level of the nerve that is on the opposite side of the hemiplegia. In this case, at the level of CN XII. The isolated cranial nerve deficit tells you the level of the lesion.

The term *Inferior Alternating Hemiplegia* aptly explains the syndrome of a CN XII deficit on one side and UMN signs from the neck down on the contralateral side. It is *inferior* because it is in the medulla. The most common scenario for this lesion would be an occlusion of the anterior spinal artery or vertebral artery which leads to medial medullary syndrome. In addition to the inferior alternating hemiplegia, the occlusion usually compromises the medial lemniscus which would lead to a contralateral loss of dorsal columns (vibration, proprioception, two-point discrimination) (Fig. 20.2).

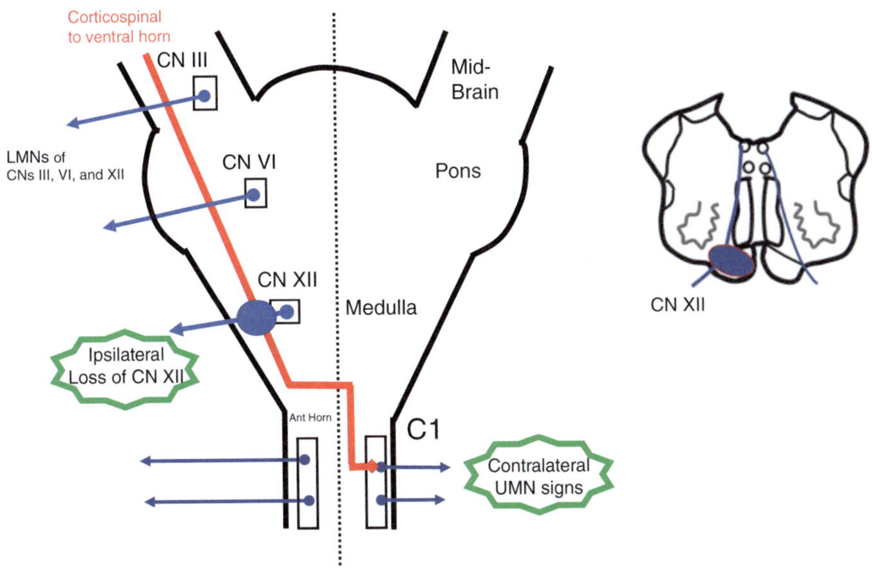

Fig. 20.2 Inferior alternating Hemiplegia. Lesion affects corticobulbar tract and LMNs of CN XII [12, 13]

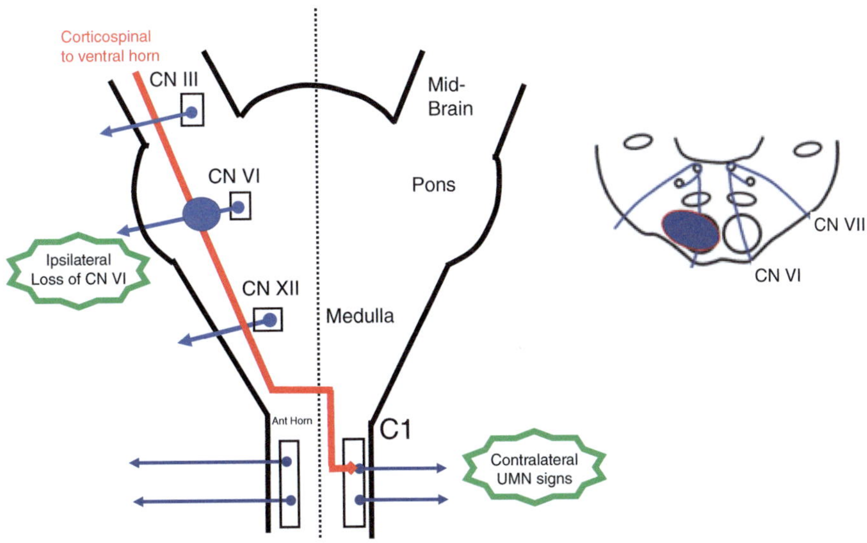

Fig. 20.3 Middle alternating Hemiplegia. Lesion affects corticobulbar tract and LMNs of CN VI [12, 13]

Middle Alternating Hemiplegia

We are moving the lesion up the ladder to the pons. In this case, the lesion will compromise the LMNs of CN VI and the corticospinal and corticobulbar tracts. This leads to an ipsilateral medial strabismus, and contralateral upper motor neuron signs to the limbs. Again, if you see a patient with a hemiplegia on one side, and just one, or two, cranial nerve defects on the contralateral side, then you think alternating hemiplegia, and the lesion will be at the level of the cranial nerve deficit, which in this case is CN VI, which is in the caudal pons. Thus, the term middle alternating hemiplegia. Cranial nerve VII is also found at this level and is close to CN VI thus a patient could also have a CN VII deficit (Fig. 20.3).

Superior Alternating Hemiplegia

We are now moving the lesion up the ladder to the midbrain where it damages the corticospinal and corticobulbar tracts and the LMNs of CN III. The patient will have an ipsilateral lateral strabismus and contralateral UMN signs—hemiplegia-from the neck down. This is usually the result of a stroke in a paramedian branch of the posterior cerebral artery as it wraps around the cerebral peduncle (Fig. 20.4).

All three alternating hemiplegic patients: superior, middle, and inferior, have the same signs from the neck down, but one has a third nerve palsy (superior), one has a sixth nerve palsy (middle), and one has a twelfth nerve palsy (inferior).

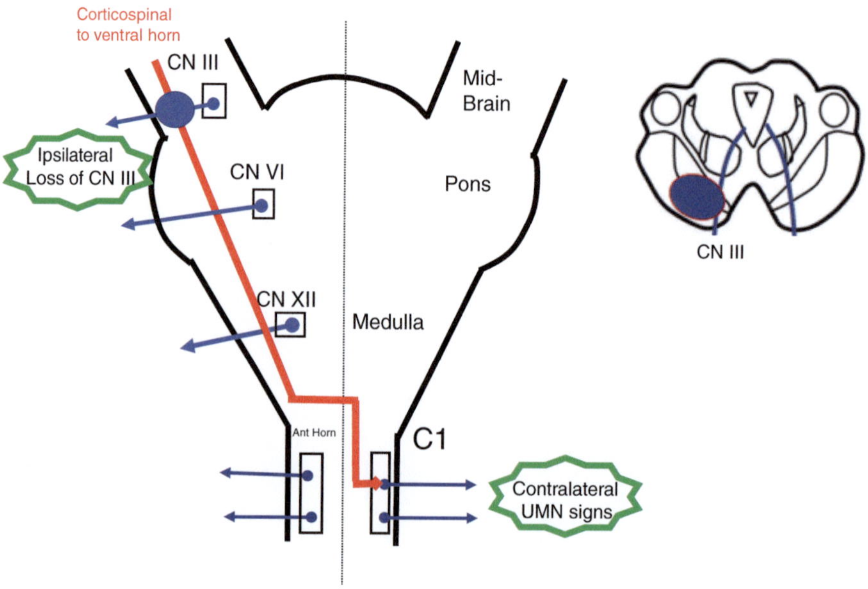

Fig. 20.4 Superior alternating Hemiplegia. Lesion affects corticobulbar tract and LMNs of CN III [12, 13]

Rule of Fours

In a masterful 1995 paper, Peter Gates presented a straightforward way for the non-neurologist to think about brainstem lesions. His "Rule of Fours" points out that in the brain stem there are four Midline structures beginning with the letter "M," and there are four structures on the Side beginning with "S." Four Ms., and four Ss. In addition, there are four cranial nerves in the medulla: IX, X, XI, and XII; four cranial nerves in the pons: V, VI, VII, and VIII; and four in the midbrain and above: I, II, III, and IV (Fig. 20.5).

The four **Ms** on the medial side are the **M**otor pathway (corticospinal and corticobulbar tracts), the **M**edial lemniscus, the **M**LF, and the **M**otor Cranial Nerves—either CNs XII, VI, or III, depending on where you are. The motor cranial nerves on the medial side are CN XII in the medulla, CN VI in the lower pons, and CN III in the midbrain. Sound familiar? This relates to an inferior alternating hemiplegia in the medulla, middle alternating hemiplegia in the pons, and superior alternating hemiplegia in the midbrain. On the lateral side are the four **S**s—the **S**pinothalamic, the **S**pinal nucleus of V, the **S**ympathetics (descending sympathetics), and the **S**pinocerebellar (dorsal spinocerebellar pathway travelling in the inferior cerebellar peduncle).

Using the Rule of Four's helps one to think through the lateral versus medial brainstem injuries. *Lateral pontine* and *lateral medullary syndromes* both damage the four Ss. Both syndromes share a set of signs and symptoms including: an ipsilateral loss of pain and temperature sensation to the face because the spinal nucleus of V is damaged; a contralateral loss of pain and temperature to the limbs because the spinothalamic is damaged; Horner's syndrome because the descending hypothalamic fibers are affected; and balance problems because the dorsal spinocerebellar tract is damaged. The difference between the two syndromes comes down to which cranial nerves are affected. Think back to the idea of the brainstem as a ladder. Lateral Medullary Syndrome affects cranial nerves lower on the ladder—CNs IX and XII. While Lateral Pontine Syndrome affects CNs higher up on ladder—CNs V, VII, and VIII.

Medial syndromes, such as medial medullary, medial pontine, and medial midbrain syndrome damage the corticospinal and corticobulbar tracts and various cranial nerves, giving us either inferior, middle, and superior alternating hemiplegia, depending on where the lesion is.

Now for the details of each syndrome.

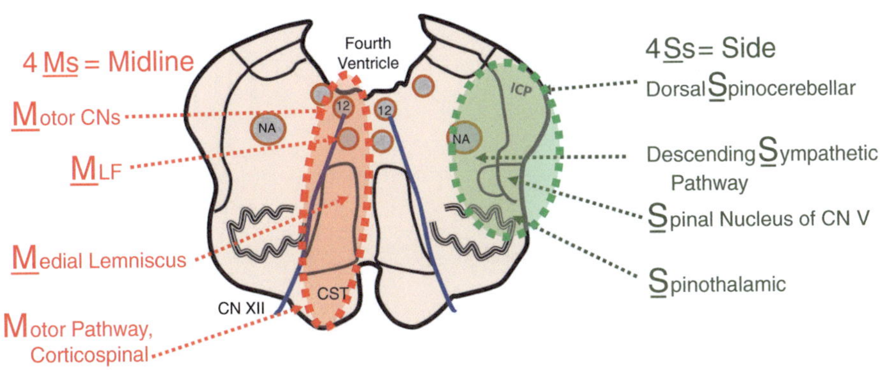

Fig. 20.5 Rule of fours [12, 13]

Lateral Medullary Syndrome

In lateral medullary syndrome there is a stroke to the lateral side of the medulla usually due to an occlusion of either the vertebral artery or posterior inferior cerebellar artery. A hallmark of this lesion is an ipsilateral loss of pain and temperature to the face, and a contralateral loss of pain and temperature to the limbs. The loss of ipsilateral pain and temperature sensation results from damage to the spinal nucleus and tract of V. Running right next to spinal nucleus of V is the spinothalamic tract, and lesions to the spinothalamic tract result in a contralateral loss of pain and temperature to the limbs (Fig. 20.6).

There are other aspects to the syndrome. The inferior cerebellar peduncle is damaged so there is ipsilateral ataxia. Because we are low down on the ladder, the lower cranial nerve structures are affected. The lesion compromises nucleus ambiguus which is sending LMNs to the muscles of the pharynx and larynx on branches of CNs IX and X, which will lead to dysphagia and dysarthria. If the vestibular nuclei are compromised then nystagmus could be present. In addition, the patient will have ipsilateral Horner's syndrome due to lesioning the descending hypothalamic fibers traveling down through the lateral brainstem on their way to the lateral horn at T1.

It is important to pay attention to what is not affected in this scenario. Note that the lesion spares the pyramids, the medial lemniscus, and the nucleus and fibers of CN XII.

Medial Medullary Syndrome

Medial medullary syndrome is the result of an occlusion to either the vertebral or the anterior spinal artery. The patient will have a contralateral loss of motor function from the neck down and an ipsilateral loss of CN XII. In addition, they will have a contralateral loss of the dorsal columns/medial lemniscus modalities. The other name for this is inferior alternating hemiplegia. These patients will not have Horner's syndrome, since the descending hypothalamic fibers in the dorsal longitudinal fasciculus (DLF) are located laterally in the brain stem (Fig. 20.7).

Structure	Symptoms
Inferior Cerebellar Peduncle	Ipsilateral Ataxia. Patient fall towards the lesion side
Nucleus Ambiguus	Dysphagia, Dysarthria
Spinothalamic	Contralateral loss of pain and temperature from body (neck down)
Inferior Vestibular Nucleus	Vomiting, Dizziness. Nystagmus
Spinal Nucleus of V	Ipsilateral loss of pain and temperature from face
Descending Hypothalamics	Horner's Syndrome

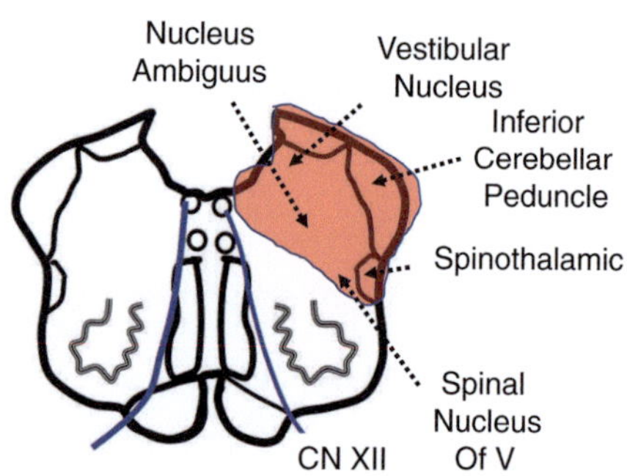

Fig. 20.6 Lateral medullary syndrome. Due to occlusion of posterior inferior cerebellar artery, or vertebral artery [12, 13]

Structure	Symptoms
Hypoglossal Nucleus	Ipsilateral tongue deficit
Medial Lemniscus	Lose of dorsal columns on contralateral side
Pyramid (Corticospinal)	Contralateral upper motor neuron signs

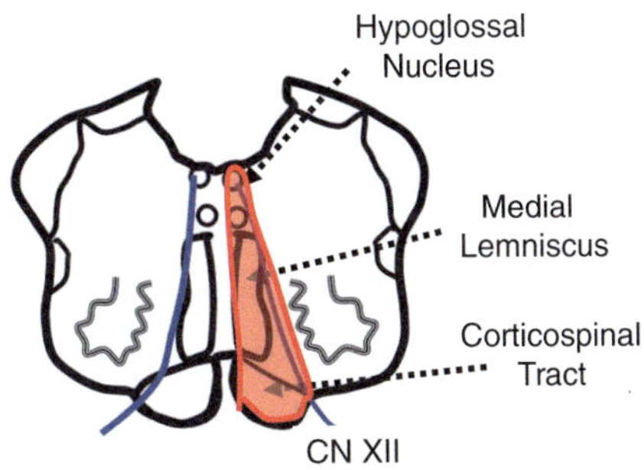

Fig. 20.7 Medial medullary syndrome [12, 13]

Lateral Pontine Syndrome

This is like lateral medullary syndrome, just a bit higher up on the ladder, and is due to an occlusion of the anterior inferior cerebellar artery. Like lateral medullary syndrome, the patient will have an ipsilateral loss of pain and temperature to the face due to damage to the spinal nucleus of V, and contralateral loss of pain and temperature to the body due to damage to the spinothalamic pathway. But since the lesion is in the pons, in the middle of the ladder, the middle cranial nerves, such as CNs V, VII or VIII may be affected. Horner's syndrome will also typically be present.

Medial Pontine Syndrome

In medial pontine syndrome there is a deficit to the corticospinal and corticobulbar tracts traveling through the pons which will lead to a contralateral UMN deficit. Crossing these tracts and running horizontally are LMN fibers from the nucleus of CN VI. Damage to these fibers will lead to an ipsilateral CN VI palsy (one eye is affected). However, if the lesion is large enough it could also damage the nucleus of CN VI which would lead to a paralysis of ipsilateral horizontal gaze (both eyes are affected). In addition, if the lesion is large enough it could also compromise CN VII which would lead to an ipsilateral CN VII deficit. The problematic arteries in medial pontine syndrome are the perforating branches of the basilar artery.

The LMNs come out of the abducens nucleus and travel through the pons to exit ventrally. As the fibers travel though the pons there are three potential lesions in the ventral pons to the nerve or nucleus of CN VI. The explanation below is based on first understanding the pathway from the cortex to the FEF and then to the lateral and medial rectus muscles, which was explained earlier. All these lesions involve damage to the lower motor neuron fibers of CN VI between the nucleus and their exit from the brainstem at the pontomedullary junction (Fig. 20.8).

1. Raymond's Syndrome: CN VI palsy (CN VI fibers) plus contralateral hemiparesis (corticospinal tract). This is a lesion to the ventral pons that damages the fibers of CN VI and their close neighbor, the corticospinal tract. This will lead to ipsilateral CN VI palsy plus a contralateral hemiparesis.
2. Millard-Gubler Syndrome: CN VI palsy (CN VI fibers) plus CN VII and contralateral hemiparesis (corticospinal tract). This is like the lesion above, but it is larger and now hits the fibers of CN VII.
3. Foville's Syndrome: Lateral Gaze Palsy (CN VI nucleus), plus CN V, VII, and VIII palsies, ipsilateral Horner's syndrome, and contralateral hemiparesis (corticospinal tract). Note that this lesion has moved posterior and now damages the nucleus of CN VI which results in lateral gaze paralysis. Remember that a lesion to the nucleus of CN VI will affect both eyes.

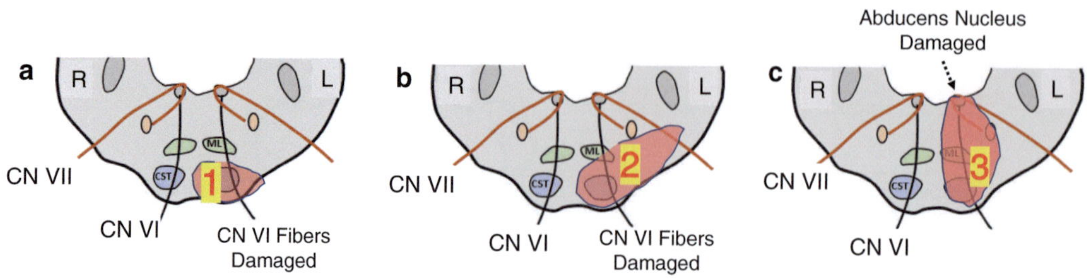

Fig. 20.8 Medial pontine syndromes—variations on a theme. All three lesions disrupt the corticospinal tract and some portion of CN VI. Panel (**a**) Lesion #1 leads to contralateral UMN signs from neck down and ipsilateral CN VI palsy. Panel (**b**) Lesion #2 leads to contralateral UMN signs and ipsilateral CN VI and CN VII palsies. Panel (**c**) Lesion #3 leads to contralateral UMN signs and paralysis of horizontal gaze. Note that lesion #1 and #2 damage the fibers of CN VI, while Lesion #3 damages the abducens nucleus [12, 13]

In terms of CN VI, Raymond's and Millard Gubler are similar in that in both cases, the *LMN fibers* of CN VI are damaged before leaving the pons and in both cases the corticospinal tract is damaged. Foville's on the other hand involves damage to the *nucleus* of CN VI which leads to lateral gaze paralysis. Note that for these three lesions, as a medical student, it is *not* critically important to remember the names of the lesions. Think of them all as variations on medial pontine syndrome. It is much more important to understand the reasoning behind the symptoms, which comes down to knowing the neighboring structures of CN VI within the CNS. You should realize that CNVI lies near the corticospinal tract and CNs, V and VIII, so that these neighbors can also be affected if there is damage to CN VI in the pons.

Medial Midbrain Syndrome

Running laterally, or horizontally, across the cerebral peduncle is the posterior cerebral artery on its way to the occipital lobe. As it passes by the peduncle, it sends branches into the medial midbrain perfusing the cerebral peduncle housing the corticospinal and corticobulbar tracts along with the accompanying oculomotor nerve. Damage here will lead to contralateral upper motor neuron deficits from the lesion down, and an ipsilateral CN III palsy. A CN III palsy will lead to the eye going down and out (lateral strabismus). Because the preganglionic fibers coming from Edinger-Westphal on their way to the ciliary ganglion are also affected, the patient will have a dilated pupil and droopy eyelid (Fig. 20.9).

What happens to this patient's face? You really do not need information about the face to determine where the lesion is in this patient but, in case it is mentioned, you should understand the logic of the facial deficits. We need to focus on the corticobulbar fibers that are damaged at the peduncle. Because the lesion is at the level of CN III, we know that we are at the top of the ladder. Meanwhile, CN VII is lower down on the ladder and sits at the level of the pons. Thus, the lesion at the level of CN III hits corticobulbar fibers that have not crossed over yet to CN VII. At the level of the lesion the corticobulbar fibers are still traveling down, through the lesion, and will eventually cross over below the lesion—at the level of CN VII. And the nucleus of CN VII is divided into half, with the upper part getting a bilateral input, and the lower part getting a contralateral input. Thus, in medial midbrain syndrome, the contralateral lower face is affected (Fig. 20.10).

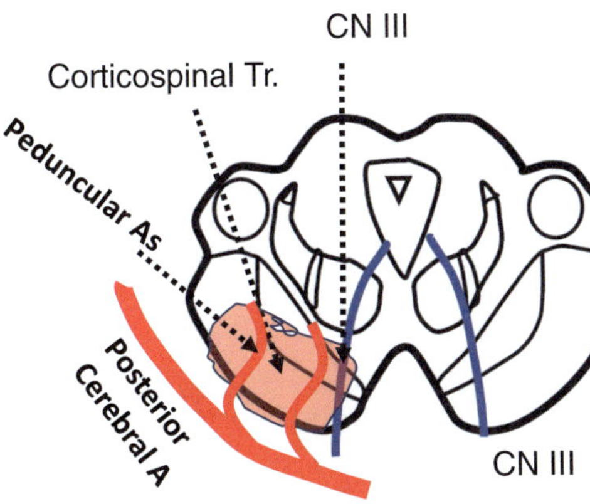

Structure	Symptoms
CN III	Ipsilateral deficit CN III
Corticospinal Tract	Contralateral upper motor neuron signs
Corticobulbar Tract	Contralateral lower facial paralysis

Fig. 20.9 Medial midbrain syndrome. Due to occlusion of peduncular branches of the posterior cerebral artery [12, 13]

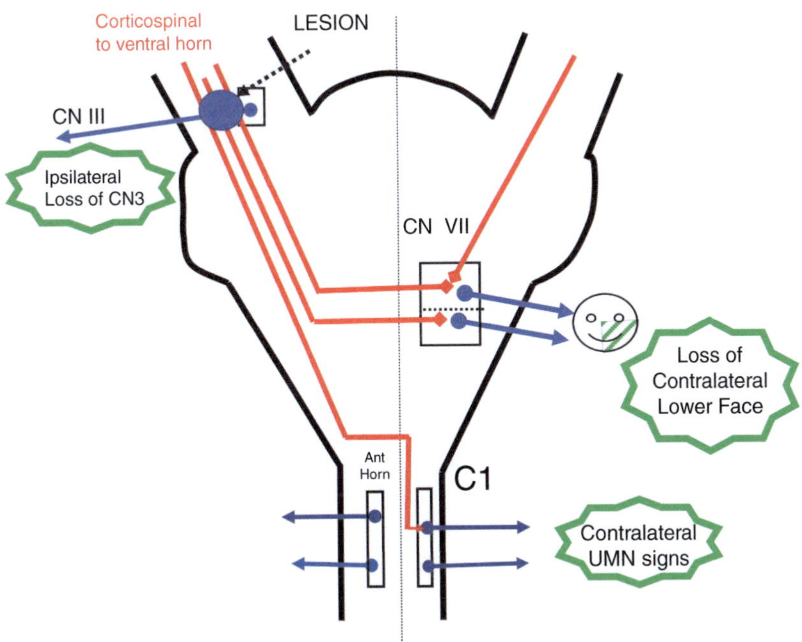

Fig. 20.10 Medial midbrain syndrome and the face. The lesion at the level of CN III, damages the corticospinal tract heading towards the opposite side of the body. It also damages the corticobulbar fibers heading to the contralateral lower face. The upper part of the face will be intact because of its bilateral corticobulbar input [12, 13]

Benedikt's Syndrome

Benedikt's syndrome involves a lesion to the red nucleus and its surrounding structures. Coming out of the red nucleus is the rubrospinal tract which projects to the contralateral LMNs. It is related to the cerebellum, so a lesion here will result in a contralateral tremor. Running through the red nucleus are the fibers of CN III so a lesion here will also result in an ipsilateral CN III palsy. If the lesion is large enough it can compromise the medial lemniscus, sitting next to the red nucleus, leading to contralateral dorsal column symptoms. And the lesion could potentially compromise the spinothalamic tract leading to a contralateral deficit of pain and temperature (Fig. 20.11).

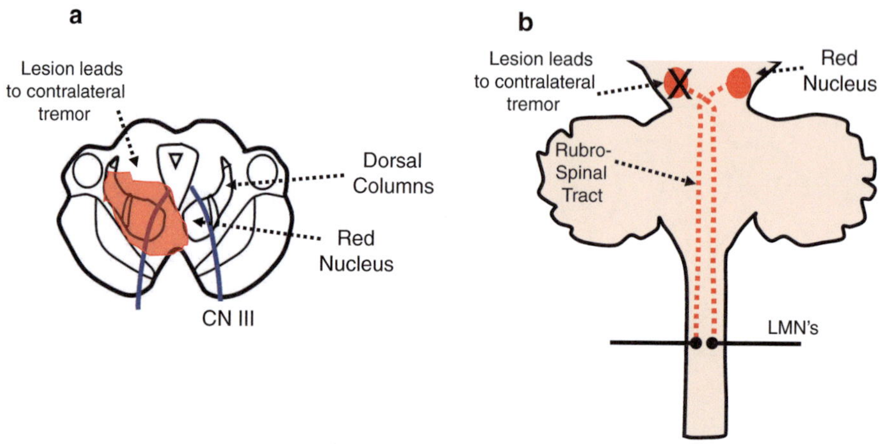

Fig. 20.11 Benedikt's syndrome. Panel (**a**) shows a lesion to the red nucleus and surrounding structures in cross section. Panel (**b**) shows the longitudinal view of the rubrospinal tract emerging from the red nucleus. A lesion to the red nucleus leads to a tremor on the contralateral side [12, 13]

Locked-In Syndrome

The basilar artery travels along the center of the pons and terminates by bifurcating into the two posterior cerebral arteries—like a "T." Along the way the basilar artery sends branches into the pons. A lesion to the top of the basilar artery can lead to locked-in-syndrome, which is a loss of all motor function, except for limited eye movements. Higher cortical functions are all intact. In 1995, Jean-Dominique Bauby, a 43-year-old magazine editor, was driving to work and had a stroke of his basilar artery. He lost all motor function except for his ability to blink. He subsequently authored the book, The Diving Bell and the Butterfly by blinking out the letters. At night he would plan what he wanted to say, and then in the day he would dictate the text. On the wall in his hospital room was a poster of the alphabet. His stenographer would stand by the poster and slowly slide a finger along the alphabet, and Bauby would blink when the stenographer's finger was on the letter he wanted. The stenographer would then move onto the next letter. Baudy's analogy was that his body was like a diving bell that could not move, and mind was like a butterfly that could effortlessly glide through his memories. The day after his book was published, a heroic work, he died.

Superior Cerebellar Peduncle Lesion

The superior cerebellar peduncle is perfused by the superior cerebellar artery. Occlusions will typically result in an: ipsilateral tremor because the superior cerebellar peduncle which carries the dentatothalamic fibers will be damaged; a contralateral loss of pain and temperature because the spinothalamic tract will be damaged; and a bilateral diminution of hearing because the lateral lemniscus will be damaged; and a nystagmus.

Cranial Nerve III Lesions

Cranial nerve III palsies are common to see in a clinical encounter or on an exam. However, just knowing that there is a lesion to CN III does not answer the question: Where is the lesion? A lesion to CN III could be at multiple sites along its pathway, thus we need to look at what other symptoms the patient would have Fig. 20.12.

Lesion #1 is to CN III as it travels through the red nucleus which would result in Benedikt's Syndrome. The patient will have an ipsilateral CN III deficit and a contralateral tremor.

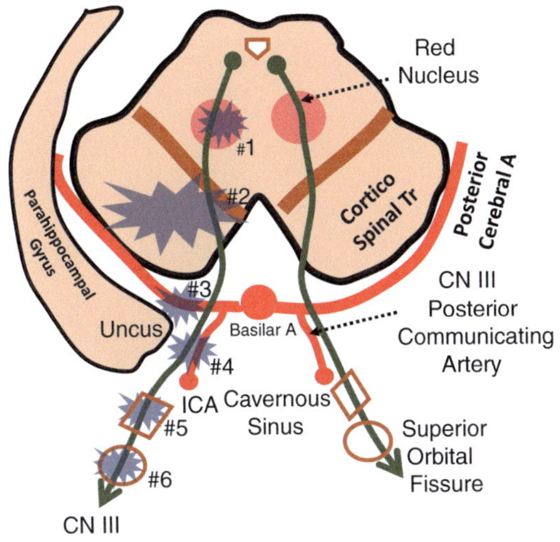

Lesion	In Addition to CN III Findings
1 Benedikt's Syndrome	Contralateral tremor
2 Medial Midbrain Syndrome	Contralateral spastic paralysis
3 Uncal Herniation	Ipsilateral or contralateral spastic paralysis, Contralateral homonymous hemianopia
4 Posterior Communicating A.	Pupillary defect
5 Cavernous Sinus	Deficits with CNs III, IV, VI, and V1 and V2
6 Superior Orbital Fissure	Ophthalmoplegia

Fig. 20.12 Six Lesions to CN III. All six lesions shown on the figure result in a CN III palsy. In addition, each lesion has other signs and symptoms depending on which structure is damaged. *ICA* Internal carotid artery [12, 13]

Lesion #2 is to the cerebral peduncle right near the corticospinal and corticobulbar pathways which would result in contralateral UMN signs. The artery involved is typically the posterior cerebral.

Lesion #3 is an uncal herniation. The typical scenario involves someone getting hit to the head. Take a baseball player who was hit by a ball to his left skull and brought to the ER with a subdural hematoma. The pressure from the hematoma can lead to the left medial temporal lobe, particularly the uncus, herniating out of the skull at the tentorium cerebelli. The left uncal herniation will compress the left oculomotor nerve resulting in a dilated pupil, often referred to as a *blown pupil*, which leads to the eye deviating down and out. As the left uncus herniates it can put pressure on the left corticospinal tract and lead to contralateral UMN signs.

However, there is another scenario that can also occur. As the uncus herniates out on the left it can push the brain stem towards the right. On the right side the tentorium will compress the right cerebral peduncle with the corticospinal tract. The impression made by the tentorium on the peduncle is known as Kernohan's notch. Compression on the right corticospinal tract will lead to left side UMN signs. Thus, the eye deficit will be on the same side as the UMN signs. The left UMN sign is sometimes referred to as a false localizing sign, as it is opposite the typical alternating hemiplegia. In short, with an uncal herniation, in terms of the UMN signs, they could be found on the ipsilateral or contralateral side of the herniation.

And in addition, in some cases, the herniated uncus can put pressure on the posterior cerebral artery which will lead to a contralateral homonymous hemianopia (Fig. 20.13).

And last but least, the pressure on the pons and medulla can stretch and lacerate the arteries deep within these structures, which are known as *Duret's hemorrhages*.

Lesion #4 is due to an aneurysm of the posterior communicating artery which compresses the third nerve and can result in a blown pupil. To understand the progression of symptoms when CN III in this region is compromised it is important to understand how the various nerve fibers in CN III are organized. In the center of the nerve are the motor fibers, while on the periphery of the nerve are the parasympathetic fibers.

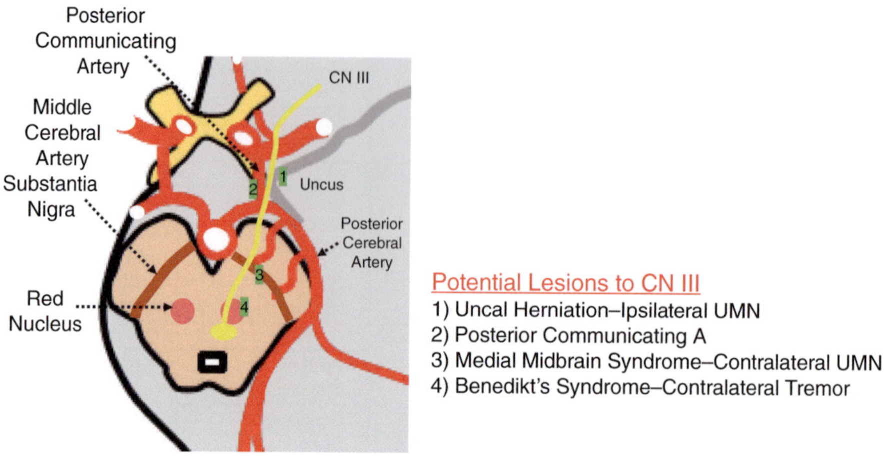

Fig. 20.13 Close up of Brainstem and CN III. On the close-up view you can see four possible lesions to CN III [12, 13]

In the initial stages of the aneurysm, these peripherally located parasympathetic fibers will be compressed leading to a pupillary dilation. At least in the initial stages, the motor fibers will be spared. As the aneurysm expands the motor fibers will also be compressed which will lead to the lateral strabismus.

The other side of this scenario is compromised blood flow to the very small arteries supplying the central part of the third nerve. In a diabetic patient for instance these arteries will be compromised. In this case, the patient will have lost the extraocular muscles supplied by CN III but the pupil will still function normally. Interestingly, in this scenario the patient will have ptosis because they lose the function of the levator palpebrae superioris, but the pupil will be spared. (Fig. 20.14).

Lesion #5 occurs to CN III as it travels though the cavernous sinus. An infection on the face can travel back along the deep facial veins and eventually enter the cavernous sinus. Traveling through the sinus are all the nerves associated with the eye: III, IV, VI, plus V1 and V2. Thus, the patient will have ophthalmoplegia. However, because CN VI is located deeper in the sinus, while the other nerves are on the lateral wall, the initial eye deficit will be a CN VI palsy with a medial strabismus. Eventually, as the lesion enlarges, and all the eye muscles are affected, the patient will have full complete ophthalmoplegia.

Interestingly, as CN VI passes through the cavernous sinus the postganglionic sympathetic fibers traveling to the eye travel with CN VI (they hitchhike) for a moment. They shortly jump from CN VI to V1 (ophthalmic division of V) on their way to the eye. Thus, a patient presenting with an ipsilateral CN VI deficit and an ipsilateral Horner's syndrome most likely has pathology in the cavernous sinus. The presence of both an ipsilateral CN VI palsy and Horner's syndrome is referred to as *Parkinson Sign* (Not to be confused with Parkinson's disease).

Lesion #6 is a mass in the superior orbital fissure. The superior orbital fissure can be subdivided into two parts by the tendinous origin of the eye muscles. One part is in the SOF but outside the tendinous insertion. The second part is with both the tendinous insertion and the SOF. A saying for the nerves travelling through the SOF is LFT 36 N. The LFT part stands for **l**acrimal, **f**rontal and **t**rochlea, all of which travel in the SOF, but outside the tendinous insertion. The 36 N stands for CN 3, CN

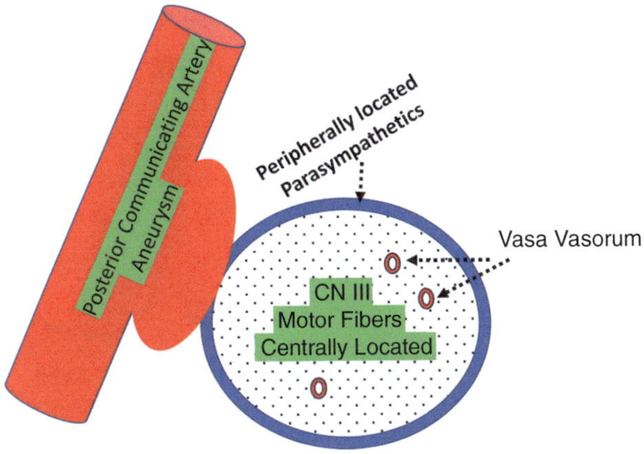

Fig. 20.14 Cranial nerve III organization of fibers. The parasympathetic fibers involved with the pupil are located on the periphery of the nerve. An aneurysm of the posterior communicating artery will initially compress the parasympathetic fibers. The motor fibers are located centrally and are perfused by the vasa vasorum. Patients with compromised perfusion of the vasa vasorum will present with eye movement deficits [12, 13]

6 and the nasociliary nerve (a branch of V1) which all travel through the SOF but also within the tendinous insertion. A lesion in the fissure will lead to ophthalmoplegia. Note the optic nerve does not travel through the SOF, so visual acuity is not affected.

Trochlear Nucleus

We discussed CN IV with eye movements but one thing to note with CN IV is that the LMNs of CN IV decussate before leaving the CNS. Let us think about it from the lesion's point of view. We know that if we lesion the right trochlear nerve the head will tilt to the left—the right nerve goes to the right superior oblique which is an intorter. If we lose that intorter, the right eye will be extorted, so to compensate we lean away from the damaged side which is to the left. In other words, we are doing with our head and neck what we cannot accomplish with the eye muscle. However, if we lesion the right nucleus, keep in mind this is going to the left nerve, so the left eye is extorted, and we will lean to the right. The condensed version: With a trochlear *nerve* lesion the patient leans to the opposite side, but with a trochlear *nucleus* lesion the patient leans to the same side. (Fig. 20.15).

Arteries to Brainstem

The two vertebral arteries travel up through the foramen transversarium of C6-C1 and enter the skull through the foramen magnum and unit to form the single basilar artery. Right before joining, they give off the right and left posterior inferior cerebellar arteries (PICA) that supply the cerebellum and brain stem and are one of potential arteries to be involved with lateral medullary syndrome. Coming off the basilar close to its origin is the anterior inferior cerebellar artery (AICA) which is involved with lateral pontine syndrome.

Close to the termination of the basilar artery are the right and left superior cerebellar arteries (SCA), followed by the posterior cerebral arteries (PCA). The posterior cerebral arteries wrap around the cerebral peduncle and send branches into the midbrain. These branches of posterior cerebral arteries are involved with medial midbrain syndrome. The posterior cerebral arteries also give off the posterior communicating arteries that join the circle of Willis. The superior cerebellar arteries are thought to be involved with trigeminal neuralgia. Compression by the artery primarily affects V1 and V2. All the branches mentioned above were discussed in more detail with the various brain stem lesions (Fig. 20.16).

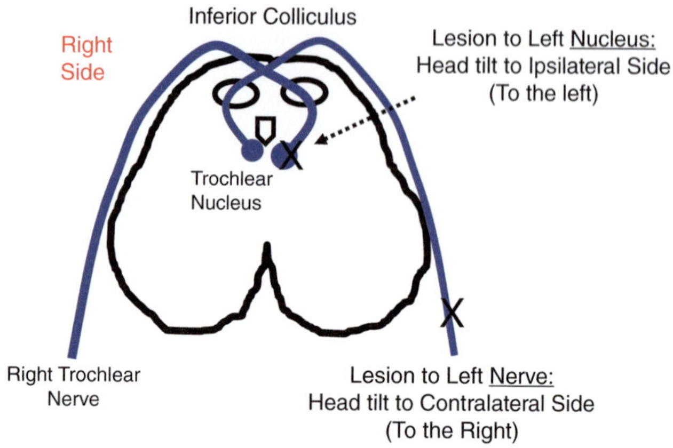

Fig. 20.15 Decussation of CN IV LMNs. This is the only time where a LMN decussates before leaving the CNS. The right trochlear nucleus goes to the left superior oblique. A lesion to the trochlear nerve will lead to a head tilt to opposite side. A lesion to nucleus will lead to an ipsilateral head tilt [12, 13]

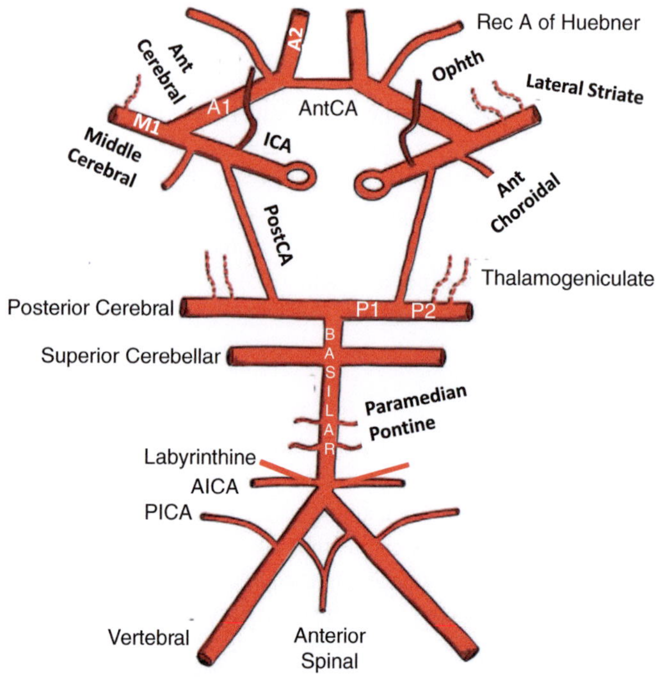

Fig. 20.16 Circle of Willis and its named branches. *AntCA* anterior communicating artery. *PostCA* posterior communicating artery. *PICA* posterior inferior cerebellar artery. *AICA* anterior inferior cerebellar artery. *ICA* internal carotid artery. Note that arising from the basilar artery there are also short and long circumferential As which are not shown in the picture [12, 13]

Two Abducens Cases

There are two cases below. They are similar, however there are several significant differences between the two that are important when it comes to localizing the lesion.

Abducens Nerve Case

A 70-year-old right-handed female was brought to the office by her children because this morning she fell while trying to get out of bed. She had difficulty walking and dragged her right leg while walking. On exam you find that her right upper extremity is weak when she tries to grasp objects for support. She is drooling from the left side of her mouth. There are no sensory deficits.

When asked to look to the right, up, and down, she could not move her left eye laterally. When she was asked to smile, the right side moved appropriately while the left side remained immobile. She also had difficulty closing her left eye. Babinski's sign was present on the right. The right upper extremity was slightly flexed at the elbow, and the slightly extended right lower extremity moved slowly and stiffly when the patient attempted to walk.

Abducens Nucleus Case

A 70-year-old right-handed female was brought to the office by her children because this morning. This morning she fell while trying to get out of bed and she had difficulty walking and dragged her right leg while walking. On exam you find that her right upper extremity is weak when she tries to grasp objects for support. She was drooling from the left side of her mouth. There were no sensory deficits.

When asked to look to the right, up, and down, *she could not look to the left with either eye.* When she was asked to smile, the right side moved appropriately while the left side remained immobile. She also had difficulty closing her left eye. Babinski's sign was present on the right. *Pinprick testing revealed a loss of pain and temperature on the right side of her body.* The right upper extremity was slightly flexed at the elbow, and the slightly extended right lower extremity moved slowly and stiffly when the patient attempted to walk (Fig. 20.17).

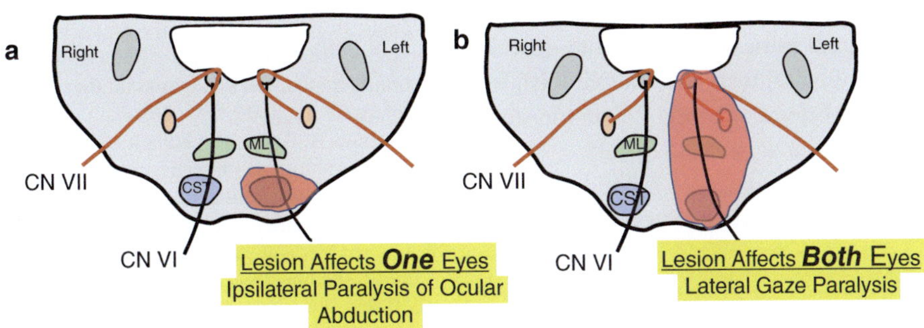

Fig. 20.17 Two medial pontine cases: in panel (**a**) the lesion is affecting the corticospinal tract and the fibers of CN VI traveling through the CST. Because only the *fibers* of CN VI are affected the patient only has a deficit with one eye. In panel (**b**) the lesion is slightly larger and is moved ventrally to the point where it is damaging the *nucleus* of CN VI. Because the nucleus is damaged the patient will have a lateral gaze palsy when looking to the left—neither eye can look left. Both patients will have contralateral UMN signs from the neck down [12, 13]

Localization of the Two Lesions

In both cases the lesions are in the basis pontis, and in both cases the corticospinal tract on the left is compromised so the patient has right side UMN signs. In the first case, the patient only has a deficit with the abduction of the left eye which tells us that the abducens nerve is affected.

In the second case, the patient has a lateral gaze palsy to the left (both eyes are affected). This tells us the lesion is not just damaging the nerve but is affecting the nucleus. Because this lesion extends from the ventral side all the way to the dorsal side of the pons, it is also affecting the spinothalamic tract resulting in a right-side deficit of pain and temperature.

Historical Snippet: Proustian Moment

One of the more famous insights into memory, and its close relationship to olfaction, came from Marcel Proust, who in 1907 observed that certain odors trigger autobiographical memories. He noticed that a certain kind of dessert (Madeline cakes) triggered memories about his aunt. For a modern reference to the Proustian moment see the 2019 movie *Ratatouille*, in which the snobby anxious restaurant critic, who is used to upscale French cooking, is given the simple dish of Ratatouille, the French version of a simple stew. At first, he is aghast at the idea of such a simple dish, but the first taste releases a flood of happy childhood memories, and he is won over.

Ondine's Curse

If the lesion is in the medulla the patient may develop *Central Hypoventilation Syndrome,* also known as *Ondine's Curse*. This is an exceedingly rare form of sleep apnea that is typically the result of a genetic defect and usually discovered early in life—around 2-years old. It is often fatal, In some cases though it occurs following an upper cervical cord injury. The name of the syndrome comes from a German fairy tale about Ondine, a nymph, who fell in love with a human. After finding out the human had an affair, Ondine cast a spell on him causing him to stop breathing every time he fell asleep, so the story goes. In the real world, the syndrome results in a buildup of carbon dioxide and low levels of oxygen during sleep.

Further Reading

1. Afifi AK, Bergman RA. Functional neuroanatomy: text and atlas. London: McGraw-Hill; 1998.
2. Balami JS, Chen RL, Buchan AM. Stroke syndromes and clinical management. Q J Med. 2013;106:607–15.
3. Bauby JD, Leggatt J. The diving bell and the butterfly: a memoir of life in death. New York: Vintage; 1998.
4. Blumenfeld H. Neuroanatomy through clinical cases. 2nd ed. Wiley-Blackwell; 2010.
5. Brazis PW. Ocular motor abnormalities in Wallenberg's lateral medullary syndrome. Mayo Clin Proc. 1992;67:365–8.
6. Brazis PW, Masdeu JC, Biller J. Localization in clinical neurology. Philadelphia: Lippincott, Williams, and Wilkins; 2016.
7. Campbell W, Barohn RJ. Dejong's the neurological examination. Philadelphia: Lippincott, Williams, and Wilkins; 2019.
8. Danchaivijitr C, Kennard C. Diplopia and eye movement disorders. J Neurol Neurosurg Psychiatry. 2004;75(Suppl IV):iv24–31.
9. Fuller G. Neurological examination made easy. 6th ed. London: Elsevier; 2019.
10. Gates P. The rule of 4 of the brainstem: a simplified method for understanding brainstem anatomy and brainstem vascular syndromes for the non-neurologist. Intern Med J. 2005;35(4):263–6.
11. Hartman B, Kremer I, Gutman I, Krakowski D, Kram J. Cavernous sinus infection manifested by Horner's syndrome and ipsilateral sixth nerve palsy. J Clin Neuroophthalmol. 1987;7(4):223–36.
12. Leo J. Medical neuroanatomy for the boards and clinic: finding the Lesion. 2nd ed. Cham: Springer; 2024a.
13. Leo J. Clinical anatomy and embryology: a guide for the classroom, clinic, and clinic. 2nd ed. Cham: Springer; 2024b.
14. Manconi M, Mondini S, Fabiani A, Rossi P, Ambrosetto P, Cirignotta F. Anterior spinal artery syndrome complicated by the ondine curse. Arch Neurol. 2003;60:1787–90.
15. Splittgerber R. Snell's clinical neuroanatomy. 8th ed. Philadelphia: Lippincott, Williams, and Wilkins; 2018.
16. Young PA, Young PH, Tolbert D. Basic clinical neuroscience. Philadelphia: Lippincott, Williams, and Wilkins; 2015.

21 Cerebral Cortex Lesions

Introduction

There are two major lines of demarcation in the cerebral cortex. The first is the central sulcus, running from superior to inferior, which divides the frontal lobe from parietal lobe. The second is the lateral fissure, running from anterior to posterior, which separates the temporal lobe from the frontal and parietal lobes. The temporal lobe is below the lateral fissure.

The frontal lobe includes the prefrontal cortex with the orbitofrontal cortex. One of the more famous patients in neurology is Phineas Gage. Phineas was working on the railroad tracks when an explosion sent a steel rod through the left side of his skull damaging his prefrontal cortex, inadvertently leading to one of the first lobotomies. Although he lost vision in his left eye he could still see with his right eye, he could still hear, and his somatosensory cortex was still intact. But while his senses were intact, Phineas was not quite the same person as he was prior to the accident. With damage to his prefrontal cortex, he had lost his inhibitions and was prone to saying whatever came to his mind—something that can lead to trouble in run of the mill day-to-day communications. His condition provided some of the first insights into the role of the frontal lobe in controlling inhibitions and our ability to function in society.

As mentioned in the chapter on the limbic system, the orbitofrontal cortex on the inferior surface of the frontal lobe receives a sample of information from all the different senses coming into our nervous system. It is thought that the orbitofrontal cortex integrates this information and, along with the hippocampus and amygdala, is involved in decision making.

The central sulcus is bounded anteriorly by the precentral gyrus, also known as the primary motor cortex, and posteriorly by the postcentral gyrus, also known as the primary sensory cortex. Both these gyri are organized topographically with the superior portion being the lower limb territory, and the inferior portion being the face and upper limb territory. Think of upside-down stick figures on each gyrus. If you look at the medial side of the cortex (aka a midsagittal cut), a small portion of each gyrus can also be seen. This small parcel of cortex with a sliver of the central sulcus on this medial view is named the paracentral lobule—it represents the primary motor and primary sensory regions for the contralateral lower limb. Lesions here will naturally affect motor and sensory function to and from the lower limb on the opposite side (Fig. 21.1). If you saw a patient in your office with contralateral loss or motor and sensory function to the lower limb, you might think of a deficit in the thoracic spinal cord. However, a lesion to the thoracic cord would affect motor on one side and sensory on the other side. In contrast, a lesion to the paracentral lobule would affect motor and sensory on the same side (which is contralateral to the lesion) (Fig. 21.2).

J. Leo, *Gross Anatomy, Neuroanatomy, and Embryology for Medical Students*,
https://doi.org/10.1007/978-3-031-87151-1_21

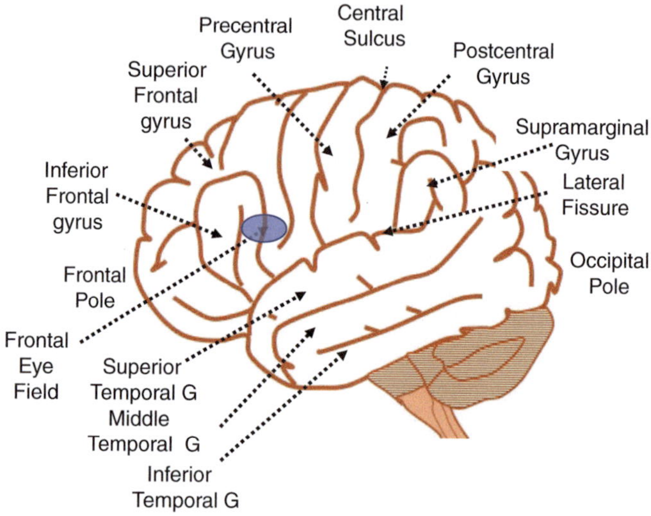

Fig. 21.1 Cerebral cortex. Anterior to the central sulcus is the precentral gyrus also known as primary motor cortex. Posterior to the central sulcus is the post central gyrus also known as primary sensory cortex [6, 7]

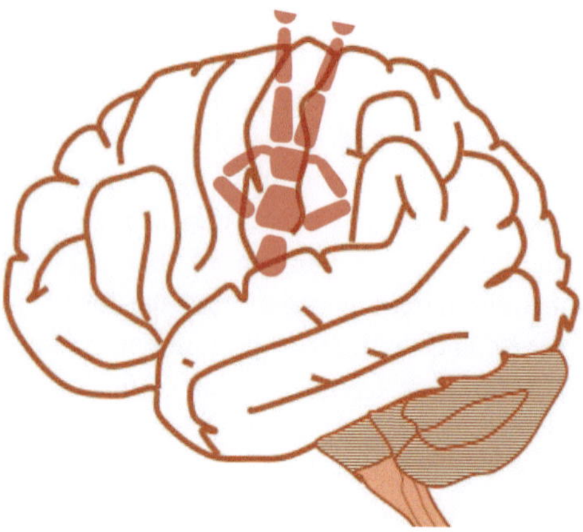

Fig. 21.2 Topographical organization. Both the pre- and post-central gyri are organized topographically such that the lower limb territory is more superior, while the face region is more inferior [6, 7]

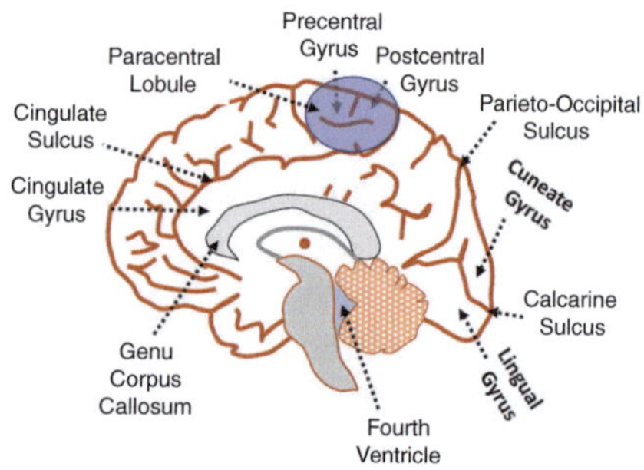

Fig. 21.3 Midsagittal section of cerebrum. The paracentral lobule is a small piece of cortex on either side of the central sulcus on the medial side. It represents primary motor and primary sensory to the contralateral lower limb [6, 7]

On the midsagittal view, one can see the occipital lobe with the calcarine sulcus being a major dividing line. Superior to the calcarine sulcus is the cuneate gyrus, and inferior to it is the lingual gyrus. If you follow the lingual gyrus anterior, it turns into the parahippocampal gyrus (Fig. 21.3).

Broca's Aphasia

In most humans (80–90%), language is located on the left side of the cortex. There are two important regions for language: Broca's and Wernicke's. To carry on a normal conversation these two regions need to work together. You need to understand what that person is saying to you, and you need to verbalize back to that person in complete sentences so that they understand you.

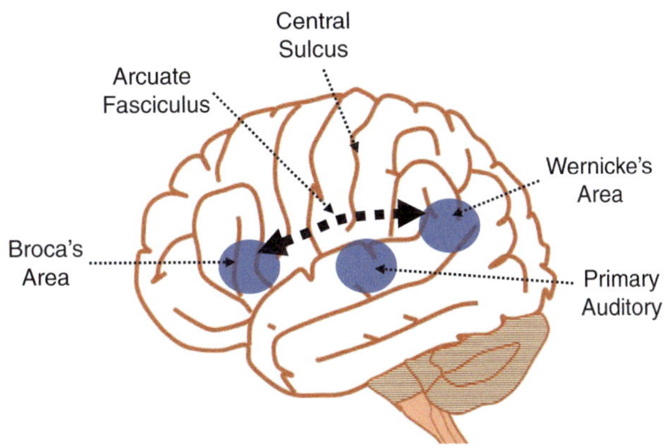

Fig. 21.4 Language regions. Broca's area is located on the inferior frontal gyrus. Wernicke's is in the temporal lobe. The two regions communicate with each other through the arcuate fasciculus [6, 7]

Broca's area lives on the inferior frontal gyrus and is responsible for the speaking or motor component of language (Fig. 21.4). In other words, it takes all the various parts of a sentence: verb, subject, objects, and prepositions and puts them together to make a coherent sentence. Lesions here will result in "Broken Speech" meaning that when a patient speaks, all they can do is say a word here and there. When the words come out, the words are not organized into coherent sentences. If you ask the patient about getting up this morning, they understand the question, and they want to give you a full explanation of their morning, but they can only manage to say a couple of words. Their speech is considered non-fluent, or "broken." Instead of saying something like, "my alarm went off at 7 am, I hit the snooze button, slept for another 15 minutes, and then got out of bed" they say "alarm…bed….day." Again, their speech is "broken."

Wernicke's Aphasia

Wernicke's area is in the left temporal lobe and is responsible for comprehending speech—it is the part of your brain that you are using right now as you read this page. Lesions here will result in "word salad." Think of a tossed salad with all the components present but just tossed into a salad bowl with little organization. Patients with Wernicke's aphasia can speak, but their sentences are jumbled and mixed up. When they tell you about their day, they keep right on talking, but their sentences are jumbled and incoherent. While they are "fluent," but they do not make sense.

Conduction Aphasia

In a healthy individual, during a normal conversation, Wernicke's and Broca's areas talk to each other via the *arcuate fasciculus.* Lesions of the arcuate fasciculus result in a conduction aphasia. A conduction aphasic sounds like a Wernicke's patient because they are both fluent but do not make sense. However, in contrast to the Wernicke's patient, the conduction aphasic understands you. If two aphasiac patients are sitting in your office and one has Wernicke's and one has conductive aphasia, they will both sound similar. They are both fluent but make little sense, so how do you tell them apart? If you give both the same directions to follow, the conduction patient will understand you and follow through with the directions, but the Wernicke's patient does not follow through. If you tell both to get up, go to the back of the room, turn the light on and off, and then come back and sit down, it is the conduction aphasiac who can follow the directions. The conduction aphasiac understood you, but the Wernicke's patient did not.

Frontal lobe patients will often shuffle their feet and take short steps—*Marche a Petit Pas.* Their gait closely resembles Parkinson's patients who also have a short shuffling gait, however Parkinson's patients will tend to lean forward, while frontal lobe patients stand upright. Frontal lobe patients exhibit frontal release signs such as the grasp, Moro, and rooting reflexes. These are reflexes common in infants that may return in frontal lobe patients.

Cortical Blood Supply

The internal carotid artery enters the skull through the carotid canal and crosses the foramen lacerum and enters the cavernous sinus where it does an 180^0 turn to form the genu of the internal carotid artery. At this bend, the internal carotid artery gives off the ophthalmic artery, which in turn gives off the central artery of the retina. After the bend, as the internal carotid artery approaches the ventral surface of the brain, it splits into the middle and anterior cerebral arteries.

The blood supply to the cerebral cortex comes from the middle, anterior, and posterior cerebral arteries. If you imagine placing your hand on your brain, you are covering the territory of the middle cerebral artery (Fig. 21.5). Your hand is covering the lateral surface of the cortex except for the edges. The superior edge is perfused by the anterior cerebral artery, while the inferior edge and the occipital pole are perfused by the posterior cerebral artery.

The first branches of the middle cerebral artery are the lateral striate arteries which travel deep into the cerebrum and perfuse the internal capsule. Strokes in these arteries can lead to a "Pure Motor deficit." (See the section on the internal capsule for more details). The middle cerebral artery heads towards the lateral side of the cortex as the M1 branch. As it approaches the lateral fissure, it splits into two M2 branches. One of these M2 branches, the superior division, continues superiorly up to the frontal lobe, and the inferior division descends to the temporal lobe. The superior division supplies Broca's area and the face and upper limb territory of the precentral gyrus. A stroke to the superior branch will lead to Broca's aphasia, plus contralateral motor deficits to the upper limb and face (brachiofacial paralysis). Keep in mind that this patient will not have Babinski's sign because the lower limb region of the precentral gyrus is typically not affected. A lesion to the inferior division of the middle cerebral artery will lead to Wernicke's aphasia and in some cases a contralateral superior quadrantanopia (pie in the sky) (Fig. 21.6). The M2 branch can be seen at the insula and is considered the insula branch. The M3 branches travels out towards the surface where they split into M4 branches, or cortical branches.

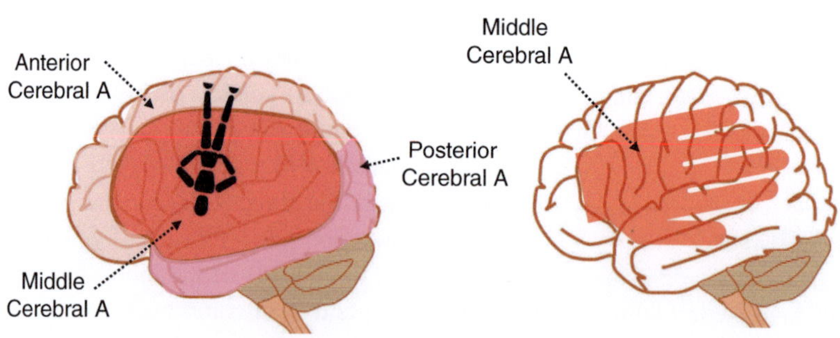

Fig. 21.5 Arteries to cerebral cortex. The middle cerebral artery covers the central part of the lateral surface. The edges of the cortex are perfused by the other two. Imagine placing your hand on your brain. Your hand Is overlying the territory of middle cerebral artery. The edges of the brain—surrounding your hand—are the territories of two other arteries—the posterior and anterior cerebral arteries [6, 7]

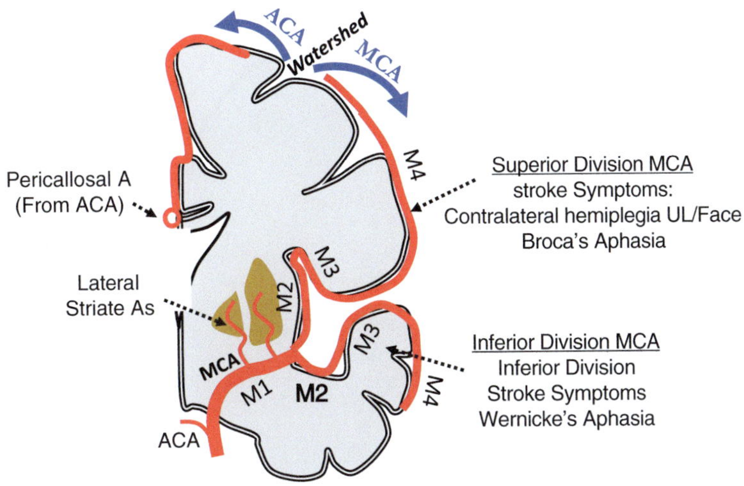

Fig. 21.6 Branches of anterior and middle cerebral arteries. M1 is the horizontal portion heading laterally. M1 divides into M2 at the insula. M3 is the opercular portion, and M4 is the cortical portion. Note there is also the designation of superior and inferior portions or MCA. The superior division heads up onto the frontal lobe which includes Broca's area. The inferior division heads down to where the temporal lobe meets the parietal lobe and includes Wernicke's area [6, 7]

From the origin of the *anterior cerebral artery* to the anterior communicating artery is the A1 segment of the anterior cerebral artery. The first branches coming off this A1 segment are the small medial striate arteries perfusing parts of the internal capsule. The A2 segment then continues and splits into the pericallosal and callosomarginal arteries. The callosomarginal artery travels superior to the cingulate gyrus, while the pericallosal artery travels between the corpus callosum and the cingulate gyrus. The callosomarginal artery sends branches to the medial surface of the cerebral cortex, including the paracentral lobule. Remember, the paracentral lobule is this small region on the medial surface of the cortex that includes the ends of the precentral and postcentral gyri, which is the territory for motor and sensory information for the contralateral lower limb. Lesions of the callosomarginal artery, or the anterior cerebral artery itself, can lead to a motor and sensory deficit to the contralateral lower limb. Along with the motor and sensory deficits, the patient may present with incontinence because the nerves to the pelvic region can be compromised.

The *posterior cerebral arteries* arise from the basilar artery, then travel along each cerebral peduncle towards the occipital cortex. Along the way they give two or three peduncular arteries that travel into the midbrain to supply the cerebral peduncles. From the origin of the posterior cerebral artery to the posterior communicating artery, is the P1 segment. The thalamoperforating arteries arise from the P1 segment. The thalamogeniculate arteries arise from the P2 segment and perfuses the VPM and VPL of the thalamus. The posterior cerebral artery then continues to supply the inferior temporal lobe, and via the calcarine artery supplies the calcarine cortex of the occipital lobe. The posterior cerebral artery also gives off the splenial artery (also referred to as the posterior pericallosal artery) which supplies the splenium of the corpus callosum. The splenial artery meets up with the pericallosal artery from the anterior cerebral artery (Fig. 21.7).

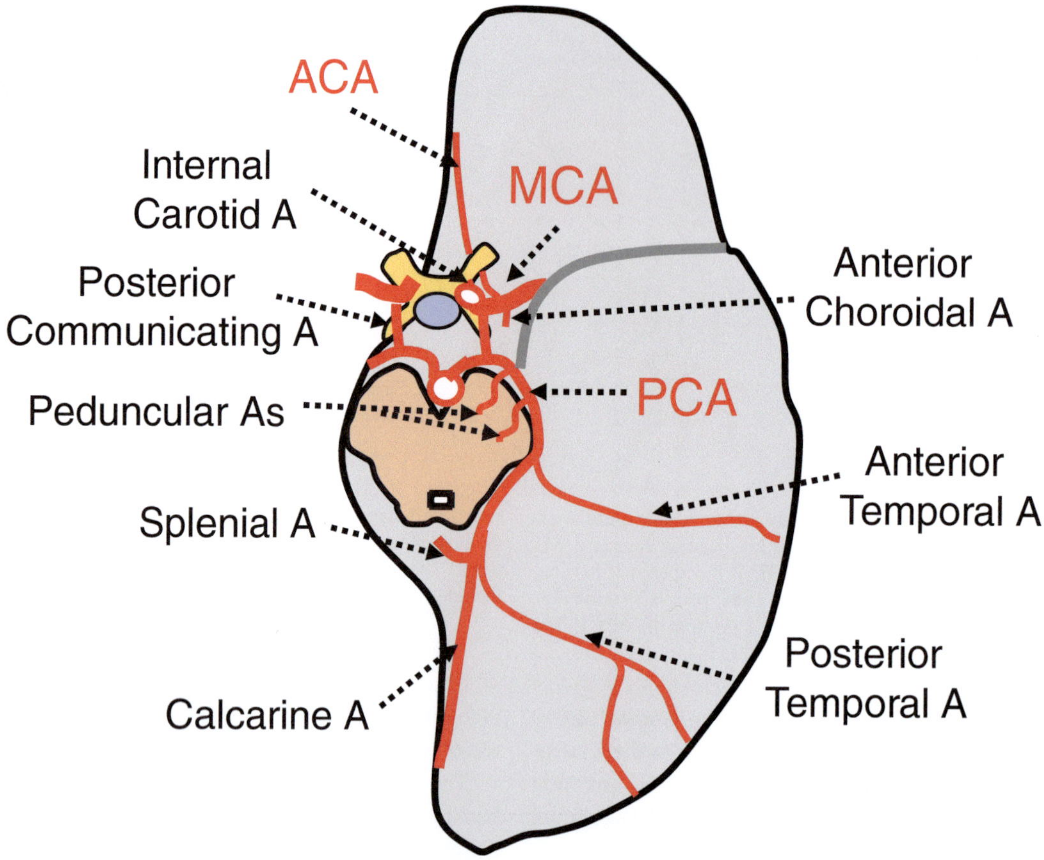

Fig. 21.7 Ventral view of three major cerebral arteries. The internal carotid artery splits into the anterior cerebral artery (ACA) and the middle cerebral artery (MCA). The anterior choroidal artery comes off the MCA. The posterior cerebral artery (PCA) gives off the peduncular arteries that supply the medial midbrain. The PCA continues to supply parts of the inferior temporal lobe and the occipital lobe [6, 7]

Top of Basilar Artery Stroke

Occlusions at the top of the basilar artery can lead to several deficits due to loss of blood flow to the posterior cerebral arteries. Because the posterior cerebral arteries come off right at the top of the basilar artery, the patient will have visual field deficits and cortical blindness because the occipital cortex is supplied by the PCA. In addition, because the posterior cerebral artery goes to the thalamus the patient will have a sensory deficit like a patient with thalamic pain syndrome. And because the PCA perfuses the inferior temporal lobe the patient may have memory and behavior disturbances and even Korsakoff's like symptoms. Motor function is usually not affected in these patients.

Alexia Without Agraphia

A patient with alexia but not agraphia can write but not read. To understand how a stroke can lead to a patient who can write but not read we need to talk about several cortical areas and their connections. When we read something, we are seeing the words with our occipital cortex, but we need to do more than just "see" the letters—just "seeing" the letters or symbols is not enough. To make sense of these letters we need to send the information from both the right and left occipital lobes to Wernicke's area on the left. Remember, Wernicke's is the region of the brain that understands language. The left occipital lobe has a short, straight projection to Wernicke's that does not have to go through the corpus callosum. But the right occipital cortex needs to send its information across the corpus callosum. This information from the right occipital lobe makes its way to Wernicke's on the left side by way of splenium of the corpus callosum. Wernicke's area then turns these letters into words and into meaningful language.

The posterior cerebral artery (PCA) supplies the occipital cortex, but it also supplies the splenium of the corpus callosum. A lesion to the left PCA will damage the left occipital cortex and the splenium, which results in a patient who can write but cannot read. When the patient is shown a written sentence, they can "see" the letters with their right occipital lobe because the information travels along their optic nerves, tracts, and radiations to the right occipital cortex. But they cannot see the words with the left cortex since it has been compromised. For the patient to understand the words that made their way back to their right cortex, they need to send the information from the right cortex across to Wernicke's area, but since the splenium is damaged, they cannot do this. Thus, while they can *see* the words with the right occipital cortex, they cannot *understand* the words since the information cannot move from the right occipital cortex to Wernicke's area on the left (Fig. 21.8).

If the damage is on the right side, they would not have this deficit. They would see the words on the page with the left cortex, and since it is a direct connection from left occipital cortex to left Wernicke's area—the information does not need to go through the splenium- and they would still be able to read and write. And not to overcomplicate it too much, but if we are talking about an individual with language on their right side, then the scenarios would be reversed—if the stroke was on the right side, they would have alexia without agraphia, and if it was on the left, they would not have this deficit.

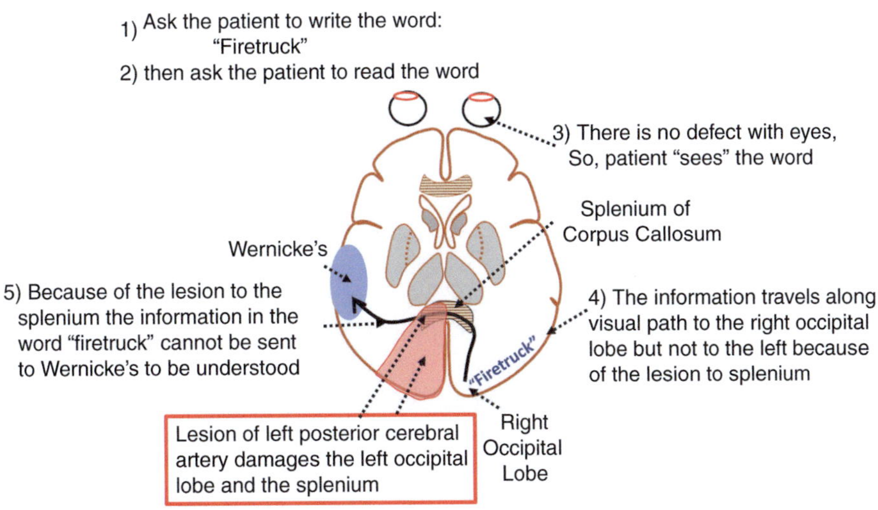

Fig. 21.8 Alexia without agraphia [6, 7]

Parietal Lobe

The parietal lobe is considered an association cortex. It receives information from various regions of the cerebral cortex and then integrates this information. Lesions to the right parietal lobe result in patients with left side neglect. If you ask the patient to draw a clock, they will accurately draw just the right side of the clock but not the left side. Or if you give them a plate of food, they will eat everything on the right side and then ask for more. You simply turn the plate, and they continue eating. This patient scenario does not arise from a visual field deficit but from an inability to consolidate various inputs to the cortex. It is also an example of how we do not completely understand the brain.

The right parietal lobe is also the site of our ability to sense tone, rhythm, intonation, and the deeper meaning of language—referred to as prosody. The easiest way to understand prosody is to think about the communication between a mother and her toddler. When a toddler hears their mother call them by name, the child can tell if the mother is happy, sad, mad, proud, worried, etc. Likewise, when the mother hears the toddler call her by name, she can sense the state of mind of the toddler. There is more to just stating the name. There is an important meaning in the tone. Likewise, the mother can sense the nuances of meaning when the child says "mom." Lesions to the parietal lobe can lead to prosodic deficits.

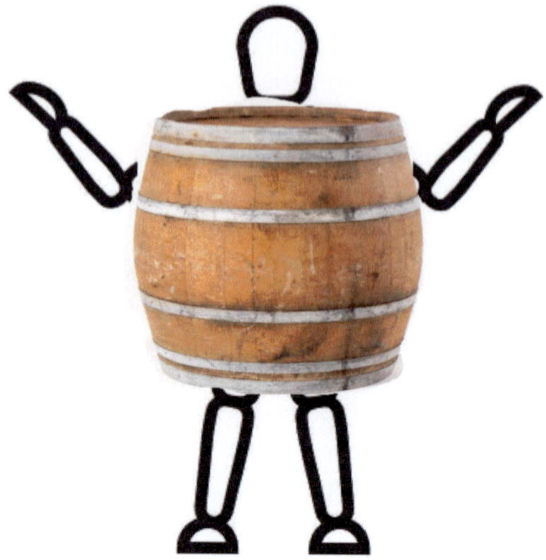

Fig. 21.9 Man in a barrel. The barrel represents the area compromised in hypotensive patients [6, 7]

Man-in-a-Barrel

Watershed zones are problematic for those with low pressure or hypotensive moments (Fig. 21.9). The anterior and middle cerebral arteries territories meet on the lateral surface of the cerebral cortex and form a watershed zone. A lesion here, where the middle and anterior cerebral arteries meet, will result in a syndrome which is sometimes referred to as "Man-in-a-Barrel." Think of a person with a barrel dropped over them and covering up the middle part of their body. The barrel covers the region of the body that is deficient due to loss of perfusion of the watershed area on the cortex. You need to understand the topography of the precentral gyrus and postcentral gyrus to understand these symptoms. Imagine standing with a barrel around your midsection. In these patients, their face is intact, their lower limb is intact, and their hands can be intact. Their deficit is in their midsection.

Gerstmann's Syndrome

Gerstmann's syndrome results from lesions, usually strokes, in the region of the angular gyrus of the non-dominant parietal lobe (usually on the left). The typical Gerstmann's patient will exhibit four classic symptoms: *acalculia*—inability to do simple math calculations; *finger agnosia*—cannot identify their own fingers; *agraphia*—cannot write; and *right-left disorientation*. The most universal finding in these patients is finger agnosia, and in some cases, it may be the only symptom. One way to think of the parietal lobe is to associate it with the hand. Symptoms of parietal lobe damage often lead to dysfunction of movements that we associate with the hands such as drawing or writing. In addition, parietal lobe patients will often present with apraxia and agnosia.

Temporal Lobe

The medial temporal lobe houses the amygdala and hippocampus. Lesions in this area are discussed in more detail with the limbic system. A lesion in the temporal lobe is exemplified by the case of the composer George Gershwin who died from a glioblastoma in his temporal lobe. Prior to his death, he reported that several times while he was playing the piano, he just forgot the music—like a short circuit. He also noted that prior to these events he smelled a "pungent odor" like burning rubber. The tumor was aggravating both his hippocampus which led to memory issues, and his amygdala, which caused him to complain of noxious odors (uncinate fits). Gershwin's medical file did not mention a superior homonymous quadrantanopia, but this has been reported in similar types of patients.

Cingulate Gyrus

One hypothesis of the neuropathology of *Obsessive-Compulsive Disorder* (OCD) is that there is a disruption in the anterior portion of the cingulate gyrus and its connection with the orbitofrontal cortex.

Hydrocephalus

CSF is produced by the choroid plexus in the lateral and third ventricles. Starting in the lateral ventricle, CSF comes down through the foramen of Monroe into the third ventricle and then through the cerebral aqueduct into the fourth ventricle. From the fourth ventricle it goes out the single midline foramen of Magendie and the two laterally located foramen of Luschka, where it now enters the subarachnoid space which surrounds the brain. There are several regions of the subarachnoid space that have specific names such as: the pontine cistern, the cisterna magna, the interpeduncular cistern, or the quadrigeminal cistern. Once in the subarachnoid space, the CSF eventually makes its way to the arachnoid granulations, adjacent to the superior sagittal sinus, which absorb the CSF. There are several types of hydrocephalus. The two main categories are communicating or non-communicating.

With *non-communicating hydrocephalus* (or obstructive hydrocephalus) there is a blockage somewhere between where the CSF is made and where it is absorbed. Because the CSF cannot be absorbed, its volume increases, putting pressure on the system. The most common site for the blockage is in the cerebral aqueduct. This leads to the CSF backing up in the lateral and third ventricles leading to hydrocephalus.

With a *communicating hydrocephalus* there is no blockage, but instead there is either too much CSF being made, or not enough being absorbed. Meningitis or a subarachnoid hemorrhage can lead to a failure of reabsorption of CSF. Tumors of the choroid plexus can lead to overproduction of CSF.

Hydrocephalus ex-vacuo occurs following a stroke or other disease that leads to loss of cortical tissue and a subsequent empty space. The once occupied space is now filled in by CSF.

Normal pressure hydrocephalus (NPH) can occur in an elderly patient whose has enlarged lateral ventricles. The enlarged ventricles fill with fluid and put pressure on the cerebral cortex which can lead to incontinence, confusion, and ataxia, also known as: *Wet, Wacky, and Wobbly*. A shunt from the lateral ventricle to the peritoneum is likely to relieve the symptoms. To test whether the shunt will work, a spinal tap, basically a temporary shunt, can be performed. The spinal tap should relieve some of the pressure on the cortex. If the patient improves then they are a suitable candidate for a permanent shunt.

Apraxia

Patients with apraxia have a motor deficit, even though the motor pathway is intact. My analogy is to a computer program that is working perfectly, but the password is wrong, and you cannot access the program. There are several types of apraxia but let us start with a patient who has damaged the anterior portion of the corpus callosum (the anterior cerebral artery) who has *transcortical apraxia*. This patient cannot follow a simple command to move their left hand, but they can move their right hand. When you ask this person to move their left hand, they hear you and understand what you are asking, because Wernicke's region is intact. Furthermore, they want to follow your command to move their left hand, but to do this they need to send the information from Wernicke's on the left to the right precentral gyrus. Remember the right precentral gyrus controls the left hand. However, the information from Wernicke's cannot cross to the right side of the brain because the corpus callosum is damaged.

They can successfully move their right hand because the information from Wernicke's goes straight to the left precentral gyrus without having to go through the corpus callosum. You also might notice that, while they cannot move their left hand following a command, during the exam they might reach up and spontaneously scratch their head with their left hand. This is because scratching their head is not based on the connection from Wernicke's to the motor cortex. It is just a simple reflex-like activity. Again, there is no deficit with the precentral gyrus, or the corticospinal pathway, or the peripheral nerves, or the muscles—the entire program is intact. The deficit is with gaining access to the program—Wernicke's cannot get the password over to the precentral gyrus to turn it on.

Childhood Apraxia of Speech (CAS) or verbal apraxia is a developmental disorder where the child understands you and wants to communicate but has difficulty making a sentence. In contrast to dysarthria, which typically involves difficulty speaking because of a nerve or muscle deficit, CAS is thought to be caused by a cortical issue. Speech is affected but not intelligence.

With lesions to the cerebral cortex, or cerebrum, think of the A's: Aphasia, Agnosia, Apraxia, Anopsia, Asomatognosia, Alexia, and Agraphia. This contrasts with patients with lesions to the brainstem who often exhibit one or more of the four "D"'s. Dysphagia is a swallowing deficit, and Dysarthria is a deficit with speaking. Both are found in patients with lesions to nucleus ambiguus. Diplopia or blurred vision is found in patients with deficits to CNs III, IV, or VI. Dysmetria or past pointing is found in patients with cerebellar involvement. Lateral brainstem injuries often lead to cerebellar symptoms because of involvement of the cerebellar peduncles.

Coup Contrecoup Lesions

Traumatic blows to the skull can put pressure on the underlying cortical tissue that leads to neuronal damage– the coup lesion. In addition, the impact can also push the brain against the other side of the skull leading to damage on the other side of the brain—the contrecoup lesion. In many cases this contrecoup lesion is worse than the coup lesion.

Cerebral Cortex Gray Matter Layers

If you look at a section of gray matter from the cerebral cortex under the microscope you will see six layers. This is the case for any wedge of cerebral cortex; however, the size of these various layers will vary depending on which cortical lobe the tissue came from. We do not need to talk about each of the six layers, but instead focus on two layers:

1. *Layer IV* is the major input layer, and since the major input to the cerebral cortex is from the thalamus, it is the thalamocortical tracts that project to layer IV. Thus, a piece of cortex from the postcentral gyrus will have a large layer IV. You cannot distinguish one layer from another with your naked eye—you need a microscope—with one exception. In the occipital cortex, because there is so much information from the lateral geniculate bodies, in a cross section from the occipital pole you can see, with the naked eye, the fibers projecting to the layer IV. These fibers stand out as a white line, referred to as the *line of Gennari*, which are the myelinated fibers carrying visual information. This is why the visual cortex is also referred to as the striate cortex.

2. *Layer V* is the major output layer. It is here where the *pyramidal cells of* Betz are located. These are the cell bodies of the corticospinal and corticobulbar tracts projecting down to the spinal cord. Thus, the best place to see a prominent layer V would be the precentral gyrus.

Historical Snippet: London Cabbies and the Hippocampus

Eleanor Maguire, a memory researcher, spent years studying the role of the hippocampus in *animals*. She also produced an ingenious idea for studying it in *humans* and she realized that there is no better group for this than London Cab Drivers who are famous for their encyclopedic memory of the street map of London. The test to become a London cabbie is referred to as "The Knowledge" and it requires memorizing the entire map of London—a total of 25,000 streets. During a series of oral exams, they are given two points in the city and then must describe how to get from point A to point B. One would surmise that that they have exceptional visual-spatial abilities, and Maguire showed that the cabbies had a larger than normal hippocampus. An obvious question about the size of their hippocampus relates to age-old nature-versus-nurture-debate. Did the cabbie job attract people with a large hippocampus, or did the hippocampus become larger as the trainees studied for the exam? Maguire showed that at the start of their four-year training program, the trainees had normal sized hippocampi. However, by the end of their four years of training their hippocampi had become larger.

Further Reading

1. Afifi AK, Bergman RA. Functional neuroanatomy: text and atlas. New York: McGraw-Hill; 1998.
2. Blumenfeld H. Neuroanatomy through clinical cases. 2nd ed. Hoboken: Wiley-Blackwell; 2010.
3. Brazis PW, Masdeu JC, Biller J. Localization in clinical neurology. Philadelphia: Lippincott, Williams, and Wilkins; 2016.
4. Campbell W, Barohn RJ. Dejong's the neurological examination. Philadelphia: Lippincott, Williams, and Wilkins; 2019.
5. Fuller G. Neurological examination made easy. 6th ed. Barcelona: Elsevier; 2019.
6. Leo J. Medical neuroanatomy for the boards and clinic: finding the lesion. 2nd ed. Cham: Springer; 2024a.
7. Leo J. Clinical anatomy and embryology: a guide for the classroom, clinic, and clinic. 2nd ed. Cham: Springer; 2024b.
8. Ray S. Basilar artery ischemic syndromes – a brief discussion of current concepts. J Neurol Stroke. 2017;7(6)
9. Splittgerber R. Snell's clinical neuroanatomy. 8th ed. Philadelphia: Lippincott, Williams, and Wilkins; 2018.
10. Swanson PD. Signs and symptoms in neurology. Philadelphia: Lippincott Williams and Wilkins; 1984.
11. Young PA, Young PH, Tolbert D. Basic clinical neuroscience. Philadelphia: Lippincott, Williams, and Wilkins; 2015.

22 Neurophysiology

Excitable Cells

The ability of two neurons to talk to each other starts with the resting membrane potential (RMP), which in turn allows neurons to propagate action potentials. To explain the RMP we start with two fluid-filled compartments separated by a semi-permeable membrane. These two fluid-filled compartments represent the inside and outside of the cell. On one side of the membrane is the intracellular space, and the other side is the extracellular space. The membrane wall itself is impermeable to sodium and potassium but within the membrane, sodium and potassium leak channels allow these two ions to move down their gradients. In addition, the membrane is *impermeable* to the anions, which leads to the sequestration of these anions on the intracellular side of the membrane. This model was worked out in the early 1950s by Alan Hodgkin and Andrew Huxley (Fig. 22.1).

Leak Channels

There are two forces acting on the flow of ions: (1) the concentration gradient, and (2) the electrical gradient. Again, keep in mind that the negatively charged anions are sequestered on the intracellular side.

To start, let us look at equilibrium potential of sodium and potassium separately, and then when the two are combined. Starting with sodium first, there is a higher concentration of sodium outside of the cell, thus the concentration gradient drives the sodium from the extracellular to the intracellular side. As the positively charged sodium ions build up on the intracellular side, the electrical gradient drives sodium back across the membrane from the intracellular to the extracellular side. Eventually, like a tug of war, the concentration gradient and the electrical gradients reach equilibrium, which in the case of the sodium ion is $ENa^{+} = +65$ mV (Fig. 22.2).

J. Leo, *Gross Anatomy, Neuroanatomy, and Embryology for Medical Students*,
https://doi.org/10.1007/978-3-031-87151-1_22

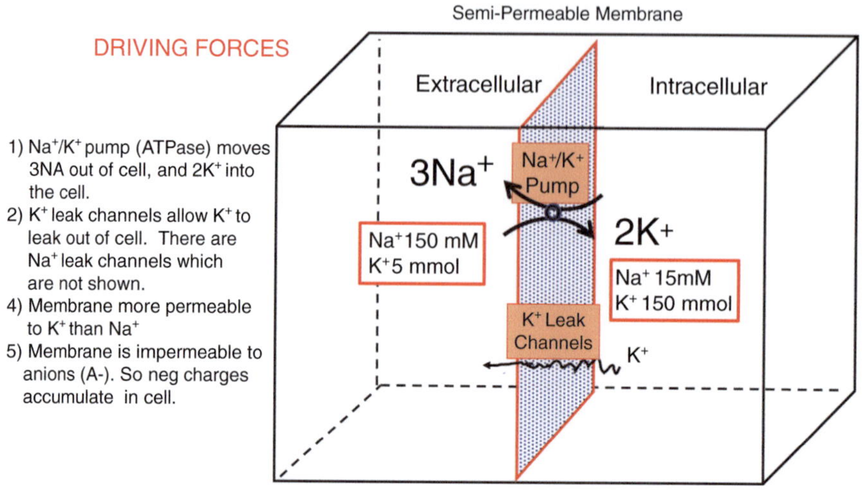

Fig. 22.1 Resting membrane potential. The intracellular and extracellular compartments are separated by a semi permeable membrane. Embedded in the membrane are the NA^+/K^+ pumps. For every 3 Na^+ ions moved extracellularly, 2 K^+ ions are moved intracellularly. As the ion concentrations build up on their relative sides of the membrane, leak channels allow the ions to move back against there gradients. The membrane is impermeable to anions which build up on the intracellular side [4, 5]

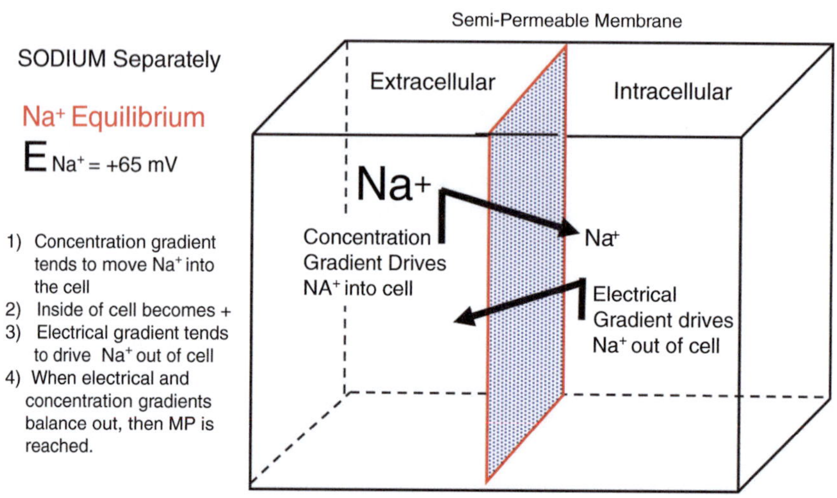

Fig. 22.2 The effect of just sodium on the RMP [4, 5]

Meanwhile, similar forces are at work on potassium ions but in the opposite direction. The concentration gradient for potassium is driving the ions from the intracellular to the extracellular side. And in turn, the electrical gradient drives the potassium ions from the extracellular to the intracellular side. When the two forces equilibrate the RMP of potassium is $EK^+ = -90$ mV (Fig. 22.3).

The final RMP of the cell is based on the equilibrium of both sodium and potassium together. However, the sodium and potassium leak channels are not equal. The potassium leak channels are significantly "leakier" than the sodium channels. Thus, considering both sodium and potassium together, the resting membrane potential ends up closer to the resting membrane potential of potassium. In other words, because the potas-

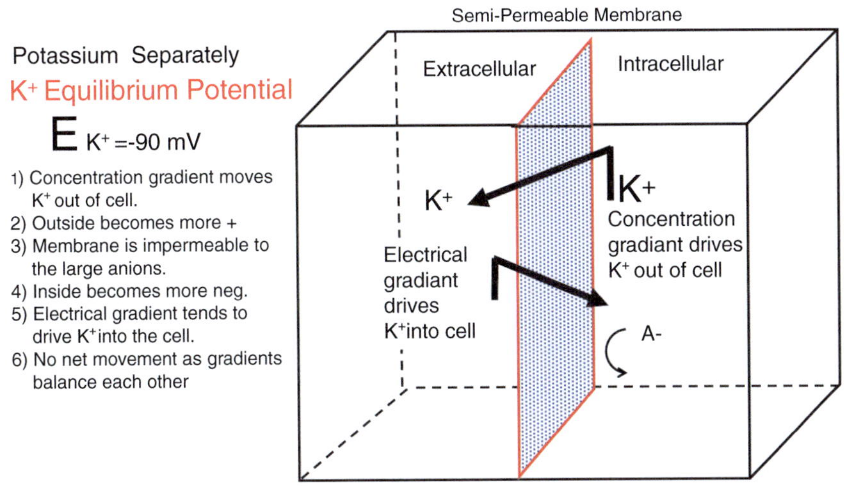

Fig. 22.3 The effect of just potassium on the RMP [4, 5]

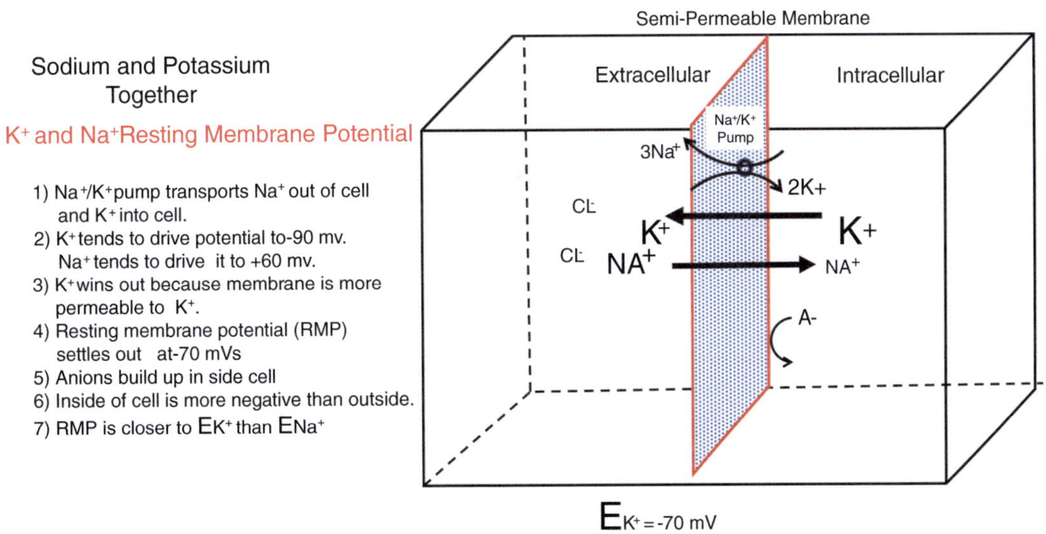

Fig. 22.4 The combined effect of sodium and potassium on RMP. Because the membrane is much more permeable to K⁺ than Na⁺ the final RMP lies closer to the equilibrium potential of potassium than to sodium [4, 5]

sium leak channels are more permeable than the sodium leak channels, potassium has a greater effect on the final resting membrane potential of the cell which settles at −70 mV. At rest, the inside of the cell is now negative compared to the outside of the cell. As we will see, the subsequent movement of ions in one direction or the other will alter the charge. If there is rush of positive ions from the outside to the inside of the cell, the cell will become more positive—or depolarized. If there is a rush of negatively charged ions from the outside to the inside of the cell, then the cell will become more negative—or hyperpolarized (Fig. 22.4).

Sodium-Potassium Pump

Because of the leak channels, the ions will tend to flow down their concentration gradients—in a downhill direction. To maintain the RMP, there is an energy-dependent sodium-potassium pump

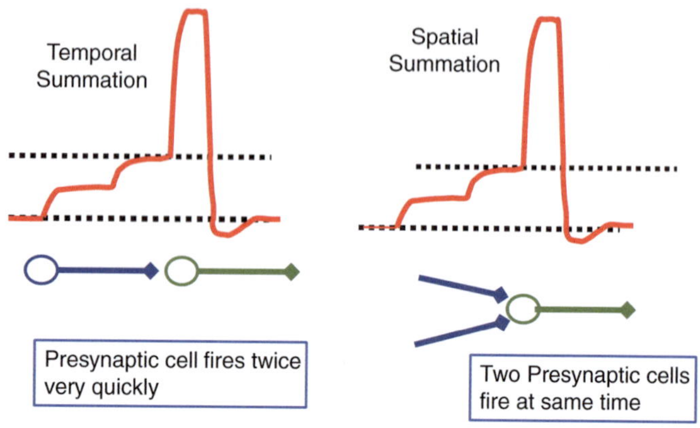

Fig. 22.5 Temporal and spatial summation [4, 5]

embedded within the membrane that moves the ions against their gradients—in an uphill direction. The pump moves sodium from the intracellular to the extracellular side. And in turn, potassium is moved in the opposite direction—from the extracellular side to the intracellular side. Specifically, three sodium ions are moved out of the cell, and two potassium ions are moved into the cell for every molecule of ATP consumed.

Graded (Local) Potentials

With the cell sitting at rest with a −70 mV RMP, it can now respond to a stimulus. A graded potential is just a temporary change in the voltage which depends on the size of the stimulus and whether it leads to a depolarization or a hyperpolarization. An excitatory event that leads to depolarization is referred to as an excitatory postsynaptic potential (EPSP), while an inhibitory event that leads to a hyperpolarization is referred to as an inhibitory postsynaptic potential (IPSP). These graded potentials are summative based on time and space. In the case of temporal summation, a single presynaptic cell fires a burst of signals very quickly and each signal builds on its predecessors. In the case of spatial summation, several presynaptic neurons meet the postsynaptic cell at different points. If just one presynaptic cell fires it leads to a small postsynaptic depolarization, but when several presynaptic cells fire together the effect is additive leading to a larger depolarization of the postsynaptic cell (Fig. 22.5).

Action Potentials

In contrast to graded potentials, action potentials operate on the "all or none principle" meaning that if the membrane potential reaches a threshold limit, then the action potential will be triggered. Slight changes in the membrane potential (subthreshold) that do not reach threshold will not trigger an action potential. And likewise, a change in the membrane potential higher than the threshold (suprathreshold) will not produce a larger or stronger action potential.

When the threshold level is reached there is a rapid opening of voltage gated Na^+ channels leading to an influx of Na^+ into the cell. This increased level of Na^+ leads to an increase in the membrane potential to approximately +40 mVs. At the point where the membrane potential is reaching its apex, these voltage gated Na^+ channels start to close. At the same time, voltage gated K^+ channels are opening leading to efflux of K^+ out of the cell. These positively charged K^+ ions now lead to the membrane potential reversing and heading back towards its RMP. As the membrane potential approaches the threshold level, the voltage gated K^+ channels close which slows down the movement of K^+ out of the cell. During this time (about 3–4 ms), the cell is unable to respond to another presynaptic input no matter how strong the input. This period where the cell is unable to respond is referred to as the absolute refractory period and is due to the inactivation of the Na^+ channels. As the Na^+ channels start to recover, there is a brief time called the relative

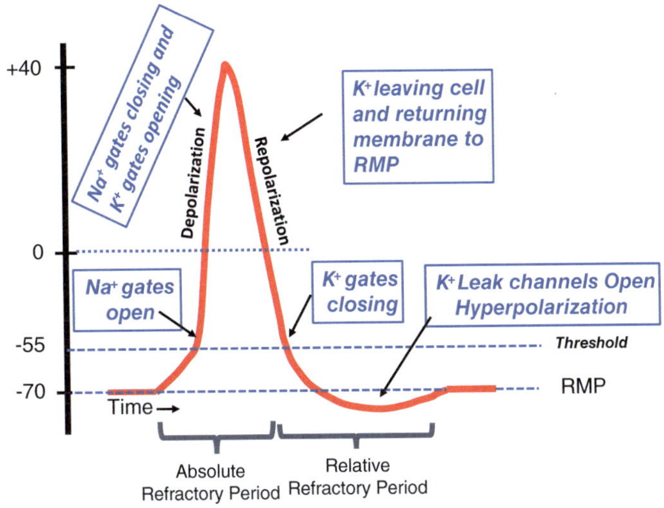

Fig. 22.6 Action potential. During the rising phase of the AP, the voltage gated Na + gates are open. This influx of Na^+ makes the inside of the cell positive compared to outside. During the falling phase, the Na^+ channels are closed but the voltage gated K^+ channels are open allowing K^+ to leave the cell and return the RMP to negative. However, for a moment, the cell is slightly more negative than the RMP. This is due to time lag of the K^+ gates closing. Eventually the K^+ gates are all closed, and the cell returns to the RMP [4, 5]

refractory period where the cell can depolarize again if the input is strong enough (Fig. 22.6).

For a moment, the membrane potential dips below the threshold level—it undershoots. This is due to the K^+ leak channels being open, and some of the voltage gated K^+ channels still being open. At this point, the cell can respond to a presynaptic input, but it will need a stronger input to generate an action potential. This is referred to as the relative refractory period. Eventually, all the K^+ channels close, the cell returns to its RMP, and the cycle can start again. The mechanism of action for certain antiepileptics, such as phenytoin (Dilantin) is to extend this relative refractory period by blocking the voltage gated sodium channels in their inactive state.

One feature of the absolute refractory period is that it prevents the action potential from moving in reverse along an axon. At the point on the neuron where the AP fires, the Na^+ channels are closed and cannot open; thus, the action potential cannot move into this region of closed channels. But the channels located downstream are free to open so the AP continues forward, or downstream towards the axon. After several milliseconds, the adjacent upstream membrane can depolarize, but by then the action potential has moved along further down the axon, where the channels are open (Fig. 22.7).

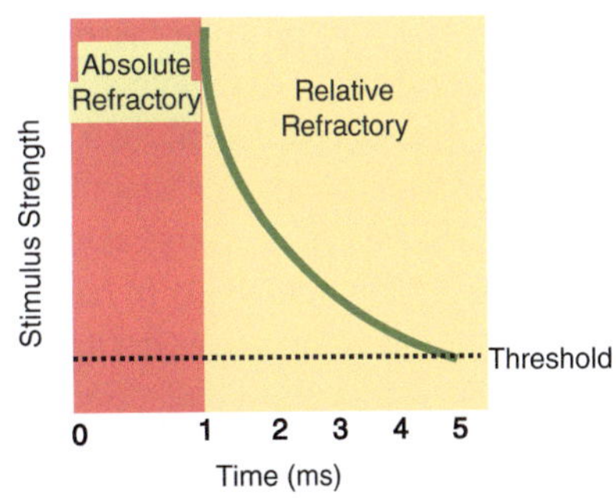

Fig. 22.7 Absolute vs. relative refractory period. During the absolute refractory period there is no way to elicit an action potential. During the relative refractory period, a stronger than normal stimulus can elicit a response. At the start of the *relative* refractory period a stronger stimulus is needed compared to later. As the Na^+ channels close the stimulus strength needed to elicit a response is less [4, 5]

Differences Between Graded and Action Potentials

As mentioned above, graded potentials can respond to spatial and temporal summation. This is not the case with action potentials which operate on an all or none property. Likewise, with graded potentials there is no refractory period, while action potentials have an absolute and relative refractory period. The graded potentials arise from ligand gated channels, while the action potentials utilize voltage gated channels. And finally graded potentials can occur on dendrites, cell bodies or sensory receptors, while action potentials are found on axons.

Action Potential Propagation

Action potentials (APs) move along the axon very quickly; however, because the membrane is "leaky," as ions leak back across the membrane, this slows down the action potential. Larger axons have less relative membrane area which leads to these larger axons having a faster conduction velocity. For instance, type 1a fibers are the largest fibers with a diameter of 13–20 um, and a conduction velocity of 80–130 m/s. On the other hand, type IV fibers are much smaller with a diameter of 0.2–15 um and a subsequent velocity of 0.5–2.0 m/s.

There comes a point where simply increasing the axon diameter becomes unworkable. There is just not enough room in the body to handle large fibers. One solution is to add an insulator to the axon, which increases the conduction velocity while keeping the fiber at a manageable size. Myelin serves as an insulator and reduces membrane capacitance by thickening the membrane wall which leads to more separation between the intracellular and extracellular ions. This increases the conduction velocity by decreasing the number of times the myelinated neuron must produce APs. Myelin is produced by Schwann cells and enwraps the axon. The node of Ranvier is the point where the myelin from one Schwann cell meets the myelin from another Schwann cell. The AP in a myelinated cell then moves from one node of Ranvier to the next node, to the next node, and so on, in a process called saltatory conduction. From the neuron's point of view, this is also an energy saving device, since with fewer ions crossing the membrane, and less ion pumping by the Na^{+}/K^{+} pump, less ATP is used.

Local analgesics, such as lidocaine, are membrane stabilizers and lead to a reduction in the ability of Na^{+} to cross the cell membrane which in turn makes it more difficult for the cell to depolarize. And these analgesics have an easier time working on small unmyelinated fibers than large unmyelinated fibers.

Fiber Classification

Nerve fiber classification is very confusing for several reasons: there are different classification systems; there is overlap between the categories; and there is variation in species. All of this leaves a student to ponder how much of this relates to clinical medicine and how much do I need to know. The most important characteristic is that speed or *conduction velocity* is based on both fiber diameter and whether the fiber is myelinated or not. The thicker the fiber, the faster the conduction velocity. And fibers enclosed by myelin have much faster conduction velocity. If we think about what information we want to get to our CNS as fast as possible, it is proprioceptive information. As we move our muscles, we need feedback quickly to make postural adjustments. On the other hand, while pain is obviously important, we do not need to transmit it to our cortex as fast as proprioceptive information.

Nerve fibers are categorized into three main groups: A, B and C. Group A are large diameter and myelinated, both of which give them the highest conduction velocity. Group B fibers are myelinated but have a smaller diameter. Because of this smaller diameter they have a slower conduction velocity. They are the preganglionic fibers of the autonomic nervous system. Group C are unmyelinated, with a small diameter giving them the lowest conduction velocity. They carry pain information (mechanical, thermal, and pain) (Fig. 22.8).

Group A fibers can be further subdivided into A alpha, beta, A gamma, and A delta.

A alpha (Aα) are the alpha motor neurons that innervate extrafusal muscle fibers and are responsible for muscle contraction. They have a high

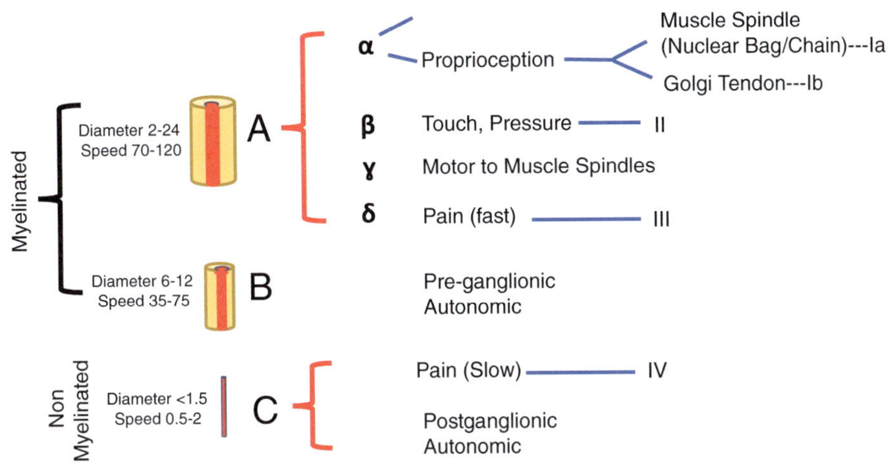

Fig. 22.8 Categories of nerve fibers [4, 5]

conduction velocity. They are also the afferents from the muscle spindles and Golgi tendons.

1a coming from muscle spindles monitoring the length of the tendon.

1b from Golgi tendons monitoring tensions of the tendon.

A beta (Aβ) carry sensory information for touch and pressure.

A gamma (Aγ) are the efferent fibers to intrafusal muscle spindles. These are the thickest, fastest fibers carrying information from Golgi tendon organs and muscle spindles.

A delta (Aδ) carry information about pain perception. A delta are small, myelinated fibers carrying pain information (mechanical and thermal). If you step on a tack, you immediately feel a sharp pain via your myelinated A delta fibers. This will be followed in a moment by a more diffuse, dull pain, which is being transmitted on non-myelinated C fibers.

B Preganglionic autonomic nerves.

C slow pain, diffuse and deep pain, postganglionic autonomic nerves, olfaction.

Deep Tendon Reflexes

When you tap on a tendon you are testing the reflex circuit between the muscle spindles, the spinal cord, and the muscle. If you see hyperreflexia or hyporeflexia then this suggests pathology. Muscle spindles are the intrafusal fibers within the muscle belly that respond to stretch—for muscle Spindles think Stretch. As an example, take the patella tendon reflex. When you tap at the knee, the muscle spindles, either nuclear bag or nuclear chain fibers, sense the elongation (they are stretched) and send afferent signals travelling on Type 1a and Type II afferent fibers to the dorsal roots. At the L4 level, the fibers enter the cord, travel through the dorsal horn, and then detour to the ventral horn to make a direct projection onto the large alpha motor neurons that will project out the ventral roots, and then onto the femoral nerve to stimulate the *extrafusal fibers* of the knee extensors (Figs. 22.9 and 22.10).

Situated deep inside the muscles belly (extrafusal fibers) are the encapsulated muscle spindles made up of intrafusal fibers which sense the state of muscle contraction. There are two categories of intrafusal muscle fibers (Fig. 22.9):

1. *Nuclear bag fibers* are multinucleated fibers that sense stretch. The nuclei are gathered in the center of the fiber giving it a swollen or bag-like appearance. There are also two subdivisions of nuclear bag fibers: (1) static and (2) dynamic.
2. *Nuclear chain fibers* are also multinucleated, but their nuclei are lined up in rows, like a chain.

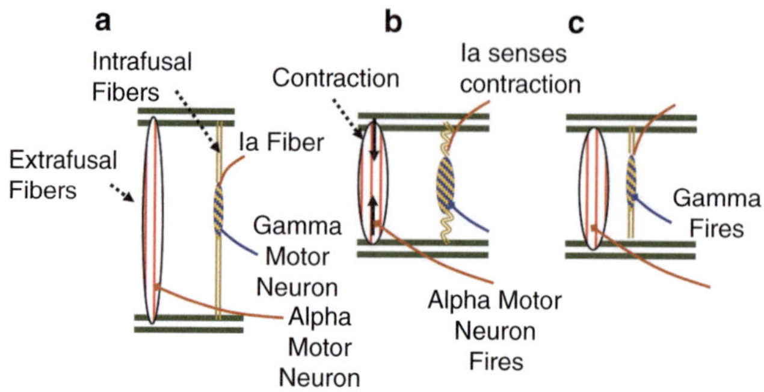

Fig. 22.9 Muscle spindles. In panel (**a**) the extrafusal muscles are relaxed and the muscles spindles are tight. In panel (**b**) the alpha motor neurons have stimulated the extrafusal fibers to contract. The intrafusal fibers are now loose which is sensed by the Ia afferents. In panel (**c**) the gamma motor neurons have responded by contracting the intrafusal fibers [4, 5]

A typical muscle spindle usually has 2–3 nuclear bag fibers and 4–5 nuclear chain fibers. There are also two types of afferent fibers (Ia) emerging from a muscle spindle. The *annulospiral endings* get their name because they wrap around the central part of the spindle like a coil. They emerge from the central part of the spindle. The *flower spray endings* get their name because they resemble the shoots from the stem of a plant, and they emerge from the ends of the muscle spindle. The Ia afferent fibers carry information about stretch from the muscle to the nucleus proprius in the dorsal horn of the spinal cord.

Looking at the reflex arc, in addition to this alpha motor neuron activity to the extrafusal fiber, the small unmyelinated gamma motor neurons will send information to the *intrafusal* muscle fibers. Note that the reflex arc is a monosynaptic pathway consisting of one sensory or afferent fiber, one motor or efferent fiber, and just one synapse between the two in the gray matter of the spinal cord.

Concurrent with the muscle activity in the quadriceps, the antagonist muscles of the hamstrings will be inhibited via a polysynaptic pathway. In this case, the afferent information comes into the cord, and goes to an inhibitory interneuron, which then inhibits the hamstrings (flexors at the knee). The inhibition of the antagonist muscle group is referred to as reciprocal inhibition.

Golgi Tendon Organs

Golgi tendon organs are in the tendons, and they measure tension. When stimulated, they lead to relaxation of the muscle to prevent excessive strain on the muscle fibers—the inverse myotatic reflex. Golgi tendon organs are small capsules embedded with free nerve endings that sense tension. Once a Golgi tendon organ is stimulated, it sends signals into the spinal cord on a 1b fiber, which then contacts an interneuron projecting to the alpha motor neuron, leading to relaxation of the muscle under strain. For Golgi **T**endon organs think **T**ension (Fig. 22.10).

The clasp-knife reflex is a sign of UMN pathology. During the neurological exam it occurs when the examiner attempts to flex a joint. There is an initial resistance against the movement, which suddenly gives way, the muscles relax, and the limb moves freely—like when you close a pocketknife, and you push the blade a bit to get it started, but then all of sudden the knife snaps shut. This sudden closing is due to the action of the Golgi tendon organ sensing the tension and leading to relaxation of the muscles.

In summary, in a typical mixed nerve there are three types of motor fibers coming into a muscle:

1. Alpha motor neurons to the extrafusal fibers
2. Gamma motor neurons to the intrafusal fibers

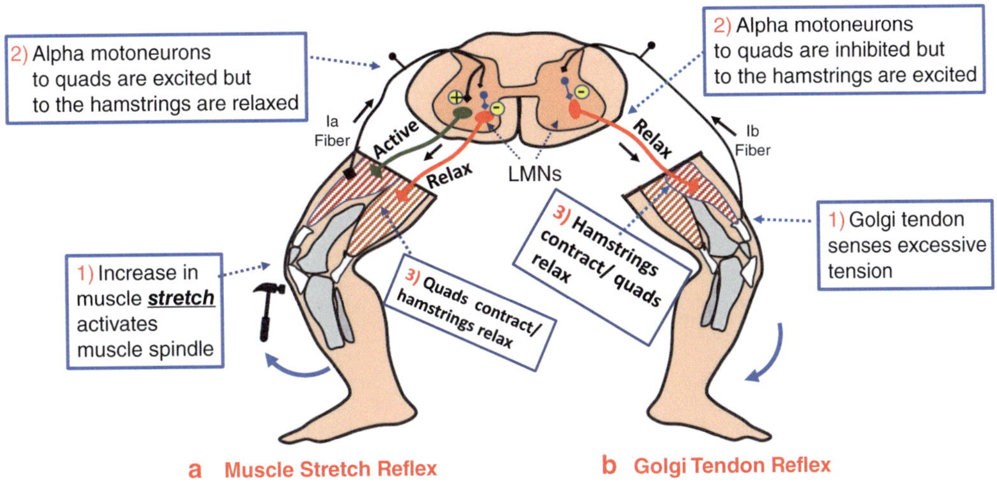

Fig. 22.10 Muscle stretch reflex and golgi tendon. Panel (**a**) On the patient's right side, when the tendon is tapped, the muscle spindles sense *stretch* which leads to the quadriceps firing and extension at the knee. Panel (**b**) On the patient's left side, excessive *tension* on the muscle is sensed by the Golgi tendon organs which leads to flexion at the knee [4, 5]

3. Unmyelinated C fibers, which are postganglionic autonomic efferent fibers.

And there are three types of sensory fibers leaving the muscle:

1. 1a fibers originating from nuclear bag and nuclear chain fibers in the muscle spindles.
2. 1b fibers originate in the Golgi tendon organs.
3. various fibers from the tissue surrounding the muscle.

Hypotonia, which is either a diminished or absent muscle tone, occurs when a peripheral nerve (LMN) is cut. *Hypertonia*, which is increased muscle tone, occurs when the corticospinal tract (UMN) is cut.

Superficial Reflexes

In contrast to the hyperactive DTRs, in patients with UMN injuries the superficial reflexes such as abdominal, cremaster, and corneal will typically be absent. The abdominal reflexes are stimulated by stroking gently on the abdomen from lateral to medial and looking for contraction of the abdominal muscles. The umbilicus should move towards the side of the scratching. However, the clinical utility of these reflexes are debatable. The *presence* of the reflexes is a healthy sign, but their *absence* does not necessarily indicate a lesion. The reflexes are absent in a fair number of healthy individuals, the elderly, patients who have had surgery, and women who have delivered children. The mechanism of these abdominal reflexes is also up for debate.

Gate Control Theory of Pain

The gate-control theory of pain postulates that the large diameter Aβ fibers which do not carry pain sensation, can reduce pain sensation from the periphery by blocking the electrical input from the pain fibers at the dorsal horn. This is why when you stub your toe you reach down and massage your foot. It is also the basis for transcutaneous electrical nerve stimulation (TENS). It is thought that by stimulating the large fibers, that this "closes the gate" in the dorsal horn which diminishes the pain perception. Over time there is a tendency for the large fibers to adapt, which leads to opening the gate. It is thought that

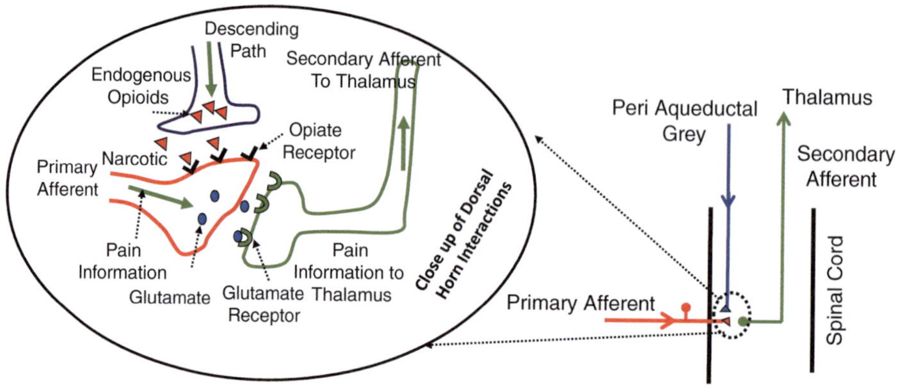

Fig. 22.11 Descending control of pain. The primary afferent carrying pain sensation from the periphery enters the dorsal horn. At the dorsal horn it synapses with the secondary afferent to carry impulse to the thalamus. The descending pathway from the periaqueductal grey (PAG) projects to the dorsal horn. It release enkephalins that bind to the presynaptic cells to decrease the pain signal by inhibiting the release of glutamate. Narcotics can also be used to block the pain sensation by inhibiting the presynaptic cell [4, 5]

scratching or itching around the injury is one way to circumvent this adaptation and keep the gate closed.

The **periaqueductal gray (PAG)** surrounds the cerebral aqueduct and is also involved in the descending control of pain. Intuitively, it makes sense to think of pain as a signal coming in from the periphery to higher centers, but there are also descending pathways involved in the pain response. These pathways can either heighten or lessen pain perception. The dorsal raphe has also been implicated in the descending pain pathway. It has an excitatory serotonergic projection to enkephalin interneurons in the dorsal horn. These enkephalin interneurons are in turn inhibitory to the primary afferents (Fig. 22.11).

The PAG sends a descending projection down to the rostral ventral medulla (RVM) which in turn projects down to the dorsal horn of the spinal cord. This descending pathway uses endogenous opioids to inhibit the incoming pain pathways. The endogenous opiates such as enkephalins, β-endorphins, and dynorphins are found in high concentrations in the structures involved in the descending control of pain (Fig. 22.11).

Blood-Brain and Blood-CSF Barriers

There are several compartments located in the skull: (1) One compartment is the brain interstitial tissue containing neurons, glia, and cerebral vessels; (2) the second compartment is made up of the cerebral vessels with their endothelial walls. Note that this second compartment—composed of the blood vessels—is buried within the first compartment—the interstitial tissue. Between the blood vessels and the interstitial fluid is the blood brain barrier; and (3) a third compartment is the CSF. Between the interstitial fluid and the CSF are ependymal cells. However, there are also specializations of these cells in several locations; there is *choroid plexus* where CSF is produced, and *arachnoid granulations* where CSF is reabsorbed (Fig. 22.12).

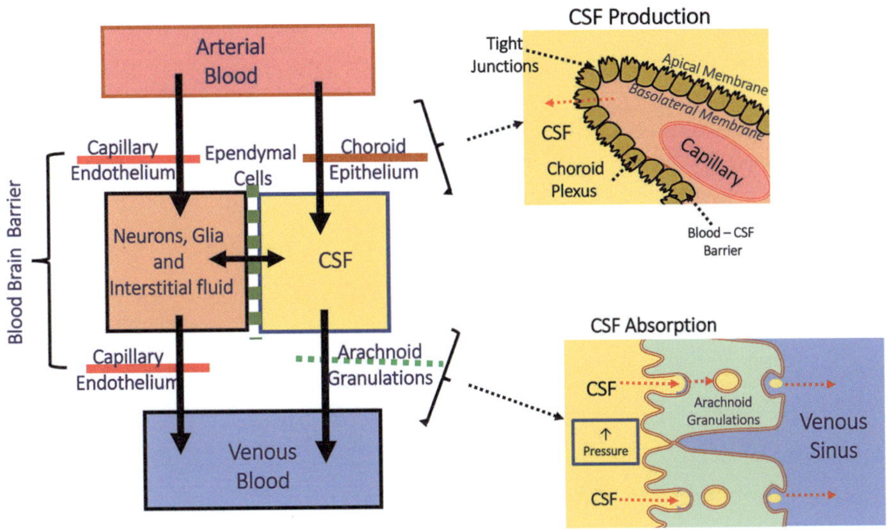

Fig. 22.12 Compartments in and around the brain. The choroid epithelium is the site of the blood CSF barrier. There are tight junctions between the choroid epithelial cells. Between the arterial blood vessels and the interstitial fluid is the BBB. CSF is reabsorbed at the arachnoid granulations by pinocytosis. The CSF pressure is higher on the apical side of the arachnoid granulations than the venous sinus. Thus, movement of CSF is to the venous sinus [4, 5]

Choroid Plexus and CSF Production

Choroid plexus (CP) is a specialization of the choroid epithelium that surrounds a highly fenestrated capillary. The choroid plexus and its associated capillary resembles the villus in the jejunoileum surrounding the blood vessels and lacteals. CSF is produced by the choroid plexus. The choroid plexus is also the site of the blood-CSF barrier. Specializations along the borders of the CP allow for the movement of ions and other materials from the blood into the CSF. The apical border of the choroid plexus faces the CSF while the basolateral border faces the interstitial tissue (Fig. 22.12).

On the apical surface of the CP are Na^+/K^+ pumps moving Na^+ into the CSF, while also moving K^+ into the CP. The K^+ then moves along to the basolateral border where it is excreted into the venous channels. Thus, there is a net movement of Na^+, Cl^-, HCO_3, and H_2O from the serum to the CSF, while there is a net movement of K^+ in the other direction- from CSF to the interstitial fluid. Because the capillaries within the tufts of choroid plexus are fenestrated the material moving from the CSF into the interstitial fluid can then move into capillaries. Likewise, ions can move from the capillaries, across the basolateral and apical borders of the CP and into the CSF. For instance, moving from the CSF across the choroid plexus and into the blood stream are waste products, ions, and amino acids. Moving out of the blood vessels and into the CSF are Na^+, Cl^-, HCO_3, and Mg^{2+}.

CSF is normally colorless. Cloudy CSF could be the result of white blood cells from meningeal inflammation or encephalitis. The white cloudy look could also be due to increased protein levels found with tuberculosis, meningitis, or poliomyelitis. If CSF has a red color to it, this could be from a subarachnoid hemorrhage, or a leaky spinal tap site. If there is a hemorrhage, then several hours later the CSF will typically be yellow from the oxyhemoglobin. With acute bacterial meningitis, glucose levels will decrease, while in the case of viral meningitis, the glucose levels would be normal (Fig. 22.13).

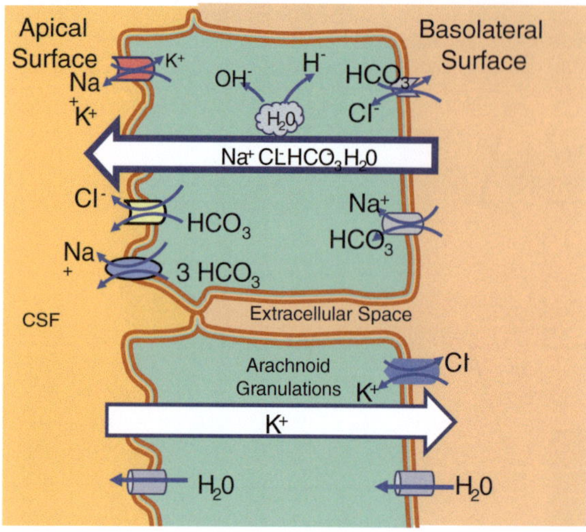

H2	CSF	Serum
Water	99%	93%
Protein(mg/dl)	35	7000
Glucose	60	90
Sodium	138	138
Potassium	2.8 →	4.5
Calcium	2.1	4.8
Magnesium	0.3	1.7
Chloride	119	← 102
pH	7.33	7.41

Fig. 22.13 Movement across choroid plexus. Note that the Na^+/K^+ pump is located on the apical surface, note the basal surface, thus the net secretion of Na^+ into CSF. The Cl^-HCO_3 exchanger is on the basal surface. HCO_3 moves across basal and apical surface via co-transport with Na^+ to enter CSF. K^+ moves concentration gradient into the extracellular fluid [4, 5]

CSF Reabsorption

At the arachnoid granulations, materials can move from the CSF into the venous system. Because about 500 ml of CSF is produced per day, and the compartment itself only holds 150 ml, this naturally leads to increased pressure in the CSF compartment, resulting in continuous reabsorption of the CSF by the arachnoid granulations. Besides the pressure gradient driving ions through one-way valves into the venous network, there is also transport via pinocytosis that moves vacuoles across the arachnoid granulations.

Blood Brain Barrier

Capillaries in other parts of the body are fenestrated so that material can move from the vessel into the tissue. However, in the brain, the capillary endothelial cells are adherent to their neighbors via tight junctions which prevent material easily moving from the vessel into the brain tissue. The tight junctions are maintained by the astrocyte end feet that enwrap the vessel. An injection of dye into these vessels will not travel across the blood brain barrier, thus the dye will not get into the interstitial fluid (Fig. 22.14).

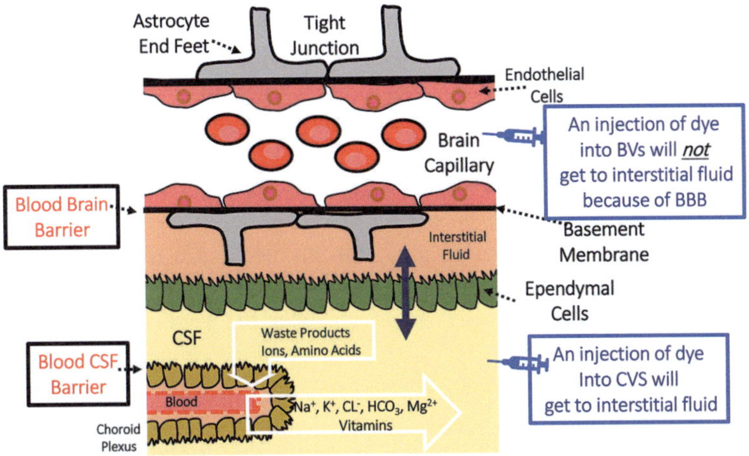

Fig. 22.14 Blood brain barrier. The blood vessels in the brain are unique in that they have the blood brain barrier (BBB), which allows the vessels to control what crosses from the blood stream to the brain parenchyma. Whereas normal blood vessels are fenestrated, the vessels in the brain have tight junctions between apposing endothelial cells. While the tight junctions are the site of the BBB, the barrier is maintained by the astrocyte end feet that encase the capillary. Both the endothelial cells and the astrocytes contribute to the basement membrane between them. If you inject it into blood vessels the dye will not get into the extracellular space because of the BBB [4, 5]

The **area postrema** is in the medulla near the vagal trigone at the base of the fourth ventricle. The endothelial cells in this area lack tight junctions, which enables them to monitor the bloodstream. It is involved in the vomiting response.

Virchow Robbin Spaces

The arteries running along the surface of the brain sit between the pia mater and the arachnoid in the subarachnoid space. As these arteries cross the pia, they send penetrating branches into the brain tissue. The initial segment of these penetrating arteries are still encased by pia. This creates small spaces referred to as the Virchow Robbin spaces which are continuations with the subarachnoid space. With aging, these spaces can enlarge. They can also be enlarged in various pathological conditions. On an MRI, these enlarged spaces can look like dots because of the CSF signal (Fig. 22.15).

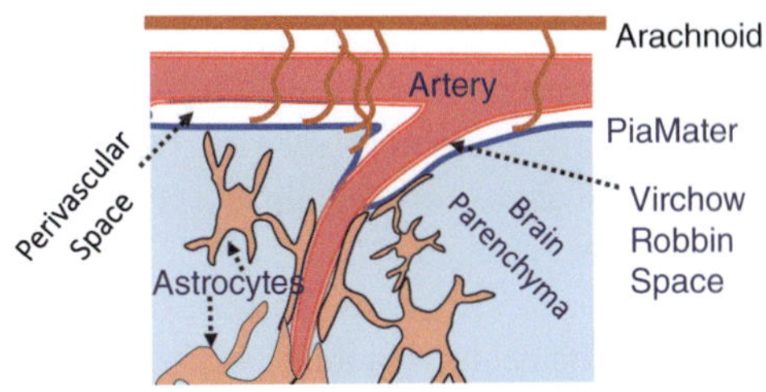

Fig. 22.15 Virchow robbin spaces. Arteries on the surface of the brain send penetrating vessels into the parenchyma which are covered by pia mater. Proteins move from the capillaries into the brain parenchyma. These spaces tend to widen with age [4, 5]

Supporting Cells

In addition to the neurons, there are several types of supporting cells found in the nervous system:

1. *Astrocytes* are star shaped cells with several functions. As mentioned above they are involved with maintaining the blood barrier.

They also surround the synapse and absorb glutamate and GABA. There are also K^+ channels in the astrocyte membrane to absorb the K^+ released from neurons. They also play a role in the brain's response to an injury. Reactive astrogliosis is generally considered to be indicative of a neuropathological event. Near an insult the astrocytes become larger and produce glial fibrillary acidic protein (GFAP) which can lead to the formation of a glial scar. During development, radial glia, a form of astrocytes, contribute to the scaffolding that migrating neurons use. Astrocytes are also the site of glucose storage in the brain. There are glucose transporters on the astrocyte membrane that transport glucose into the cell. The glucose can then be stored as glycogen in the astrocytes. Healthy neurons do not store glycogen, but when the brain needs extra energy, glycogen in the astrocytes can be metabolized into lactate. The lactate is then transported into the neurons where it is converted into pyruvate which in turn is metabolized to ATP.
2. *Microglia* are immune cells of the nervous system and are responsible for maintaining the microenvironment.
3. *Oligodendrocytes* are responsible for myelination of the neurons in the CNS.

Multiple sclerosis affects the oligodendrocytes.

4. *Schwann cells* are responsible for myelination in the PNS.

Historical Snippet: The Discovery of Acetylcholine

In 1981, the Spanish neuroscientist Santiago Ramón y Cajal (1852–1934) proposed that the nervous system was made up of thousands of individual neurons that communicated with each other to make up an extensive interconnected network. From that point on, the search was on to understand the physiological basis for neuron-to-neuron communication.

In 1920, one night after falling asleep, the pharmacologist Otto Loewi (1873–1961) had a dream about an experiment. He woke up, and quickly jotted down some notes and headed to the lab to set up the experiment he had visualized in the dream. He took two frog hearts and put each in a separate perfusion chamber. In one chamber, the heart had an intact vagus nerve, but in the second chamber, the heart did not have a vagus nerve. In the first chamber, he confirmed what had already been known for some time; namely, that stimulation of the vagus nerve slowed down the heart rate. But he went a step further and then took the perfusate from this first chamber with a stimulated heart and added it to the second chamber. He found that in the second chamber the heart also slowed down. This showed that the vagus nerve was secreting a chemical into the perfusate that slowed down the heart. Loewi called this chemical *vagusstoff* (vagus stuff in English), which eventually came to be known as acetylcholine. In 1936, Loewi shared the Nobel Prize with Henry Dale (Fig. 22.16).

Yet, even after this discovery, from the end of the 1930s to the mid-1960s, there was still a healthy debate over whether nerves communicated via electrical activity or by chemicals. This debate, that some have referred to as the war of the soups and the sparks, was between the pharmacologists and the physiologists. Much of the debate occurred in Europe during WWII. At one point Loewi, who was Jewish, was banished from the University of Vienna and had to leave the country. The neuropharmacologists won the debate, and we now know that when two neurons communicate there is a small space or cleft between them (not withstanding gap junctions) and that the neurons communicate by neurotransmitters. Besides neuron-to-neuron communication, there is also the motor end plate where neurons communicate with muscle tissue.

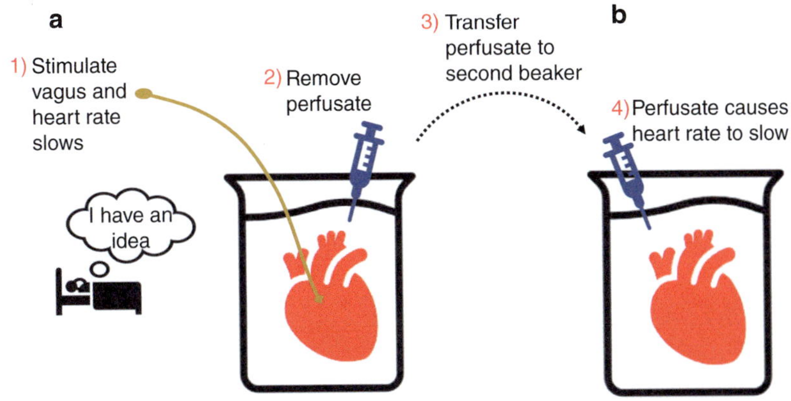

Fig. 22.16 Otto Loewi's Dream. In the middle of the night, Loewi had an idea about an experiment. In panel (**a**) the heart is attached to the Vagus nerve. In panel (**b**) there is no Vagus nerve. If the Vagus is stimulated in panel (**a**) the heart slows down, and if perfusate from here is transferred to the second beaker the heart also slows down. Therefore, the Vagus must cause the heart to release a chemical. Loewi called this chemical, *Vagus Stuff*, which eventually came to be known as acetylcholine [4, 5]

Further Reading

1. Barkhof F. Enlarged virchow robbin spaces: do they matter? Neurol Neurosurg Psychiatry. 2004;75(11):2316–7.
2. Blumenfeld H. Neuroanatomy through clinical cases. 2nd ed. Hoboken: Wiley-Blackwell; 2010.
3. Drake RL, Vogl AW, Mitchell A. Gray's anatomy for medical student's. 4th ed. Elsevier; 2019.
4. Leo J. Medical neuroanatomy for the boards and clinic: finding the lesion. 2nd ed. Cham: Springer; 2024a.
5. Leo J. Clinical anatomy and embryology: a guide for the classroom, clinic, and clinic. 2nd ed. Cham: Springer; 2024b.
6. Leo J, Huether SE. Pain, temperature, sleep and sensory function. In: McCane KL, Huether SE, editors. Pathophysiology: the biological basis for disease in adults and children. New York: Mosby; 1998.
7. McCoy A, Tan SY. Otto Loewi (1873-1961): dreamer and Nobel laureate. Singapore Med J. 2014;55(1):3–4.
8. Woodburne RT, Burkel WE. Essentials of human anatomy. 9th ed. Oxford: Oxford University Press; 1994.

23 Neuroanatomy Atlas

Atlas Overview

The best way to look at the atlas, at least when you first start studying neuroanatomy, is to follow individual tracts one at a time, either rostral or caudal (up or down) the CNS from section to section. As you do this, watch how the tract can move position, how it can change shape, and most importantly where it decussates. For the motor tracts, it makes sense to start in the cortex and follow the tracts downward—they are descending tracts. For the sensory tracts, it makes sense to start at the sacral cord and move up through the CNS into the cortex—they are ascending tracts. The following discussions assume that you have read the pertinent chapters on these tracts and understand the terminology and function of the tracts. We are now looking at their locations.

Spinothalamic In Slides 23.2 and 23.3 you can see the primary afferents for pain and temperature entering the cord and then synapsing in the dorsal horn. From the dorsal horn, the secondary fibers decussate by crossing in the anterior white commissure and then enter the contralateral spinothalamic tract. (note that these primary afferents can first travel up a segment or two in Lissauer's tract before synapsing, but for the purposes of the illustration, I am showing the fibers entering and decussating at the same level.)

As you move up the cord, at each level, fibers join the spinothalamic tract. Looking at Slide 23.3, for instance, you see fibers from the thoracic, lumbar, and sacral cord levels. As you move to Slide 23.4 the tract now also contains all these same fibers, plus cervical fibers. Moving to Slide 23.6, you can now see how the tract has moved more laterally. Keep in mind that if you lesion the spinothalamic tract in the medulla, pons, or midbrain that the patient's signs and symptoms will be on the contralateral side of the body. In the pons, the spinothalamic tract, also known as the spinal lemniscus, is seen just lateral to the medial lemniscus. And then lateral to the spinothalamic tract is the lateral lemniscus carrying auditory fibers to the inferior colliculus. So, in a row, going from lateral to medial, is the lateral lemniscus, spinal lemniscus, and medial lemniscus.

Moving to the midbrain, the spinothalamic has become more condensed and is just lateral to the medial lemniscus, just like the pom-pom on top of a stocking hat mentioned in earlier chapters. Moving to the thalamus, the spinothalamic tract can then be seen terminating in the ventral posterior lateral (VPL) nucleus of the thalamus.

J. Leo, *Gross Anatomy, Neuroanatomy, and Embryology for Medical Students*,
https://doi.org/10.1007/978-3-031-87151-1_23

Dorsal Columns

The primary afferents carrying vibratory, proprioception, and two-point discrimination information from the lower limb enter at the sacral and lumbar cord levels and immediately enter the fasciculus gracilis. At this point, there is no fasciculus cuneatus. These primary afferents do not synapse in the cord but travel up the ipsilateral cord. As you move up to the sections of the upper thoracic and cervical cord, the fibers carrying the same information from the upper limb enter the spinal cord above T6 and travel up the fasciculus cuneatus. So above T6 the dorsal columns includes both fasciculus gracilis and fasciculus cuneatus; but below T6 there is only fasciculus gracilis. In Slide 23.4, for instance, you can see fasciculus gracilis and cuneatus.

Once the fibers reach the lower medulla, they terminate in the nucleus gracilis and cuneatus. The second order fibers now come out of these two nuclei as the internal arcuate fibers and travel horizontally across the medulla (the decussation) to enter the contralateral medial lemniscus (Slide 23.6). As they enter the medial lemniscus, they are making a 90° turn to now travel vertically and ascend the brainstem. At this point, the fibers are arranged in the medial lemniscus as cervical, thoracic, lumbar, and sacral and they are sitting on top of the corticospinal tract, or pyramid.

As you move up the CNS, take Slide 23.11 as an example, one can see that the medial lemniscus is condensing and slightly moving position. The sacral fibers are moving off to the lateral side, and the cervical fibers are moving medially—the medial lemniscus has twisted a bit.

As we move up to the midbrain—Slide 23.17—the fibers are now sitting on top of the red nucleus like a stocking cap. These fibers will then terminate in the ventral lateral nucleus of the thalamus—Slide 23.19.

Corticospinal Tract

The corticospinal tract begins as cell bodies in layer five of the cerebral cortex. These are upper motor neurons whose fibers come together as the corona radiata, which resembles a fan, and then merge—like a funnel—to turn into the internal capsule. In Slide 23.21 we can see the corona radiata beginning to turn into the internal capsule. At this point, the corticospinal fibers are between the caudate and putamen. We can follow the fibers down the CNS and on Slide 23.17 we can see the corticospinal tract sitting in the middle one-third of the cerebral peduncle. In Slide 23.13 we can see the fibers in the basis pontis, and in Slide 23.9 we can see them in the medullary pyramid. The fibers travel down the pyramid—they still have not crossed by this point so a lesion to the pyramid would lead to contralateral signs and symptoms. As we get to the bottom of the pyramid, at Slide 23.5 we can see the corticospinal fibers crossing from right to left at the motor decussation. In Slides 23.1, 23.2, 23.3, and 23.4 we now see the corticospinal tract in the lateral cord. As we travel down the spinal cord, at each level of the cord, like exit ramps off a highway, upper motor neuron fibers are leaving the lateral corticospinal tract to reach the lower motor neurons in the ventral horn.

Orientation to MRIs Versus Cross Sections

Most students are aware of the radiological view of MRIs. From the examiner's point of view, the patient is lying down on their back with their feet towards you. But long before there were neuroradiologists, there were anatomists, and anatomists described images from a slightly different orientation. In some cases, they even just used random orientations, but in other cases the images are reversed from the now used clinical view. They called this the anatomical orientation, which involved the patient lying down on their stomach with their head towards the examiner. Thus, for better or worse, in contrast to the MRI view, the image that is most often used when looking at *slices* of the CNS is the anatomical orientation.

In the atlas pictures shown here the patient is lying down on their stomach—take Slides 23.1, 23.2, 23.3, and 23.4 as an example. The dorsal columns are at the top of the slide, and the ventral horns at the bottom of the slide. And the patient's head is facing you, the viewer. Before panicking, when discussing lesions, if I use the term ipsilateral or contralateral, it should not really matter whether it is the patient's right or left. For instance, in slide two, if you lesion the corticospinal tract, you should know that the patient will have ipsilateral motor symptoms. And if you lesion the spinothalamic tract at the same level, the patient will have contralateral loss of pain and temperature. Obviously knowing the side is important when you are dealing with a patient, but for our purposes of understanding the tracts and where they decussate it is not essential. You will note that on some of the slides I designate which side is which.

Cranial Nerves

We will start with the lower motor neurons of three important cranial nerves, all located medially. At the level of the midbrain in Slides 23.16 and 23.17 we can see the nucleus of CN III situated near the periaqueductal gray area. Coming out of the nucleus are the LMN fibers that travel through the interpeduncular fossa. At the level of the caudal pons in Slides 23.10 and 23.11, we can see CN VI traveling from the nucleus located dorsally, to the fibers exit on the ventral side. Also at this level, you can see the fibers of CN VII coming out its nucleus, heading dorsally, and then doing a U-turn and traveling around the nucleus of CN VI to eventually exit on the ventral side. In the medulla, in Slides 23.7, 23.8, and 23.9, you can see the hypoglossal nucleus near the fourth ventricle. Coming out of the nucleus are the LMN fibers which exit ventrally between the pyramid and the inferior olive.

On the lateral side of the brainstem, you can see the beginnings of CNs V, VIII, IX, and X. Starting with the lateral medulla, in Slide 23.5 one can see the prominent spinal nucleus of V, which is nothing more than the superior extension of the substantia gelatinosa of the spinal cord. The primary afferents for pain and temperature from the face, traveling on V1, V2, and V3 of the trigeminal nerve synapse here in the spinal nucleus of V. After synapsing, the second order fibers then decussate to join the ventral trigeminothalamic tract (VTT) and travel to the ventral posterior medial nucleus of the thalamus.

The nucleus ambiguus, in Slides 23.6 and 23.7, is the start of the LMNs for cranial nerves IX and X which travel to the muscles of the larynx and pharynx. Close to the nucleus ambiguus is the nucleus solitarus which is the sensory nucleus for the fibers carrying taste information from CNs VII, IX, and X. Remember that for nerves like CN IX and X, which have motor, sensory, and parasympathetic fibers, each set of fibers is associated with a different brainstem nucleus. Take CN X as an example, the motor fibers in CN X that go to the palate, pharynx, and larynx come from nucleus ambiguus, while the dorsal motor nucleus sends parasympathetic fibers to CN X, and the taste fibers on CN X travel back to the nucleus solitarus.

Moving to the rostral medulla, in Slide 23.8, one can see the various nuclei associated with CN VIII. The dorsal cochlear nucleus is evident on slide eight. One can also identify the inferior vestibular nucleus by its stippled or dotted appearance. The "dots" are the fibers descending from the lateral vestibular nucleus down through the inferior vestibular nucleus. And just medial to the inferior vestibular nucleus is the medial vestibular nucleus (Slides 23.12, 23.14, 23.15, 23.18, 23.20, 23.22, 23.23, 23.24, 23.25, and 23.26).

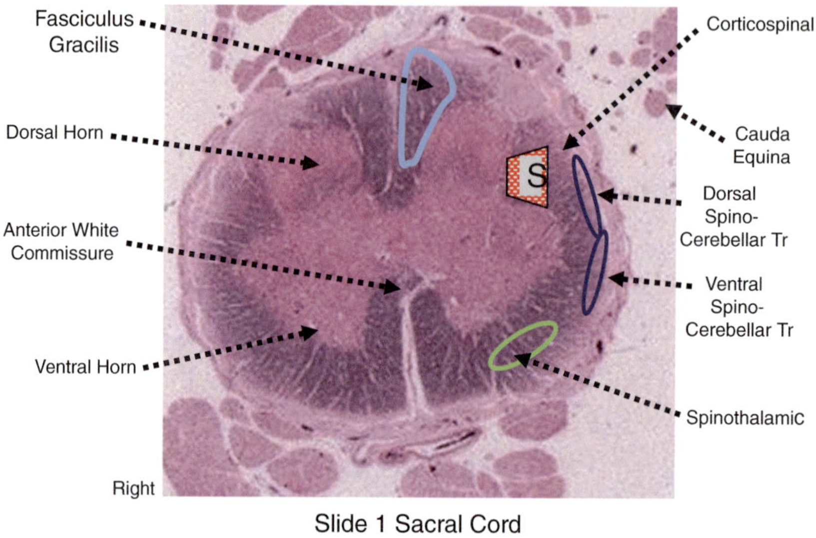

Slide 23.1 The corticospinal, spinothalamic, and dorsal columns are all labelled and color coded. The same colors will be used as we ascend through the CNS. Since this cut is below T6, we are only seeing the fasciculus gracilis and not fasciculus cuneatus. The dorsal spinocerebellar tract carries information about unconscious proprioception to the cerebellum via the inferior cerebellar peduncle. In the corticospinal tract at this point there are only sacral fibers

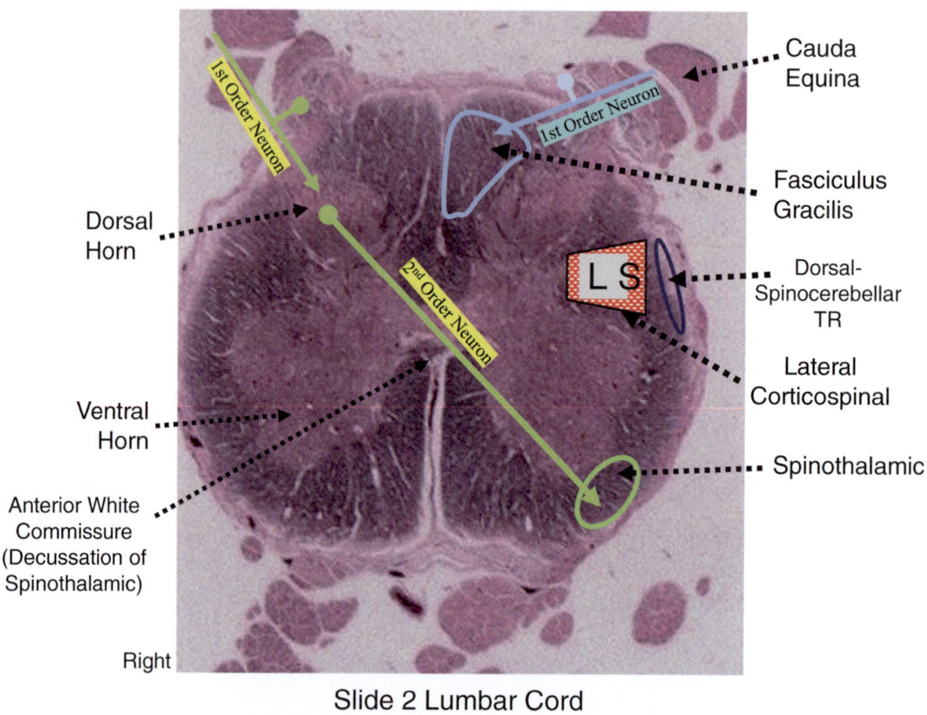

Slide 23.2 We have moved up the cord from the previous slide so that the white matter has enlarged. Note that the first order neuron of the DC/Medial lemniscus pathway enters the cord, does not synapse, and travels up the cord on the ipsilateral side. The first order neuron of the pain/temperature pathway enters the cord and synapses in the dorsal horn. The second order neuron decussates at the anterior white commissure and travels up the contralateral cord in the spinothalamic pathway. In the corticospinal tract at this level there are lumbar and sacral fibers

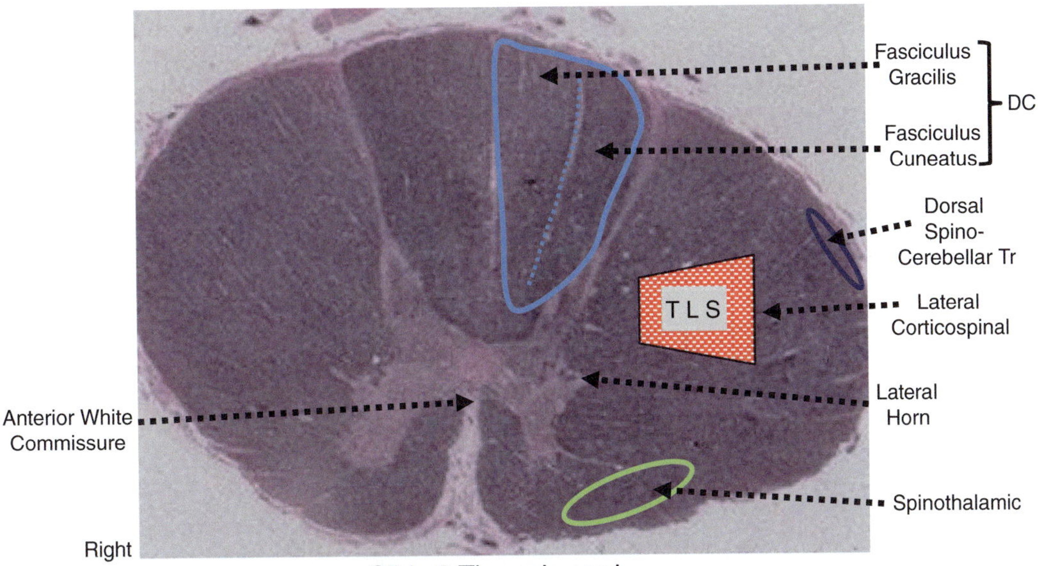

Slide 3 Thoracic cord

Slide 23.3 This cut is above T6, so the dorsal columns (DC) include both the fasciculus gracilis and cuneatus. The amount of white matter is significantly larger compared to the sacral cord image. In the corticospinal tract there are now thoracic, lumbar, and sacral fibers. The lateral horn is found between T1 and L2 and is the site of the cell bodies of origin for the preganglionic sympathetic neurons

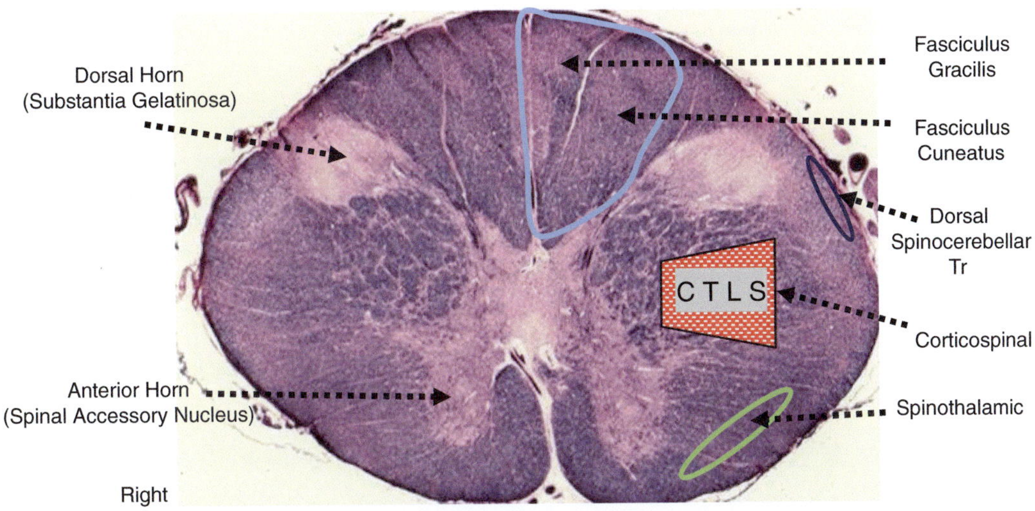

Slide 4 Cervical Cord

Slide 23.4 We are now at the top of the spinal cord where the cord is about to transform into the lower medulla. At this point, the anterior horn is the spinal accessory nucleus. The substantia gelatinosa is visible as a subdivision of the dorsal horn, and it will shortly become the spinal nucleus of CN V. In the corticospinal tract there are now cervical, thoracic, lumbar, and sacral fibers

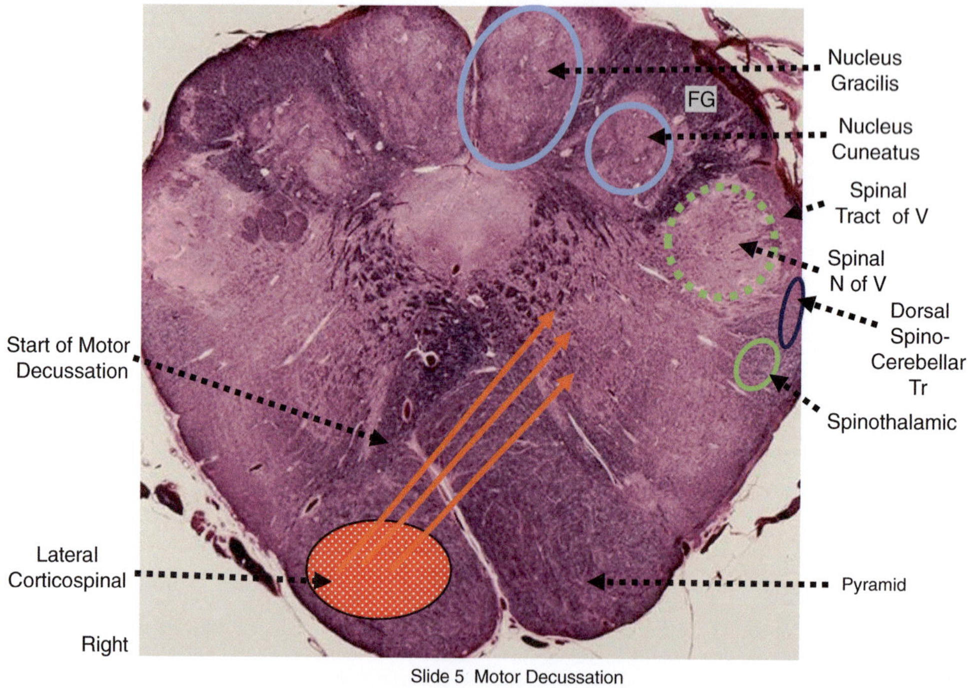

Slide 23.5 We are now at the motor decussation at the level of the closed medulla. The descending corticospinal fibers are starting to cross from one side to the other. The substantia gelatinosa has now become the spinal nucleus of V. The *fasciculus* gracilis and cuneatus have now become the *nucleus* gracilis and cuneatus. There is still a small piece of fasciculus gracilis (FG) evident

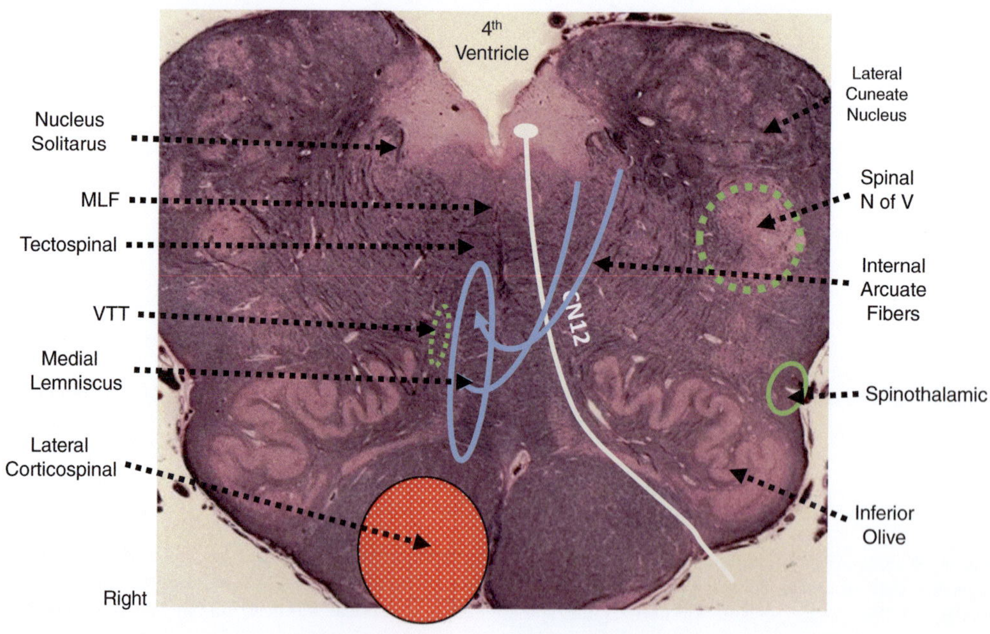

Slide 23.6 Sensory Decussation. We are seeing the sensory decussation (just a bit higher than the motor decussation) in this slide. The internal arcuate fibers are heading over to the contralateral medial lemniscus. In addition, fibers from the spinal nucleus of V are decussating to the opposite side to become the ventral trigeminothalamic tract (VTT). They assume a position just lateral to the medial lemniscus. The hypoglossal nerve can be seen emerging from the hypoglossal nucleus and traveling between the pyramid and the inferior olive. Sitting on top of the medial lemniscus is the tectospinal tract and medial longitudinal fasciculus

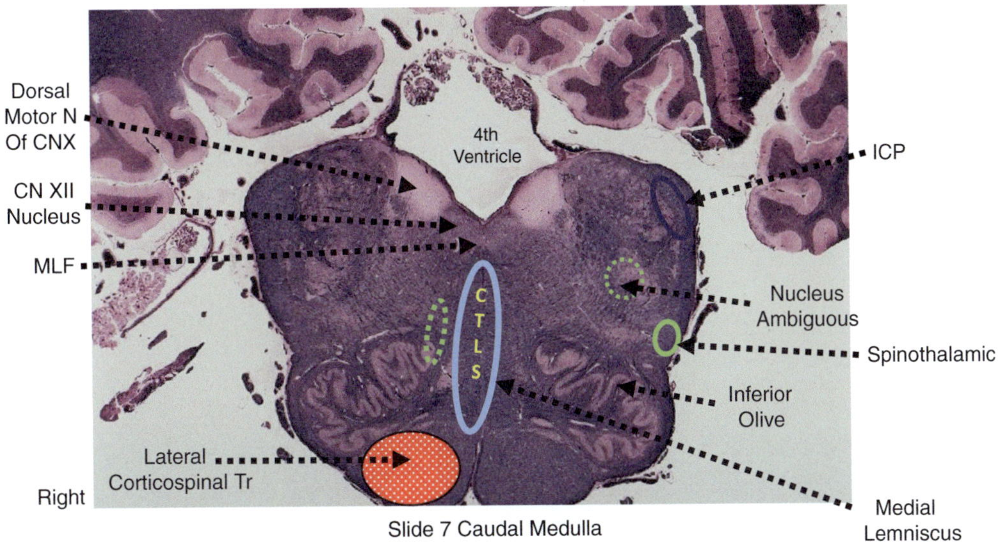

Slide 7 Caudal Medulla

Slide 23.7 This slide is slightly higher than the previous one. We can see the dorsal motor nucleus of CN X. The nucleus ambiguus (NA) is not visible but we know that it lives halfway between the inferior olive and the inferior cerebellar peduncle (ICP). A lesion to the NA would lead to dysphagia and dysarthria. The fibers in the medial lemniscus are organized topographically going from posterior to anterior as Cervical, Thoracic, Lumbar, and Sacral. In other words, the lower limb fibers in the medial lemniscus sit atop the corticospinal tract

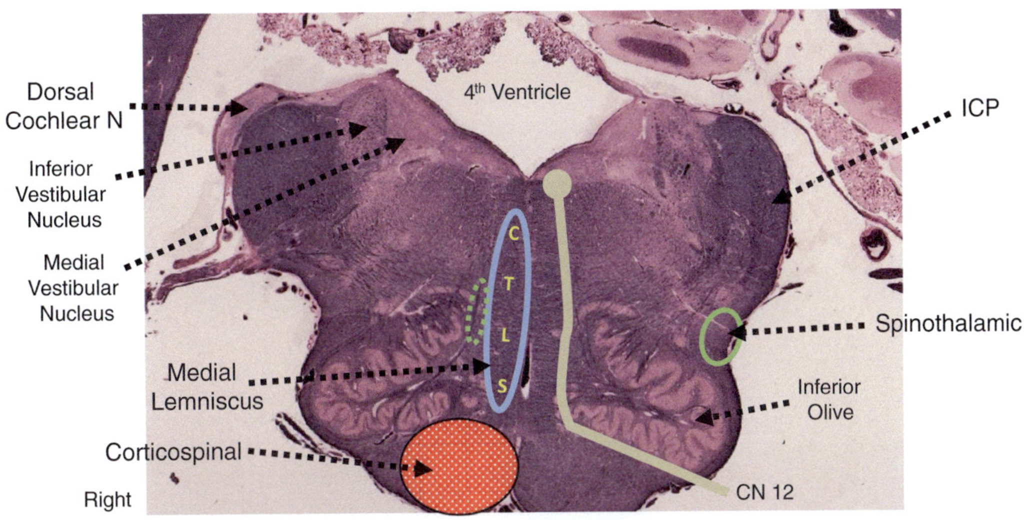

Slide 8 Caudal Medulla

Slide 23.8 We can now see the vestibular nuclei on both sides and the dorsal cochlear nucleus on one side. The inferior vestibular nucleus is identified by its stippled (or dotted) look to it. This is because the lateral vestibulospinal tract is traveling through it. Medial to the inferior vestibular nucleus is the medial vestibular nucleus. In this picture we can also see the inferior cerebellar peduncle (ICP) which is carrying the fibers from the dorsal spinocerebellar tract into the cerebellum. Note that in the previous slide (7) we can also see the ICP although it is slightly smaller. We can also see it in the following slide (9). In this slide we can see the fourth ventricle

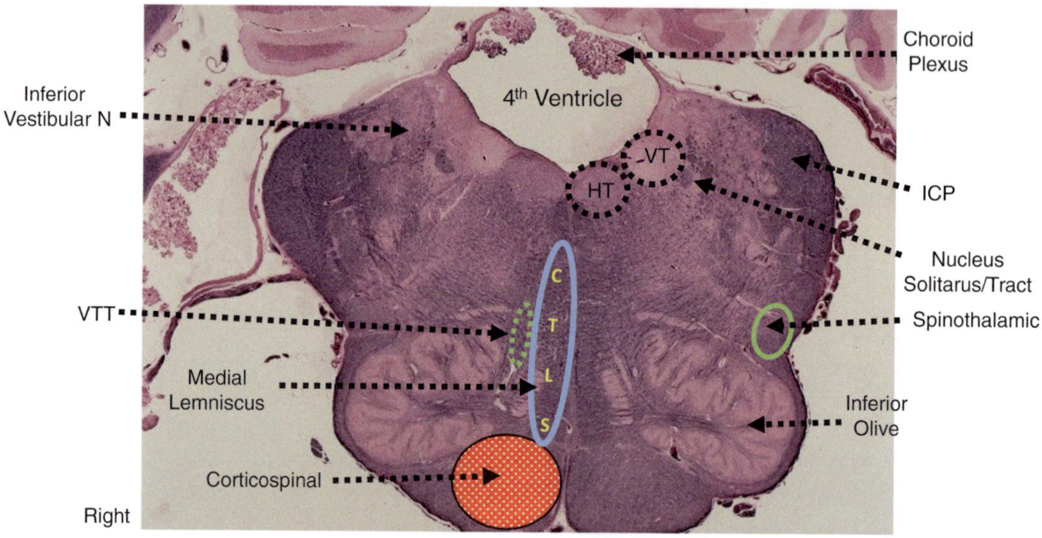

Slide 9: Caudal Medulla

Slide 23.9 In this slide we can see the nucleus solitarus and tract. The hypoglossal trigone (HT) and vagal trigone (VT) can be seen on the floor of the fourth ventricle. On the roof of the fourth ventricle are some cells of the choroid plexus, which produce CSF. The medial lemniscus is still sitting atop the pyramid. We can also see the VTT just lateral to the medial lemniscus. And most lateral, is the inferior cerebellar peduncle. Sitting just lateral and ventral to the ventral trigone is the solitary nucleus and its tract. Note that the tract is more centrally located, while the nucleus is lateral. If you think of it like a donut, the hole of the donut is the tract, and the nucleus is the doughy part of the donut

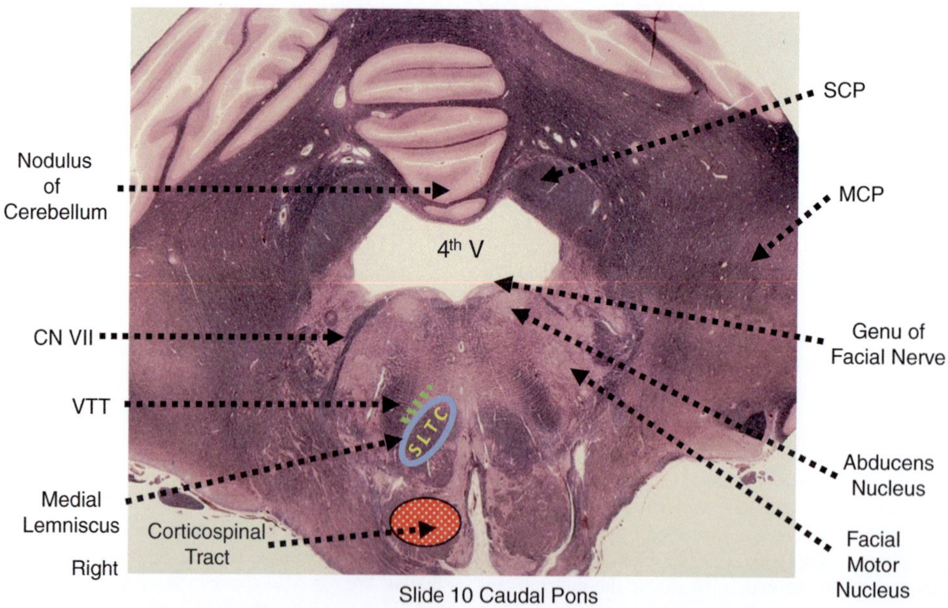

Slide 10 Caudal Pons

Slide 23.10 On the floor of the fourth ventricle is a protuberance—the facial colliculus—which is made up of the fibers from CN VII (the genu) wrapping around the nucleus of CN VI. See the next slide for a close-up view of the facial and abducens nerves. We have lost the ICP in this slide because we are above it, but we now see the MCP and SCP. The MCP) is carrying pontocerebellar fibers to the cerebellum, and the SCP is carrying fibers from the cerebellum to the thalamus. Compared to the previous slide the fourth ventricle is starting to get smaller, This is because as we move rostrally, the fourth ventricle is becoming the cerebral aqueduct

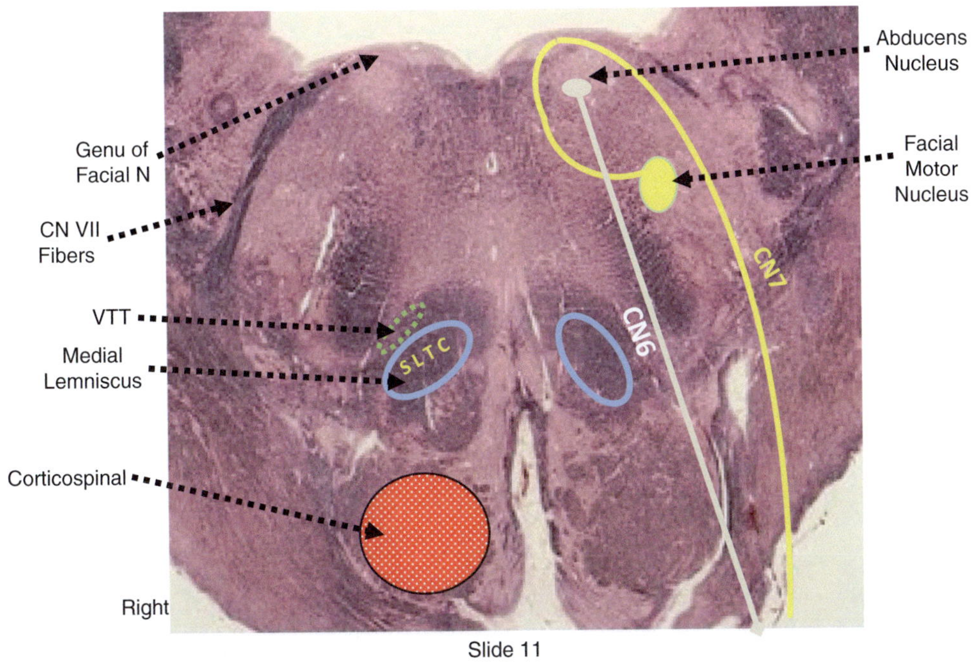

Slide 23.11 Close-up from Slide 23.10. On the floor of the fourth ventricle is the genu of the facial nerve which is made up of the fibers from CN VII wrapping around the nucleus of CN VI

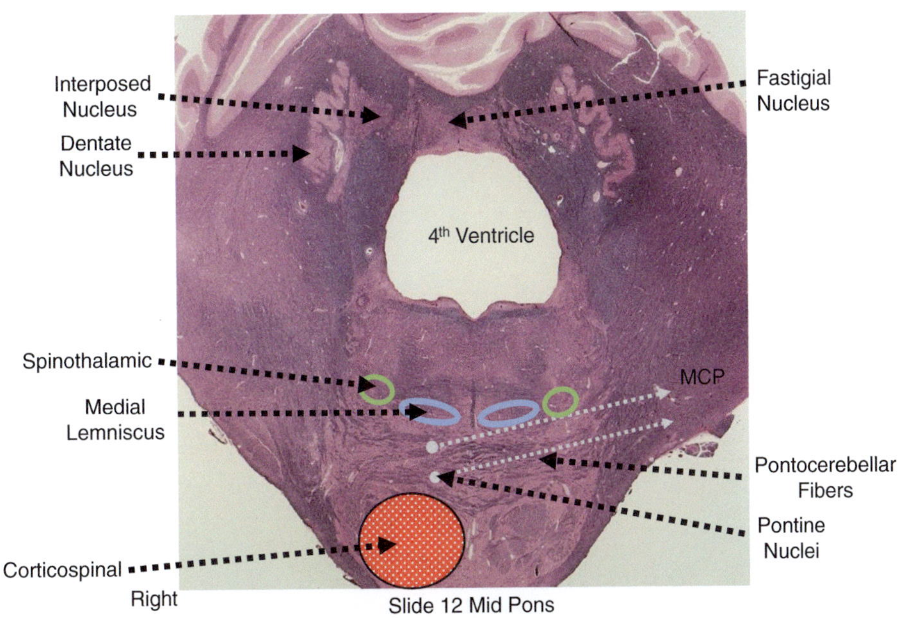

Slide 23.12 In this cut we can see the middle cerebellar peduncle (MCP). The deep cerebellar nuclei: fastigial, interposed (globose, and emboliform), and dentate are visible. The ponto-cerebellar fibers are traveling from the pontine nuclei to the contralateral cerebellum in the MCP

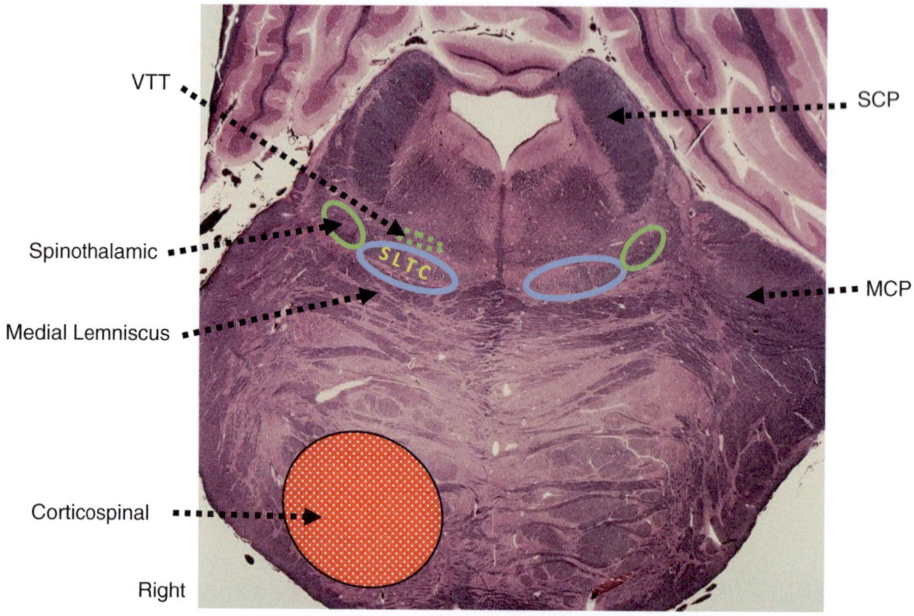

Slide 13 Mid Pons

Slide 23.13 In addition to the MCP we can now see the superior cerebellar peduncle (SCP). Running in the SCP are the fibers from the dentate nucleus on their way to the contralateral thalamus (dentatothalamic fibers), specifically the contralateral ventral lateral nucleus of the thalamus

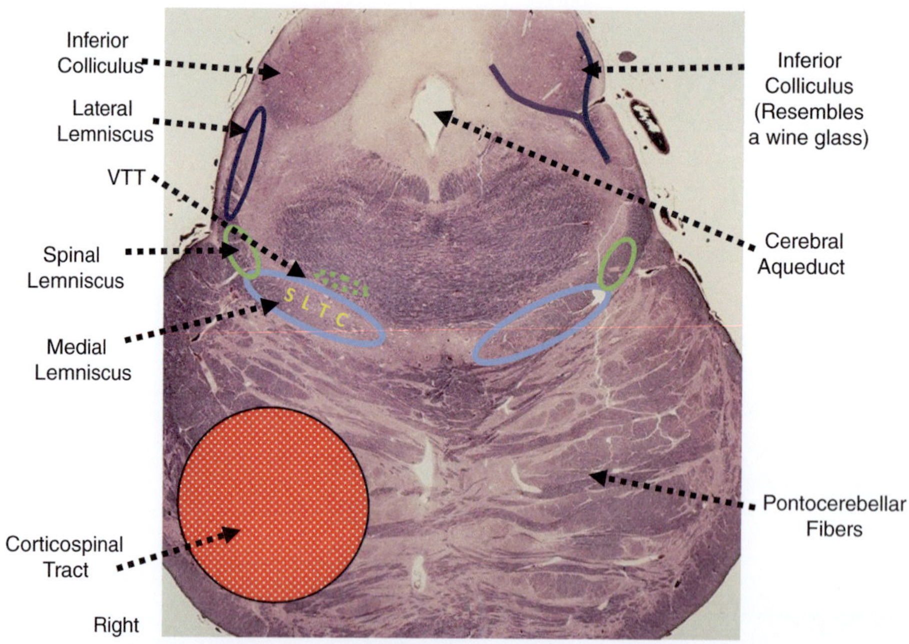

Slide 14 Superior Pons

Slide 23.14 The lateral lemniscus carrying fibers from the auditory system is about to terminate in the inferior colliculus. Note that the inferior colliculus is shaped like a wine glass (goblet) with the stem being the lateral lemniscus and the cup being the inferior colliculus.

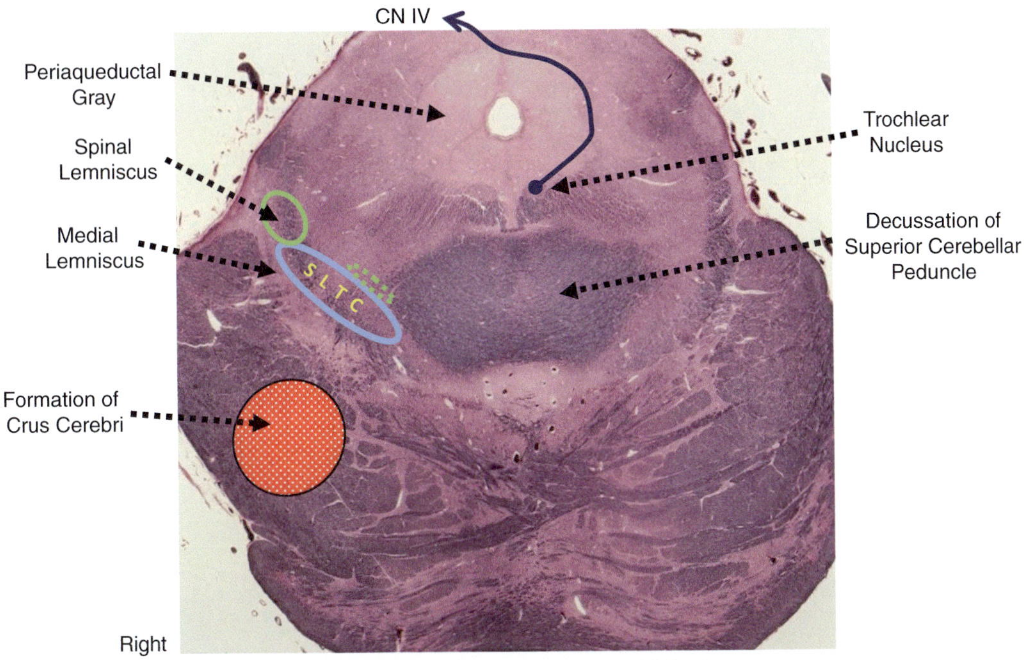

Slide 15 Superior Pons, Lower Midbrain

Slide 23.15 The superior pons is turning into the inferior midbrain. The dentato-thalamic fibers coming out of the cerebellum and traveling through the superior cerebellar peduncle are destined for the contralateral thalamus. They can be seen crossing as the decussation of the superior cerebellar peduncle. The trochlear nucleus can also be seen. CN IV comes out of the trochlear nucleus and heads to the contralateral superior oblique muscle

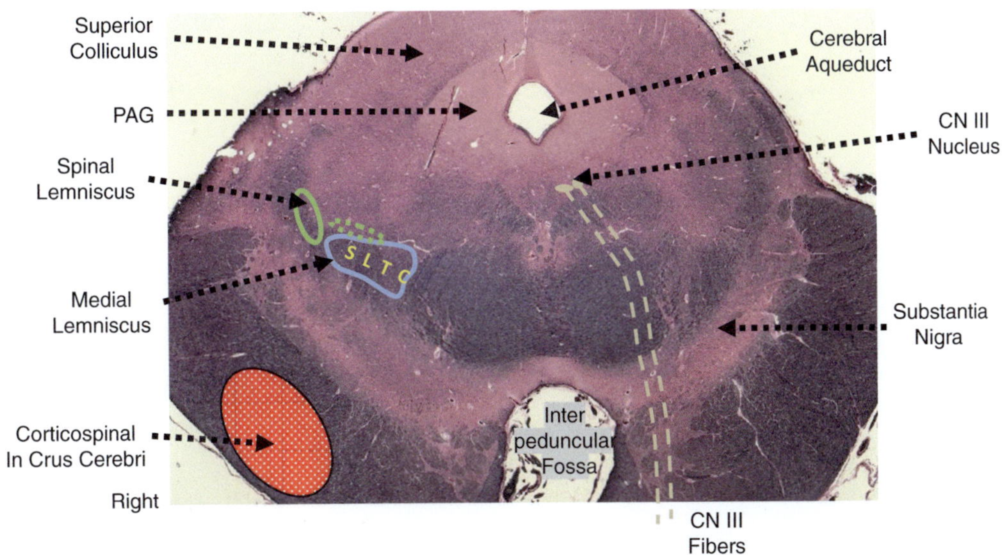

Slide 16 Caudal Midbrain

Slide 23.16 The superior colliculus can be seen. The nucleus of CN III and some of the fibers of CN III (slight wisps of fibers) can be seen traveling from the nucleus to their exit point near the interpeduncular fossa. The corticospinal tract is in the middle one third of the crus cerebri. The superior colliculus is also evident.

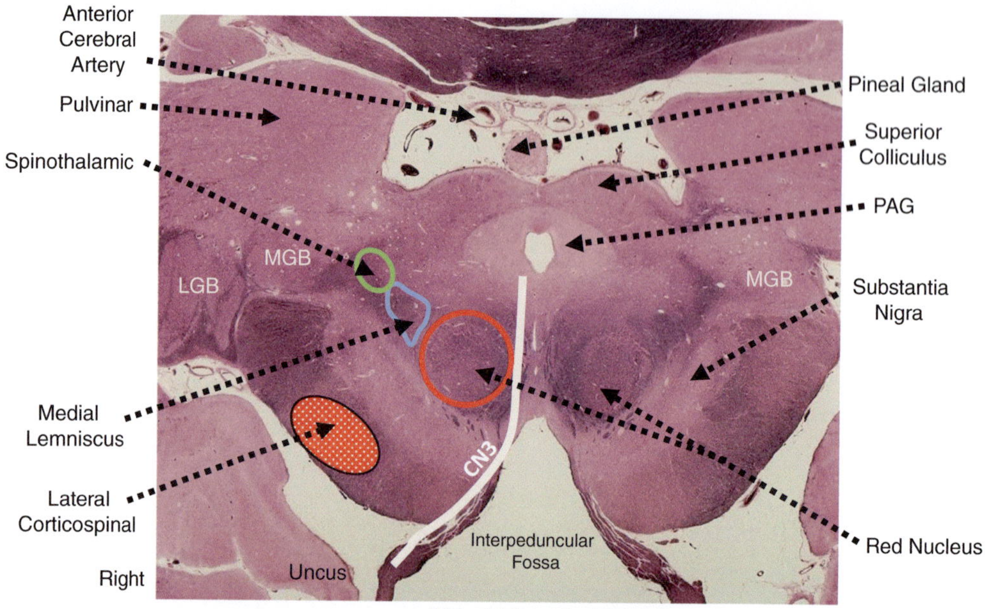

Slide 17 Superior Midbrain

Slide 23.17 We can now see the back (caudal) end of the thalamus—the pulvinar nucleus. Jutting off the caudal end of the pulvinar are the medial (MGB) and lateral geniculate bodies (LGB). The pineal gland is also visible. Surrounding the cerebral aqueduct is the periaqueductal gray which is involved with the descending control of pain. Coming out of the red nucleus is the rubrospinal tract headed to the contralateral spinal cord. The uncus is the medial temporal lobe near CN III. It is easy to see how an uncal herniation can compress these fibers. At the top of the picture is the corpus callosum

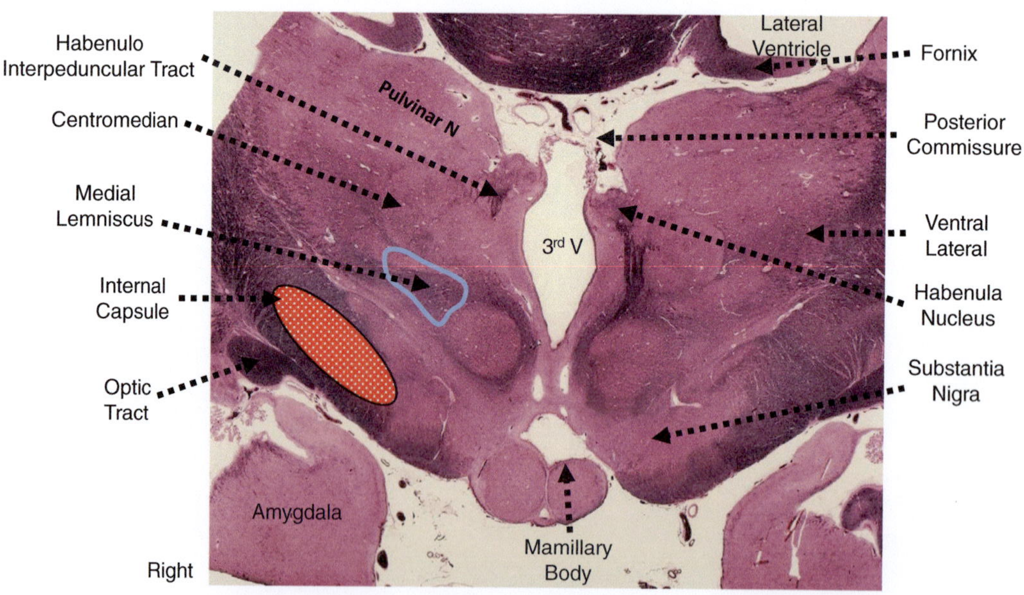

Slide 18 Caudal Thalamus

Slide 23.18 The amygdala is seen as a solid mass of gray matter. The habenula nucleus and start of the habenulointerpeduncular tract is evident. The medial lemniscus is turning into the ventral lateral nucleus. The fornix—the outflow of the hippocampus—can be seen separating the lateral ventricle and third ventricles on its way to the mamillary bodies. A small piece of the optic tract is seen. The fibers in the optic tract are running along the cerebral peduncle

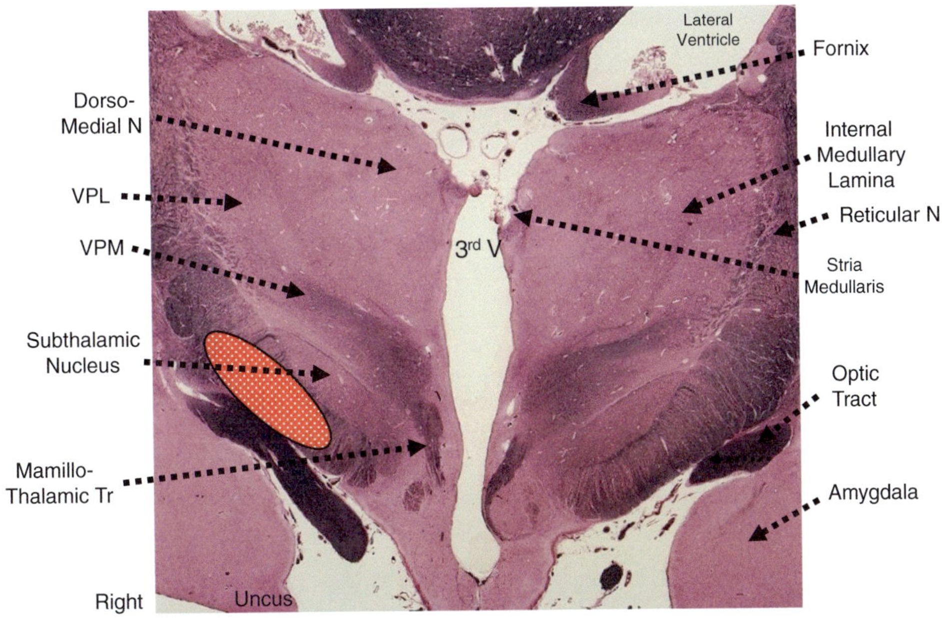

Slide 19 Mid-Thalamus

Slide 23.19 The dorsomedial nucleus is seen surrounding the third ventricle. The subthalamic nucleus is an oval shaped structure near the internal capsule. The internal medullary lamina is between the dorsomedial and ventral lateral nucleus. Both the ventral posterior lateral (VPL) and ventral posterior medial (VPM) nuclei of the thalamus can be seen

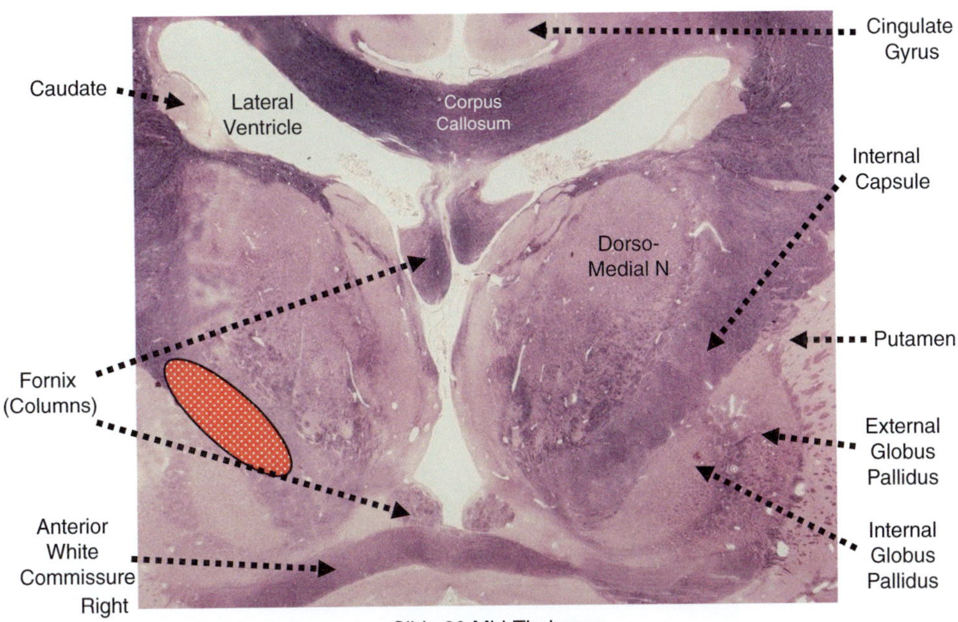

Slide 20 Mid-Thalamus

Slide 23.20 The internal and external globus pallidus and the putamen together all form a triangular shaped structure pushing into the internal capsule. The body of the fornix has turned into the columns of the fornix which are dropping down towards the mammillary bodies near the anterior white commissure. Above the corpus callosum is the cingulate gyrus. The caudate nucleus is small and abuts the lateral ventricle

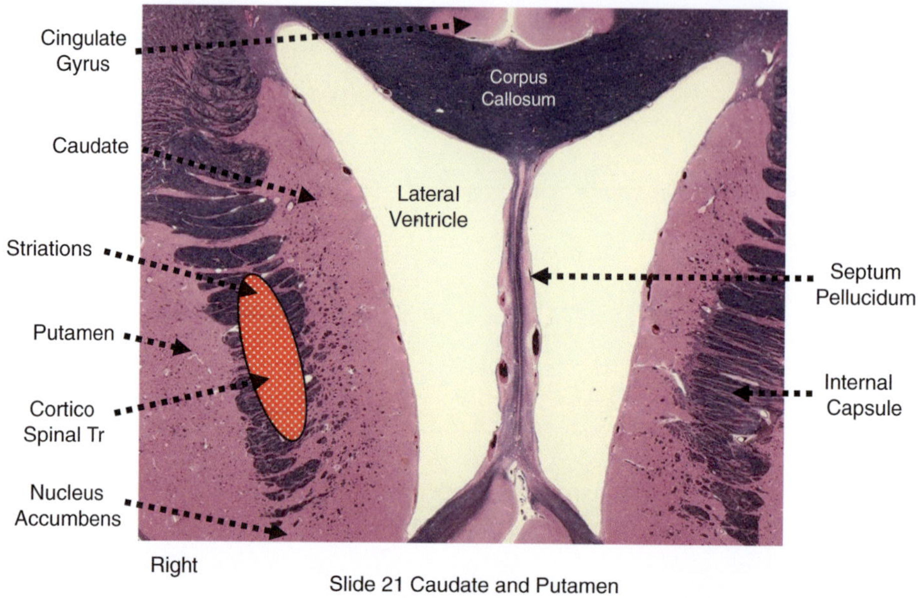

Slide 23.21 The caudate and putamen together are referred to as the striatum. At the rostral end of the caudate and putamen the two structures are connected by fibers which look like striations. In this picture it is clear how it got its name. The caudate borders the lateral ventricle. The septum pellucidum is in the midline

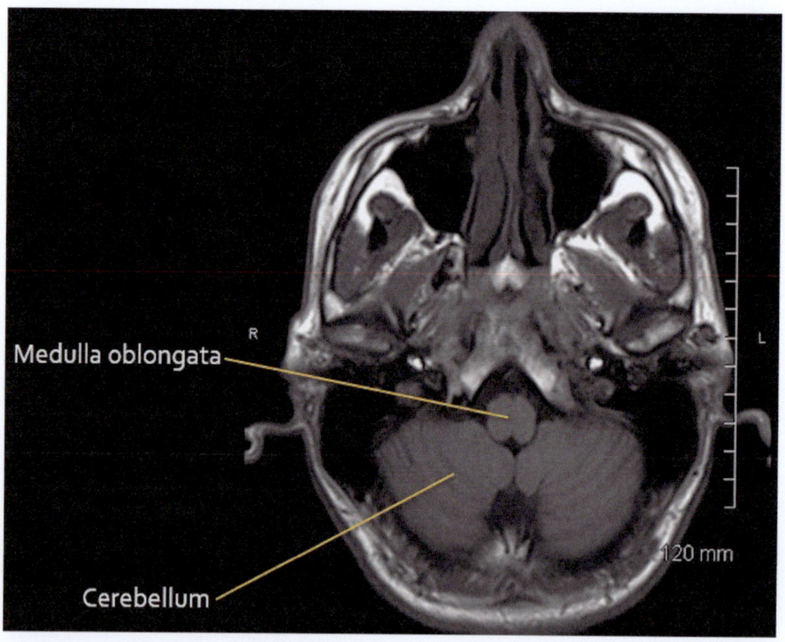

Slide 23.22 MRI through Medulla. The cerebellum can be seen in the posterior cranial fossa. The maxillary sinuses can also be seen just lateral to the nasal cavity

Slide 23.23 MRI Through Pons. Just behind the pons is the fourth ventricle. The internal carotid artery can be seen just before it is about to split into anterior and middle cerebral arteries. The middle cerebellar peduncle is carrying fibers from the pons to the cerebellum

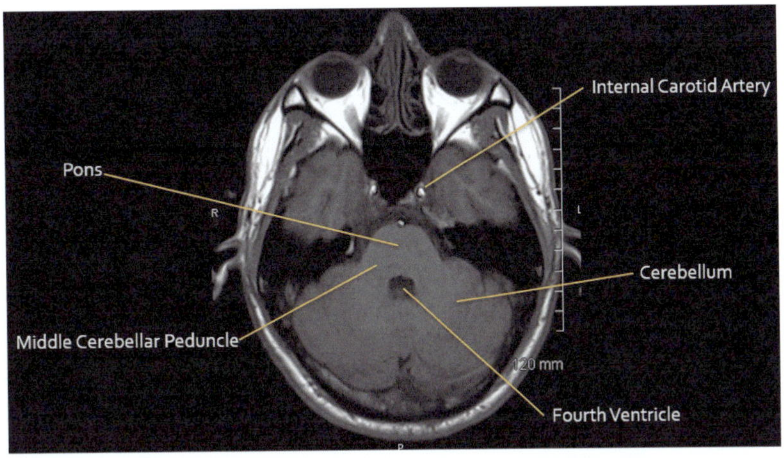

Slide 23.24 MRI through the Midbrain. The quadrigeminal cistern is between the colliculi and the cerebellum. Between the two cerebral peduncles is the interpeduncular fossa or cistern. Within the cerebral peduncle is the lateral corticospinal tract

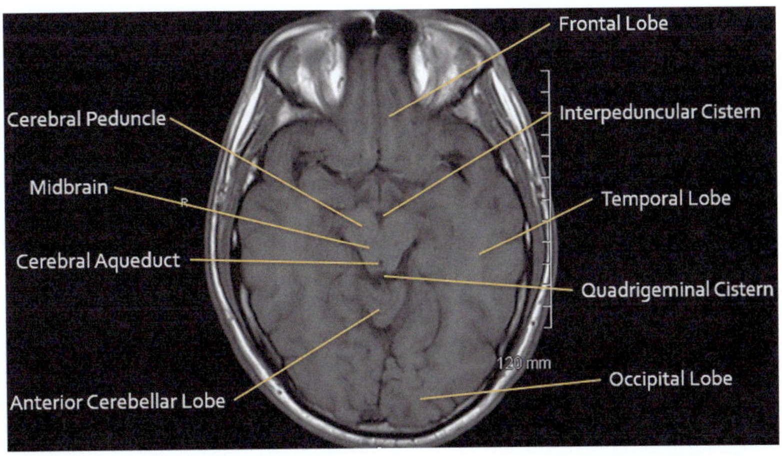

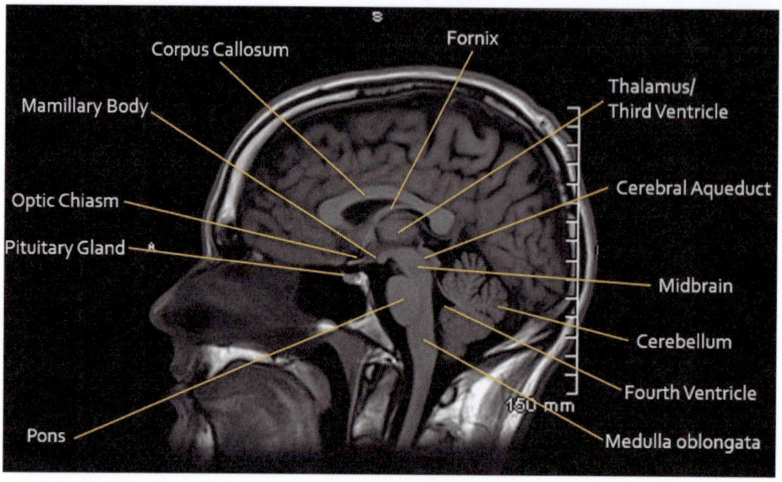

Slide 23.25 Mid Sagittal MRI. If you start with the medulla you can move up the CNS and into the pons and then midbrain. Between the pons and the cerebellum is the fourth ventricle. Sitting just atop the midbrain is the thalamus and the third ventricle. The fornix is the outflow tract of the hippocampus on its way to the mammillary body. Posterior to the midbrain is the cerebral aqueduct

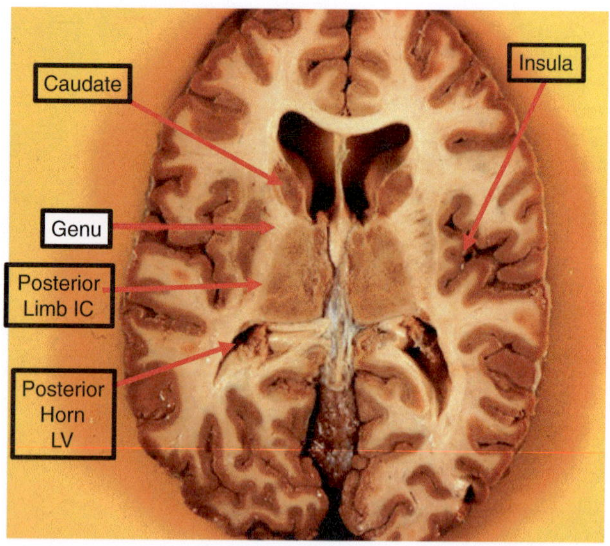

Slide 23.26 Axial Section of Cerebral Cortex. The internal capsule with the anterior and posterior limbs and the genu are all clearly seen. The caudate is pushing into the lateral ventricle. Coming back into the occipital cortex is the posterior horn of the lateral ventricle (VL)

Further Reading

1. Haines DE, Hutchins JB, Lynch JC. Medical neurobiology: do we teach neurobiology in a format that is relevant to the clinical setting? Anat Rec. 2002;269:99–106.

Lesion and Blood Vessel Test 24

Lesion and Blood Supply Test

Each picture below represents a lesion scenario. For each patient, list the symptoms, the tract involved, and the cell body of origin for the compromised fibers. If it is a vascular incident, list the artery involved.

Lesion #1

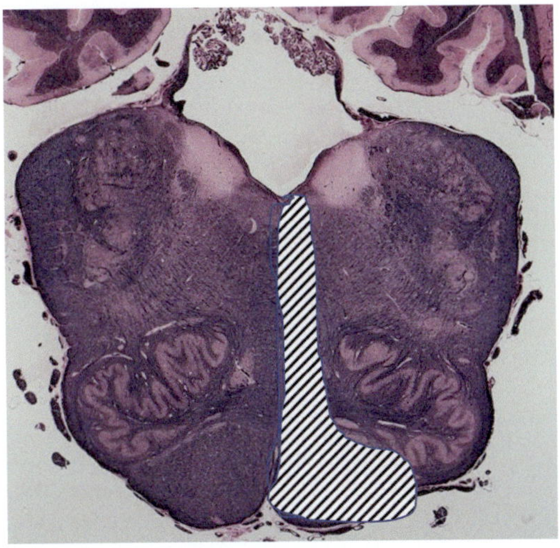

Syndrome:
Artery:

Symptom	Tract	Cell body of Origin

 # Lesion 2

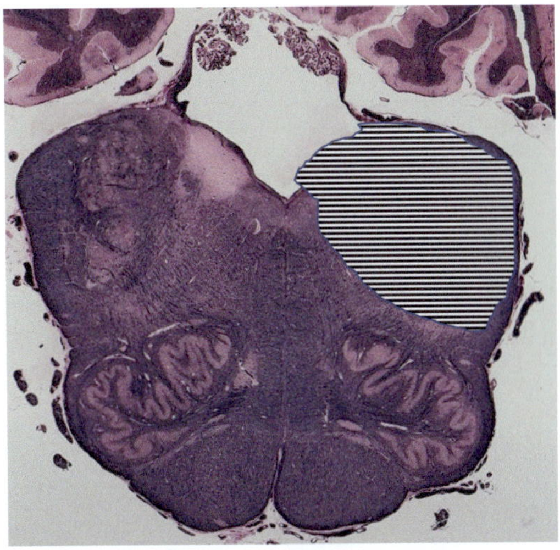

Syndrome:
Artery:

Symptom	Tract or Nucleus Compromised	Cell body of Origin (for tracts)

J. Leo, *Gross Anatomy, Neuroanatomy, and Embryology for Medical Students*,
https://doi.org/10.1007/978-3-031-87151-1_24

Lesion #3

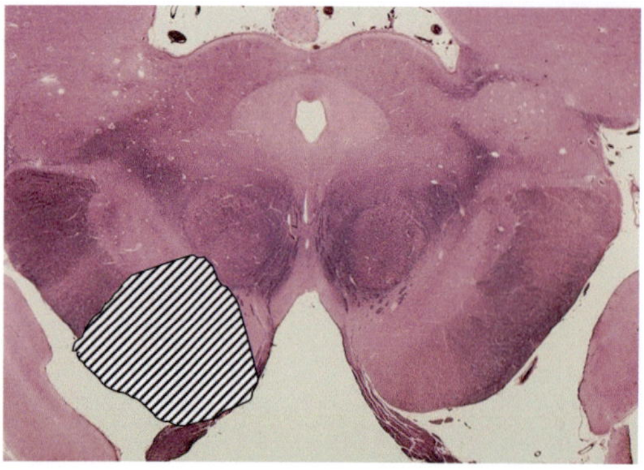

Syndrome:
Artery:

Symptom	Tract	Cell body of Origin

Lesion #4

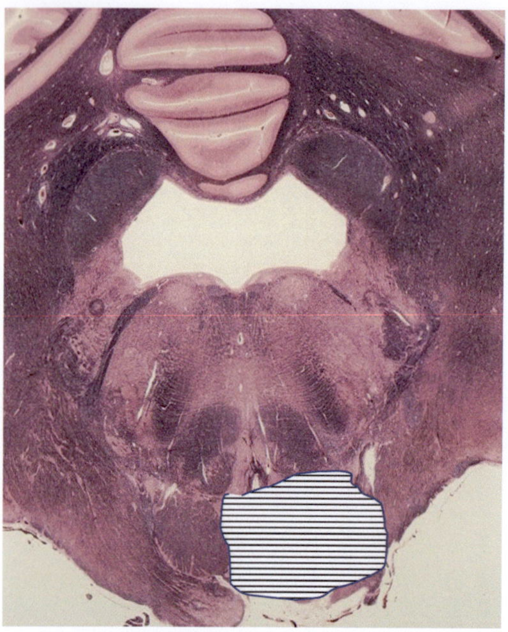

Syndrome:
Artery:

Symptom	Tract	Cell body of Origin

Lesion #5 (Hint, there Is a Subtle Difference Between 4 and 5)

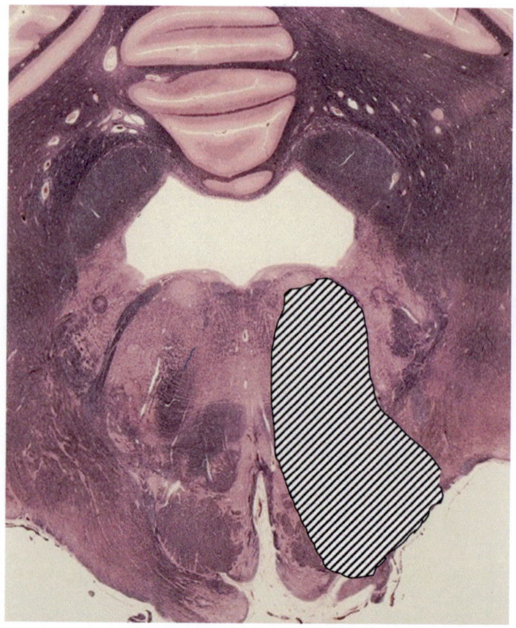

Syndrome:
Artery:

Symptom	Tract	Cell body of Origin

Lesion #6

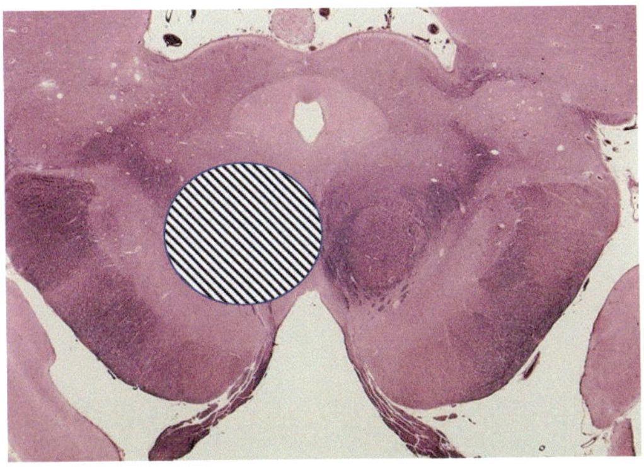

Syndrome:
Artery:

Symptom	Tract	Cell body of origin

Lesion #7

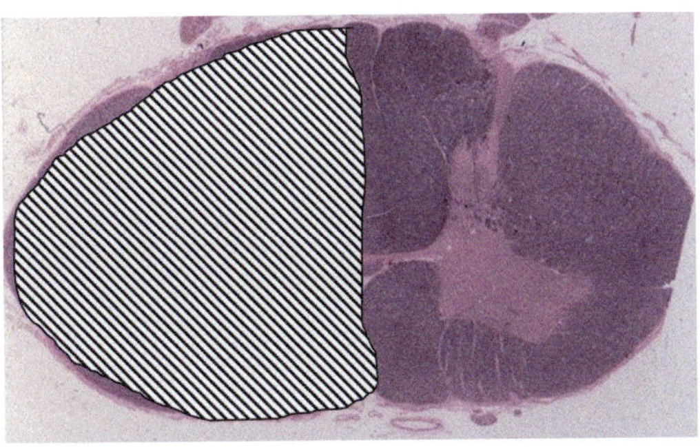

Syndrome:

Symptom	Tract	Cell body of Origin

Lesion #8

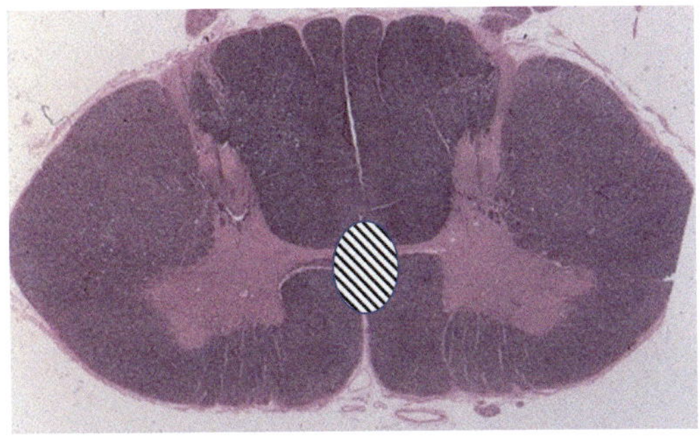

Syndrome:

Symptom	Tract	Cell body of Origin

Answers to Lesion Test

Lesion #1 Key

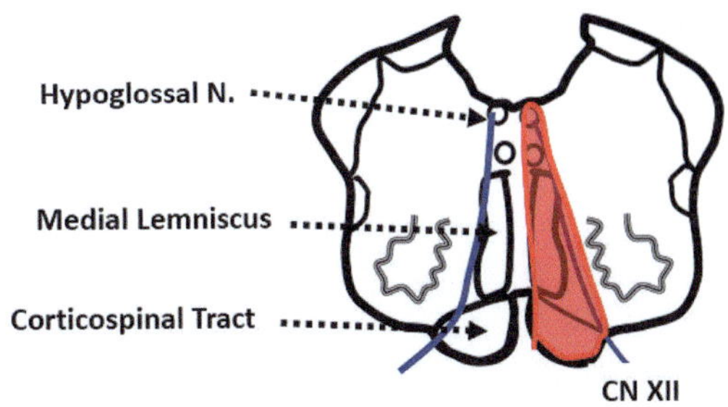

Syndrome: Medial Medullary Syndrome
Artery: Vertebral Artery, Anterior Spinal Artery

Symptom	Tract	Cell body of origin
Contralateral UMN sign	Corticospinal	Precentral gyrus
Contralateral dorsal column signs	Medial lemniscus	Nucleus cuneatus and gracilis
Ipsilateral CN XII deficit	CN XII	Hypoglossal nucleus

Lesion #2 Key

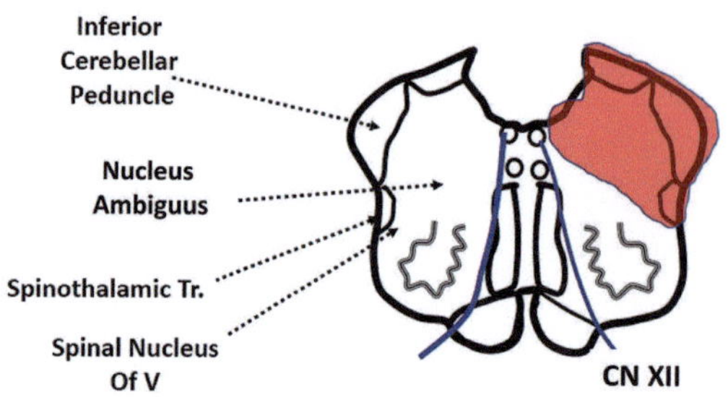

Syndrome: Lateral Medullary Syndrome
Artery: Posterior Inferior Cerebellar

Symptom	Tract or Nucleus compromised	Cell body of origin (for tracts)
Ipsilateral loss of pain and temp to face	Spinal nucleus of V and spinal tract of V	Trigeminal ganglion of spinal nucleus of V
Contralateral loss of pain and temp to limbs	Spinothalamic tract	Dorsal horn
	Nucleus Ambiguus CN 9 and 10	Nucleus Ambiguus
Ipsilateral ataxia	Inferior cerebellar peduncle	Dorsal nucleus of Clark
Horner's syndrome	Descending Hypothalamics	Hypothalamus
Nystagmus	Vestibular nucleus	

Lesion #3 Key

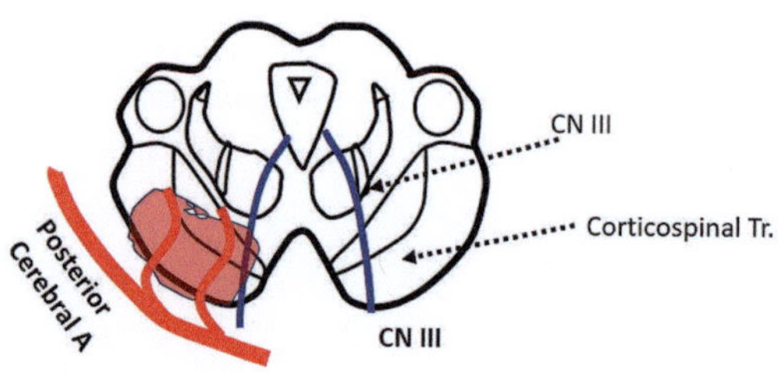

Syndrome: Medial Midbrain Syndrome
Artery: Posterior Cerebral

Symptom	Tract	Cell body of origin
Contralateral UMN	Corticospinal	Precentral gyrus
Ipsilateral CN III deficit	CN III	Oculomotor nucleus
Ptosis, dilated pupil	CN III	Edinger Westphal nucleus
Contralateral lower face weakness	Corticobulbar	Precentral gyrus

Lesion #4 Key

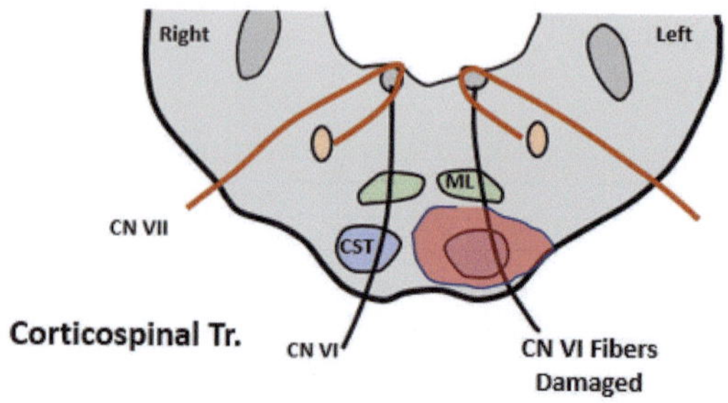

Syndrome: Medial Pontine/Raymond's Syndrome
Artery: Paramedian branches of basilar

Symptom	Tract	Cell body of origin
Contralateral UMN signs	Corticospinal	Precentral gyrus
Ipsilateral CN VII deficit	CN VII	Facial motor nucleus
Ipsilateral medial strabismus	CN VI	Abducens nucleus

Lesion #5 Key

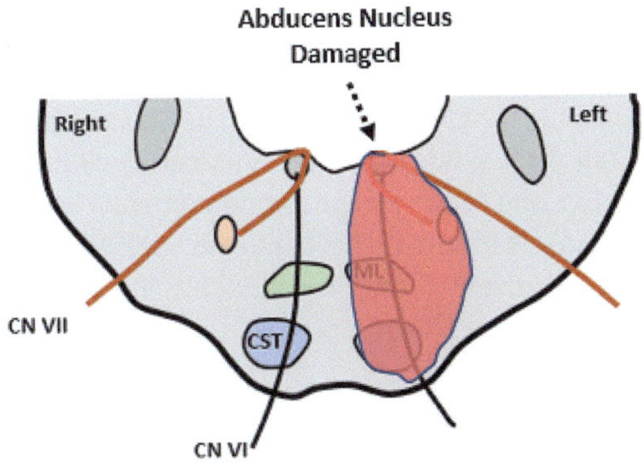

Syndrome: Medial Pontine Syndrome/Foville's Syndrome

Symptom	Tract	Cell body of origin
Contralateral UMN signs	Corticospinal	Precentral gyrus
Ipsilateral loss of facial expression	CN VII	Facial motor nucleus
Lateral gaze paralysis	Abducens nucleus	Abducens nucleus

Note that 4 and 5 are almost identical, except that patient 4 has a lesion to the abducens nerve so only the ipsilateral eye is affected—paralysis of ipsilateral ocular abduction. While patient 5 has a lesion to the abducens nucleus so both eyes are affected—lateral gaze paralysis.

Lesion #6 Key

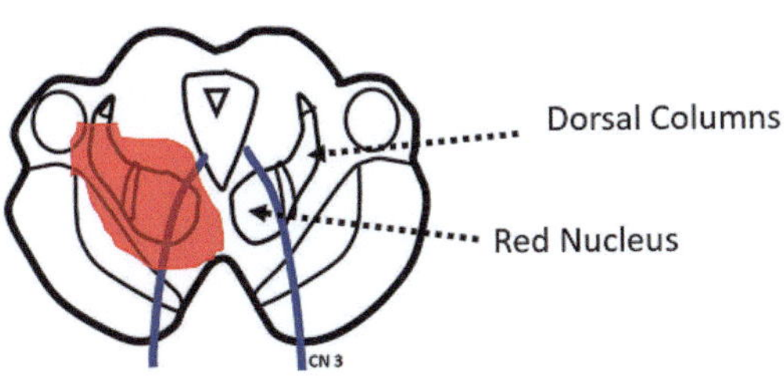

Syndrome: Benedikt's Syndrome
Artery: Perforating branches of posterior cerebral

Symptom	Tract or Nucleus	Cell body of origin
Contralateral tremor	Red nucleus	Red nucleus
Ipsilateral CN III palsy	CN III	Oculomotor nucleus
Ptosis, dilated pupil	CN III	Edinger Westphal nucleus

Lesion #7 Key

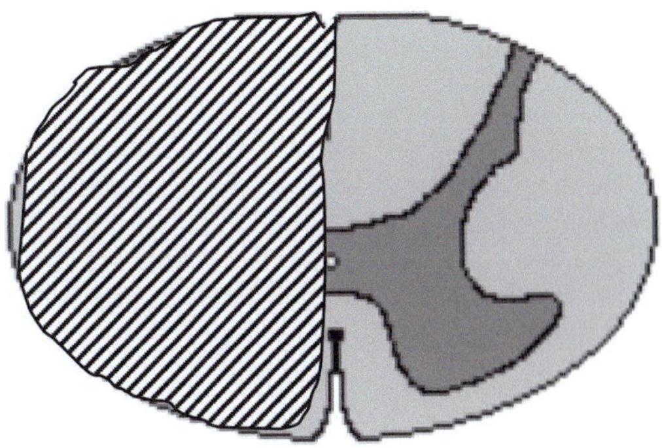

Syndrome: Hemisection of cord at C5

Symptom	Tract	Cell body of origin
LMN signs at C5	Anterior horn	Anterior horn
UMN sings in lower limb	Corticospinal	Precentral gyrus
Contralateral loss of pain and temperature in from C5 down	Spinothalamic	Dorsal horn
Ipsilateral loss of pain and temperature at C5	Tract of Lissauer	DRG
Horner's syndrome	Descending Hypothalamics	Hypothalamus
Ipsilateral dorsal column signs	Fasciculus gracilis and cuneatus	DRG

Lesion #8 Key

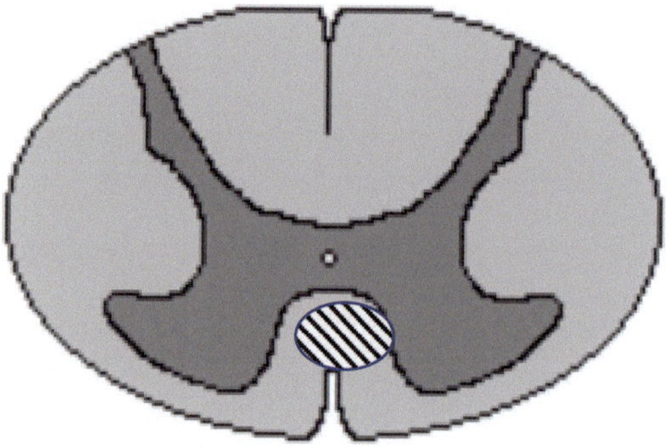

Syndrome: Syringomyelia

Symptom	Tract	Cell body of origin
Bilateral loss of pain and temperature to upper limbs	Anterior white commissure	Dorsal horns, bilateral
LMN signs in hands	Anterior horns	Anterior horn

Review of Blood Supply to Nervous System

The first picture of the circle of Willis is not labeled. The goal is to attempt to label each artery on your own. Note that the next picture includes the name of the arteries. And then the table that follows includes the name of the symptoms or clinical scenarios associated with each artery. In addition, there is a column in this table with a summary of the main findings that go along with each syndrome. Keep in mind that all these syndromes are addressed within the various sections of the book in much more detail. The purpose of this table is to jog your memory, not to explain in detail each syndrome. If the clinical signs listed next to one of the symptoms do not make sense, then this is time to go back into the book and read in more detail (Figs. 24.1 and 24.2; Tables 24.1 and 24.2).

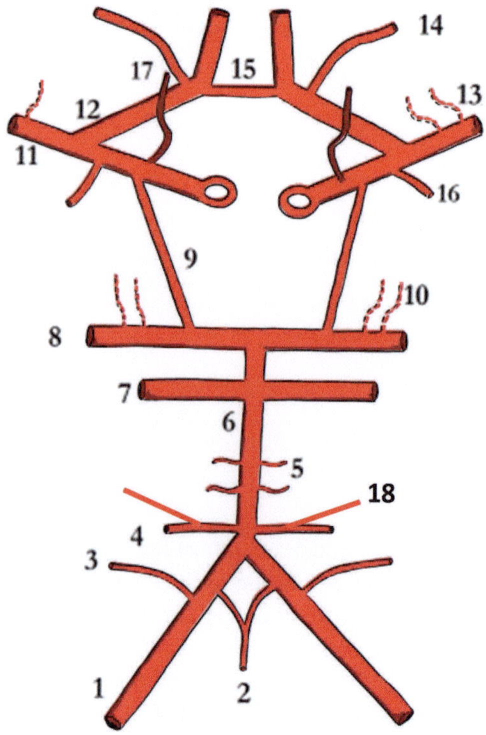

Fig. 24.1 Circle of Willis. You can test yourself by filling in the names and major syndromes associated with each artery

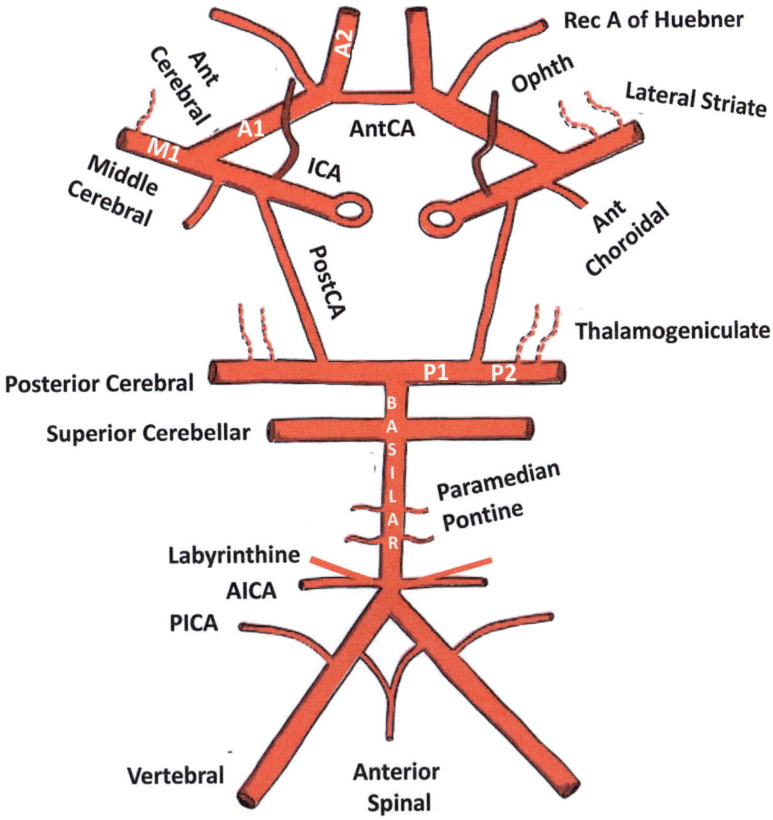

Fig. 24.2 Circle of Willis and its Named Branches. *AntCA* anterior communicating artery, *PostCA* posterior communicating artery, *PICA* posterior inferior cerebellar artery, *AICA* anterior inferior cerebellar artery, *ICA* internal carotid artery. Note that arising from the basilar artery there are also short and long circumferential As which are not shown in the picture

Table 24.1 Summary of Lesions arising from compromised branches of the circle of Willis

Key	Artery	Syndrome	Deficits
1	Vertebral A	Medial Medullary Syndrome (sometimes anterior spinal A)	Contralateral hemiplegia and DC symptoms, ipsilateral CN XII palsy
2	Anterior spinal A (at level of spinal cord)	Anterior spinal artery syndrome	Bilateral loss of CST and Spth below the lesion. Sparing of DCs. Bladder dysfunction. T4-T8 is most vulnerable region so lower limbs would be affected, but not upper limbs typically.
3	Posterior inferior cerebellar A	Lateral medullary syndrome	Ipsilateral anesthesia face (VTT), contralateral anesthesia body (Spth), ipsilateral CN IX and X palsies (nucleus Ambiguus), ipsilateral ataxia (dorsal spinocerebellar Tr). Vertigo, vomiting (vestibular nucleus), Horner's (descending Hypothalamics)
4	Anterior inferior cerebellar A.	Lateral pontine syndrome	Ipsilateral anesthesia face (VTT), contralateral anesthesia body (Spth), ipsilateral CN V, VII, VIII palsies. Horner's
5	Paramedian branches of basilar	Medial pontine syndrome	Contralateral hemiplegia, hemianesthesia, ipsilateral CNs VI and VII palsies
6	Basilar A	Locked-in syndrome	Quadriplegia – bilateral loss of all motor function in the body
7	Superior cerebellar A	Trigeminal Neuralgia	Pain from face. The artery is compressing the trigeminal nerve. Not an infarct
8	Posterior cerebral artery (at least 3 potential lesions)	Medial midbrain syndrome Alexia without agraphia Pie in the sky	Contralateral hemiplegia, ipsilateral CN III palsy Lesion to splenium of corpus callosum Lesion to Meyer's loop
9	Posterior communicating A	CN III deficit	Blown pupil
10	Thalamogeniculate as	Thalamic pain Syndrome	Severe pain from contralateral body
11	Middle cerebral A	Cortical infarct	*Superior division:* Broca's aphasia, eyes deviate towards lesion side, upper limb affected, lower limb spared. Brachiofacial paralysis *Inferior division:* Wernicke's aphasia, hearing deficit
12	Anterior cerebral A	Cortical infarct (medial) Anterior corpus callosum	Contralateral loss of primary motor and contralateral sensory loss to lower limb Trans cortical apraxia
13	Lateral striate as	Pure motor deficit Post limb IC	Contralateral hemiplegia and contralateral corticobulbar symptoms
14	Recurrent artery of Huebner	Recurrent A of H Syndrome	Abulia, contralateral hemiplegia
15	Anterior communicating A	Visual field deficit	Amnesia, confabulations
16	Anterior choroidal A	Anterior choroidal syndrome	Contralateral hemiplegia and hemianesthesia, homonymous hemianopia
17	Ophthalmic A	Blind in one eye	Blind, cherry red spot
18	Labyrinthine A	Infarct (travels to ear through internal acoustic meatus)	Loss of hearing and balance ipsilateral

Table 24.2 This is just a summary of arteries and syndromes. This table is just meant to jog your memory. There are potential variations in all these syndromes from one patient to another. In addition, the table does not include the subtle details. See the text for more details for each syndrome

1	Syringomyelia	1	Bilateral loss of pain and temperature at the level of lesion. Possible LMN deficit in upper limbs. Cavitation of central canal
2	Hemisection of spinal cord	2	Contralateral loss of pain from lesion down, ipsilateral UMN signs from lesion down, ipsilateral loss of DCs from lesion down. Belt like loss of P/T at level of lesion. Horner's if above T1
3	Tabes dorsalis	3	Three "Ps" pain, paresthesia, and polyuria. Most likely a Romberg sign. Argyll Robertson pupil
4	Anterior spinal artery occlusion in cord	4	Bilateral paresis and bilateral loss of pain to the lower limbs. Most common site of pathology is artery of Adamkiewicz. Usually occurs at T9–12 level. Side effect of aortic surgery or spine surgery
5	Posterior spinal artery occlusion	5	Damages dorsal columns on one side. Ipsilateral deficit of conscious proprioception
6	L4 radiculopathy	6	Sensory loss on medial foot and leg; patellar tendon weak, quadriceps weakness
7	L5 radiculopathy	7	Sensory loss on dorsum of foot, no good reflex test, dorsiflexion of toes
8	S1 radiculopathy	8	Sensory loss on lateral foot, weakened Achilles' tendon reflex, plantar flexion
9	Dentate nucleus projection	9	VL, VA of thalamus and red nucleus
10	Gerstman Syndrome	10	Acalculia, finger agnosia, agraphia, R/L disorientation, posterior lobule of parietal lobe, particularly the angular and supramarginal gyri
11	Three layers of cerebellar gray matter	11	Molecular, Purkinje, granule
12	Pinpoint pupils	12	Pontine lesion, or opioids
13	Vestibular nerve lesions	13	Fast nystagmus to contralateral side
14	Medial midbrain syndrome	14	Ipsilateral CN deficit, contralateral UMN deficit to body and contralateral lower face. Posterior cerebral artery
23	Medial medullary syndrome	23	Ipsilateral CN XII deficit, contralateral UMN signs on body. Contralateral DC signs. No Horner's syndrome. Anterior spinal or vertebral artery
16	Benedickt's Syndrome	16	Contralateral tremor, ipsilateral CN III deficit, maybe contralateral dorsal column signs
17	Dorsal midbrain syndrome	17	Paralysis of upward gaze. Hydrocephalus. Parinaud syndrome. "Setting sun sign"
18	Lateral medullary Syndrome	18	Ipsilateral loss of pain and temperature on face, contralateral loss of pain and temperature on body, ataxia, dysphagia, dysarthria, nystagmus. Ipsilateral Horner's. Most likely PICA or vertebral artery
19	Uncal herniation	19	Compresses CN III. Ipsilateral CN III deficit, contralateral homonymous hemianopia, and ipsilateral UMN signs (most likely, but could be contralateral UMN signs). Books will vary on UMN side. Cerebral peduncle is compressed at Kernohan's notch
20	Posterior communicating artery aneurysm	20	Compresses CN III. Dilated pupil, possibly ophthalmoplegia
21	Meyers loop	21	"Pie in the sky," superior quadrantanopia
22	Pie on the floor	22	Parietal lobe. Inferior quadrantanopia
23	Alexia without agraphia	23	Splenium of corpus callosum. Lesion to occipital artery on dominate side that damages left occipital lobe and splenium. Typically *left* posterior cerebral
24	Lingual gyrus lesion	24	Contralateral inferior quadrantanopia with macular sparing
25	Cuneate gyrus lesion	25	Contralateral superior quadrantanopia with macular sparing
26	RAPD	26	Paradoxical dilation of pupil. Due to lesion of optic nerve or retina.

(continued)

Table 24.2 (continued)

27	Adie's pupil	27	Parasympathetic deficit. Dilated pupil
28	Craniopharyngioma and visual defect	28	Bitemporal visual field defect. Starts in superior field than moves inferiorly
29	Adenoma and visual defect	29	Bitemporal visual field defect. Starts in inferior field and moves superiorly
30	Cherry red spot	30	Occluded central artery of retina
31	Lesion to non-dominant parietal lobe	31	Contralateral neglect, think clock face picture
32	Tumor in pterygopalatine fossa, what CN nerve?	32	V2 and its branches
33	Medial pontine lesion	33	Paralysis of lateral gaze to ipsilateral side (CN VI nucleus), ipsilateral facial palsy (CN VII fibers), contralateral hemiparesis (corticobulbar tract). At rest, eyes will drift towards the paralyzed side of body– "Wrong way eyes." Paramedian branch of basilar artery
34	Decorticate Rigidity	34	Bilateral lesion above red nucleus. Upper limbs flexed at elbow
35	Decerebrate rigidity	35	Bilateral lesion below red nucleus, but above vestibular nucleus. Upper limbs extended at elbow
36	Cold water in right ear. Which way is slow deviation?	36	Right
37	Spinning chair test and post rotatory movement. Which direction is slow deviation at stop after spinning?	37	In direction of spinning
38	Argyll Robertson pupil	38	Pupil reacts to accommodation but not light. Neurosyphilis patients
39	Thalamic pain Syndrome	39	Contralateral loss of pain followed by excreting pain emanating from contralateral side of body—Thalamogeniculate arteries
40	Basal ganglia. Direct and indirect pathways are from which nucleus?	40	Caudate and putamen
41	Hemiballismus	41	Subthalamic nucleus
42	Dopamine drives movement by driving the direct or indirect pathway?	42	Direct, although the direct pathway is inhibitory. Dopamine increases output of direct pathway, so inhibition is increased.
43	Wernicke's Symptoms	43	Ataxia, ophthalmoplegia, confusion (triad)
44	Korsakoff's symptoms	44	Confabulation, hallucinations
45	Wernicke-Korsakoff's site of pathology	45	Mammillary bodies, dorsomedial nucleus of thalamus
46	Kluver-Bucy	46	Medial temporal lobe, placidity, loss of fear hypersexuality, hyperorality
47	Amygdala	47	Responsible for response to fear
48	Nucleus basalis of Meynert	48	Degeneration of cholinergics, Alzheimer's
49	Cell bodies of fibers in optic tract	49	Ganglion cells of retina
50	Locked-in syndrome	50	Lesion to basilar artery. Patient loses all motor control except for ability to blink
51	Lesion at Stylomastoid foramen	51	Loss of muscles of facial expression.
52	Lesion in Facial Canal	52	Loss of muscles of facial expression plus a dry eye, hyperacusis, and loss of glands to palate and mouth
53	Lesion to inferior cerebellar peduncle	53	Ipsilateral ataxia
54	Lesion at genu of internal capsule	54	Loss of contralateral corticobulbar input to CNs. Loss of contralateral lower face
55	Anoxia, most sensitive part of hippocampus	55	CA1—Somer's sector

(continued)

Table 24.2 (continued)

56	Wilson's Disease	56	Genetic, Hepatolenticular degeneration. Copper builds up in putamen and globus pallidus
57	Carbon monoxide poisoning	57	Globus Pallidus
58	Methanol poisoning	58	Putamen
59	Superior division of MCA occlusion	59	Broca's aphasia, contralateral UMNs to face and arm. Lower limb spared
60	Inferior division of MCA occlusion	60	Wernicke's aphasia. Possible contralateral homonymous hemianopia
61	Normal pressure hydrocephalus	61	Wet, wacky, wobbly
62	Facial colliculus	62	Facial nucleus and fibers of CN VI. Significant because CN VI and VII are so close
63	Which thalamic nucleus is in limbic circuit	63	Anterior
64	Thalamic pain syndrome, artery?	64	Contralateral pain, Thalamogeniculate A.
65	NMDA receptor	65	Ligand and voltage gated. Involved in LTP
66	Scottie dog's collar	66	Pars Interarticularis
67	Asking the patient to adduct the eye and then look inferior tests the	67	Superior oblique
68	Expected response of a comatose patient with an intact brain stem to cold water in the left ear?	68	Slow eye deviation toward the left ear. The fast-phase of nystagmus is absent
69	Lesion to the left MLF. What happens on attempted gaze to the left, and to the right?	69	Normal gaze to the left. On gaze to the right, inability to adduct the left eye, nystagmus in right eye–contralateral effort nystagmus
70	Expected response of a comatose patient with an intake cortex to warm water in right ear	70	No eye movements
71	Bilateral Bow Tie Atrophy	71	Optic chiasm
72	Orbitofrontal Lobe	72	Decision making
73	Phineas Gage	73	Railroad accident. First frontal lobotomy
74	Horner's with upper or lower brachial plexus injury?	74	Lower
75	Clockface picture	75	Parietal lobe on non-dominant side
76	CN IX Parasympathetics travel on?	76	Auriculotemporal nerve, a branch of V3
77	Area Postrema	77	Vomiting
78	Jet lag	78	Suprachiasmatic nucleus, melatonin receptors
79	Ventral tegmental area VTA	79	Motivation, reward, behavior. Behaviors associated with drug use. High concentration of dopamine receptors
80	Obsessive compulsive disorder	80	Cingulate gyrus
81	Locus Coeruleus	81	Principal site for norepinephrine, thought to be involved with ADHD
82	Dorsal raphe	82	Principal site for serotonin, thought to be involved in clinical depression
83	Periaqueductal gray	83	High concentration of opioid receptors. Involved in descending control of pain
84	Disc herniation between L4-L5. Root exiting at that level or level below? And what root?	84	Nerve exiting one level below. L5 root
85	Disc herniation between C5 and C6. Root exiting at that level or one level below? And which root	85	Root exiting at that level. C6 root
86	Disc herniation. Which ligament gives way?	86	Posterior longitudinal ligament. On lateral edge

(continued)

Table 24.2 (continued)

87	Right IV nerve palsy. Which way head tilt?	87	Left
88	Cavernous sinus. Which CNs travel though it? And symptoms of compression?	88	All nerves associated with eye movement: CN III, IV, VI. Plus, V1 and V2. So ophthalmoplegia and V1 and V2 territory. Not V3
89	Horner's syndrome found in medial or lateral brain stem injury?	89	Lateral
90	Trigeminal neuralgia, artery?	90	Superior cerebellar artery
91	Anterior choroidal artery	91	Contralateral hemiparesis, contralateral homonymous hemianopia
92	Watershed infarct in cerebral cortex	92	Between MCA and ACA. Effects upper-limb territory, spares lower limb and face territory "man in a barrel"
93	Guillain-Barre	93	Autoimmune, often follows respiratory or intestinal infection. Symptoms begin in lower limbs and ascend to upper limbs and face: Weakness, ataxia, paresthesia, eventual paralysis
94	LTP, what, where	94	Long term potentiation, hippocampus, learning and memory
95	Damage to medial temporal lobe following a CVA	95	CA1 of hippocampus
96	Coma due to loss of?	96	Reticular activating system (RAS)
97	Central cord syndrome	97	Motor deficits more than sensory. Upper limb. Lower limbs spared usually
98	Conus Medullaris Syndrome	98	Combination UMN + LMN signs to lower limb
99	Optic tract lesion	99	Contralateral homonymous hemianopia, contralateral RAPD, contralateral bow tie atrophy
100	Friedreich ataxia	100	Loss of DC and DRG. Ataxia. Usually die from cardiomyopathy. Inherited.

Neuroanatomy Word Association

100 Neuroanatomy Buzz Words to Know the First Day of Your Neurology Rotation

In the left-hand column below, you will find 100 words that should trigger a response. With a blank sheet of paper cover up the answers on the right and test yourself by seeing what the words on the left trigger. These are 100 high yield facts that you should be familiar with before a clinical rotation or an exam. Each buzzword is explained in the book

Part III

Embryology

Introduction

As a student, it is important to focus on the first 3 weeks of development since this is when the early germ layers and various supporting structures are formed. After the first 3 weeks, it is important to focus on each organ system with an emphasis on congenital defects. When a child is born with an anomaly, you want to be able to explain what happened during development. The first 2 weeks are the germinal period, and then from week 3 to week 8 is the embryonic period. To birth starting with week 4 the organs will start to develop. The nervous system with the formation of the neural tube is the first organ to develop. By the end of week 8 all the structures for each organ have been formed. Starting with week nine and continuing to birth is the fetal period.

Testes, Ovaries, and Gametogenesis

25

Germ Cell Formation

The haploid gametes are the result of the germ cells dividing by meiosis. The diploid zygote comes from the haploid gametes joining together. Early in development the primordial germ cells migrate to the genital ridges where they form the sex cords, which in turn go onto become either the seminiferous tubules or the follicles. The progression of the germ cells through meiosis is referred to as either spermatogenesis or oogenesis. In males, this progression continues without interruption, while in females the progression is arrested at various stages.

Meiosis

Meiosis involves one cell dividing twice to form four daughter cells, each with half a complement of chromosomes. *Ploidy* refers to the number of complete sets of chromosomes in a somatic cell (n). Human somatic cells are diploid (2n), meaning that we carry two copies of each chromosome. However, gametes are haploid (1n). In meiosis I, DNA replication results in two sets of chromosomes in the cell. During prophase 1, the two copies of a chromosome will unite, and it is here that bits of DNA can be exchanged between the chromosomes. In metaphase I, these chromosome pairs line up along the equator of the cell. In anaphase I, the chromosomes are then pulled apart to end up on opposite sides of the cell. Note that at this point the sister chromatids are together. The cell then pinches off and we are left with two cells that each have 23 chromosomes (23 pairs of chromatids).

In meiosis II, these two cells undergo a second division. At this point, there is no replication of DNA, instead the 23 chromosomes line up along the equator which is metaphase II. In anaphase II the chromatids now pull apart, the cell pinches in two as it divides, so we are left with four daughter cells, each with 23 chromosomes (1n) (Fig. 25.1).

J. Leo, *Gross Anatomy, Neuroanatomy, and Embryology for Medical Students*,
https://doi.org/10.1007/978-3-031-87151-1_25

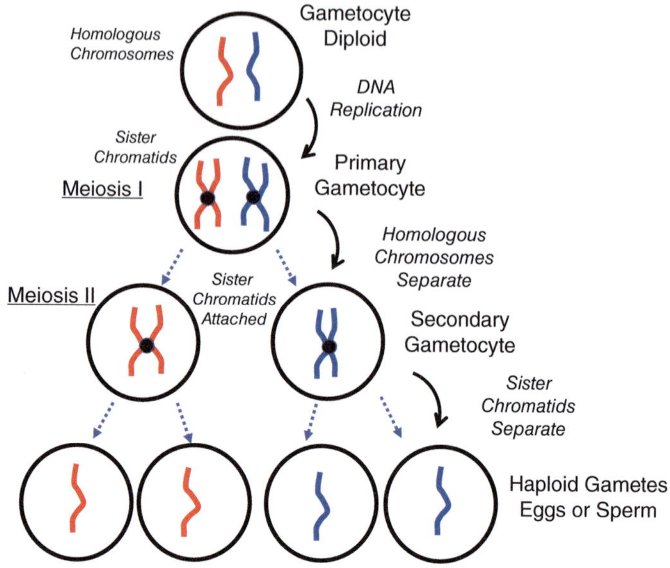

Fig. 25.1 Meiosis. In the first step, the homologous chromosomes replicate their DNA which produces the primary spermatocytes or oocytes which then enters meiosis I. These cells then divide, and the homologous chromosomes separate to produce secondary gametocytes. These then enter Meiosis II, and the sister chromatids separate to produce haploid gametes [5, 6]

Formation of Spermatozoa in the Testes

The *tunica albuginea* is a thick, tough, white-colored layer surrounding the testes. Extensions or septa of the tunica albuginea penetrate the testes dividing it into compartments which house the seminiferous tubules. The sperm develop within the seminiferous tubules.

When you look at a cross section under the microscope, the tubules are surrounded by interstitial tissue. The sperm start their development on the outer edge of the tubules and, as they mature they move towards the lumen. On the outer edge of the tubules are Type A spermatogonia which are the stem cells. These Type A spermatogonia divide by mitosis to give rise to spermatogonia B. It is the Type Bs that will eventually grow and develop into sperm, while the As stay on the edge to give rise to more Bs. As the Type B spermatogonia divide, they slowly progress towards the lumen where they will eventually form *spermatozoa* that separate from the mass of developing cells to enter the duct system (Fig. 25.2).

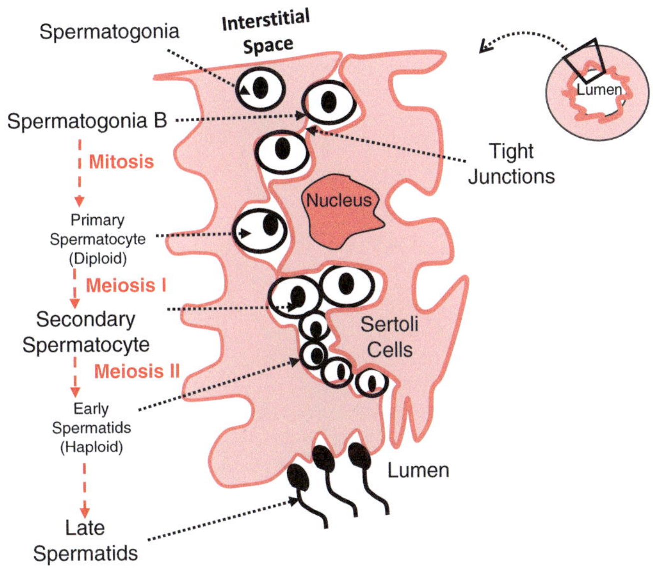

Fig. 25.2 Spermatogenesis. The proliferative stage involves spermatogonia A differentiating into spermatogonia B, which then divide by mitosis to produce primary spermatocytes. The meiotic phase involves primary spermatocytes entering meiosis I to produce secondary spermatocytes and then Meiosis II produce spermatids. Spermiogenesis involves the maturation of the spermatids. There is no cell division in spermiogenesis [5, 6]

Leydig and Sertoli Cells

Leydig cells are located within the interstitial tissue and surround the seminiferous tubules. Luteinizing hormone (LH) from the anterior pituitary stimulates the Leydig cells to produce testosterone. The Sertoli cells, also called nurse cells, surround and encircle the spermatogonia that are dividing and moving towards the lumen. The membranes of the neighboring Sertoli cells meet each other to form the blood-testis barrier which protects these dividing spermatogonia. Follicle stimulating hormone (FSH) released by the anterior pituitary stimulates the Sertoli cells to produce androgen binding protein (ABP).

Testosterone from the Leydig cells is released into the blood stream and has access to every organ in the body. The ABP from the Sertoli cells binds to the testosterone to maintain an even higher level of testosterone in the testes. In males, FSH levels are low up until puberty. At puberty, the levels increase. In an adult, elevated levels of FSH can result from chemotherapy, radiation, infection, or alcohol. Low levels of FH can be due to a disorder of the hypothalamus or pituitary. Leydig cell tumors, which are rare, will lead to precocious puberty and gynecomastia—an enlargement of the breast tissue (Fig. 25.3).

Spermatogenesis

As the developing sperm move from the edge of the tubules towards the lumen they go through a series of divisions and growth to transform from a diploid spermatogonia to haploid spermatozoon. One spermatogonia will give rise to four spermatozoa.

Spermatogonia Type B: As the spermatogonia B (immature gametes) mature and grow by mitotic division, they move towards the lumen of the seminiferous tubules. After about 16 days, a Type B spermatogonia will replicate its DNA and then enter meiosis I. Just prior to entering meiosis I, the cell is now a primary spermatocyte (2n, 4C) with twice the normal number of chromosomes.

Primary Spermatocytes: Primary spermatocytes are diploid cells entering meiosis I. The 46 homologous chromosomes have replicated so there are 46 × 2 chromosomes. At metaphase of meiosis I, the homologous chromosomes are paired together. As the cell divides, the homologous chromosomes separate to form secondary spermatocytes.

Secondary Spermatocytes: The secondary spermatocytes are haploid (n) cells with 23

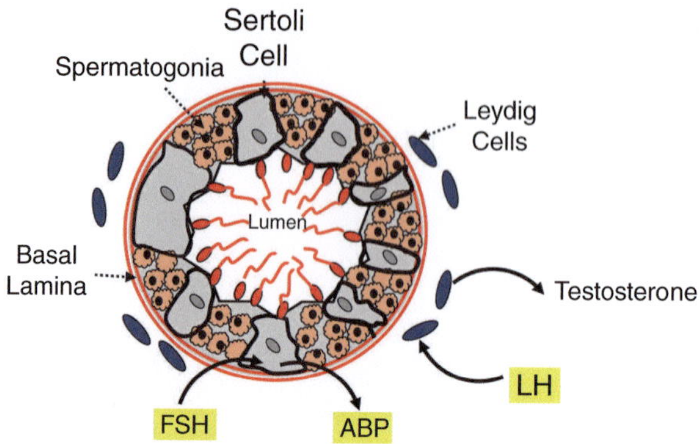

Fig. 25.3 Leydig cells and sertoli cells. The Sertoli cells are within the seminiferous tubules. Follicle stimulating hormone (FSH) stimulates them to produce Androgen Binding Protein (ABP). The Leydig sells live outside the seminiferous tubules in the interstitial tissue. Luteinizing hormone stimulates the Leydig cells to produce testosterone. Testosterone enters the blood stream to act on various organs. In the testes, ABP binds to testosterone to maintain high levels of testosterone within the testes [5, 6]

chromosomes (1n, 2C)—each secondary spermatocyte has just one homologous chromosome, but two copies of whichever one it is.

Spermatids: To go from secondary spermatocytes to spermatids (1n, 1C), the cells go through meiosis II and the sister chromatids (copies) separate. The spermatids are immature sperm that are about to break loose from the mass of cells and enter the lumen of the seminiferous tubules. Along their migratory path, the spermatids will mature into spermatozoa through a process referred to as spermiogenesis.

Spermiogenesis

During spermiogenesis the haploid spermatids transform from round spermatids, incapable of movement, into mature spermatozoa with a flagellum, so that they are now capable of movement. Several changes to the spermatids occur so that they become mature spermatozoa. Remember sperma*tids* are just *kids* and they still need to mature into spermatozoa. There are four stages of spermiogenesis:

1. In the *Golgi phase*, the Golgi complex starts the formation of the hydrolytic enzymes that will eventually be deposited into the acrosome, located at the head. The mitochondria congregate at the other end, where the distal centriole starts the formation of the tail—the flagella.
2. In the *cap phase*, the acrosome becomes more prominent and is referred to as the acrosomal cap.
3. Meanwhile, the *formation of a tail* continues as the tail becomes more prominent.
4. In the *maturation stage*, the remaining cytoplasm is destroyed by Sertoli cells.

At the end of this stage, the tails project into the lumen. The spermatozoa then break free and begin their journey towards the epididymis. During this initial part of their trip through the straight tubules, the rete testes, and efferent ductules, the spermatozoa are still immotile, and they are moved along by muscular contractions of the various ducts. In the tail of the epididymis the spermatozoa become motile.

At ejaculation, the mobile spermatozoa are almost ready to fertilize an egg, however there is one more step which takes place in the female reproductive tract. In *capacitation*, the protective coat over the acrosomal vesicle is removed so that the hydrolytic enzymes can penetrate the ova particularly the corona radiata and the zona pellucida. In addition, in the tail region, increased motility of the tail is achieved by an increase in intracellular Ca^{++}.

Female Gonads and Oogenesis

In the ovary the oogonia divide mitotically to produce primary oocytes, which progress through the stages of meiosis to produce a secondary oocyte arrested in metaphase II which is ovulated.

Primary Oocytes: Female germ cells divide mitotically to produce primary oocytes in the embryonic stage of development—when the child is still in the womb. At birth, the oocytes are arrested in prophase of meiosis I. At this point there are 46 chromosomes. The nucleus of a primary oocyte is referred to as a germinal vesicle. The primary oocyte is within a primordial follicle.

Secondary Oocytes: At the end of meiosis I, there is one polar body and one secondary oocyte. At ovulation, the secondary oocyte is arrested in meiosis II.

Mature Oocyte: If the cell is fertilized, meiosis II produces three polar bodies, and one mature ovum.

Folliculogenesis

The ovary is also surrounded by a tunica albuginea. In women of child-bearing age, within the ovary are follicles in various stages of development, either primordial, primary, secondary, tertiary (or graafian). Note that another way to look at the process is to divide follicle development by looking at the presence or absence of an antrum. Primordial, primary, and secondary follicles are sometimes referred to as preantral, while tertiary (or graafian) follicles are referred to as antral.

Within the developing follicle there are ovaries in various stages of development. The primordial follicles contain primary oocytes arrested in prophase I. As the follicle matures to a primary follicle, and then secondary follicle, it still contains a primary oocyte arrested in prophase I. In the graafian follicle just prior to ovulation the oocyte completes meiosis I, enters meiosis II and become arrested in metaphase II.

During folliculogenesis, follicle stimulating hormone (FSH) stimulates the development of the follicle. About halfway through the cycle, due to a negative feedback loop, FSH levels will drop. At this point, there will be a luteinizing hormone (LH) surge which leads to rupture of the follicle, also referred to as ovulation.

Primordial follicles. The primordial follicles develop in the fetus in the third trimester (in utero). At birth, the ovary contains approximately 400,000 primordial follicles. Each one is surrounded by a single, thin layer of squamous granulosa cells. These primordial follicles each contain a primary oocyte arrested in prophase of miosis I, and there is no zona pellucida surrounding the primary oocyte. The primordial follicles can remain in this stage for four decades or more (Fig. 25.4).

Primary follicles. Starting at puberty, and once a month from that point on, about 20 primordial follicles will start to develop and become primary follicles. Only one will fully mature. Primary follicles enlarge and become surrounded by cuboidal granulosa cells. FSH receptors will appear on the walls of the granulosa cells. At this point, the oocyte is surrounded by a zona pellucida. As the follicles progress through the next stages, the granulosa cells will increase in number and size. Note that the oocyte itself is not dividing at this point.

Secondary Follicle. In a secondary follicle, the granulosa cells thicken and a new layer called *the theca* appears and surrounds the granulosa cells. The theca and the granulosa cells both have receptors for FSH and LH. The oocyte at this point is a primary oocyte (4 N DNA) that has completed its first meiotic division.

Tertiary or Graafian Follicle. A graafian follicle is characterized by a significant increase in size. At the end of this stage the follicle will ovulate. In preparation for ovulation, it will migrate to the periphery of the ovary. The graafian follicle is characterized by a large fluid-filled antrum surrounded by a layer of granulosa cells and an outer layer of

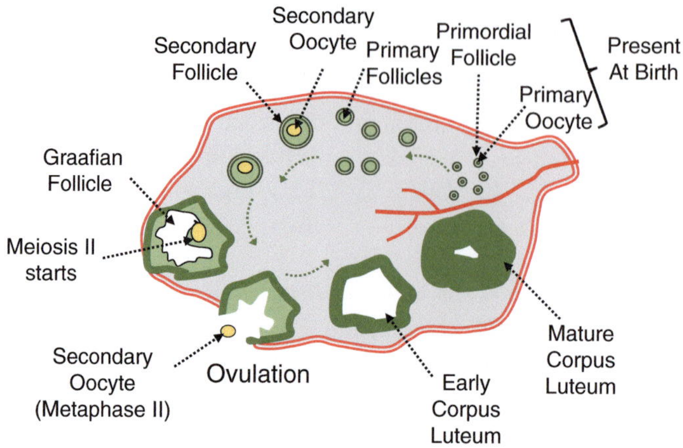

Fig. 25.4 Ovary and oogenesis. At birth there are 400,000 primary oocytes housed in primordial follicles. At this point, the primary oocytes are arrested in prophase of Meiosis I. Once a month, one will become a primary follicle. Primary oocytes will then enter meiosis and produce one oocyte and three polar bodies (not shown). At ovulation, it is a secondary oocyte arrested in metaphase II. If fertilization occurs, the graafian follicle will become a corpus luteum. With no fertilization it will become a corpus albicans [5, 6]

theca cells. The fluid in the antrum is referred to as follicular fluid. The oocyte itself is surrounded by the corona radiata and has a projection to the granulosa cells referred to as the cumulous oophorous (follicular cells). At the start of the graafian follicle stage, the oocyte starts the second meiotic division. At ovulation, the graafian follicle ejects a secondary oocyte arrested in metaphase of meiosis II (2 N DNA). At ovulation, the corona radiata is attached to the oocyte, and deep to the corona radiata is the zona pellucida. If the egg is not fertilized it will not finish its second meiotic division.

In females, high FSH levels may be a sign of *Primary Ovarian Insufficiency, Polycystic Ovary Syndrome*, an *ovarian tumor*, or *Turner Syndrome*. If FSH is low, it could be a sign of problems with the pituitary, hypothalamus, or being underweight. At puberty both FSH and LH levels increase.

The First 3 Weeks

When it comes to the first 3 weeks there is a simple rule to follow. At the end of week one, there is one germ layer, and one supporting membrane; at the end of week two, there are two germ layers and two supporting membranes; and at the end of week three, there are three germ layers and three supporting structures. Before looking at the specifics, consider the following statement from the view of the *tissue types*:

1. There are four types of tissue in the adult: Muscle, Connective, Nervous and Epithelial. Muscle tissue comes from mesoderm; Nervous tissue comes from ectoderm; Connective tissue comes from mesoderm, and Epithelia tissue comes from endoderm, mesoderm, and ectoderm.

And another statement from the view of the *three germ layers*:

Fig. 25.5 Overview of embryology [5, 6]

Big Picture

All three germ layers give rise to some epithelia:
Endo : Epithelium
Mesoderm : Connective, Muscle, Some Epithelia
Ectoderm : All Nervous Tissue, Some epithelia
Note that mesoderm lines some organs of cardiovascular, reproductive and urinary systems.

or look at it another way,

There are four kinds of tissue that come from :
1) Nervous : Ectoderm
2) Connective : Mesoderm (Neural crest in the head)
3) Muscle : Mesoderm
4) Epithelia : Endoderm, Ectoderm, Mesoderm

2. There are three germ layers: endoderm, ectoderm, and mesoderm. All three germ layers will give rise to epithelial tissue: Endoderm will give rise to epithelial; Ectoderm will give rise to nervous tissue and some epithelial; and Mesoderm will give rise to connective tissue, and some epithelial tissue. As one example, mesoderm gives rise to the epithelial tissue that lines some of the structures of the heart, kidney, and reproductive systems (Fig. 25.5).

Ovulation and Fertilization

Week one starts with fertilization and ends at implantation. Therefore, ovulation occurs right before week one. At ovulation, the ovary ejects a secondary oocyte arrested in *metaphase II*. At this point, the oocyte is surrounded by a thick barrier—the *zona pellucida*. And outside the zona pellucida are several layers of cells—*the corona radiata*. At ovulation, the secondary oocyte crosses the peritoneal cavity and is swept up by the fimbria to enter the fallopian tube. In some cases, the oocyte is fertilized while it is in the peritoneal cavity, which leads to an ectopic pregnancy.

After being swept up by the fimbria, as the oocyte travels along the fallopian tube it moves into the ampulla. If a spermatocyte is present, then it will attach to the oocyte, typically in the ampulla. For the sperm to attach to the oocyte it must travel through the corona radiata, and then reach the zona pellucida. On the head of the sperm the acrosome will release its hydrolytic enzymes and burrow through the zona pellucida. The membranes of the spermatocyte and oocyte fuse, and the oocyte then completes meiosis II. This is followed by the intermingling of the chromosomes from the male and female pronuclei to form the zygote. The mitochondria from the sperm does not enter the secondary oocyte, so an individual's mitochondria is derived from the maternal side. In addition, once the DNA from the sperm enters the oocyte, the cortical reaction occurs and there is an electrical depolarization of the egg's membrane which prevents any subsequent sperm from entering the oocyte. This is day one, the starting line (Fig. 25.6).

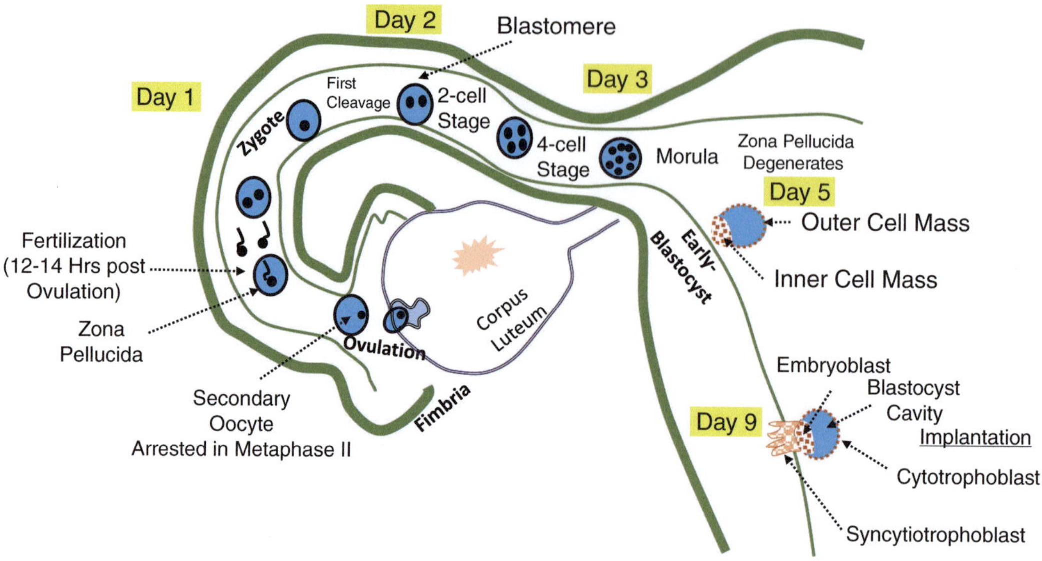

Fig. 25.6 First week. The secondary oocyte arrested in metaphase II is ovulated. Fertilization occurs in the ampulla of the uterine tube. The zygote is formed and starts dividing. Just prior to implantation, the zona pellucida degenerates. At this point, the inner cell mass and the outer cell mass have formed with the blastocyst cavity between them. Note that implantation occurs at Day 9 which is the start of the second week [5, 6]

Week One

The zygote will now start to divide. As the developing fetus divides into a 2-cell, then 4-cell, then 8-cell stage, etc. this is referred to as cleavage, and during these divisions the fetus does not get any larger. Instead, each cell gets smaller and smaller to fit into the same sized space. This makes sense from the host's point of view, because during cleavage the fetus is still in the fallopian tube on its trip to the uterus. If it kept growing with each division, it would soon be too large for the fallopian tube (Fig. 25.6).

While still in the fallopian tube, the zygote will now enter the 16-cell stage where it is referred to as a morula. By day three, the fetus is in the early morula stage, and by day 4 it is in the later morula stage—32 cell stage. The morula, at least to outward appearance, is an undifferentiated mass of cells. In Latin, morula means a bunch of grapes.

At day 5, as the morula approaches the uterus the cells will start to differentiate. A portion of the cells of the morula will migrate towards one end forming the inner cell mass. The remaining cells will form the outer cell mass, which will become the trophoblast. Between the inner cell mass and the outer cell mass is the blastocyst cavity (blastocoele). The morula has now become the blastula. At this point, the zona pellucida is degenerating and being sloughed off so that the blastula can implant in the uterine wall. The inner cell mass is a source of undifferentiated embryonic stem cells which is now referred to as the embryoblast. At day 7, the blastula is ready to implant into the uterine endometrium.

In summary, remember that at the end of week one, think of the number ONE. We have one germ layer– the embryoblast, one extraembryonic support structure- the trophoblast, and one cavity—the blastocyst. At this point, the trophoblast starts secreting human chorionic gonadotropin (B-HCG) which will instruct the corpus luteum to secrete progesterone. Think of HCG as the signal for the mother that she is pregnant. It is also the basis for several types of pregnancy tests as it is present in blood and urine.

Clinical Scenarios

Hydatidiform Mole

In normal conception, sperm, either a haploid 23X or 23Y, is injected into the oocyte to meet with a maternal 23X to form the full diploid complement of 46XX or 46XY. A molar pregnancy refers to a noncancerous tumor that develops in this early stage when the sperm and ovary first meet. Instead of the normal joining of the maternal and paternal DNA, the embryo only contains paternal DNA, at least in the case of a complete mole. Moles can be categorized as complete or incomplete moles. A complete mole consists of abnormal placental tissue and fluid filled cysts. An incomplete mole has a combination of normal and abnormal placental tissue along with fluid filled cysts. *Choriocarcinomas* can happen after any pregnancy but are more likely to occur with hydatidiform moles (Fig. 25.7).

There are several variations on the formation of a hydatidiform mole (Fig. 25.7):

1. *Monospermic Complete Mole.* The DNA from the male (23X) enters the oocyte and the 23X from the female is ejected from the oocyte. The 23X from the male then replicates to from 46 XX but all the DNA is from the male. There is no fetal tissue present.
2. *Dispermic Complete Mole.* Two sperm attach to the egg and inject their DNA– either a 23X a 23Y or a combination—into the oocyte. The maternal DNA is ejected resulting in a 46 XX or 46 XY which all come from the father. There is no fetal tissue present in this type of mole.
3. *Partial Mole.* Unlike the examples above, with a partial mole there will still be some maternal DNA. Two sperm inject their DNA -either a 23X or a 23 Y-which meets with the 23X from the mother resulting in a 69 XXX, 69 XXY, or 69 XYY. There will be some fetal tissue present.

Twins

Twins can be classified according to both *zygosity* and *chorionicity*. Zygosity refers to the type of conception.

Dizygotic twins (fraternal or non-identical twins) are formed by two different sperm and two different eggs (multiple ovulation). They account for approximately 70% of twins. In this scenario, there will be two amniotic cavities, and two chorionic cavities—dichorionic and diamniotic. The twins will develop independent of each other and have the same genetic relationship as developing siblings. They share on average 50% of genes (range between 34% and 61%) (Fig. 25.8).

Monozygotic (identical twins) come from the splitting of a zygote and share 100% of their genes. The later the zygote splits, the more embryonic structures they share (Fig. 25.9).

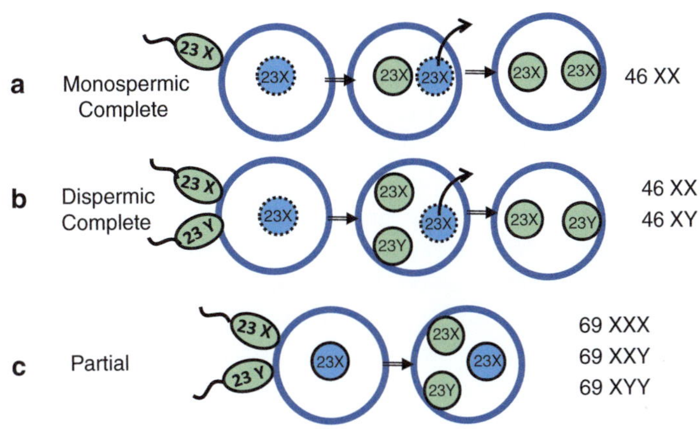

Fig. 25.7 Hydatidiform mole. Panels (**a, b**) are complete moles where the maternal DNA has been ejected from the egg and replaced with paternal DNA. Panel (**c**) is a partial mole where some maternal DNA remains [5, 6]

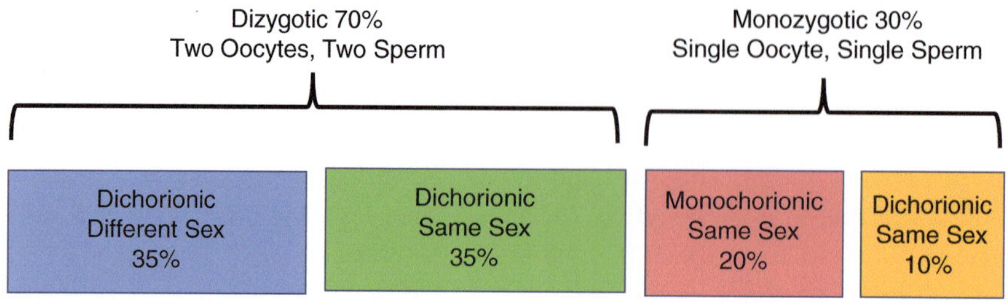

Fig. 25.8 Twin types and percentages. Seventy percent of all twins are dizygotic; 30% are monozygotic. All the dizygotic twins are dichorionic and diamniotic. Dizygotic twins have an equal chance of being male or female. Monozygotic twins will be the same sex, and 20% are monochorionic, while 10% are dichorionic [5, 6]

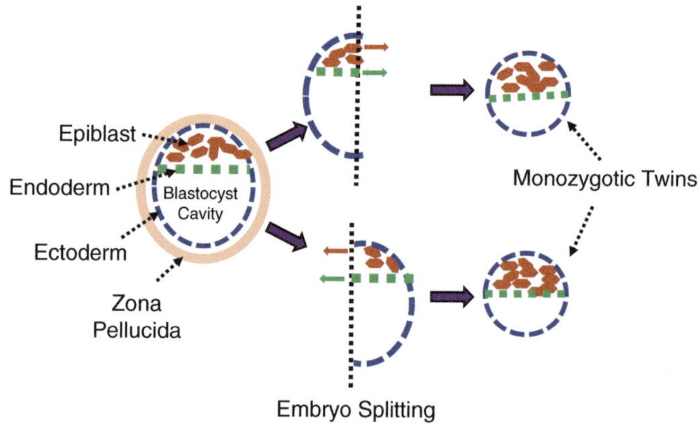

Fig. 25.9 Twinning at blastocyst stage. The blastocyst is seen splitting into two halves. Cells from each lineage then replace themselves to form two embryos—or monozygotic twins [5, 6]

Chorionicity refers to the type of placenta—is it a single, shared placenta or are there two placentas? The key to making sense of the different scenarios is to look at the normal timing of the development of the chorion and amnion. First, consider dizygotic twins, which because they arise from two eggs, two sperms, and two zygotes, will always have two chorions and two amnions—dichorionic/diamniotic. It is the monozygotic scenario that is more complicated to keep straight. We need to think through this step-by-step. The chorion normally develops at day 3 so if the split occurs before day 3, typically at the 2-cell stage, then two separate chorions and amnions will develop. If the split is after day 3 then there will only be one chorion. The amnion on the other hand does not develop until day 8 (just before the primitive streak develops) so if the split occurs before day 8 then two amnions will develop, and if it occurs after day 8 then one amnion develops. Twin formation (the splitting of zygote) after day 8 is rare but if it happens then there will be one chorion and one amnion. This monochorionic and monoamniotic scenario carries a high chance of complications such as twin-twin transfusion (Fig. 25.10).

On either ultrasounds or MRIs, the dichorionic-diamniotic scenario is indicated by the lambda sign (λ) or the twin peak sign. On an image, one can see placental tissue extending between the two chorions. It is widest at the base and then tapers towards where the two placentas oppose each other—the resemblance to lambda. The lambda sign disappears by the start of the second trimester.

The "T" sign, on the other hand, which is really the lack of the twin peaks sign, is indicative of the monochorionic-diamniotic scenario. This is because since there is only one chorion, there is no space for the placental tissue to migrate into (Fig. 25.11).

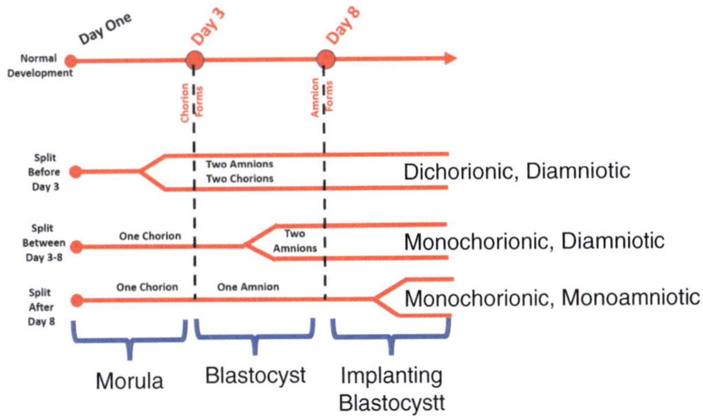

Fig. 25.10 Monozygotic twins and supporting structures. The chorion develops at Day 3, and the amnion develops at day 9. If the split occurs before day 3 there will be two chorions and two amnions. If it occurs between day 3 and 9, then there will be one chorion and two amnions. If it occurs after day 9 there will be one amnion and one chorion [5, 6]

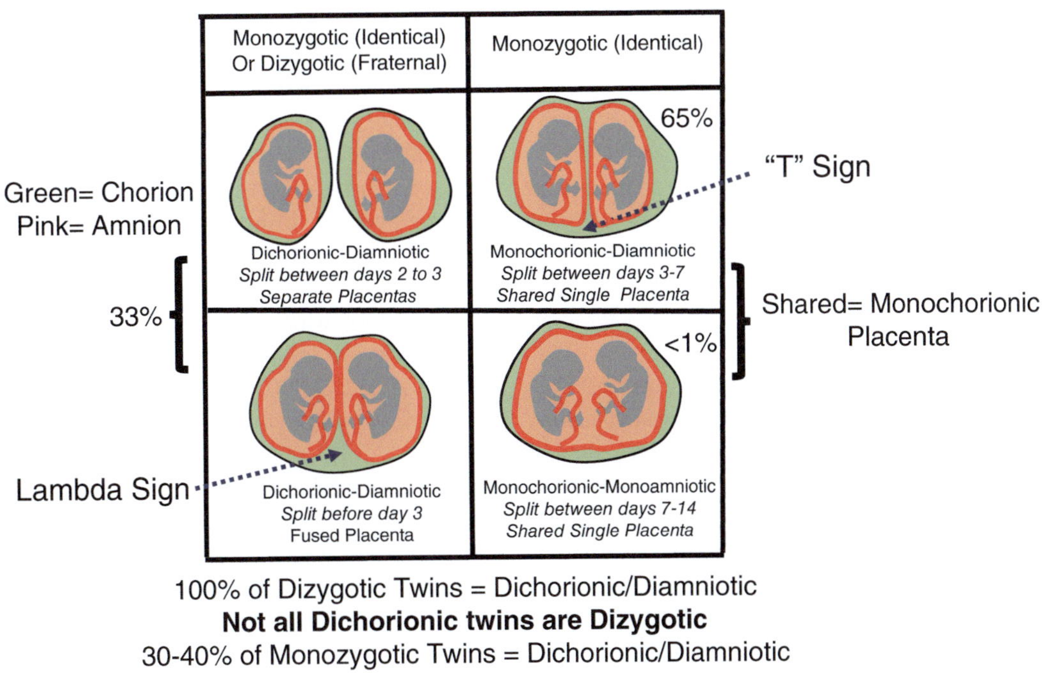

Fig. 25.11 Twins and their membranes. Monozygotic twins can be either monochorionic or dichorionic. Shared chorions pose the greatest risk for twins. The lambda sign is indicative of dichorionic-diamniotic, while the "T" sign is indicative of monochorionic—diamniotic [5, 6]

Stem Cells: Totipotent, Pluripotent, and Oligopotent

The critical issue with stem cells is the timing of when the cells are harvested—undifferentiated cells have the most potential to differentiate into other cells. For a researcher, when it comes to harvesting stem cells, the earlier the better, because as time goes on the cells become more differentiated. At the zygote stage there is no differentiation. At the morula, there is some differentiation, and by the time the fetus reaches week three, with three germ layers, there is even more differentiation. The term *totipotent* refers to an undifferentiated cell that technically has the potential to give rise to all the future cells of an embryo along with the extraembryonic supporting structures. A zygote is considered a totipotent cell. A *pluripotent* cell has the potential to give rise to all the future cells of the embryo but not to the extraembryonic supporting structures. The inner cell mass of a morula is considered a pluripotent cell. As development proceeds, and the cells become more differentiated, the stem cells are considered *oligopotent.* For instance, a lymphoid cell can give rise to T-cells and B-cells but not to red blood cells.

Week Two and Differentiation of Trophoblast and Embryoblast

In short, during the second week of development the embryoblast will give rise to two germ layers: the *epiblast* and *hypoblast*; the trophoblast will give rise to two layers: the *cytotrophoblast* and *syncytiotrophoblast*; and two supporting structures, the *amnion* and *chorion* will have formed. Think of "The Rule of Twos."

As the blastula attaches to the uterine wall, the inner cell mass is facing the uterine wall and will burrow into the endometrial layer of the uterus. Implantation typically occurs on the posterior superior portion of the uterus. *Placenta previa* is when the placenta covers the cervix. Vaginal bleeding during the second or third trimester is one sign of placenta previa.

The trophoblast now differentiates into the *cytotrophoblast* and *syncytiotrophoblast.* Both these structures plus the extraembryonic somatic mesoderm will become part of the chorion. The chorion is the fetal contribution to the placenta:

1. The *cytotrophoblast* is the site of mitotic activity.
2. The *syncytiotrophoblast* is the structure that burrows into the uterine wall. It also produces HCG which doubles every 24 h during early pregnancy. Alterations in HCG levels serve as an indicator of pathology. Elevated levels of HCG are associated with a hydatidiform mole, and low levels are associated with an ectopic pregnancy. The syncytiotrophoblast will meet the maternal blood system.

The decidua is the maternal contribution to the placenta which comes from the uterine endometrium which is referred to as the *functionalis layer.*

Epiblast and Hypoblast

The inner cell mass will now form the bilaminar disk composed of the epiblast and hypoblast. The epiblast is a cuboidal layer of cells that will eventually give rise to all three germ layers. At this point, the epiblast will also give rise to cells that move laterally and surround the future amniotic cavity sitting just above the epiblast. Below the epiblast is the hypoblast layer, composed of tall columnar cells surrounding the developing yolk sac.

The epiblast also gives rise to the extraembryonic mesoderm which in the initial stages surround the developing embryo. By the end of the second week, this extraembryonic mesoderm will split into two layers:

1. The *extraembryonic* <u>*somatic*</u> *mesoderm* surrounds the cytotrophoblast.
2. The *extraembryonic* <u>*visceral*</u> *mesoderm* surrounds the yolk sac and developing embryo. Note that the extraembryonic coelom now lies between the extraembryonic somatic and visceral mesoderm. The visceral layer of mesoderm is also the site of early hematopoiesis.

The connecting stalk is where the visceral and somatic layers meet. At this point in time the placenta is more prominent. Note that the placenta is a joint production of the mother and the fetus (Fig. 25.5).

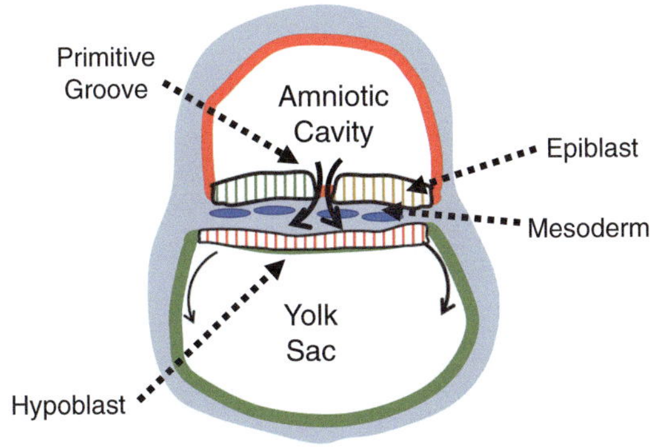

Fig. 25.12 Gastrulation. The epiblast cells migrate towards the midline located primitive groove. When they reach the midline, they drop down to the hypoblast where they push the hypoblast cells off to the sides. This becomes endoderm. Some cells from the epiblast land in the middle layer and become mesoderm. The cells that stay in the epiblast become ectoderm [5, 6]

Week Three and Gastrulation

In week three, the two germ layers will differentiate into three germ layers via gastrulation. This process starts with the development of the primitive streak in the midline. The epiblast cells will give rise to all three germ layers (Fig. 25.12).

1. *Endoderm.* The epiblast cells migrate towards the primitive streak. At the primitive streak, they will then migrate down towards the hypoblast cells and displacing them by pushing them to the sides. The original hypoblast cells are now pushed aside by the epiblast cells which have now become the endoderm.
2. *Mesoderm.* In some cases, the epiblast cells that migrate towards the primitive streak also come to land between the epiblast and hypoblast to become the mesoderm. This is a mesenchymal layer, meaning that in contrast to the cells lined up in rows like the endoderm, these mesoderm cells are secreting substances that will surround each cell and separate each one from their neighbors.
3. *Ectoderm.* Not all the epiblast cells will migrate down at the primitive streak. Those that stay will become the ectoderm (Figs. 25.11 and 25.12).

Body Folding

In addition to longitudinal folding, there is also a lateral folding of the embryo. There are several goals of the folding (Fig. 25.13):

1. To transform from a small dorsally located amnion sac to a much larger cavity surrounding the entire embryo. As the somatopleure migrates laterally, it is also migrating ventrally such that the two pieces will meet and fuse in the midline.
2. To transform from a yolk sac to the gut tube. As the mesoderm migrates laterally, the two pieces meet in the midline and form the midgut, made up of endoderm, which in turn is surrounded by the mesoderm. The midgut is now connected via the *vitelline duct* during development to the yolk sac which is now outside the embryo. Within the embryo, the midgut is now connected to the ventral and dorsal walls by the ventral and dorsal mesenteries.
3. To surround the embryo with ectoderm, which will eventually give rise to the skin. The interior of the amniotic cavity at week 3 is surrounded by ectoderm. As the mesoderm migrates laterally it drags with it the edges of the amnion to eventually meet and close in the midline leaving the ectoderm to surround the embryo.

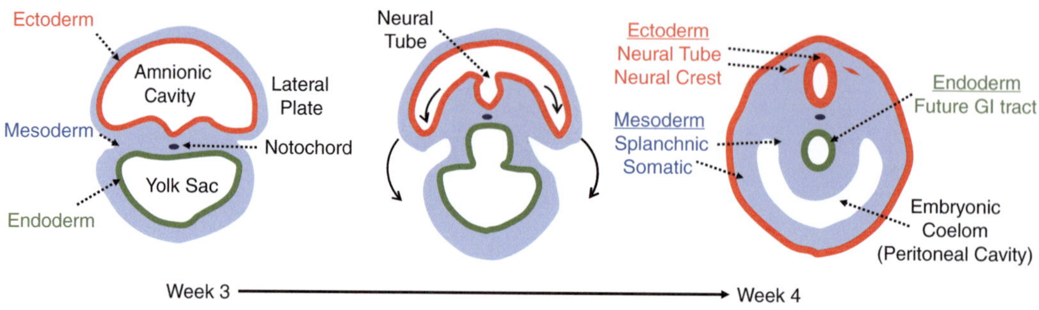

Fig. 25.13 Body folding. Starting at week three, the amniotic cavity and mesoderm start curling around to pinch off the yolk sac. At the same time, the neural tube is forming. At the end of week four, you can see three tubes: the yolk sac, the neural tube, and the coelom. Red = ectoderm, Blue = mesoderm, and Green = endoderm [5, 6]

Historical Snippet: Heteropaternal Superfecundation

Heteropaternal superfecundation is the rare scenario where a woman gives birth to twins, but the twins are from two different fathers. Two events must occur for this to happen. First, the woman must ovulate at least two eggs in a single cycle, and second, the woman must have sexual intercourse with two different men during this time. This creates the scenario where two eggs are fertilized at the same time by the sperm from two different fathers and the woman gives birth to twins with different paternal DNA. Besides this scenario, it can also occur as an accident with *in vitro* fertility equipment, where the sperm from two fathers is mixed. On average, these types of twins will share 25% of their DNA. Also, as an aside, this is common in dogs or cats, where half a litter can come from one male and the other half of the litter from another male. Again, in humans this is extremely rare—almost nonexistent- and I have only mentioned it because it aids in understanding the nature of the process of how twins are formed.

Further Reading

1. Calvo-Garcia MA. Guidelines for scanning twins and triplets with US and MRI. Ped Radiol. 2016;46(2):155–66.
2. Carlson B. Human embryology and developmental biology. 6th ed. New York: Elsevier; 2018.
3. Condic ML. Totipotency: what it is and what it is not. Stem Cells Dev. 2014;23(8):796–812.
4. Graham A, Richards J. Development and evolutionary origins of the pharyngeal apparatus. Evol Dev. 2012;3(24)
5. Leo J. Medical neuroanatomy for the boards and clinic: finding the lesion. 2nd ed. Cham: Springer; 2024a.
6. Leo J. Clinical anatomy and embryology: a guide for the classroom, clinic, and clinic. 2nd ed. Cham: Springer; 2024b.
7. Moore KL, Persaud TVN. The developing human: clinically oriented embryology. 11th ed. New York: Saunders; 2019.
8. Sadler TW. Langman's medical embryology. 14th ed. New York: Lippincott Williams and Wilkins; 2018.
9. Sweeney L. Basic concepts in embryology: a student's survival guide. New York: McGraw-Hill; 1997.

26 Development of Major Organs

Neurulation: Plate, to Groove, to Tube

The nervous system starts to develop in the third week of development with the formation of the notochord within the mesoderm. The ectoderm above the notochord will condense into the *neural plate*—at this point, just a flat piece of tissue. The edges of the neural plates then rise to form the *neural groove*. The edges of the groove then start to come together forming the *neural tube*. The neural tube will drop down into the embryo to become surrounded by mesoderm. The ventral surface of the neural plate also gives rise to neural crest cells which migrate down towards the notochord. The *neural crest* cells give rise to numerous cell types, one of which is the dorsal root ganglia cells lying alongside the neural tube. As the neural tube is closing, the ends, referred to as *neuropores*, are the last structures to close—think of two zippers starting in the midline and moving towards the ends to close the tube. The rostral neuropore closes at day 25, and the caudal neuropore closes at day 27 (Fig. 26.1).

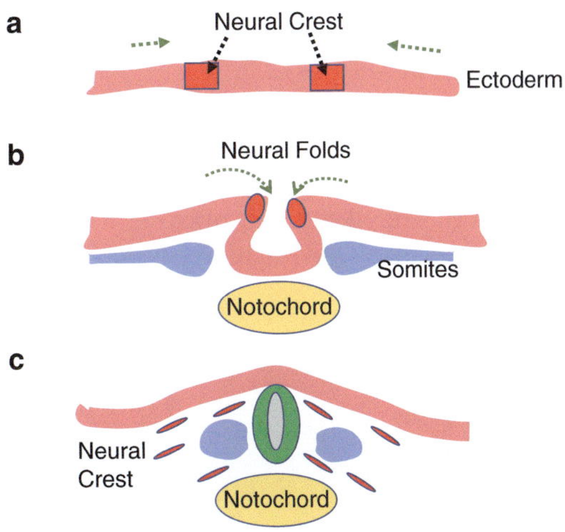

Fig. 26.1 Neurulation. (**a**) Ectoderm cells migrating towards the midline. (**b**) Neural folds forming. (**c**) Neural Tube has formed. Neural crest cells dropping down into mesoderm to form ganglia and other cells [5, 6]

J. Leo, *Gross Anatomy, Neuroanatomy, and Embryology for Medical Students*,
https://doi.org/10.1007/978-3-031-87151-1_26

Neural Tube Defects

Failure of the neuropores or the neural tube to close leads to congenital defects. The defects below are listed in order of least severe to most severe (Fig. 26.2).

1. *Spina bifida occulta* is a failure of the vertebrae around the spinal cord to develop. It can go undetected for years as it is often asymptomatic. Other than a tuft of hair over the defect there may be no obvious symptoms. Because the meninges are intact, there is no alteration in alpha fetoprotein (AFP) levels. The word "occulta" means hidden.
2. *Spina bifida with meningocele* is a failure of the vertebrae and the meninges to develop in the region of the defect. The meninges typically protrude through the defect. There is an increase in AFP.
3. *Spina bifida with meningomyelocele* is a failure of the vertebrae, meninges, and spinal cord to develop. The spinal cord can protrude through the defect. It often occurs with Arnold-Chiari type 2 malformation.
4. *Spina bifida with myeloschisis* is the most severe of the spina bifidas and leads to the spinal cord being present on the back. There will be an increase in AFP.
5. *Anencephaly* is a failure of the anterior neuropore to close resulting in failure of the cerebral hemispheres to develop. There will be an increase of AFP.

In the section above, it is clear that AFP is increased in some of the conditions but not all. AFP is normally present around the fetal spinal cord. Only tiny amounts of AFP will be found in the amniotic cavity of a healthy embryo. With open neural tube defects, the AFP leaks out of the defect and into the amniotic cavity. This is why in spina bifida occulta, there is no increase in AFP, but in the other neural tube defects there is an increase in AFP.

The term *spina bifida cystica* encompasses the neural tube defects with a cyst on the back. Spina bifida with either a meningocele, a meningomyelocele, or a myeloschisis are considered types of spinae bifida cystica.

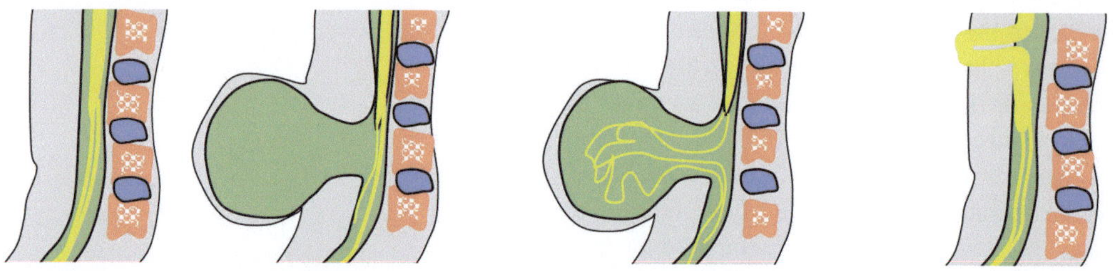

Fig. 26.2 Neural tube defects [5, 6]

Pituitary Development

The pituitary gland develops from two different regions of ectoderm. The posterior pituitary arises from an outpocketing of neural tube forming the third ventricle. The anterior pituitary comes from Rathke's pouch which is an outpocketing of ectoderm from the roof of the mouth. Rathke's pouch normally closes. In some cases, it fails to close and leaves a craniopharyngeal canal which is a small connection between the sphenoid bone and the sella turcica. The adult pituitary comes to lie inferior to the optic chiasm. Pituitary adenomas and craniopharyngiomas both aggravate the optic chiasm.

Early Heart Development

The heart starts pumping blood at day 21 or 22. Just before that, around day 18, mesoderm in the cardiogenic area, a horseshoe-shaped structure near the head starts to develop into the future heart. It starts with two strands known as the cardiogenic cords. These cords of mesoderm then differentiate into an outer wall which is the vessel wall, and an inner layer of blood cells. At this point they are referred to as endocardial tubes. Eventually the two endocardial tubes fuse to make a single tube. The pericardial cavity meanwhile is developing around the heart tube. The tube is connected to the pericardial cavity via the dorsal mesocardium.

Heart Development

The heart starts as a simple tube, but then goes through a series of foldings to become the adult heart. To make sense of the folds, it is best to follow the flow of blood through the early tube. The blood first comes into the tube at the sinus venosus. From here it goes to the primitive atrium, then the primitive ventricle, then the bulbus cordis, and finally the truncus arteriosus. The simple tube then starts rotating to the right and ventrally. At the end of its rotation the ventricles lie mostly ventral and caudal to the atria. The outflow tracts end up in the midline (Figs. 26.3 and 26.4).

Errors in the normal looping process can lead to *situs inversus* (organs are mirror image of normal), *dextrocardia* (heart is pointed to the right side instead of left), and *ventricular inversion* (normal position of ventricle is switched).

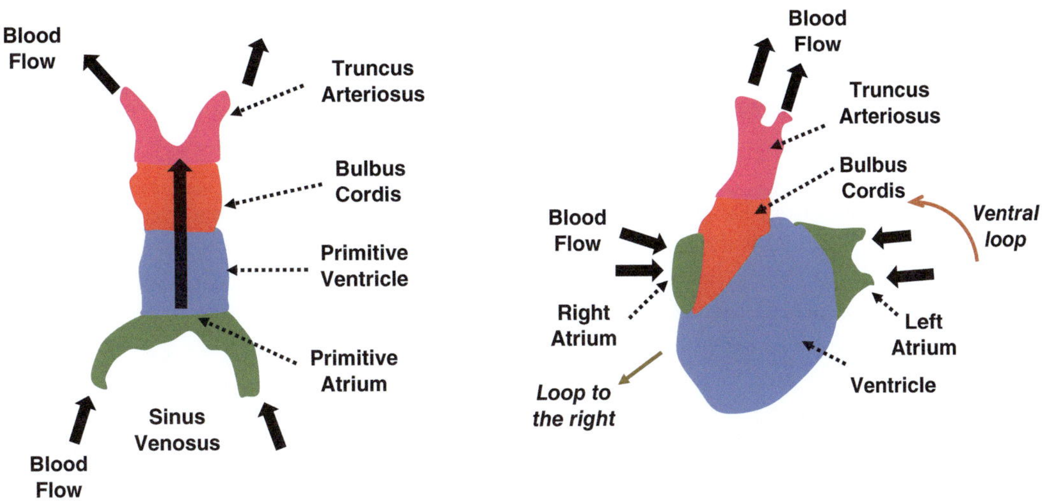

Fig. 26.3 Heart development. The early heart is a tube. Blood enters at the sinus venosus, then moves through the primitive atrium, primitive ventricle, bulbus cordis, and truncus arteriosus. The tube rotates to the right and ventrally. In the adult, for the most part, the ventricles become mostly ventral and caudal to the atria, with the outflow tracts ending in the midline [5, 6]

Blood FLow (↑)

Embryonic Structure	Adult Structure	
Truncus Arteriosus	Aorta and Pulmonary Trunk	
Bulbous Cordis	Conus Arteriosus and Aortic Vestibule	*Smooth Part of Rt Lt Ventricle*
Primitive Ventricle	Muscular Part Rt and Lt Ventricle	Muscular Part of Rt and Lt Ventricle
Primitive Atrium	Pectinate Muscle of Rt and Lt Atria	
Sinus Venosus	Smooth part Right Atrium, Coronary sinus	*Smooth Part of Rt Lt Atrium*

Fig. 26.4 Embryonic heart structures. Note that the primitive ventricle and the primitive atrium give rise to the muscular parts of the atria and ventricles. Blood enters at the sinus venosus which becomes the smooth part of the atrium, and the coronary sinus. Blood exits at the bulbous cordis which becomes the smooth part of the right and left ventricles [5, 6]

Fetal Circulation

Blood from the placenta enters the fetus via the umbilical veins. There are three bypasses in fetal circulation:

1. The first bypass is at the *ductus venosus*. Since the blood does not need to go through the fetal liver, blood bypasses the liver and goes into the inferior vena cava. In the adulthood, the ductus venosus becomes the *ligament venosum*.
2. As the blood continues in the inferior vena cava past the liver it enters the right atrium and moves superiorly towards the *foramen ovale* to bypass the lungs. The foramen ovale is an opening between the right and left atria. In the adult, the foramen ovale becomes the *fossa ovalis*.
3. Since some blood from the right atrium gets into the right ventricle it moves through the *ductus arteriosus* which is a connection between the pulmonary trunk and the aorta. In the adult, the ductus venosus becomes the *ligamentum arteriosum*.

The blood coming from the placenta is high in O_2 (80%), but it meets with the fetal blood coming from the inferior vena cava (IVC). Past the liver, the O_2 concentration is now at 65% which is right before the IVC enters the right atrium, Meanwhile the blood from the superior vena cava (SVC) is descending from the head to also enter the right atrium. Note that the O_2 concentration is lower in the SVC than the IVC as the two channels enter the right atrium. And in the right atrium, we have a crossing of the two channels. The blood from the IVC heads towards the foramen ovale, while the blood from the SVC is channeled towards the tricuspid valve to go into the right ventricle. The blood now coming into the right atrium has two channels to exit:

1. The blood coming from the IVC enters the inferior portion of the right atrium and then travels through the foramen ovale, bypassing the right ventricle, to enter the left atrium. It then goes to the left ventricle and from there to exit the heart on the aorta.
2. The blood coming down from the SVC goes into the right atrium through the tricuspid valve, and then into the right ventricle. From there it heads out the pulmonary trunk. At this point, since the blood does not need to go into the lungs it bypasses the lungs by going through the ductus venosus to enter the aorta.

Also note that the O_2 concentration in the proximal aortic arch is different than the distal portion. Coming out of the heart, the blood in the first part of the aorta is high in O_2 at about 65%. The advantage of this is that the brain via the common carotid arteries gets blood with a high concentration of O_2 to feed the brain's high metabolic rate. Note that the ductus venosus joins the aortic arch just distal to the first three branches of the aorta,

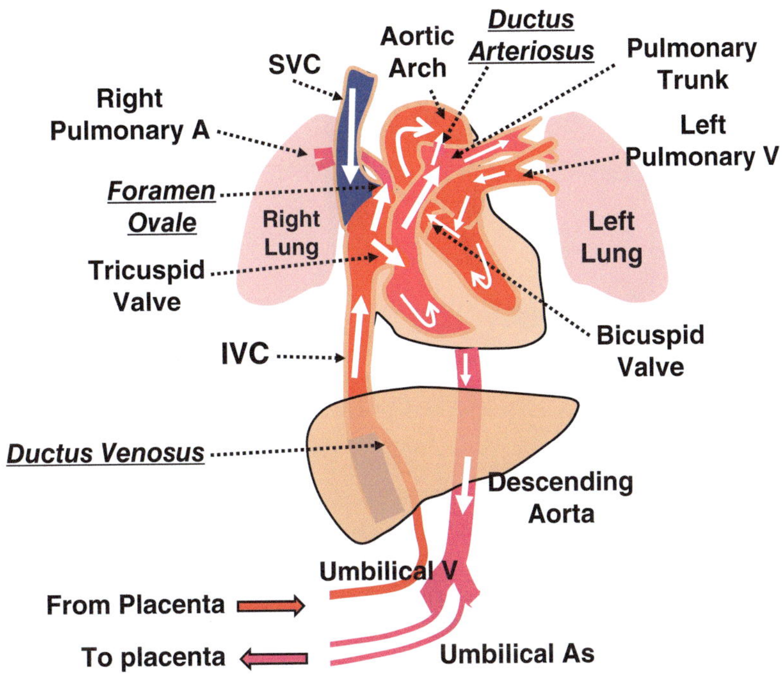

Fig. 26.5 Fetal circulation. The three bypasses are underlined and italicized. Blood from the placenta bypasses the liver via ductus venosus. It then joins the inferior vena cava and enters the right atrium. From here it crosses foramen ovale to enter the left atrium and travels to the left ventricle. From the left ventricle it passes via the aortic arch to the descending aorta. However, some of the blood entering the right atrium will pass to the right ventricle and go out the ductus arteriosum to bypass the lungs [5, 6]

which dilutes the O_2 concentration in the blood traveling down the descending aorta to approximately 60% (Fig. 26.5).

Development of the Atrial Septum

The primitive atrium is open between the right and left sides. During week 3, the septum primum starts as an outgrowth of the superior portion of the atrium. It is a which came from the neural crest cells. The endocardial cushions will go from a round mass to form the cross shaped valves in the center of the heart. As the septum primum descends towards the endocardial cushions there is still an opening between the right and left atria which is the foramen primum. The developing heart needs this communication between the two atria.

Eventually the septum primum will reach the endocardial cushions to seal off the communication between the two sides. Fortunately, just as the septum primum reaches the endocardial cushions, along the superior portion of the septum primum, small openings start to appear which soon come together to form one larger opening—the foramen secundum. Without the foramen secundum forming there would be no communication between right and left atria. Note that both the foramen primum and foramen secundum are openings in the septum primum. The presence of foramen secundum allows the right and left atria to still communicate. At this point, the septum secundum now forms. It is another wall (the second wall) that is in the right atrium, and it now moves inferiorly, parallel to the septum primum, to close off the foramen secundum.

During development, this opening is a one-way flap that allows blood to be shunted from the right atrium across to the left atrium. At birth as pressure rises on the left side, the flap closes. The *fossa ovalis* is where the septum primum and septum secundum meet. In the adult, if you are in the right atrium, you will see the fossa ovalis which is a thin sheet resembling a door, and on the superior surface of this door is a ridge—the limbus of the fossa ovalis. Conversely, if you are in the left atrium, you are looking at the valve of the foramen ovale which is the remanent of the septum primum (Fig. 26.6).

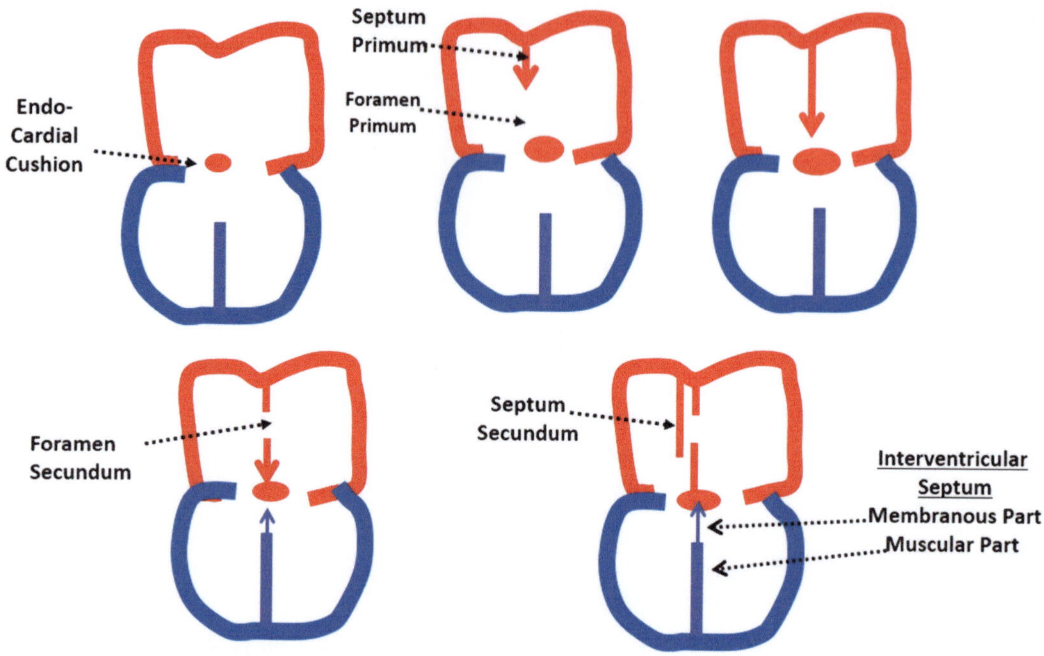

Fig. 26.6 Septal development. The septum primum grows towards the endocardial cushions. The opening between the two atria is now the foramen primum. As the septum primum and endocardial cushions fuse, the foramen secundum then opens in the septum primum. The septum secundum then grows down to cover the foramen secundum [5, 6]

Development of the Ventricular Septum

At the same time the atrial septum is forming, the ventricular septum is forming. There is a larger muscular portion which ascends from the apex to divide the ventricle into right and left sides. In addition, descending from the endocardial cushions is the membranous portion of the interventricular septum. The muscular portion and the membranous portions fuse to form the wall between the right and left ventricles.

Left-to-Right Shunts

The most common heart defect is a membranous interventricular septal defect, which leads to a left-to-right shunt. There are several types of atrial septal defects. Because the interatrial septum starts superiorly and moves inferiorly towards the endocardial cushions there are several opportunities for defects along the wall, either superiorly or inferiorly. Primum defects are down low by the endocardial cushions, while the secundum defects are higher on the wall:

1. If the septum primum fails to meet up and fuse with the endocardial cushions, there is an *ostium primum defect*. These occur in the inferior portion of the wall.
2. If there is excessive resorption of the septum primum, or a failure of the septum secundum then this is an *ostium secundum defect*. These occur on the superior portion of the wall.
3. A *patent foramen ovale* is a failure of the foramen ovale to close which allows blood to be shunted from left to right.

Septal defects will result in left-to-right shunts because the pressure is higher on the left side of the heart. Over time, this increased pressure will lead to pulmonary hypertension. As the pressure on the right side rises, eventually the shunt will reverse and turn into a right-to-left shunt. This is referred to *Eisenmenger's complex*.

A *patent ductus arteriosus* (PDA) occurs when the ductus arteriosus does not close at birth. When this happens blood will be shunted from the aorta to the pulmonary trunk because of the higher pressures in the aorta. Maternal rubella infections are a predisposing factor to the development of a PDA. PDA is also more common in babies born at high altitudes (above 8000 feet). Patients will have a machine-like diastolic murmur heard at the left upper chest.

Right-to-Left Shunts

There are several right-to-left shunts. Because the blood is shunted away from the liver, these patients will be cyanotic.

Tetralogy of Fallot results from an abnormal migration of neural crest cells which leads to failure of the truncus and conus to separate which results in an anterior placed aorticopulmonary septum leading to the following defects (think IHOP).

1. **I**nterventricular septal defect
2. **H**ypertrophied right ventricle
3. **O**verriding Aorta
4. **P**ulmonary Hypertension

The patient will have a boot shaped heart. At birth, these babies will often have a bluish tint to their skin. They will also have rounded nail beds (clubbing of the fingers). As they reach 2–4 months of age, they will often have TET spells, which typically occur after eating. They will turn blue, become agitated, and cry. They will often assume a squatting position to increase the blood flow to the lungs. Surgery can repair the defect.

Persistent truncus arteriosus occurs when the truncus arteriosus fails to separate into the aorta and pulmonary trunks which allows oxygenated and deoxygenated blood to mix which leads to cyanosis.

Transposition of the great vessels occurs when the aorta and pulmonary trunk come from the wrong sides. The blood going out the aorta will then not be carrying oxygen to the body. Surgery must be performed immediately. It is often associated with maternal diabetes, rubella, and viral illnesses.

Coarctation of the Aorta

The closing of the ductus arteriosus involves a complicated signaling pathway. In some cases, a small portion of the aortic arch can get caught up in this process and become constricted. It can happen either just proximal or just distal to the ductus arteriosum and can lead to increased blood pressure in the head and upper limb regions, but conversely a reduced pulse in the lower limbs (Fig. 26.7).

1. With a *preductal coarctation*, which is seen in infants, the ductus remains open which means blood can still reach the lower body, but this blood will have lower than normal O_2 levels.
2. With a *postductal coarctation*, which is seen in adults, because of the various anastomoses, the blood will travel down the internal thoracic arteries, to the anterior intercostal arteries, to the posterior intercostal arteries and then into the descending aorta. With time the intercostal arteries will become large and burrow into the inferior borders of the ribs which can be seen as *rib notching* on images.

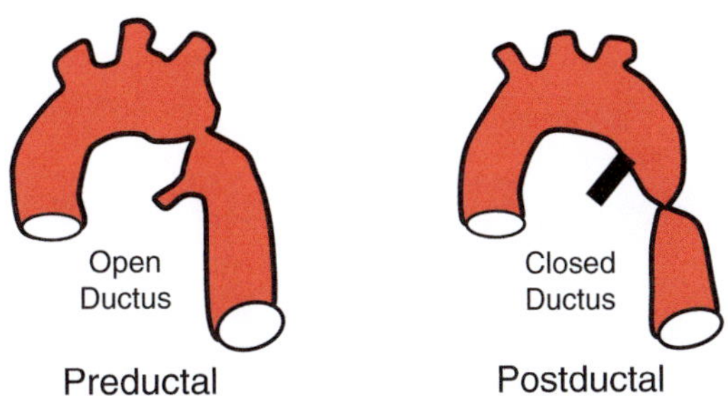

Fig. 26.7 Coarctation of the aorta. With the preductal version the constriction is proximal to the ductus arteriosus which remains patent. In a post ductal version the ductus closes [5, 6]

Development of the GI Tract and Associated Organs

The GI tract starts as a tube of endoderm which can be divided into foregut, midgut, and hindgut endoderm. The tube becomes suspended by dorsal and ventral mesentery which is attached to the ventral and dorsal walls. During week four, the stomach becomes dilated due to differential growth rates of various regions. In addition, this differential growth leads to the tract rotating. The dorsal side rotates to the left and the ventral side rotates to the right. By week 5 the midgut has also elongated to the point where it must leave the abdominal cavity and move into the yolk stalk. At the point where the midgut makes a U-turn and comes back into the abdominal cavity the vitelline duct which opens into the yolk sac is present.

Within the ventral mesentery, the liver starts to form as a liver diverticulum. The ligament between the anterior body wall and the liver is the falciform ligament. The ligament between the liver, the stomach, and the duodenum is the lesser omentum (hepatogastric and hepatoduodenal ligaments). These ligaments are discussed in detail in Chap. 3 (Fig. 26.8).

Within the dorsal mesentery, the spleen and kidney start to develop. The splenorenal ligament connects the spleen and the kidney, while the gastrosplenic ligament connects the stomach and spleen. Here is a way to think about these ligaments and determine if a certain ligament in the adult is a remnant of either the dorsal or ventral mesentery. If you look at an adult ligament, ask yourself if it is attached to the liver. If it is attached to the liver in the adult, that means it came from the ventral mesentery. For instance, the falciform ligament is attached to the liver, so it came from ventral mesentery. But the splenorenal ligament is not attached to the liver in the adult so it came from dorsal mesentery.

Development of the Pancreas and Liver

At the start of week 5, the ventral and dorsal pancreatic buds (endoderm) appear on the right and left sides of the foregut just distal to the stomach. The ventral bud gives rise to the uncinate process of the pancreas. The dorsal bud gives rise to the head, the neck, body, and tail of the pancreas. As the gut rotates, the ventral bud rotates posteriorly, while the dorsal bud rotates anteriorly. If the pancreas does not rotate correctly, it can form a loop around the intestine. This *annular pancreas* can block the GI tract (Fig. 26.9).

As the pancreas is developing, the small intestine is also changing. At the start of week 4 the duodenum has a patent lumen. The duodenum grows so quickly that at the start of week 6 its

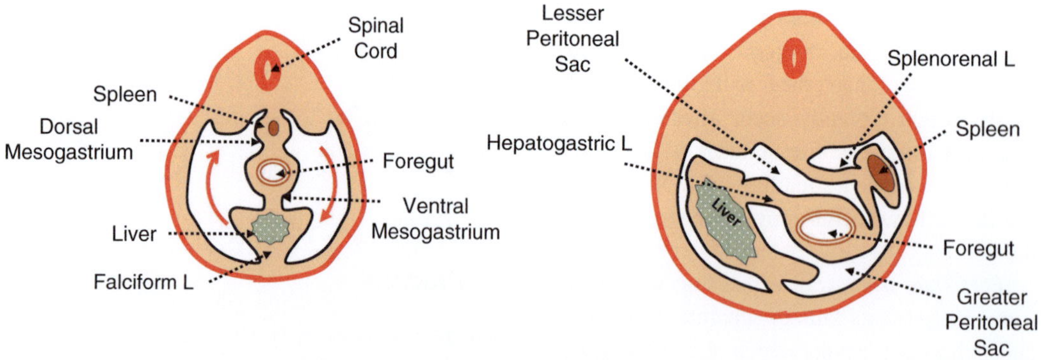

Fig. 26.8 Development of mesenteries. The liver develops in the ventral mesentery as an outgrowth of foregut endoderm. The falciform ligament runs from liver to anterior abdominal wall. The spleen develops in the dorsal mesentery from mesoderm. The splenorenal ligament connects the spleen to the posterior wall [5, 6]

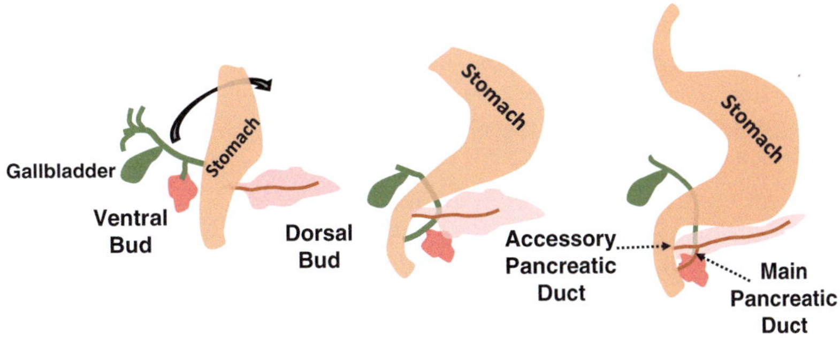

Fig. 26.9 Pancreas development. The pancreas develops from the ventral and dorsal pancreatic buds [5, 6]

lumen closes, and it stays closed for several days. However, it eventually recanalizes. Duodenal atresia refers to a failure of the duodenum to recanalize. Stomach contents will then back up in the stomach and the proximal duodenum, which can be seen as a double-bubble-sign on radiographs. Jejunal atresia results in a triple-bubble-sign.

Clinical Scenarios

A *Meckel's diverticulum* results from a failure of the vitelline duct to close. What remains is a short piece of tissue projecting from the ileum. Think of the Rule-of-Two's. The diverticulum is found 2 feet from the ileocecal junction, it is typically 2 inches long, there are two types of tissue—gastric and pancreatic, and 2% of those with the diverticulum develop complications.

Gastroschisis is a herniation through the abdominal wall just to the side of the umbilicus through the rectus abdominus. It usually occurs on the right side. It enters the amniotic cavity.

An *omphalocele* is a failure of the normally herniated midgut to come back into the abdominal cavity. It occurs in the midline at the yolk stalk and is covered by amnion, this is because the umbilical cord itself is normally covered by amnion. In most cases there are other congenital anomalies (Fig. 26.10).

Hirschsprung's disease is caused by a failure of neural crest cells to migrate into the descending colon. Normally this neural crest tissue will give rise to the postganglionic parasympathetic ganglia. Without ganglia and the parasympathetic nerves, there is no peristalsis. The affected section of the GI tract will tightly constrict so fecal material cannot move through it. This will lead to a build-up of material in the proximal bowel (megacolon), usually in the transverse colon.

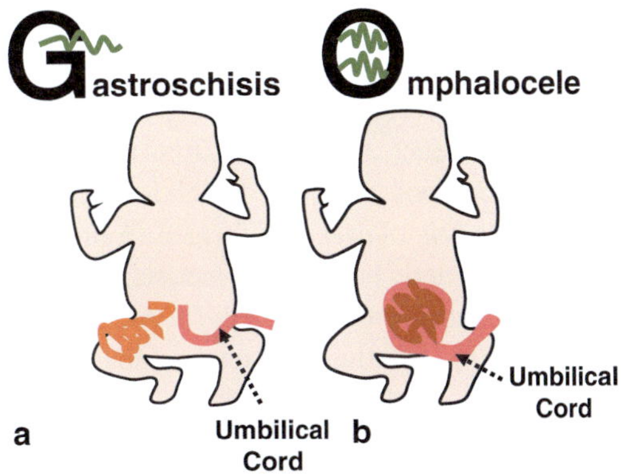

Fig. 26.10 Gastroschisis versus omphalocele. (**a**) Gastroschisis is a herniation of the intestines through the abdominal wall, usually to the right of the umbilicus. The herniation is into the amniotic sac so the herniated tract is now covered by amniotic fluid. AFP will be increased. Think of a "**G**" with an opening for the contents to slip through. (**b**) With an omphalocele**,** the contents herniate through the intestinal wall at the umbilicus and enter directly into the umbilical cord and are within a sac or an "**O**" and covered by amniotic membrane [5, 6]

Malrotation of the midgut involves a failure of the gut to rotate leading to misplacement of the gut.

The Kidney

Think of kidney development as a Broadway show with three acts. Act one, or the first stage of kidney development, involves the formation of the pronephros. The pronephros is short lived and degenerates by the end of week four.

Act two involves the formation of the mesonephric ducts and mesonephric tubules during week four. The *mesonephric tubules* are derived from mesoderm and take the place of the pronephros. Also forming from the mesoderm are the *mesonephric ducts* that grow and descend to meet up with the urogenital sinus. By the end of week 8, the mesonephric tubules degenerate, however the mesonephric ducts remain to eventually go on to become part of the male reproductive tract.

Act three involves an interaction between the two main actors—really two pieces of mesoderm. The *ureteric bud* is an outgrowth of the mesonephric duct, so it arises from mesoderm. Meanwhile, along the posterior abdominal wall the *metanephric blastema* is formed from mesoderm. The ureteric bud and the metanephric blastema then form the adult kidney. The metanephric blastema will form the nephrons and the tract up to where the collecting ducts start. The ureteric bud will form the outflow tract from the collecting ducts on out (Fig. 26.11).

In some cases, the kidneys do not form—*renal agenesis*. As long as one kidney is present then this will not be an issue, however if neither kidney develops this is incompatible with life. During the pregnancy there will be an oligohydramnios. Normally, the kidneys produce amniotic fluid. Without them, there will be a lack of

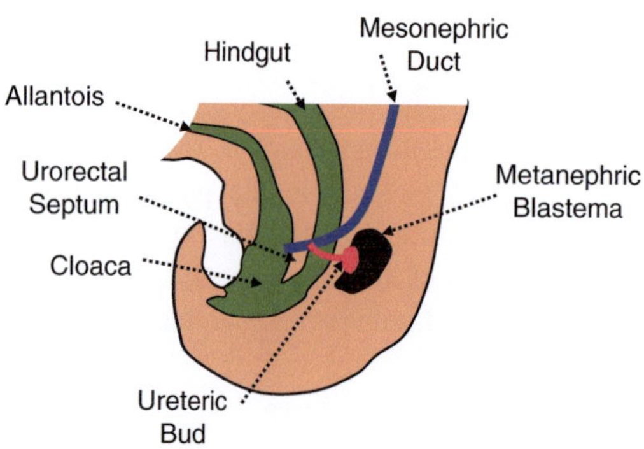

Fig. 26.11 Development of Kidney. The kidney arises from the (1) ureteric bud which is an outgrowth of the mesonephric duct, and (2) the metanephric blastema which arises from mesoderm. The cloaca is the common opening for the bladder and the hindgut. Note the urorectal septum is growing down the urogenital sinus to divide it into the bladder and anal canal [5, 6]

fluid. Without the protective function of the amniotic fluid, increased pressure on the fetus will lead to a flattened face. The amniotic fluid is also essential for normal lung development so without the fluid there will be *pulmonary hypoplasia*—reduction in the size of the lung. The patient will typically have clubbed fingers. The combination of all these symptoms together is referred to as *Potter's sequence*.

A *horseshoe kidney* refers to a failure of the kidney to ascend because it gets caught up around the inferior mesenteric artery. Instead of two kidneys there is one horseshoe shaped kidney.

Urogenital Sinus

The urogenital sinus is an outpocketing of endoderm from the cloaca. Think of it as a warehouse sending out parts to various regions of the body. The upper part of the sinus gives rise to the epithelial lining of the bladder. During development, the mesonephric ducts form the muscular wall of trigone of the bladder and the ejaculatory ducts. The detrusor muscle which forms the wall of the bladder comes from mesoderm.

In males the urogenital sinus also gives rise to the to the prostatic and membranous urethra. The prostatic urethra in turn gives rise to the prostate gland.

Also emerging from the urogenital sinus is the *allantois,* which in birds is used to process waste products. In humans, the blood vessels in the allantois are taken over by the embryo and used as the umbilical blood vessels. The umbilical veins carry oxygen rich blood from the placenta to the fetus, and the umbilical arteries carry oxygen poor blood from the fetus back to the placenta. In the adult, the *medial umbilical ligaments* are from the obliterated umbilical arteries; the *median umbilical ligaments* is from the obliterated *urachus*—the connection between bladder and allantois; and the *lateral umbilical ligaments* house the inferior epigastric arteries and veins.

If the urachus does not close off like it should, and instead remains patent, then urine can drain at the umbilicus. This is referred to as a patent or persistent urachus.

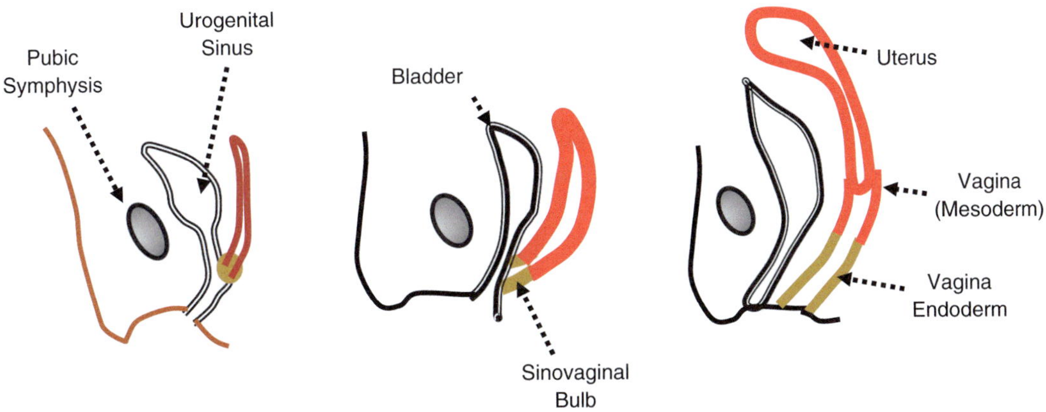

Fig. 26.12 Development of Vagina. The uterus come from the paramesonephric ducts which fuse in the midline. The ducts are connected to the bladder wall at the sinovaginal bulb. The sinovaginal bulb pulls away from the bladder to give rise to lower 2/3rds of the vagina. The upper 1/3 of the vagina comes from the mesoderm of the paramesonephric ducts [5, 6]

Development of Vagina and Uterus

The adult vagina is derived from both endoderm and mesoderm. During week 9 of development, the paramesonephric ducts, which are mesoderm, attach to the sinovaginal sinuses at the sinovaginal bulb, which is endoderm. As development proceeds, the paramesonephric ducts and sinovaginal bulbs pull away from the urogenital sinus to form the adult vagina. The uterus also develops from the fusion of the paramesonephric ducts. If the paramesonephric ducts fail to fuse correctly this can result in a bicornuate uterus (sometimes referred to as a heart shaped uterus). There are typically no symptoms with a bicornuate uterus, and the woman will be unaware of it unless she becomes pregnant. It does increase the chance of a miscarriage. The prostatic utricle in the male is the remanent of the paramesonephric ducts and is homologous to the uterus. (Figs. 26.11 and 26.12).

Canal of Nuck

The paramesonephric ducts unite in the midline to form the uterus. At the same time the gubernaculum is shrinking and pulling the ovaries towards the labia majora. As the ovaries descend, the gubernaculum on each side will attach to the horn of the uterus giving rise to a round ligament and ovarian ligament. Meanwhile, a piece of peritoneal cavity runs alongside the gubernaculum—the canal of Nuck. This will eventually degenerate during the first year of life. If it remains, this persistent canal of Nuck can lead to hernias along its path (Figs. 26.13 and 26.14).

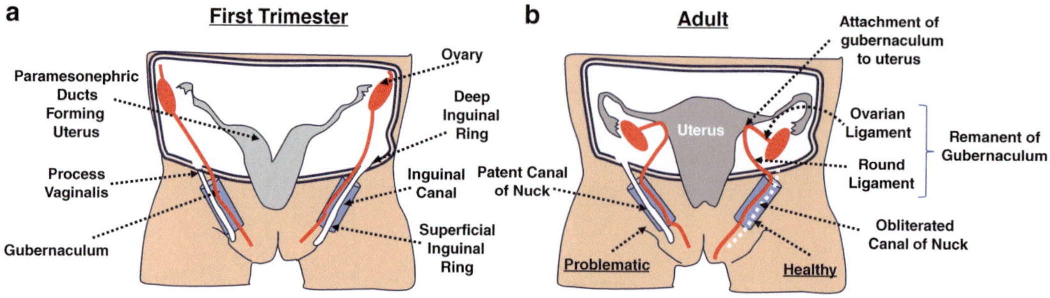

Fig. 26.13 Gubernaculum and process vaginalis. Panel (**a**): During development, the gubernaculum runs from the labia majora to the ovary. As it shrinks, it pulls the ovary down towards the pelvis. The process vaginalis is an out pocketing of peritoneal cavity that accompanies the gubernaculum. Panel (**b**): in the adult, the gubernaculum has become the round ligament and the ovarian ligament. The process vaginalis should regress and become obliterated. If it does not, then it remains as a patent canal of Nuck. The round ligament then connects the labia majora to the uterus. [5, 6]

Development of Sexual Characteristics

During development, if the Y chromosome is present, the embryo will proceed the formation of male structures. Without the Y chromosome the female structures will develop. On the short arm of the Y chromosome is the SRY gene which produces testes determining factor which promotes the development of the testes and testosterone. The 5- alpha reductase 2 enzyme converts testosterone to dihydrotestosterone (DHT). DHT is much more potent than testosterone. The descent of the testes is dependent on DHT.

In the biological world, the term hermaphrodites refers to an organism that has both types of reproductive organs. While common in the plant word, there are no examples of mammalian hermaphrodites. However, in humans, the term pseudohermaphrodites refers to a mismatch between their gonadal tissue and secondary sexual characteristics. Due to either abnormal hormone levels or abnormalities in their receptors, the external genitalia of one sex accompanies the gonads of the other sex. The older term *pseudohermaphrodites* is now more commonly seen as *pseudointersexuality*.

In *female pseudointersexuality,* the individual (XX) has ovaries but a male appearance.

Congenital adrenal hyperplasia, results in an excess of androgens that lead to male secondary sexual characteristics (virilization) such as an enlarged clitoris, facial hair, and suppressed breast development. There are five steps in the production of cortisol. A defect in any of these steps can result in congenital adrenal hyperplasia but a deficiency in 21-hydroxylase accounts for 90% of the CAH cases.

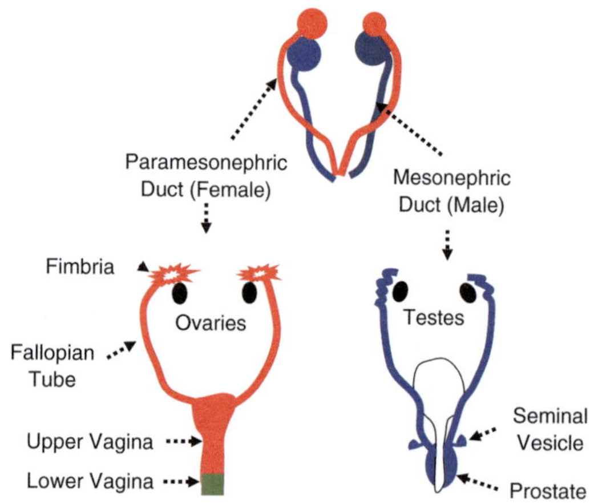

Fig. 26.14 Development of male/female reproductive tracts. In females the paramesonephric ducts give rise to the fallopian tube, cervix, and upper part of the vagina. In males the mesonephric ducts give rise to the seminal vesicle, epididymis, ejaculatory duct, and ductus deferens [5, 6]

In *male pseudointersexuality*, the testes are present, but the individual resembles a female.

One example of male pseudointersexuality is 5-alpha reductase 2 deficiency syndrome which was first described in several small villages in the Dominican Republic and involves an apparent shift of sex from female to male at puberty (güevedoces). In this instance, testosterone is not converted to DHT and without the potency of DHT, the (46:XY) individual starts with female characteristics, with the testes remaining in the inguinal canal. But then at puberty the increased levels of testosterone lead to masculinization, and the individual shifts from a female to male (an infertile male) in outward appearance. The testes can also descend into the labia majora.

In complete androgen insensitivity syndrome (CAIS), previously referred to as testicular feminization syndrome, the individual(46:XY) has testes, and produces testosterone but the cells do not respond to the testosterone due to a defect in the androgen receptor gene. With no receptor for testosterone, this leads to feminization of the outward appearance. There is a short blind-ended vagina and no uterus. The testes are usually in the inguinal canal or abdomen. It is usually first detected at puberty when there is no menstruation. The individual has female secondary characteristics but is a male genotype (46:XY).

Head and Neck Region

During the third week of development, neural crest cells migrate into the head to form the pharyngeal arches. At this early stage there are six arches. The arches form a tube with the inside of the tube coming from endoderm and forming pouches, while the outside of the tube comes from ectoderm and forms the pharyngeal grooves (or clefts). Pharyngeal groove one forms the epithelium of the external auditory tube, and pharyngeal pouch one forms the middle ear canal and auditory tube. Pharyngeal pouch two forms the epithelium of the palatine tonsil. Pharyngeal pouch three gives rise to the inferior parathyroid and thymus. Pharyngeal groove four gives rise to the superior parathyroid and ultimobranchial body (Fig. 26.15).

To organize the arches, you want to think of the nerves. Arch 1 is CN V, arch 2 is CN VII, arch 3 is CN IX, arch 4 is part of CN X, specifically the pharyngeal and superior laryngeal branches, arch 5 is going to disappear, and arch 6 is the recurrent laryngeal nerve a branch of CN X (Fig. 26.16).

There are issues that can occur due to disruptions with the arches, grooves, and pouches:

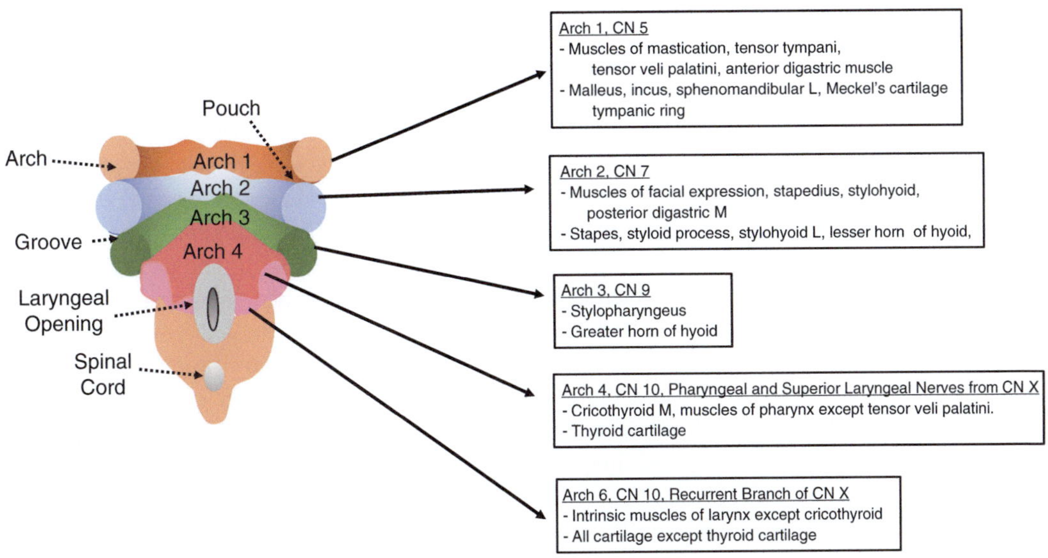

Fig. 26.15 Pharyngeal arches [5, 6]

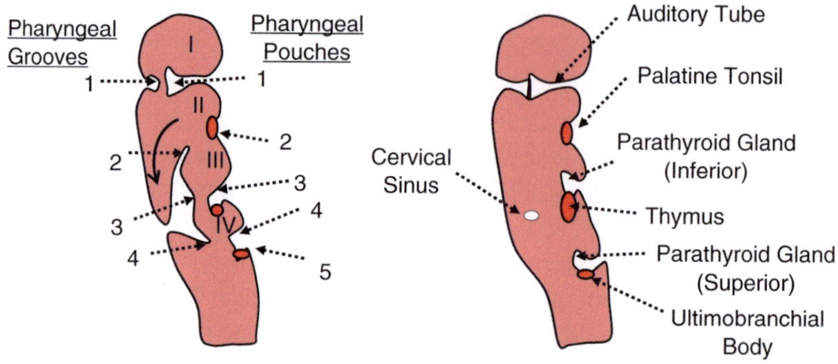

Fig. 26.16 Pharyngeal pouches and grooves. Pharyngeal *groove* 1 forms the external ear canal. Pharyngeal *pouch* 1 forms the epithelial lining of the auditory tube and middle ear. Pharyngeal *arch* 2 overgrows grooves 2, 3, and 4. Sometimes a cervical cyst remains. Pharyngeal *pouch* 2 forms the epithelial lining of the palatine tonsil, *pouch* 3 forms the inferior parathyroid gland and thymus. Pharyngeal *pouch* 4 forms the superior parathyroid gland and the C-cells of the thyroid [5, 6]

First arch syndromes involve faulty development of the first arch which leads to facial anomalies. *Treacher Collins Syndrome* includes agenesis of the mandible, poorly developed eyelashes of the lower medial lid, abnormalities of the external and middle ear, deafness, and a drooping of the outer angle of the eye. *Pierre-Robbins Sequence* involves a sequence of events, meaning that each event causes the next event. It starts with a small mandible, which in turn leads to downward displacement of the tongue, which in turn leads to obstruction of the airway, all of which leads to a failure of the palate to form—*a cleft palate.*

Normally arch 2 grows over clefts 2, 3, and 4. When it does this, it will leave behind an ectodermal covered sinus, which will eventually be absorbed. In some instances, this structure remains which can lead to sinuses, cysts, or fistulas in the neck, usually parallel to the sternocleidomastoid muscle.

DiGeorge Syndrome arises from a microdeletion on the long arm of chromosome 22 and leads to defects with the arches and pouches of 3 and 4. Symptoms vary from one patient to another but often include heart defects, a cleft palate, a high face, small teeth, low set ears, and immune deficiencies.

The thyroid gland does not develop from the pharyngeal arches, but instead arises from foregut endoderm at the back of the tongue at the foramen cecum. The tissue then migrates inferiorly through the neck to end in the adult position. Along its migratory pathway it leaves a trail called the thyroglossal duct which is eventually reabsorbed. If this duct persists the patient will have a thyroglossal cyst that can be found along this pathway.

Epstein pearls are sometimes present in the mouths of newborns. They are small white nodules that in some cases look like small teeth. They are harmless and will go away on their own.

Development of the Facial Bones

The face starts development in week four by a combination of the neural crest cells and mesoderm from the first arch. Specifically, the *frontonasal prominence* comes from neural crest cells, and the *maxillary* and *mandibular prominences* come from the mesoderm. The maxillary prominences start laterally and then expand medially to fuse with the midline located *nasal prominence.* Coming off the maxillary prominences are the palatal shelves which both expand medially to fuse in the midline. A *cleft lip* is the result of a failure of the medial nasal prominences to fuse with the maxillary prominence. A *cleft palate* is a failure of the two *palatine shelves* to fuse (Fig. 26.17).

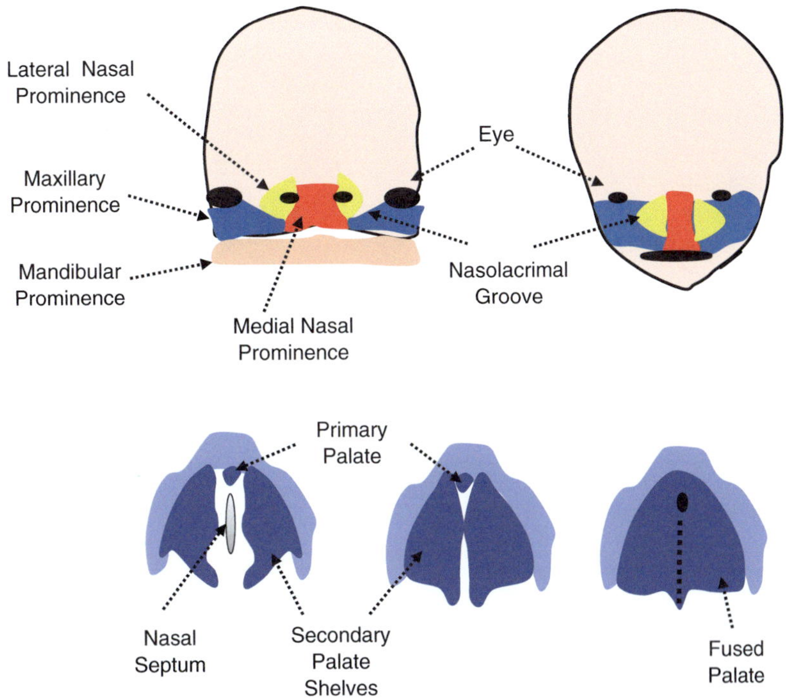

Fig. 26.17 Development of facial bones and palate [5, 6]

Polyhydramnios Versus Oligohydramnios

Amniotic fluid is produced by the kidneys and excreted into the amniotic cavity. The fetus then swallows the amniotic fluid. Congenital anomalies that result in a blockage of the intestinal tract will cause an increase in the amniotic fluid since the fetus cannot swallow it—*polyhydramnios*. If the kidneys do not develop then there will be no amniotic fluid—*oligohydramnios*.

Development of the Trachea

At week four, the developing lung arises as the respiratory diverticula from the foregut endoderm which results in one tube becoming both the esophagus and the future lung. This respiratory diverticula will then divide into two bronchial buds to form the right and left lungs. The trachea eventually separates from the esophagus to form its own tube. In some instances, this separation leads to defects. The most common one being a *tracheoesophageal fistula* with esophageal atresia. In this case the esophagus ends as a blind tube, usually along the distal 1/3rd of the esophagus, while the terminal esophagus maintains its connection with the trachea. This results in symptoms such as: polyhydramnios, cyanosis after eating, and reflux of stomach contents into the lungs (Fig. 26.18).

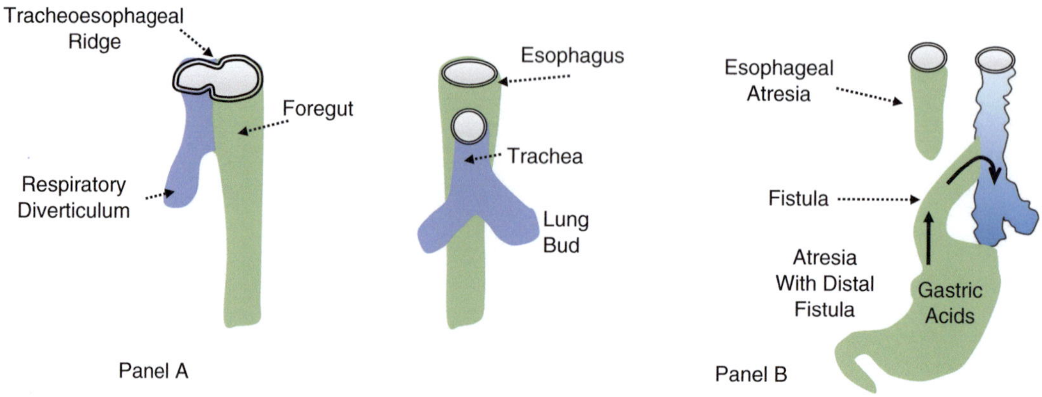

Fig. 26.18 Development of lungs and trachea. The lungs start as a respiratory diverticulum, an outgrowth of foregut endoderm. As it separates from the foregut, the tracheo-esophageal ridge separates the trachea from the foregut. In some cases, there is an esophageal atresia with a tracheo-esophageal fistula between the distal esophagus and trachea [5, 6]

Ectoderm

The ectoderm gives rise to two divisions, (1) *surface ectoderm*, which gives rise to the skin of the body and (2) *neural ectoderm*, which forms the neural tube and the neural crest tissue:

1. The *neural ectoderm* arises in the midline over the notochord. The neural tube gives rise to the CNS which includes the brain, spinal cord, optic nerve, and retina. This also includes neurohypophysis, the pineal gland, astrocytes, oligodendrocytes.
2. The *neural crest cells* are mesenchymal cells that migrate to several different regions. They give rise to all the ganglia in the PNS, which includes the dorsal root ganglia, the postganglionic autonomic ganglia, and the adrenal medulla. But they also migrate to several other body regions. In the head, they migrate into the pharyngeal arches to give rise to some of the bones and cartilage of the skull. They also give rise to the parafollicular cells of the thyroid gland. Around the brain they become the pia and arachnoid. They also migrate into the skin to give rise to melanocytes. And they migrate to the heart to give rise to the atrioventricular septum. The *surface ectoderm* gives rise to the hypodermis (not the dermis) and the hair, nails, enamel of the teeth, and Rathke's pouch. Remember from the discussion on the development of the face, that the first groove gives rise to the epithelium of the external ear, and the first pouch gives rise to the epithelium of the inner ear. Note that parotid gland comes from ectoderm. Also note that the entire pituitary comes from ectoderm, but that the anterior pituitary comes from Rathke's pouch, while the posterior pituitary comes from the neural tube (Fig. 26.19).

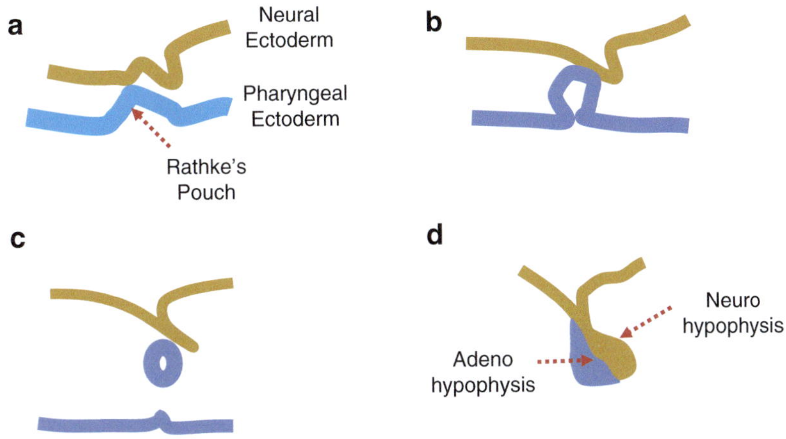

Fig. 26.19 Development of the pituitary. The pituitary comes from two different sources of ectoderm. One is pharyngeal ectoderm, Rathke's pouch. The second source is neural ectoderm [5, 6]

Endoderm

The endoderm gives rise to the epithelial lining of the GI tract, divided into foregut, midgut, and hindgut. And from the foregut endoderm comes the respiratory diverticulum which gives rise to the parenchyma of the lungs and the epithelium lining the trachea. Also from the foregut endoderm are the submandibular and sublingual glands, plus the thyroid gland. Remember the thyroid gland arises at the back of the tongue at the foramen cecum. In the ventral mesentery the liver starts as a diverticulum from the midgut, and this liver diverticula also gives rise to the gallbladder, biliary system, and pancreas. The spleen starts off in the dorsal mesentery, but it comes from mesoderm. Another way to look at it, or word it, is that the artery of the foregut is the celiac trunk which goes to endoderm structures, except the spleen—which comes from mesoderm.

Moving down to the hindgut, the urogenital sinus comes from hindgut endoderm, and it in turn gives rise to the epithelium of the bladder, which in turn gives rise to the pancreas, the urethra, and lower vagina.

Note that organs whose epithelium comes from endoderm are surrounded by tissue that comes from mesoderm.

Mesoderm

During early development, the mesoderm forms the nucleus pulposus of the notochord. The mesoderm gives rise to all the muscle tissue, including smooth, skeletal, and cardiac muscle. It also gives rise to all the connective tissue, bone, serous membranes, blood, cartilage, lymph, gonads, spleen, adrenal cortex, kidneys, and ureters. Remember the ureter arises from the mesonephric duct, a mesoderm structure that also give rise to the vas deferens, and seminal vesicles, epididymis, and ejaculatory ducts. As mentioned above, the pancreas comes from the urogenital sinus which is endoderm. In the heart the mesoderm gives rise to epithelium.

In females, the paramesonephric ducts, a mesoderm derivative, gives rise to the uterus, fallopian tube, cervix, and upper part of the vagina.

Mesoderm Divisions

During week three the mesoderm divides into three sections: (1) paraxial mesoderm, (2) intermediate mesoderm, and (3) lateral plate mesoderm. Their names give away their locations. The paraxial mesoderm is just lateral to the notochord, the lateral plate mesoderm is the most lat-

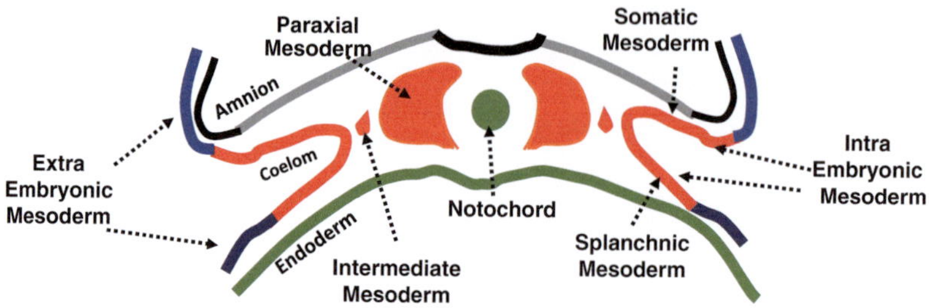

Fig. 26.20 Mesoderm and its Derivatives. The mesoderm has three divisions: (1) paraxial, (2) intermediate, and (3) lateral plate. The lateral plate, in turn, divides into two layers: the somatic and splanchnic layers [5, 6]

eral of the three divisions, and between the two is the intermediate mesoderm (Fig. 26.20).

The lateral plate mesoderm is shaped like a "Y" with one arm becoming the somatic layer of lateral plate mesoderm, or *somatopleure,* and the second arm becoming the splanchnic layer of the lateral plate mesoderm, also known as *splanchnopleure*. Located at the junction of the "Y" is the intraembryonic coelom, which is continuous with the extraembryonic coelom early in development. At the end of the lateral body wall folding, these two cavities will be separated.

1. The *somatopleure layer* of mesoderm is originally adjacent to the ectoderm which surrounds the amniotic cavity. It will go on and form the body wall and the parietal layers of the pleura, peritoneal cavity, and the pericardial cavity.
2. The *splanchnopleure layer* is adjacent to the endoderm. With the lateral folding of the body wall, the splanchnic layer will become the visceral layers of the three cavities, pericardium, pleura, and peritoneal.

As the somatopleure layer of mesoderm folds, it eventually meets in the mid-line and closes the peritoneal and pericardial cavities. In the abdomen, the meeting of the two layers in the midline gives rise to the ventral and dorsal mesentery. The ventral mesentery eventually degenerates, except for the falciform ligament and the lesser omentum. The dorsal mesentery remains to allow blood vessels to travel from the posterior wall to the various intraperitoneal organs. An *omphalocele* results from a failure of the two sides to fuse in the midline in the lumbar region. An *ectopia cordis* results from failure of the two sides to fuse in the midline in the thoracic region.

The intermediate mesoderm will give rise to the kidneys, ureter, vas deferens, and gonads. The paraxial mesoderm resembles a cord on the sides of the notochord which eventually differentiates into segmented blocks of tissue referred to as somites. The somites in turn give rise to the dermatomes (dermis and associated structures), myotomes (axial and appendicular skeletons), and sclerotomes (cartilage, tendons, bone).

The gonads start development along the mesonephric ridge.

Early Venous Drainage

Initially in early heart development, there are two sinus horns (right and left) draining into the sinus venosus. And draining into each horn are three veins:

1. The vitelline veins drain the yolk sac. They form a plexus around the duodenum (portal vein). The left vitelline vein regresses while

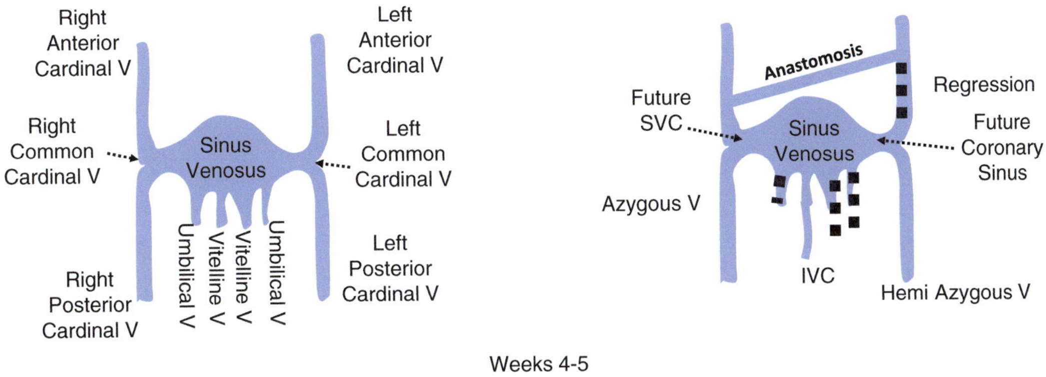

Fig. 26.21 Early venous drainage. The sinus venosus receives blood from the common cardinal, umbilical, and vitelline veins. An anastomosis forms between the right and left anterior cardinal veins which will become the left brachiocephalic vein [5, 6]

the right becomes the hepatic portion of the inferior vena cava.

2. The right and left common cardinal veins receive blood from the anterior and posterior cardinal veins and in turn drain into the sinus venosus. During the second month of development, the right and left anterior cardinal veins form an anastomosis which becomes the left brachiocephalic vein. The inferior portion of the right anterior cardinal vein becomes the superior vena cava. The proximal portion of the left anterior cardinal vein normally regresses. If it does not regress, then the patient will have a double superior vena cava. On the other hand, if the right-side regresses, the patient's superior vena cava will be on the left side. The right posterior cardinal vein forms the proximal portion of the azygous vein.
3. The umbilical vein carry oxygen rich blood from the placenta to the fetus. The right umbilical vein regresses by day 44. From day 44 onward, the left umbilical vein is responsible for delivering blood to the liver (Fig. 26.21).

Syndactyly

The most common congenital malformation in children is the presence of webbed toes or fingers—syndactyly. It can be unilateral or bilateral. It is not correlated with any other health problems. If it occurs in the fingers, surgery can be performed to separate them. If it occurs in the toes, while surgery can be performed, it is not necessary. It is thought to be due to a failure of apoptosis (Fig. 26.22).

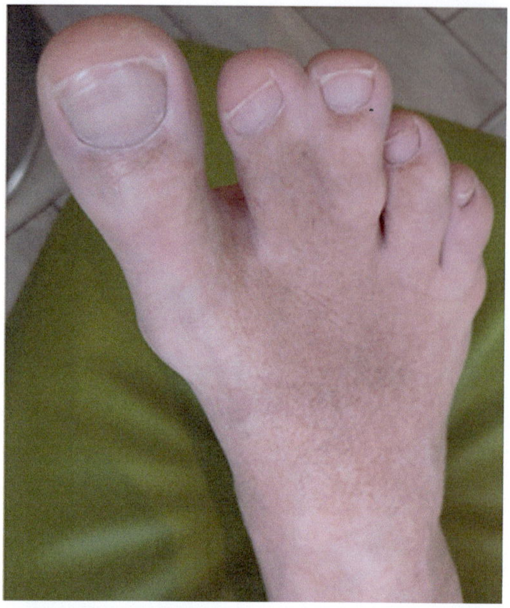

Fig. 26.22 Syndactyly

Further Reading

1. Carlson B. Human embryology and developmental biology. 6th ed. New York: Elsevier; 2018.
2. Gittenberger-De Groot AC, Bartelings MM, Deruiter MC, Poelmann RE. Basics of cardiac development for the understanding of congenital heart malformations. Ped Res. 2005;57(2):169–76.
3. Graham A, Richards J. Development and evolutionary origins of the pharyngeal apparatus. Evol Dev. 2012;3(24)
4. Hutson JM, Balic NA, Southwell BR. The role of the gubernaculum in the descent and undescent of the testis. Therap Adv Neurol. 2009;1(2)
5. Leo J. Medical neuroanatomy for the boards and clinic: finding the lesion. 2nd ed. Cham: Springer; 2024a.
6. Leo J. Clinical anatomy and embryology: a guide for the classroom, clinic, and clinic. 2nd ed. Cham: Springer; 2024b.
7. McKenzie J. The first arch syndrome. Arch Dis Child. 1958;8(1):477–86.
8. Moore KL, Persaud TVN. The developing human: clinically oriented embryology. 11th ed. New York: Saunders; 2019.
9. Sadler TW. Langman's medical embryology. 14th ed. New York: Lippincott Williams and Wilkins; 2018.
10. Saguintaah M, Eulliot J, Bertrand M, et al. Canal of nuck abnormalities in pediatric female patients. Radiographics. 2022;42:541–58.
11. Sweeney L. Basic concepts in embryology: a student's survival guide. New York: McGraw-Hill; 1997.

Appendix

The table shows the Latin word for several body parts. Many of the words here came from a video series made by the late Dr. Ronald Bergmann - an expert anatomist. I have purposefully kept the derivations simple. There is plenty of room for debate amongst etymologists about the origin of some of these words. Note that the word *fornix* refers to arches. In Rome, prostitutes used to congregate in vaulted cellars – under the arches. The word *fornix* for *arch* came to also refer to a brothel, and then fornix became *fornicis,* and eventually *fornication*. The term *sacrum* refers to *sacred* or *sacral* and gets its name because it is the last bone to decompose. Temporal refers to gray hair and is one area of the body to show your age. The term *obturator* comes from the word *obstruc*t which is thought to have been first applied to the obturator membrane which covers the obturator foramen. It has also been suggested that it refers to the obturator nerve which goes to the adductor muscles to bring the thighs together. *Jejunum* means *empty* which refers to the fact that, due to its peristaltic activity, food does not stay long in it, and at death it is usually empty. The term *pudendal* comes from the phrase, "to be ashamed of."

J. Leo, *Gross Anatomy, Neuroanatomy, and Embryology for Medical Students*,
https://doi.org/10.1007/978-3-031-87151-1

Body part	Derivation
Vomer	Plowshare
Sphenoid	Wedge
Temporal	Gray Hair
Sacrum	Last bone to Decompose
Coccyx	Bird's Beak
Cribriform Plate	Sieve
Sternum	Gladiolus (Dagger)
Crista Galli	Crest of Chicken
Radius	Circle
Phalanx	Row of Roman Soldiers
Tibia	Flute
Fibula	Toga Pin
Femur	Thigh
Dens, Odontoid Process	Tooth
Vas Deferens	Carry Away
Concha	Keel
Trochlea	Pulley
Obturator	Object, Block
Pectineus	Comb
Fibula	Brooch
Lumbricals	Worms
Callosum	Tough Body
Serratus	Saw
Hippocampus	Horse-Like Sea Monster
Labrum	Lip
Iris	Bright Colored Ring, Halo
Zygomatic	Bar, Bolt
Hyoid	The letter "U"
Longissimus	Longest
Talus	Dice
Cervix	Neck
Aorta	To Lift Up
Diaphragm	Fence
Sartorius	Tailor
Sella Turcica	Turkish Saddle
Esophagus	To Carry
Uncinate	Hooked
Modiolus	Hub of a Wheel
Scala	Stairs, Ladder

Body part	Derivation
Pterygoid	Wing
Palatine	Feudal lord
Sclera	Hard
Thalamus	Inner Chamber, Bedroom
Styloid	Pillar
Mastoid	Breast
Coracoid Process	Crow's Beak
Pons	Bridge
Raphe	Seam
Fornix	Arch, Brothel
Arcuate	Bow
Rete, Retina	Net
Petrous	Rock, as in St Peter
Rectus	Upright, straight
Gubernaculum	Helm, Rudder, Governor
Scapula	Shovel
Genu	Bend, Genuflect
Patella	Small Pan
Acetabulum	Small Cup
Peroneus	Brooch Pins
Clavicle	Key
Carotid	Deep Sleep
Splenius	Patch
Corona	Crown
Lacrimal	Tear
Limbus	Edge Border
Arytenoid	Ladle, Funnel
Thyroid	Shield
Latissimus	Widest
Meta	Change
Prostate	Protector, Guardian
Manubrium	Handle
Jejunum	Fasting
Soleus	Flat Fish, Sole of foot – Flat
Clinoid/Clinical	Four Post Bed/Bedside
Trachea	Rugged, Jagged
Condyle	Knuckle
Cochlea	Shell

Further Reading

1. Agrawal A. Musculoskeletal etymology: What's in a name? J Clin Orthopaed Trauma. 2019;10:387–94.
2. Bergman RA, Afifi AK. Anatomy: an encyclopedic reference to the language of anatomy and neuroanatomy. US: Outskirts Press; 2016.

MIX
Papier aus verantwortungsvollen Quellen
Paper from responsible sources
FSC® C105338

If you have any concerns about our products,
you can contact us on
ProductSafety@springernature.com

In case Publisher is established outside the EU,
the EU authorized representative is:
Springer Nature Customer Service Center GmbH
Europaplatz 3, 69115 Heidelberg, Germany

Printed by Libri Plureos GmbH
in Hamburg, Germany